Quick Guide

To help locate major sections of the Directory quickly, shaded tabs appear opposite the major sections listed on this page that correspond to the shaded areas found on the edge of the volume.

MEDICAL TECHNOLOGY ASSESSMENT DIRECTORY

A Pilot Reference to Organizations, Assessments, and Information Resources

Clifford Goodman, *Editor*

COUNCIL ON HEALTH CARE TECHNOLOGY
INSTITUTE OF MEDICINE

NATIONAL ACADEMY PRESS
Washington, D.C. 1988

NATIONAL ACADEMY PRESS 2101 Constitution Ave., NW Washington, DC 20418

NOTICE: This *Directory*, a project of the Council on Health Care Technology of the Institute of Medicine, fulfills in part the provision in Section 309 of Public Law 98-551 that the council serve as a clearinghouse for information on health care technologies and assessments.

Activities of the council are supported by private sector contributions and grants (see Appendix B for a list of contributors) and federal matching grants provided by grant number HS 05526 from the National Center for Health Services Research and Health Care Technology Assessment. Program representatives who consider their program, or others, to be appropriate for future revisions of the *Directory* should contact the Council on Health Care Technology, Institute of Medicine, 2101 Constitution Ave., NW, Washington, DC 20418. Subscription to the council's quarterly newsletter, *CHCT ASSESSMENT*, may be obtained for $20 per year from the same address.

The Institute of Medicine was chartered in 1970 by the National Academy of Sciences to enlist distinguished members of the appropriate professions in the examination of policy matters pertaining to the health of the public. In this, the Institute acts under both the Academy's 1863 congressional charter responsibility to be an advisor to the federal government and its own initiative in identifying issues of medical care, research, and education.

Library of Congress Cataloging-in-Publication Data

Medical technology assessment directory: a pilot reference to organizations, assessments, and information resources / Clifford Goodman, editor; Council on Health Care Technology, Institute of Medicine.

p. cm.

Prepared by the Council on Health Care Technology's Information Panel.

Includes bibliographies and indexes.

ISBN 0-309-03829-4

1. Medical technology—United States—Directories. 2. Medical technology—Directories. I. Goodman, Clifford. II. Council on Health Care Technology (Institute of Medicine). Information Panel.

[DNLM: 1. Technology Assessment, Biomedical—United States—directories. W 22 AA1 M4916]

R855.3.M43 1988

610'.28—dc19

DNLM/DLC

for Library of Congress 88-5358

CIP

Printed in the United States of America

INFORMATION PANEL OF THE COUNCIL ON HEALTH CARE TECHNOLOGY

LAWRENCE C. MORRIS
Senior Vice President, Health Benefits Management, Blue Cross and Blue Shield Association, Chicago, Illinois *(Chairman)*

GAIL L. WARDEN
President and Chief Executive Officer, Group Health Cooperative of Puget Sound, Seattle, Washington *(Co-Chairman)*

MORRIS F. COLLEN
Consultant, Division of Research, Kaiser Permanente Medical Care Program, Oakland, California

RICHARD C. FARMER
Chairman, Division of Medicine, The Cleveland Clinic Foundation, Cleveland, Ohio

MELVIN A. GLASSER
Director, Health Security Action Council, Washington, D.C.

G. MAX K. HUGHES
Vice President, Systems and Communication, Pfizer Pharmaceuticals, New York, New York

RICHARD J. JOHNS
Massey Professor and Director, Department of Biomedical Engineering, Johns Hopkins University and Hospital, Baltimore, Maryland

DONALD A.B. LINDBERG
Director, National Library of Medicine, National Institutes of Health, Bethesda, Maryland

WALTER B. MAHER
Director, Employee Benefits and Health Services, Chrysler Corporation, Detroit, Michigan

JOHN H. MOXLEY, III
President, MetaMedical Inc., Beverly Hills, California

C. THOMAS SMITH
President, Yale-New Haven Hospital, New Haven, Connecticut

GEORGE E.T. STEBBING
Director, Professional Activities, Office of the Secretary of Defense, Health Affairs, Washington, D.C.

Project Staff

CLIFFORD S. GOODMAN, Staff Officer
LESLIE M. HARDY, Research Associate
PAMELA J. SIMERLY, Research Associate

ACKNOWLEDGMENTS

A novel effort to assemble information from diverse sources, this *Directory* called for a blend of experience, original thinking, and resolve. We wish to acknowledge those who contributed these qualities to the project.

We are grateful to the members of the Information Panel for lending their experience in health plan and facility management, medicine, bioengineering, health care product development, third party payment, medical informatics, and national health policy to building a technology assessment information capacity. Of import to meeting this, the first charge of the congressional mandate for the council, is the members' ability to coalesce their sectorial interests into a group effort of needs assessment, systems design, product development, strategic planning, and marketing.

Pamela Simerly deserves special recognition for her skill and perseverance in helping to plan the project, and in assembling, reviewing, and processing information used for the assessment program profiles. Leslie Hardy collected and organized descriptive information for many of the entries in the information and data resources part of the *Directory*. Wallace Waterfall and James Gormley provided advice on editorial matters and layout.

Peter Goldschmidt's knowledge of information systems, medicine, and management made him a worthy consultant to the project. He brought systematic thinking and thoroughness to matters ranging from reviewing for relevance thousands of assessment report citations to setting the project within a long range plan. Grace McCarn provided insightful consultation regarding the needs and capabilities of the medical information community relevant to this project, including technical aspects of such matters as indexing, production, and market placement.

Since the early stages of the project, we have sought counsel from leading institutions in management of health care information systems. The staff of the National Library of Medicine has been consistently forthcoming with constructive advice. NLM's Betsy Humphreys coordinated planning sessions with key library staff to share technological expertise and to formulate strategies for development of a broadly integrated technology assessment information base. The review undertaken by NLM staff of the *Directory* provides encouraging evidence of the utility of this body of information. Guidance concerning the design and implementation of information bases for the health community was provided by Eloise Foster and staff of the American Hospital Association Resource Center and by LeRoy Walters and staff of the Kennedy Institute of Ethics, Georgetown University.

We are very pleased with the work of the TRITON Corporation, which was responsible for assembling the information base of assessment program profiles and report citations, indexing of citation records, and preparing camera-ready copy of the *Directory*. Meriting special recognition are Patricia President, who coordinated all aspects of the contractor's effort, and Linda Malcom, who had a key role in indexing a disparate and technical body of literature. This resourceful and adaptive group also included Patricia Chang and Karen Inscoe, who were responsible for programming and data entry, and corporate officer Edsel Billingy.

Finally, we thank the people associated with the organizations described in the *Directory* who completed surveys and forwarded other material incorporated here. Many of these individuals are shown as contact persons for the profiled assessment programs and the resource organizations in the *Directory*.

Lawrence C. Morris, Chairman, *Information Panel*
Clifford S. Goodman, *Staff Officer*

FOREWORD

The *Medical Technology Assessment Directory* is the first major published work of the Council on Health Care Technology. The *Directory* is an introductory vehicle that organizes recent and current assessment information from a broad though not comprehensive selection of assessment programs and related activities. With this edition, the council makes an overture to those with interests in medical technology assessment to become partners in building a wider and more integrated information network. How users respond to the *Directory* will help to determine which among a variety of ways this information capacity will evolve.

The council was mandated by the U.S. Congress in the Health Promotion and Disease Prevention Amendments of 1984 (P.L. 98-551) and by technical amendments made in 1985 (P.L. 99-117). The purpose of the council is to promote the development and application of technology assessment in health care and to review health care technologies for their appropriate use.

Provision for the council in P.L. 98-551 was the culmination of two streams of activity conducted under the auspices of the Institute of Medicine, National Academy of Sciences. The first was the initiative to create an entity, supported jointly by the private and public sectors, to enhance the assessment of medical technology. The second was a comprehensive study of the state of medical technology assessment.

In December 1982, the Institute of Medicine established the Committee to Plan a Private/Public Sector Entity to Assess Technology in Medical Care under the chairmanship of Jeremiah Barondess. The committee was charged with developing a plan for a technology assessment organization that would be based in the private sector but supported by both government and non-governmental parties[1]. This initiative grew out of an exploratory meeting convened by the Institute on June 16, 1982, in response to growing concerns in both the public and private sectors about the proliferation of technologies in medical care. These concerns were characterized by pressures to eliminate technologies that may be obsolete, harmful, or ineffective; desires to affirm the benefits of other technologies; and stringencies of the need to slow the growth of costs while maintaining and improving the quality of American medical care.

The committee completed its work on June 30, 1983. The final report, published in November 1983, recommended the creation of a medical technology assessment consortium within the Institute of Medicine. The consortium was conceived of as seeking support divided approximately evenly between governmental and non-governmental resources. It was not intended as a competitor or as a replacement for any existing entity involved in assessing medical technologies. Rather, it was to be complementary and facilitative of the efforts of others involved in responsible assessments. As a first step, the consortium was to establish and maintain an information clearinghouse for medical technology assessment. This clearinghouse function would help to build a communication network among the principal parties to technology assessment, including other technology assessment entities, third party payers, major health care providers, and others; serve to reduce unneeded or unrecognized redundancies in evaluation; establish a source of information on completed and ongoing assessments; provide a forum for all the parties at interest in the development and validation of technologies; and facilitate the dissemination of information on medical technology assessments.

Subsequent to legislation enacting the ideas in the committee's report, the Council on Health Care Technology was formed in March 1986. At its first meeting in April 1986, the council created the Information Panel to plan and establish the clearinghouse. This *Directory* is the Information Panel's first substantive product.

Another Institute committee, the Committee for Evaluating Medical Technologies in Clinical Use, under the chairmanship of Frederick Mosteller, was charged with examining the state of medical technology assessment. This study was begun following a 1980 Institute conference on linking the clinical use of biomedical technologies and the collection of evaluative data. Major areas addressed in the committee's 1985 study report, *Assessing Medical Technologies*[2], included the scope of medical technology assessment in the U.S., methods of assessment, effects of clinical evaluation on the diffusion of medical technology, the relationship of assessment and reimbursement policy, assessment activities in other countries, and papers on such topics as clinical trials, cost-effectiveness, and values and preferences in health care delivery. Also included were detailed profiles of 20 technology assessment programs in the U.S. and topics of their respective assessment reports. The work on the scope of medical technology assessment and the program profiles constituted important groundwork for this *Directory*, just as the entire study report has been a touchstone for the deliberations of our council.

On behalf of the Council on Health Care Technology, I trust you will find the *Directory* a useful working document. The council plans to expand and update the *Directory* periodically, and intends to make its information base available in a machine readable format. If you think that your organization, or another organization, has an assessment program that ought to be incorporated in an updated *Directory*, please let us know. We welcome your comments.

William N. Hubbard, Jr., *Chairman*

References

1. Institute of Medicine Committee to Plan a Private/Public Sector Entity to Assess Technology in Medical Care. *Planning study report: a consortium for assessing medical technology.* Washington, D.C.: National Academy Press, 1983.

2. Institute of Medicine Committee for Evaluating Medical Technologies in Clinical Use. *Assessing medical technologies.* Washington, D.C.: National Academy Press, 1985.

PREFACE

During the last decade, various sectors of the health care enterprise have taken a converging interest in determining the safety, effectiveness, cost-effectiveness, and social, ethical, and legal impacts of health care technologies. Each of these sectors—physicians and other health professionals, patients and other consumers, biomedical researchers, health product makers, third party payers, health plan managers, institutional administrators, academicians, public policy makers, and others—tends to rely on some familiar, though different, set of literature and information sources in an attempt to meet assessment needs.

Although more of the health care community has taken explicit interest in medical technology assessment, there remain inadequacies in the supply of good assessment information and the manner in which existing information is organized and made available to those who need it. I have learned as a committee member for the Institute of Medicine study *Assessing Medical Technologies* and from the perspective of a health care payer that the demand for assessment information is outstripping the aggregation of well conducted clinical trials, authoritative group judgments, surveillance studies, and other inquiries concerning medical technologies. Therefore, as we encourage an increase in competent assessment activity, we seek to assemble what good assessment findings there are, both from our traditional sources and from sources that are new to us. As the emerging field of medical technology assessment becomes the shared province of multiple health industry sectors, each one stands to benefit by gaining familiarity with and access to new information resources. Further, we seek to identify a coherent body of assessment literature from which all of us may benefit.

In authorizing the Council on Health Care Technology, Congress specified establishment of a clearinghouse on medical technology assessment information. The *Medical Technology Assessment Directory* is the first major step toward fulfilling this purpose. It encompasses programs that produce medical technology assessments, information and data resources, and other organizations to which inquiries about medical technology can be directed. An important contribution of the *Directory* is to make a first attempt at organizing certain valuable "gray" or "fugitive" literature, i.e. technology assessments not published in widely circulated peer reviewed medical journals or accessible through the better known citation bases such as the National Library of Medicine's (NLM) MEDLARS (Medical Literature Analysis and Retrieval System). Thus, this *Directory* describes relevant mainstream information sources, and complements them with its collection of pertinent gray literature.

Assessments cited in this first edition of the *Directory* are limited to those produced by organizations with an ongoing medical technology assessment program. Future versions, whether in hard-copy or machine readable format, will expand coverage to include more and different sources of literature. For purposes of indexing the assessment report citations, we have used NLM's MeSH (Medical Subject Headings) terms wherever possible. In the technology thesaurus particularly, we have begun to craft a controlled vocabulary that builds upon MeSH terms to make the indexing as relevant as practical to the technology assessment community.

The *Directory* is intended to be a resource to the wider technology assessment community. We hope that this edition, with alphabetical listings of organizations, contact information, descriptions of activities, list of defined acronyms, indexes, and a thesaurus of technology terms designed to lead different types of users to assessments of interest, will be a worthy guide to this multidisciplinary field. Because it assembles and organizes a strong sample of assessment activity rather than being an exhaustive compendium, we view it as a prototype for a more comprehensive, adaptive information base for medical technology assessment.

The *Directory* is the first substantive product of the council's Information Panel. In future months and years, the Information Panel plans to work with the NLM to augment the Library's MeSH vocabulary and certain files of organizational based information, produce access guides to standard literature sources, enhance and update the *Directory*, institute clearinghouse services, and establish online access to the *Directory* information base. We hope that the *Directory* will enhance communication in the assessment community, and will prompt greater participation in development of our clearinghouse activities.

Lawrence C. Morris, *Chairman, Information Panel*

CONTENTS

Part 2: Assessment Report Citations Listed by Technology

Part 3: Information and Data Resources

Part 4: Organizational Resources

Part 5: Index to Organizations

Appendices

INTRODUCTION

This introduction to the *Medical Technical Assessment Directory: A Pilot Reference to Organizations, Assessments, and Information Resources* describes the purpose of the *Directory*, its major parts, its scope and limitations, how it was compiled, and activities planned to follow up this work, including ties with the National Library of Medicine and the World Health Organization.

PURPOSE OF THE DIRECTORY

The *Medical Technology Assessment Directory* is the first substantial published guide to the field of medical technology assessment. It is intended to better define the substance of medical technology assessment, and to crystallize the emerging network of organizations, institutions, and individuals that generate and use technology assessments. The *Directory* is a reference to medical technology organizations, assessments, and information and data resources. It covers activities in the U.S. and certain other countries, including those of government agencies, private companies and associations, and research and educational institutions. It represents the first indexed bibliographic compilation devoted to medical technology assessments produced, in progress, or planned by a broad set of assessment programs spanning the public and private sectors. The *Directory* was developed to increase access to valuable health care technology assessment information, much of which is found outside standard published sources.

This is a product of the Information Panel of the Council on Health Care Technology. One of four panels of the council, the role of the Information Panel is to oversee the development and operation of an information clearinghouse for health care technologies and health care technology assessments, as called for in the congressional mandate for the council. Although the various constituencies of the council have different sets of needs regarding technology assessment, nearly all have expressed a desire for the council to collect, organize, and disseminate technology assessment report information.

As implied by the term "Pilot" in its subtitle, the *Directory* takes a leading step toward a more comprehensive capacity for information services in medical technology assessment. Though it has immediate utility in its own right, the *Directory* is an experimental compilation of information in an emerging field. The assessment report citations and other categories of information included here represent a cross-section of the field, and cover assessment activity of the recent several years of a selection of programs in the U.S. and abroad. One of the major functions of the *Directory* is to act as a hard-copy precursor of a computerized technology assessment information base. The development and testing of the *Directory* will help guide the Information Panel's clearinghouse plans.

With its extensive descriptions and contact information, the *Directory* provides ready access to assessment people, programs, and resources. It is intended for users who wish to identify available assessments and contact people currently conducting assessments of a particular technology before making a decision on medical practice, coverage, reimbursement, acquisition, or standard-setting.

Private and government third party payers, HMOs, and self-insured employers currently reviewing technologies for coverage or inclusion in their health plans may use the *Directory* to locate assessments of these technologies by regulatory bodies and physicians' groups. Physicians seeking medical consensus regarding appropriate use of technologies may find guidance from assessments indexed here. Pharmaceutical and health device and equipment makers may use the *Directory* as a reference to the processes and scope of activity of programs that are likely to assess their products. Procurement decisions for health care facilities may be more informed by reviewing assessments of devices and equipment, and by consulting organizations currently assessing new technologies. Assessors seeking information concerning such areas as postmarketing surveillance, drug utilization, or new product development may use the *Directory* to locate appropriate resources.

The *Directory* may help to advance the field in many other ways. Organizations that conduct or are considering initiating assessment activities may discern ways of strengthening their programs by examining the attributes of profiled programs. By identifying, describing, and providing contact information for assessment organizations, the *Directory* should raise the level of, and render more efficient, communication in the assessment community. Knowing the types of technologies generally assessed by programs, as well as methods used and other program characteristics, those seeking assessment information may prompt appropriate programs to undertake assessments to address specific needs. Those in the academic, research, and public policy sectors who study the field of technology assessment may contrast and compare assessment processes and consider how better to set assessment priorities and otherwise strengthen the assessment enterprise. Thus, the Council on Health Care Technology and others may use the *Directory* information base to review the capacity and products of technology assessment and to discern trends, gaps, and redundant efforts in the field.

Given that this edition could not be a comprehensive rendering of medical technology assessment and that this is an emerging field, wide dissemination of the *Directory* is crucial for building and updating its information base. The council hopes that, by reviewing the *Directory*, assessment programs and other resource organizations not already included will recognize that they conduct activities similar to certain of those described here, and will contact the council about being included in forthcoming editions.

Gray Literature for Assessment

Certainly an important step in carrying out most assessments of medical technologies is searching an information base covering the relevant peer reviewed literature in health and biomedicine. Perhaps the foremost example of such an information base is the online bibliographic citation base MEDLINE, a major component of the National Library of Medicine's MEDLARS system. MEDLINE is one of more than 70 information and data resources described in Part 3 of the *Directory*. It contains all of the citations published in *Index Medicus*. MEDLINE covers more than 5 million articles from some 3,200 biomedical journals, out of the more than 25,000 cataloged by the library.

Yet, given the rapid evolution of health care's technological portfolio and the breadth of assessment perspectives on medical technologies, valuable technology assessment information may be found outside the mainstream of published periodical literature available from traditional sources. This "gray" or "fugitive" literature is found in industry and government monographs, regulatory documents, professional association reports and guidelines, market research reports, policy and research institute studies, spot publications of special panels and commissions, conference proceedings, online services, and other sources.

Although users of the gray literature must consider that much of it has not been subject to the quality screen of peer review, it often has great utility for assessment given its scope beyond traditionally selected sets of journal literature and a currency not subject to the lag time of peer review. The border between gray and standard literature is not distinct; what is gray and what is standard may differ according to one's familiarity with and access to various sources. To be sure, some gray literature eventually passes into the standard literature. Many of the assessment reports generated by organizations profiled in this *Directory*, such as the American College of Physicians Clinical Efficacy Assessment Project, American Medical Association Diagnostic and Therapeutic Technology Assessment Program, and the National Institutes of Health Consensus Development Program, do appear in the peer reviewed literature, though months or perhaps one or two years after initial release in some gray form.

Conducting a good assessment may depend not only upon awareness of key gray literature sources, but one's ability to access them. Desired reports may be available through press releases, journal articles, or books; provided free of charge or at a fee; made available in open libraries or held as proprietary. For instance, the comparative medical device and equipment assessments published by the independent evaluator ECRI are not made available to open libraries such as the National Library of Medicine (NLM), but only to subscribing hospitals, HMOs, and other institutions because ECRI's revenues could be eroded by free or low-cost (e.g., by photocopying) access to its publications. Many of the Food and Drug Administration's (FDA) technical reports on drugs and devices are available only upon request from the FDA or from the National Technical Information Service. Certain reports on emerging and new medical technologies generated by market research firms are publicly available, though at costs ranging from a few hundred to tens of thousands of dollars.

Rather than devoting considerable effort to already organized and indexed assessment reports appearing in the peer reviewed journal literature, much of the *Directory* is addressed to gray sources, including many of the profiled assessment programs and the information and data resource descriptions. Thus, this *Directory* is the first attempt to organize gray literature sources in the field of medical technology assessment.

MAJOR PARTS OF THE DIRECTORY

Part 1 of the *Directory* includes profiles of 68 assessment programs and a total of approximately 3,200 citations of their respective assessment reports. These assessment programs are located in a variety of public and private sector organizations, including professional, scientific, and industry associations, biomedical research institutions, educational institutions, government advisory bodies, regulatory agencies, third party payers, policy institutes, and for-profit corporations. The profiled programs are primarily from the United States; among other countries represented are Canada, the Netherlands, Sweden, and the United Kingdom. These are ongoing programs that generate medical technology assessments. For the purposes of this *Directory*, a medical technology assessment is a study or inquiry, the object of which is to provide information regarding the effects of a technology that is intended to maintain or improve health, or be used as part of an intervention for such purpose, whether or not the study evaluates these effects directly.

Using a common multidimensional framework, these categorical profiles represent a systematic characterization of a diverse community of assessors. This framework was adapted from the one used to profile 20 assessment programs in the 1985 Institute of Medicine study *Assessing Medical Technologies*. The profiles address the purpose, types of technology assessed, topic selection, assessment methods, properties assessed, report dissemination, budget, contact information, and other characteristics of each program. Each profile is followed by a listing of bibliographic citations of the program's recent assessment reports (over approximately the last five years). Following the profiles is a subject index to the citations. Each of the assessment report citations is indexed using from one to five terms. For instance, a report titled "Dialysis treatment for end stage renal disease (outpatient)" is indexed under the terms *Dialysis*; *Kidney failure, Chronic*; and *Outpatients*.

Part 2 has two major sections: a technology thesaurus and a cross-listing of the assessment report citations by technology. The technology thesaurus was developed for this *Directory* to help users search for assessment reports by technology topic. It was generated based upon the technologies appearing in the titles of the assessment report citations. Where appropriate, it uses the NLM's MeSH (Medical Subject Headings) vocabulary terms. To enhance searching by all types of users, the 1,200-term thesaurus includes many synonyms, acronyms, and cross-references, and indicates broader and narrower terms to help clarify relationships among technology terms.

The cross-listing arranges the assessment report citations by technology, e.g., *Apnea monitoring, Coronary artery bypass grafting*, and *Infusion pumps*, so that all citations for each type of technology may be viewed together. Under any particular technology heading, the citations are listed in reverse chronological order to provide the newest information first. This listing is analogous to printouts of computer searches for citations involving particular technologies. In addition to bibliographic information, most citations note the general type of assessment method used, e.g., clinical trial, group judgment, and information synthesis. Because not all of the 3,200 assessment report citations have a technology term in their titles, Part 2 contains about 2,500 citations arranged by technology. Of course, the subject index to report citations at the end of Part 1 uses technology and other terms to index all 3,200 citations with respect to their source assessment programs.

It is important for users to take advantage of the technology thesaurus for searching the cross-listing of assessment report citations by technology. Unless a report citation has more than one technology in its title, it is shown only once in the cross-listing, usually appearing under its most specific technology term. For citations listed in this section, distinctions generally are made between procedures and the equipment used for them. For example, headings include *Computed tomography* as well as *Computed tomography scanners*, and *Fetal monitoring* as well as *Fetal monitors*.

Part 3 describes 73 public and private sector information and data resources that may be of value for assessing medical technologies. Arranged alphabetically by name of resource, these are of many types, including online citation bases and services; data files; compendiums, inventories, and directories; market research reports; and others. Each is described in terms of source, subject, content, compilation, and access information. The resource descriptions are preceded by a categorical chart indicating for each resource its file type (directory, bibliographic information, data set, etc.), format (hard copy, online, etc.), and degree of access (public or limited). At the end of this part is a subject index to the information and data resources.

Part 4 provides 300-word descriptions and contact information for 72 organizations that are active in affairs related to medical technology and are stakeholders in medical technology assessment. These include medical societies, scientific organizations, industry associations, and others. Although most of these organizations do not generate technology assessment reports on a regular basis, they have memberships concerned with medical technologies, conduct relevant meetings and symposiums, publish conference proceedings and other documents of note, establish standards for technologies, or are active in government, regulatory, or other policy affairs relevant to the field. At the end of this part is a subject index to these organizations.

Part 5 includes an alphabetical listing with addresses and telephone numbers for all organizations described in the *Directory*, as well as a page index to the organizations. Among the appendices to the *Directory* are a description of the council, rosters of council and panel members, a listing of organizations that have contributed financial support to the council, and the survey form used to collect information for the 68 profiles in Part 1.

SCOPE AND LIMITATIONS

This *Directory* covers many of the major national level assessment activities in the U.S. and certain significant ones from around the rest of the world. Its immediate utility as a hard-copy reference notwithstanding, the *Directory* is not a complete guide to the field or an all-encompassing information base. The set of 68 profiled programs and their 3,200 assessment report citations in Part 1, the listing of 2,500 of the assessment report citations by technology in Part 2, the 73 information and data resources in Part 3, and the 72 organizational resources in Part 4 are illustrative, not exhaustive, of the scope of technology assessment activities in the U.S. and on the international scene. The *Directory* does represent an important step toward a more comprehensive resource, as a foundation and a template for building an online medical technology assessment information base and related services.

Types of assessment programs and other assessment resources are variously represented in the *Directory*. That an assessment program or other resource is not described in the *Directory* implies nothing about its value. Rather, the breadth of the sample of those included in this first edition helps to suggest how the *Directory* information base might be expanded. For instance, of the various bureaus, institutes, divisions, and other components of the National Institutes of Health that conduct clinical trials or other assessment activities, just three are profiled here. Seventeen of the 24 member organizations of the Council of Medical Specialty Societies (CMSS) provided information for the assessment program profiles or resource organization descriptions in the *Directory*; other CMSS members may also be appropriate for addition to the information base.

Eleven university based programs are profiled; there are others worthy of note. A recent publication of the American College of Radiology noted more than 50 U.S. and international societies in the field of radiology alone; certainly, some of these organizations generate technology assessment documents or engage in other activities relevant to technology assessment.

A survey of existing inventories of health care data sets conducted for the Methods Panel of the council by intern Norma Gavin identified more than 260 data sets that meet minimum provisional criteria for inclusion in a proposed inventory of data sources for health care technology assessment. Although the data sets were identified too late in 1987 to be categorically described in this volume, that survey suggests how the set of information and data resources in Part 3 of the *Directory* could be expanded and its contents more thoroughly elucidated.

Inclusion in the *Directory* of descriptions of any assessment programs, information or data resources, or other organizations does not imply any judgment on behalf of the council, Information Panel, or staff as to the quality of those assessment resources. Similarly, inclusion of any assessment report citations in the *Directory* implies no judgment as to the validity, utility, or other aspect of the quality of the assessment reports. The bulk of the content of the *Directory* was self reported by assessment programs and other resource organizations, and this information was not independently or systematically verified. Compilation of the *Directory* was largely limited by staff awareness of assessment activities, availability of information about these, and limitations of time, personnel, and other resources available for this edition.

The technology thesaurus in Part 2 was generated based upon the technologies appearing in the titles of the assessment report citations of the 68 profiled programs. Therefore, the 1,200-term thesaurus does not encompass all medical technologies, although it may be readily augmented with additional technology terminology. The technology heading under which an assessment report citation is listed in Part 2 does not imply that the technology has been found to be safe, effective, or otherwise appropriate for the use implied by that heading. That a report citation is listed under a particular heading implies only that the technology that is the subject of that citation may have been assessed for the application represented by that heading. For instance, a particular drug may be listed under *Antineoplastics* and under *Antiarthritics*. Assessed as an antineoplastic, the drug may have been determined by a regulatory or other organization to be safe, effective, cost-effective, etc. Assessed as an antiarthritic, the drug may or may not have been found to possess one or more of these qualities. Nevertheless, it would be listed under both headings because the report citations indicate that it was assessed for both applications, regardless of the assessment findings, not because the drug was determined to be appropriate for those uses.

COMPILATION OF THE DIRECTORY

Information for the *Directory* was compiled largely from three surveys. The assessment program profiles and report citation listings of Parts 1 and 2 are based primarily upon responses to a survey of organizations with ongoing medical technology assessment programs. Many of the descriptions in Part 3 were written from responses to a survey of organizations that compile or make available data or information relevant to medical technology assessment. The organizational resources descriptions in Part 4 were drawn largely from a request for brief descriptions of professional, industry, and other organizations having interests in technology assessment.

Council staff reviewed and edited all returned survey forms. No attempt was made to verify with third parties the information provided by the organizations. Staff did not assess the quality of assessment programs, information and data resources, organizational resources, or assessments listed in the *Directory*.

Organizations known or thought to have an ongoing medical technology assessment program were identified initially from council staff files in October 1986. Additional organizations were identified by those organizations surveyed initially and by further council staff work. More than 80 organizations were sent the survey instrument, which is shown in the appendices. This survey was not applicable to organizations that may have conducted medical technology assessments but did not have an ongoing program; that cataloged, indexed, or evaluated assessments but did not produce them; or that conducted assessments but generally did not make results available outside of the organization. Due to resource constraints and because this was not an effort to assemble a library, the survey requested bibliographic citations of assessment reports and sample reports, rather than complete sets of reports from all programs.

Most of the surveys were returned to council staff fully or partially completed. In several cases, council staff and program contacts determined that a program did not constitute an ongoing assessment program, but was appropriate for inclusion in Part 4 or another part of the *Directory*. Surveys were returned to several organizations with requests for additional information or more thorough responses to portions of the survey; often such requests were for more complete citations for assessment reports. Council staff also used telephone or face-to-face interviews with assessment program staff, as well as reports and other literature submitted by the programs, to complete the surveys. Following editing by council staff and further preparation by the contractor, these descriptions were forwarded to the contact persons at each assessment program with a request to verify their factual content or make other suggestions and to return these to council staff by a deadline date, or to expect no modifications if no response was received by that date.

Staff and consultants reviewed the lists of assessment report citations provided by the programs and deleted those that did not meet the criteria of a medical technology assessment report. For purposes of deciding whether or not a report should be listed in the *Directory*, the title had to contain or suggest one or more medical technologies, or imply the consideration of medical technologies, e.g., the management of cervical cancer. Further, it had to either state or imply technology assessment, or one or more properties or attributes of a technology that could be determined by an assessment, e.g., safety, efficacy, ethical implications, or state or imply an evaluation; or be or appear to be guidelines issued by a professional body or its equivalent known by staff to conduct assessments. Staff deleted, for example, assessments of the health effects of Agent Orange because it was neither intended to be nor has it been used as a medical technology. On the other hand, staff retained in the listing assessments of the detrimental consequences of medical technologies, such as the risk of birth defects among nurse anesthetists.

Staff tended to be inclusive in determining what constituted assessment reports for listing with program profiles in Part 1. The primary reasons for this leniency were that decisions were necessarily based on limited information, i.e. report titles rather than full reports; that as a first effort, this *Directory* ought not severely circumscribe this body of literature; and that users might gain a better understanding of programs' scope by viewing fuller portfolios of their reports.

Somewhat stricter criteria were applied for including reports in the list of assessment report citations by technology in Part 2. In instances where titles were ambiguous in this regard and where full reports were on file with council staff, these reports were reviewed to determine whether they constituted assessment reports. However, staff did not make special requests to acquire reports for this purpose.

Edited survey forms were sent to TRITON Corporation, a contractor retained by the council. Using the surveys, TRITON prepared uniform descriptions, or "profiles," of ongoing medical technology assessment programs and created a record for each of their assessment report citations. Each profile has approximately 20 descriptors such as program name, address, telephone, contact person, purpose, methods, reports, etc. Descriptions were edited for consistency and to ensure, as far as possible, uniformity in detail. In creating database records for assessment citations, TRITON followed *Index Medicus* style. The base of citation records was used for two purposes: for generating the coded list of citations following each profile in Part 1, and for generating the listing of assessment report citations by technology in Part 2.

TRITON indexed each assessment report citation using from one to five subject headings, including but not limited to technology terms. Of necessity, TRITON had to rely exclusively on titles to index assessment reports. The subject headings used for indexing are taken primarily though not entirely from the National Library of Medicine's controlled biomedical vocabulary MeSH. The departure from MeSH terms occurred most often for terms related to technologies. The index to the citations appears at the end of Part 1, and is coded to citations appearing after their respective assessment programs.

The technology thesaurus that appears at the beginning of Part 2 was developed in order to arrange the listing of assessment report citations by technology that follows it. The technology thesaurus terms used as headings for Part 2 constitute, largely, a subset of the indexing terms used in Part 1, i.e., those that identify technologies. As noted above, technology terms accounted for most of the instances where indexing departed from MeSH. If MeSH did not contain a subject heading appropriate for a technology used in an assessment report citation title, one was designated based on usage in the medical technology assessment literature as determined by staff, consultants, and TRITON. In some instances, MeSH did not include a term for a particular technology. In others, the closest MeSH term may have been too broad or too narrow to adequately identify a technology, or one not commonly used or perhaps not readily recognized by users who do not have a particular medical or scientific expertise. Linkages to MeSH are retained wherever possible with the use of synonyms, acronyms, cross-references, and broader and narrower terms that are used in MeSH.

Information and data resources described in Part 3 were identified by council staff and by respondents who completed surveys for this part. About half of the descriptions of information and data resources in Part 3 were based entirely or in part on survey responses. The remainder of the descriptions was derived by staff from literature and samples received from the source organizations and telephone interviews. The copy for Part 3 that was submitted to TRITON was generated by staff.

The organizational resource descriptions in Part 4 were derived primarily from requests for narratives of 300 words or less made to organizations identified by council staff and suggested to staff by certain of these organizations. Following editing by council staff, drafts of these descriptions were forwarded to the contact persons at each organization with a request to verify their factual content or make other suggestions and to return these to council staff by a deadline date, or to expect no modifications if no response was received by that date. The copy for Part 4 that was forwarded to TRITON was generated by staff. TRITON submitted final, camera-ready copy of the *Directory* to council staff, who turned it over to the National Academy Press for printing.

PLANS OF THE INFORMATION PANEL

The Information Panel plans to develop technology assessment information products beyond this first edition of the *Directory*. Among the major proposed areas of activity are wide dissemination of the *Directory*, working with the NLM to augment the Library's MeSH vocabulary and DIRLINE (Directory of Information Resources Online) file with new information from the *Directory*, producing access guides to standard literature sources, enhancing and updating the *Directory*, instituting clearinghouse services, and establishing online access to a technology assessment information base.

Users of the *Directory* will be surveyed regarding its utility and format, and will be asked for suggestions for improvement. Additional responses will come in the form of number and distribution of sales, book reviews, and other user feedback. The Information Panel will take account of user responses in formulating its plans for further development of the *Directory* information base and related efforts.

The Information Panel plans a joint vocabulary project with the NLM to better index and thereby improve access to technology assessment information. The vocabulary effort began with the indexing of assessment report titles for the *Directory* and preparation of the technology thesaurus. From this project, the Information Panel may better determine the topical scope of the technology assessment literature, as well as the capacity of the NLM's MeSH vocabulary for indexing technology assessment topics. Instances in which current MeSH terms are found inappropriate for indexing technology assessment report titles in the *Directory* provide opportunities for augmenting MeSH with the intention of improving its utility for searching MEDLINE for assessment related information. Because the *Directory* indexes many report citations drawn from gray literature sources, it may provide a means for identifying newer terms that have not yet entered the lexicon of more traditional sources.

The vocabulary project would establish a framework for, and could begin mapping, certain existing terminology sets such as MeSH, ECRI device codes, ICD-9-CM *(International Classification of Diseases, 9th Revision, Clinical Modification)* and CPT-4 *(Current Procedural Terminology, 4th Edition)* procedure codes, and DRG (diagnosis-related group) terms to the technology topics used in the *Directory*. The mapping of vocabulary terms is consistent with the mission of the Library's Unified Medical Language System project.

Information gathered in compiling the *Directory* will be used to add, update, and modify organizational descriptions in the NLM's DIRLINE file. A component of MEDLARS, DIRLINE is accessible for all users of MEDLARS and certain commercial databases. It contains descriptive information on many organizations and resource centers in the health field. Users interested in particular subjects may enter appropriate keywords to locate information about organizations active in those areas. Adding to DIRLINE descriptive information from the *Directory* about organizations involved in technology assessment will provide broad online access to it through MEDLARS, and any services that download DIRLINE from MEDLARS.

Whereas the *Directory* deals primarily with technology assessments generated by specific assessment organizations and found to a large extent in the gray literature, the Information Panel is planning access guides that would address retrieval of technology assessment information from existing citation bases and other sources. Some of these sources, such as BIOETHICSLINE, MEDLINE, and the National Technical Information Service, are noted in the information and data resources part of this *Directory*. The purpose of these guides would be to help users extract valuable medical technology assessment information from sources that are not specifically devoted to the field or are structured in ways that are not amenable to searching for this information. The guides would describe these sources in greater detail, explain what subfiles or other aspects of each may be useful for assessment purposes, indicate how to access them, and provide examples of assessment searches.

The *Directory* information base may be developed in several major ways. Profiles of programs entered in the first edition may be updated and their new assessments indexed. Additional assessment programs may be profiled and their assessments indexed, and the technology thesaurus updated accordingly. Based upon the information and data resources in Part 3, an expanded, more detailed inventory of data sets for technology assessment could be developed using more quantitative and qualitative descriptors. This inventory would be guided in part by the survey work on data sets described above.

Of particular interest to both the Evaluation Panel and Information Panel of the council is strengthening the information base to enable tracking of new and emerging medical technologies. Such information has value to different sectors of the health care enterprise. It can be used to anticipate assessment needs and prepare timely and well informed assessments, e.g., at the time of market entry of a new drug or device, or when a reimbursement claim is made for a new procedure. Further, it may be useful for remaining apprised of the state-of-the-art in medical practice, planning clinical services, making resource allocation decisions to foster development and diffusion of promising technologies, charting trends in health care product and practice innovation, and identifying investment opportunities. Sources that might be monitored for information concerning emerging and new technologies might include status reports of biomedical research projects, patent information, medical and bioengineering conference proceedings, medical and scientific bibliographic information bases, future-oriented surveys and monographs, market research reports, financial investment sources, product development databases, annual and quarterly reports of health care product companies, news services, FDA approval documents for new drugs and devices, and health insurance claims data. Although this edition of the *Directory* has descriptions of certain information sources that fall into these categories, development of the information base could emphasize addition of information sources, indexing, and retrieval means to help meet needs for intelligence about new and emerging technologies.

The Information Panel is considering implementing selected clearinghouse services with expanded staff or under contract. Initial clearinghouse services may be established based upon the *Directory* and continued updating of its information base, and access to MEDLINE and other online information sources. With these resources, the council could begin to respond to certain types of assessment related inquiries received via written correspondence, telephone, or electronic mail. Staff assigned to this activity could also conduct special searches or generate assessment report bibliographies on topics of current interest for broad distribution. These services would be initiated on an experimental basis, and the demand for them monitored carefully. Commitments to phone answering and conducting searches would have to be adjusted according to demand and availability of resources.

The Information Panel will continue to study the feasibility of providing computer access to technology assessment information. Computer access may entail use of central information bases and distribution of the *Directory*, its updates, and related products via optical or magnetic disks. The panel has determined that appending a technology assessment information base to an existing online system would be preferable to initiating a new stand-alone system. The panel will take account of what is learned from the response to the *Directory* and other current efforts, consult with the NLM and other information base authorities, and plan accordingly.

Providing computer access to the technology assessment information base will be furthered by implementing other of the Information Panel's plans. Together, the *Directory* and access guides will account for much of the gray literature and other online and traditional sources that could be integrated in an online system. Augmenting DIRLINE and MeSH will help to make NLM's MEDLARS more useful to users concerned with technology assessment. Response to the *Directory*, which represents a hard-copy analog of certain aspects of an online system, and access guides will inform the Information Panel about the desirable content and format of assessment information compilations. Clearinghouse services would enhance the council's ability to meet, and learn more about, user needs.

NLM's review of the *Directory*, described below, and other council efforts will provide insight into the extent to which an online technology assessment information base may be linked with the MEDLARS system. One venue for such a link would be to append the *Directory* information base to the HEALTH (HEALTH Planning and Administration) file of MEDLARS, which covers citations on nonclinical aspects of health care delivery such as facilities planning and administration, manpower, insurance, financial management, regulation, and quality assurance. HEALTH is compiled primarily by the American Hospital Association using selections from MEDLINE and augmented by a variety of sources not indexed by NLM. Thus, HEALTH stands as a model of an online base formed from published literature sources as well as certain gray literature sources.

Ties with the National Library of Medicine

In devising the clearinghouse plan and developing this *Directory*, the Information Panel and staff have worked closely with the NLM to develop an information base that complements NLM resources. As indicated above, of particular interest are the extent to which the *Directory* information base identifies new indexing terminology, adds to what is known concerning descriptions of organizations that are significant in biomedical affairs, and identifies valuable sources of literature not indexed by NLM. Pursuant to these interests, NLM staff members have reviewed pertinent portions of an early draft of the *Directory* to gain preliminary measures of these characteristics of the *Directory* information base.

The NLM review indicates that the technology thesaurus terms derived from the assessment reports cited in the draft *Directory* provide some 40 potential new MeSH headings and nearly 400 potential entry terms, i.e. new synonyms for cross-references in MeSH. NLM also reviewed more than 2,500 of the assessment reports citations to determine what proportion were owned and/or indexed by the library. (Approximately 1,000 of the 3,500 report citations in the draft *Directory* were not reviewed because they were assessments in progress, were more than five years old, or were then incomplete citations.) Of the citations reviewed from the draft *Directory*, NLM found that 23 percent were owned and indexed by NLM. Of the remaining 77 percent, about half were owned but not indexed by NLM, and half were neither owned nor indexed by NLM. Since NLM was given the preliminary draft of the *Directory*, some assessment report titles were added, and a few hundred were deleted as irrelevant to medical technology assessment. Also, a few program profiles were added to the *Directory*, and the technology thesaurus was revised. These modifications would not appreciably affect the findings of the NLM review.

NLM compared approximately 190 organizational descriptions from the profile, information and data resources, and organizational resources parts of the draft *Directory* with DIRLINE records to determine the extent to which those in the *Directory* might be used to augment DIRLINE. NLM found that about 28 percent of the organizational descriptions in the *Directory* had directly comparable records in DIRLINE. Another 28 percent of the descriptions were entirely new to DIRLINE. Of the remaining 44 percent of the draft *Directory* descriptions, half were represented only at a more general level in DIRLINE. The rest of the *Directory* organization descriptions were mentioned in DIRLINE records but had no DIRLINE record of their own, were described only in part in DIRLINE records, or were part of larger organizations for which the DIRLINE records did not describe the part included in the *Directory*. Thus, most of the organization descriptions in the draft *Directory* are suitable for augmenting DIRLINE. Some 20 organizational descriptions have been added to various parts of the *Directory* since the preliminary draft was given to NLM.

NLM's review provides some insight into the extent to which the *Directory* information base may be used to complement existing NLM and other major resources for technology assessment, and will help to plan a appropriate strategy for providing this information online.

International Ties

The Information Panel seeks to incorporate valuable sources of international information on technology assessment into the *Directory* information base. This first edition of the *Directory* includes profiles and assessments of 14 programs outside of the U.S., as well as descriptions of other European and international organizations and information resources of interest to the assessment community. This represents only a sample of international sources of potential value to users in the U.S. and abroad.

Although the information concerning assessment activities in other countries was provided directly to council staff for this *Directory*, other organizations in particular countries or certain international agencies could collect such information to be shared with the *Directory* information base. In particular, the Information Panel has been planning certain of its efforts with the European Office of the World Health Organization (WHO), which has among its charges to act as a health technology assessment information clearinghouse for its member countries.

In 1987, WHO established a collaborative effort with the University of Linköping in Sweden, known as WHO/LINFO, to further this charge. The first project of WHO-/LINFO is to assemble a technology assessment information base, modeled in part after this *Directory*. The Information Panel and WHO/LINFO have agreed to coordinate their efforts by using similar information collection, indexing, and display formats to facilitate exchange of assessment information and to avoid duplicative work. As compilation of the council's *Directory* was launched prior to that of WHO/LINFO, WHO-/LINFO was able to use a modified version of the council's *Directory* profile survey to collect information about European organizations involved in assessment. Further, the council is sharing the technology thesaurus used to index the assessment report citations in the *Directory* so that WHO/LINFO may consider using similar terminology to index assessments of its participating programs. Plans concerning responsibility for ongoing collection of assessment information from European and other international sources and related collaboration will be made subject to response to the *Directory* and WHO/LINFO products.

GUIDE TO DIRECTORY'S CONTENTS

The *Directory* includes the following five major parts, described below:

- Part 1: Assessment Program Profiles and Report Citations
- Part 2: Assessment Report Citations Listed by Technology
- Part 3: Information and Data Resources
- Part 4: Organizational Resources
- Part 5: Index to Organizations.

PART 1: ASSESSMENT PROGRAM PROFILES AND REPORT CITATIONS

This part has two major sections. First are the profiles of 68 medical technology assessment programs, with citations of their approximately 3,200 completed, ongoing, and planned assessments. Second is a subject index to the citations, to be used for locating citations on particular subjects among the profiles.

Profiles and Citations

The profiles are of ongoing programs that generate medical technology assessments. For the purposes of this *Directory*, a medical technology assessment is a study or inquiry, the object of which is to provide information regarding the effects of a technology that is intended to maintain or improve health, or be used as part of an intervention for such purpose, whether or not the study evaluates these effects directly.

Most of the information for the assessment program profiles was drawn from the survey of organizations with an ongoing medical technology assessment program, reproduced in Appendix C. Entries for the information categories in each profile include responses to checklists and other questions on the survey. The survey shows these checklists and questions, as well as definitions of terms where necessary. The level of detail in the information categories across the profiles varies. Although staff worked with some assessment program representatives to complete responses to the survey, certain information was unavailable from programs.

The assessment program profiles are listed alphabetically by name of parent organization, and are arranged according to the following common format.

Parent organization and assessment program name, address, and telephone number.

Contact person(s): name, title, address, telephone number if different from the above, telex, telefax, and other numbers.

Overview provides a brief description of the parent organization's purpose, and the assessment program's purpose and origins.

Primary intended users describes the intended audience of the program's assessments. Taken from the checklist of more than 20 categories of primary intended users on page 4 of the survey in Appendix C, examples of these are: general public, patients, physicians, acute facility administrators, long-term care facility administrators, health product manufacturers, health/medical professional associations, third party payers, government regulators, biomedical researchers, and specified others.

Technologies lists the general categories of technology usually assessed by the program. The first listed, in italics, is the one assessed most often. The categories, shown and defined on page 4 of the survey, are: drug, device, medical or surgical procedure, support system, organizational or administrative system, and specified others.

Intervention lists the types of technological intervention normally assessed by the program. The first listed, in italics, is the one assessed most often. The types, shown and defined on page 5 of the survey, are: prevention, diagnosis, treatment, rehabilitation, and specified others.

Stage lists the stages in the life-cycle of technologies at which the program normally conducts its assessments. The first listed, in italics, is the stage assessed most often. The stages, shown and defined on page 5 of the survey, are: emerging, new, established or widespread practice, obsolete, and specified others.

Properties lists the properties or attributes of a technology that the program normally assesses. The first listed, in italics, is the property or attribute usually emphasized. The properties or attributes of technologies assessed, shown and defined on page 5 of the survey, are: safety, efficacy, effectiveness, cost, cost-benefit, cost-effectiveness, service requirements, acceptance/adoption level, system impact, economic implications, and ethical, legal, social implications.

Selection process describes how the program generally selects technologies for assessment. As posed on pages 9 and 10 of the survey, this may encompass who can request that an assessment be conducted, how requests for assessment are made, how and by whom assessment priorities are set, and what provisions are made for reassessing technologies.

Methods lists the broad categories of assessment methods that the program normally employs to conduct an assessment. The first listed, in italics, is the method the program relies on primarily, or exclusively if no other method is listed. The categories of assessment methods, shown and defined on page 6 of the survey, are: information syntheses, expert opinion, group judgment, modeling, cost analyses, epidemiological and other observational methods, clinical trials, and bench testing. This section also includes supplemental descriptive information encompassing: how the assessment process is conducted and by whom, the approximate (average or range of) turnaround time from selection of assessment topic to report of findings, and approximate cost per assessment.

Assessors describes the types of expertise of a program's assessors.

Assessment reports include lists the types of items generally included or addressed in a program's assessment reports. Taken from the checklist of more than 20 items listed on page 6 of the survey, examples of these are: abstract, purpose of assessment, who sponsored assessment, who conducted assessment, description of technology, how the technology works, properties assessed, sources of data/information, methods for analyzing/synthesizing data/information, limitations of findings, regulatory agency approval status, coverage/reimbursement status, and specified others.

Dissemination lists the means by which a program disseminates its assessment findings. The first listed, in italics, is the one relied on primarily. The general types of dissemination means, shown on page 6 of the survey, are: printed reports (excluding journal articles); journal articles; advisories to members/constituents;

press conferences/news releases; TV/radio broadcasts, video products; clearinghouse, data/citation bases, online services; other (specify). This section also includes supplemental information encompassing: types of assessment products, details of how assessment results are disseminated, and how to acquire copies of assessment reports.

Budget gives the program's annual budget in U.S. dollars for calendar 1986 unless specified otherwise, and the percentage from type of source. These sources, shown on page 7 of the survey, are: parent organization; government grants/contracts; foundations and other private grants; sponsors/members dues contributions; sales of assessments, consultant services, etc.; and specified others.

Use describes how assessments are used by the parent organization, who else uses them and for what purpose (and how the program knows this); documented use of assessment reports and their impact, including citation of published documents; and citations in the published literature to the program or its assessments.

Program evaluation describes the evaluations that have been conducted of the program, who did them, evaluation results, and how evaluation results have been used to improve the program.

Related activities describes additional information about the technology assessment activities of the program not covered elsewhere in a profile.

Completed Reports are listed in reverse chronological order and then in alphabetical order by author and title. For most of the profiles, the citations cover assessments generated since 1980. The completeness of bibliographic citations varies. To the extent possible, the citations are in *Index Medicus* style. If an organization sponsoring the technology assessment is not the author of the report, the organization name is enclosed within brackets. Reports issued by programs of the U.S. Government often are available from the U.S. Government Printing Office or the National Technical Information Service. Where provided by assessment programs, order numbers are included in the bibliographic citation. The report code preceding each citation (consisting of a two letter prefix and a number) is used to link the report to the index to report citations at the end of Part 1. Information in brackets following the citation indicates the type of method(s) used by the program to conduct its assessments.

Ongoing Assessments are listed in chronological order (based on expected completion date), earliest first and then in alphabetical order by author and title. The citation provides the expected date of the report, if the program provided one. Assessments for which the program did not provide a completion date are listed alphabetically by author and title after those for which it provided a completion date. Some of the ongoing assessments have been completed and made available by the time of publication of this *Directory*. Not all programs provided information about ongoing assessments.

Planned Assessments lists assessments the program expects to conduct by author and title. Some of the planned assessments may have been completed and made available by the time of publication of the *Directory*. Not all programs provided information about ongoing assessments.

Not all reports generated by the 68 programs are cited in the *Directory*. In most instances, reports dated prior to 1980 are excluded, although for certain smaller programs earlier reports are retained. The scope of activity of certain of the 68 programs does not neatly or consistently coincide with medical technology assessment. In other cases, an understanding of a program's activity does indicate that it conducts assessments of medical technologies, but pertinent report titles are not written in a manner reflecting this. Many report titles produced by certain programs mention no medical technology and/or do not indicate that an assessment was involved.

In general, to appear in the *Directory*, report citations must, in at least a broad sense, mention or imply an assessment of one or more technologies. For example, a report title reading "Evaluation of . . . " qualifies, as do titles mentioning one or more attributes or properties of an assessment such as safety, effectiveness, cost-effectiveness, or economic, ethical, legal, or social implications, or such related extensions as market analysis or analysis of variation in clinical practice. Reports that are "Guidelines for . . . " or "Standards for . . . " are also listed, although some are, strictly speaking, model practices or criteria developed based upon assessment findings.

Assessments of the effects of environmental hazards, substances, and interactions neither intended nor used as medical technologies are excluded from the *Directory*. However, interventions to prevent, diagnose, or treat the effects of these are considered medical technologies. Assessments of certain natural processes, e.g., breast feeding, are included because other interventions (e.g., infant formula, in this case) create the possibility of alternative modalities. Excluded specifically are documents describing regulatory requirements. Examples of reports generated by assessment programs but excluded from the *Directory* because they are not about medical technologies or assessments of technologies are: "Carcinogen regulation," "Effects of toxic chemicals on the reproductive cycle," "Health effects of smokeless tobacco," "Health effects of Agent Orange and dioxin contaminants," and "Smoking related deaths and financial costs."

Because the conduct and utility of technology assessments depends on the availability of suitable methods for this purpose, assessments of methods are considered within the scope of the *Directory*. Examples of reports about assessments of methods are "Assessment of double-blindness at the conclusion of the Beta-Blocker Heart Attack Trial," "Postmarketing surveillance of prescription drugs," and "The impact of randomized clinical trials on health policy and medical practice."

In certain instances where council staff was aware by discussion with assessment program representatives and familiarity with program reports, citations were included that had short titles not indicating that report content did address assessments of technologies. This is the case, for example, for certain citations of the American College of Obstetricians and Gynecologists Committee on Technical Bulletins. Reports with such titles as "Carcinoma of the endometrium," "Hemorrhagic shock," and "Osteoporosis" deal with the management of these conditions or alternative technologies for diagnosis or treatment of them, and therefore were retained in the listing of citations following the program profile in Part 1 of the *Directory*. Similarly, reports of the NIH Consensus Development Program titled "Travelers' diarrhea," "Osteoporosis," and "Health implications of obesity" are included in Part 1. Instances such as these are exceptions, however, and staff did not seek on a systematic basis to determine report content beyond what could be discerned from titles. Further, because titles such as these do not name a specific technology, they are not included in the listing of assessment report citations by technology in Part 2.

Index to Report Citations

At the end of Part 1 is an index to report citations. The index has approximately 1,900 subject terms, e.g., *Aspirin*, *Decubitus ulcer*, *Monoclonal antibodies*, and *Urinary calculi*.

These terms were compiled by indexing the titles of the assessment reports generated by the programs profiled in Part 1. Each assessment report citation is indexed using from one to five terms. The indexing terms are listed alphabetically, each followed by one or more relevant assessment report codes. Each code has a two letter prefix indicating an assessment program in Part 1, and a number indicating the report's placement in the program's list of citations. For instance, the term *Decubitus ulcer* is followed by the codes AG49, CB10, CB13, NC74, NC104, NC122, and ND19. A list of prefixes and their respective programs is shown immediately preceding this subject index.

Because each assessment report citation is indexed with from one to five terms, a particular report citation may be shown under more than one term in the index to report citations at the end of Part 1. For instance, the report code NC2, corresponding to the NCHSR Office of Health Technology Assessment report "Apheresis in the treatment of systemic lupus erythematosus (SLE)," is listed under *Apheresis* and under *Lupus erythematosus, Systemic*.

This index includes technology terms (e.g., *Dental sealants, Magnetic resonance imaging,* and *Tonometry*) as well as non-technology terms (e.g., *Esophagus, Fetus,* and *Thrombophlebitis*). For non-technology terms, the subject index to report citations relies primarily upon the National Library of Medicine's (NLM) MeSH (Medical Subject Headings) terminology. For technology terms, this index relies primarily upon the terms developed for the technology thesaurus in Part 2, which includes some MeSH terms.

PART 2: ASSESSMENT REPORT CITATIONS LISTED BY TECHNOLOGY

This part has two major sections: a technology thesaurus and a cross-listing of the assessment report citations by technology. These two sections are directly related in that the listing of assessment report citations by technology is arranged according to the terminology set forth in the technology thesaurus.

Technology Thesaurus

The technology thesaurus was developed for the *Directory* to help users search for assessment reports by technology topic. It was generated based upon the technologies appearing in the titles of the assessment report citations shown in Part 1. Where appropriate, it uses the NLM's MeSH vocabulary terms. To enhance searching, the 1,200-term thesaurus includes many synonyms, acronyms, and cross-references, and indicates broader and narrower terms to lead users to desired citations and to help clarify relationships among technology terms.

Technologies are listed at the most specific level suggested by terms used in report titles, usually the name or class of a drug, procedure, device, etc. In general, drugs are listed by generic name, and procedures, devices, etc. are listed by class, e.g., *Radiographic equipment*, in preference to individual brands or models. Thus, assessments of all brands of hydrophilic contact lenses are listed together.

The technology thesaurus lists a technology's synonyms, including abbreviations as well as alternative terms. For each synonym, the thesaurus indicates the listing term under which pertinent citations are shown, using **SEE** *(listing term)*. For each listing term, the thesaurus indicates terms from which the user may have been referred using **x** (e.g., from a **SEE** *(listing term)*); indicates which terms are broader than the listing term, using **BT**; and which terms are narrower than the listing term, using **NT**; and indicates related terms, using **SEE ALSO** *(related term)*. With respect to **BTs** and **NTs**, each indicates only one level broader or narrower. However, by referring to the next **BT** or **NT**, a user can find other terms yet broader or narrower.

Because a technology may have more than one type of application, or may be classified along a number of dimensions, two or more **BTs** may be shown for a given technology.

For example, *Ibuprofen* has as broader terms *Antipyretics* and *Nonsteroidal anti-inflammatory analgesics*, so that a user looking under either of these broader terms would be referred to assessment report citations concerning ibuprofen. *Laser angioplasty* has as broader terms *Angioplasty* and *Laser surgery*, so that a user seeking citations about means for performing angioplasty, or about applications of laser surgery, would be referred to assessment citations concerning laser angioplasty. Where assessment report citations exist of both a device and its use in practice, each is referred to the other. For example, *Fetal monitors* suggests **SEE ALSO** *Fetal monitoring*, and vice-versa.

Designation of broader or narrower terms is not intended to be complete according to some established framework, although a hierarchically arranged framework of technology terms is conceivable. The extent to which portions of such a framework appear here reflects only the need to accommodate the terms drawn from the assessment report citations included in the *Directory*.

MeSH terms are used in preference to other terms, unless a MeSH term appears to vary substantially from common usage. Thus, pertinent assessment citations are listed under *Coronary artery bypass grafting* in the *Directory* instead of the corresponding MeSH term *Aortocoronary bypass*; *Beta blockers* is used instead of the MeSH term *Adrenergic beta receptor blockaders*; and *Computed tomography* is used instead of the MeSH term *Tomography, X-ray computed*. Nevertheless, such MeSH terms are shown as synonyms so that users using these as "entry terms" will be referred to the term under which pertinent assessments are listed, so that linkages with MeSH are retained. Word form variations are consistent with the basic term, e.g., *Computed tomography scanners*. Technologies are listed by full name, in preference to an abbreviation, except where an abbreviation is used more commonly or the full name is unwieldy, e.g., *APACHE* instead of *Acute Physiology and Chronic Health Evaluation*, and *BCG vaccine* instead of *Bacillus Calmette-Guérin strain of Mycobacterium bovis*.

Assessment Report Citations by Technology

The cross-listing of assessment report citations listed by technology arranges the citations under technology terms from the thesaurus, e.g., *Cataract extraction, Heart valve prosthesis*, and *Propranolol*, so that all citations for each type of technology may be viewed together.

Citations listed are those in which the title includes one or more identifiable medical technologies. For example, a report titled "Evaluation of nadolol in treatment of hypertension" is listed under *Nadolol*. Under any particular technology heading, the citations are listed in reverse chronological order, and then in alphabetical order by author and title. In addition to bibliographic information, most citations note, in brackets at the end of the citation, the general type of assessment method used, e.g., clinical trial, group judgment, and information synthesis. Because not all of the 3,200 assessment report citations shown with the assessment program profiles in Part 1 have a technology term in their titles, Part 2 contains a subset of these, i.e. about 2,500 citations.

Given its synonyms, acronyms, cross-references, and broader and narrower terms, referring to the technology thesaurus first is the best way to search the listing of assessment report citations by technology in Part 2. Unless a report citation has more than one technology in its title, it is shown only once in the technology listing, usually appearing under its most specific technology term.

Where a title indicates that two or more specific medical technologies are assessed either individually or one in comparison to the other, the citation is listed under both terms. If two or more technologies appear to be used in combination, e.g., "Protein-calorie therapy in combination with anabolic steroids in alcoholic hepatitis," the citation is listed only once under the combined term, in this instance, *Protein-calorie therapy with anabolic steroids*. If a title is ambiguous in this respect, the report is listed under each of the medical technologies mentioned.

For citations listed in this section, distinctions generally are made between procedures and the equipment used for them. For example, headings include *Computed tomography* as well as *Computed tomography scanners*, and *Fetal monitoring* as well as *Fetal monitors*.

Where a report involves a technology to address consequences of a previously applied technology, the active technology is indexed. For instance, the title "Prevalence and pathogenesis of cholesterol gallstones in Halifax: prevention of recurrence by diet changes after medical dissolution therapy" is listed under *Diet therapy*, rather than under a technology for medical dissolution of cholesterol gallstones.

PART 3: INFORMATION AND DATA RESOURCES

This part describes 73 public and private sector information and data resources that may be useful in conducting medical technology assessments. Included are a categorical chart of all of the resources, the 73 resource descriptions, and a subject index to the resources.

At the beginning of Part 3, a categorical chart indicates which of three types of descriptors characterizes each resources. These are:

File type

directories/compendiums

bibliographic information/abstracts

reports/texts/references

data sets

news bulletins

Format

hard copy/print/microfiche

online computer

machine-readable/disk/magnetic tape

Access

public

limited.

An information or data resource may be characterized by more than one descriptor for each of the three main types. For instance, a resource may have bibliographic as well as full text files, may appear in hard copy as well as online format, or may have both public and limited access files.

The descriptions of each of the 73 information and data resources are arranged alphabetically by name of resource. Each is described according to the following common format.

Name of information or data resource.

Source gives the name, address, and telephone number of the organization that produces or makes available the information or data.

Subject indicates the general subject matter covered by the information or data resource.

Content describes the information or data contained in the resource, such as scope of coverage, file format, and descriptions of subfiles.

Compilation describes how the information or data resource is assembled, such as primary sources, when compilation began, and how often the resource is updated.

Access describes how to acquire the information or data, including subscription and use charges, limitations to public access, need for computer hook-up, etc.

At the end of Part 3 is a subject index for identifying information and data resources relevant to particular topics, e.g., market research.

PART 4: ORGANIZATIONAL RESOURCES

This part provides brief descriptions and contact information for 72 organizations that are active in affairs related to medical technology and are stakeholders in medical technology assessment. Although most of these organizations do not generate technology assessment reports on a regular basis, they have memberships concerned with medical technologies, conduct relevant meetings and symposiums, publish conference proceedings and other documents of note, establish standards for technologies, or are active in government, regulatory, or other policy affairs relevant to the field.

The organizational descriptions are arranged alphabetically by organization name. Each includes name, address, and telephone number of the organization; contact person(s), and a narrative description of the organization in 300 words or less, including discussion of medical technology related activities. At the end of Part 4 is a subject index for identifying organizations involved in particular areas, e.g., biomedical engineering.

PART 5: INDEX TO ORGANIZATIONS

This part includes an alphabetical listing with addresses and telephone numbers for all organizations described in the *Directory*, as well as a page index to the organizations.

WAYS TO USE THE DIRECTORY

DO YOU WANT TO SEE IF AN ORGANIZATION IS LISTED, OR WHAT IT DOES?

Check the index to organizations in Part 5 to find the pages on which organizations are described in the *Directory*.

DO YOU WANT TO FIND ASSESSMENT REPORTS ON A SPECIFIC TECHNOLOGY?

Check the technology thesaurus at the beginning of Part 2 on page 313. The thesaurus will inform you whether reports are listed under the technology term that you have in mind, or under a synonym or related term. Once you have located the appropriate term, you can find the pertinent report citations under that heading in Part 2.

YOU MAY BE INTERESTED IN REPORTS THAT HAVE TITLES REFERRING TO TECHNOLOGY TERMS THAT ARE BROADER OR NARROWER THAN THE ONE YOU HAVE IN MIND.

For example, if you are interested in reports about beta-blockers, you will find reports under the heading *Beta-blockers*. But, as the thesaurus indicates, additional reports are to be found under more specific names for beta-blockers, such as *Propranolol*. Except for cases in which more than one technology is shown in the title of a report citation, a citation is listed only once in Part 2, i.e. under the most specific technology heading. So, it is important to refer to the thesaurus first to get the most out of the listing of assessment report citations by technology in Part 2.

DO YOU WANT TO FIND REPORTS INDEXED BY NON-TECHNOLOGY TERMS SUCH AS COST BENEFIT ANALYSIS, PARTICULAR DISEASES, OR OTHER SUBJECTS?

Check under the desired term in the index to report citations at the end of Part 1, and use the report codes found there to look up the assessments in the indicated program profiles. Each code under that term has a two letter prefix indicating the assessment program in Part 1, and a number indicating the report's placement in the program's list of citations. A list of prefixes and their respective programs is shown immediately preceding this subject index.

Under *Cost benefit analysis*, you would find the reference numbers BA2, CP3, CU62, etc., which correspond to the numbered assessment report citations following the profiles on Battelle Memorial Institute, College of American Pathologists, Congress of the United States Office of Technology Assessment, etc. Similarly, under *Asthma*, you would find AC110, MG14, and ND86; under *Breast neoplasms* are AE15, AH4, AH6, etc.; under *Hypertension* are AG25, BA1, HN28, etc., and under *Postmarketing surveillance* are CU56, HN79, MG9, and MG10.

Because each assessment report citation is indexed with from one to five terms, a particular report citation may be shown under more than one term in the index to report citations at the end of Part 1. For instance, the 1987 report by the Medical Technology and Practice Patterns Institute, "Dialysis treatment for end stage renal disease (outpatient)," is indexed under the terms *Dialysis*; *Kidney failure, Chronic*; and

Outpatients. This means that the code for that report, MT6, is shown under each of these three terms.

For non-technology terms such as asthma, cost benefit analysis, or hypertension, the subject index to report citations relies primarily upon MeSH terminology. The actual titles of the the aforementioned three reports indexed under *Cost benefit analysis*, i.e. BA2, CP3, and CU62, include the phrases "cost-effectiveness analysis, "cost-effective," and "Allocating costs and benefits," respectively. *Cost benefit analysis* is the MeSH indexing term assigned for these. For technologies such as beta-blockers, coronary artery bypass grafting, or chorionic villi sampling, this index relies primarily upon the terms developed for the technology thesaurus in Part 2, which includes some MeSH terms. Searching for reports by technologies is best done using the technology thesaurus at the beginning of Part 2 because it shows cross-references, synonyms, and related terms.

DO YOU WANT TO FIND REPORTS THAT ADDRESS MORE THAN ONE SUBJECT?

This involves locating the set of reports common to the multiple subjects of interest. For instance, to find reports that address both cost benefit analysis and cervical cancer screening, note the reports listed under *Cost benefit analysis* in the subject index at the end of Part 1. Next, determine if any of these reports is also listed under *Cancer screening—Cervical* in the index at the end of Part 1 or the listing of assessment report citations by technology in Part 2. Remember that the thesaurus at the beginning of Part 2 is the best guide in the *Directory* for locating reports by their technology subjects. Among the reports found under both *Cost benefit analysis* and *Cancer screening—Cervical* is a report from the Congress of the U.S. Office of Technology Assessment, "Allocating costs and benefits in disease prevention: an application to cervical cancer screening."

This manual approach of looking under two or more subject headings is necessary given that the *Directory* information base is available only in hard-copy format at the time of printing this first edition. In a computer format, the "and/or" operations of Boolean algebra could be used more readily for searching reports involving such constraints as multiple subjects.

DO YOU WANT TO OBTAIN A TECHNOLOGY ASSESSMENT REPORT?

Check the subject index to assessment report citations at the end of Part 1 or the listing of assessment report citations by technology in Part 2 to find out which assessment program produced it. Find the program's profile in the alphabetical listing of assessment programs in Part 1, and see the section on *Dissemination* for ordering information. The program's address, telephone number, and other contact information are shown at the beginning of the profile.

DO YOU WANT TO GET IN TOUCH WITH AN ORGANIZATION THAT DEALS WITH A CERTAIN TOPIC?

Use the subject indexes to the different parts of the *Directory* to identify organizations active in certain areas. The index to report citations at the end in Part 1 and the listing of assessment report citations by technology in Part 2 may be used to identify profiled assessment programs, arranged alphabetically in Part 1, by the topics of their assessment reports. The information and data resources in Part 3 and the organizational resources in Part 4 are indexed by subject at the ends of those parts. For instance, under the heading *Market research* in the index to information and data resources in Part 3 are listed IMS Audits, Scrip, Market/Technology Reports (Biomedical Business International), and other resources. Under the heading *Biomedical engineering* in the index to organizational resources in Part 4 are listed the Alliance for Engineering in Medicine and Biology, American Society of Mechanical Engineers, RESNA—Association for the Advancement of Rehabilitation Technology, Institute of Electrical and Electronics Engineers, and the International Federation for Medical and Biological Engineering. Contact information and descriptions of these are arranged alphabetically.

GLOSSARY OF ACRONYMS

AABB	American Association of Blood Banks
AAD	American Academy of Dermatology
AAFP	American Academy of Family Physicians
AAMC	Association of American Medical Colleges
AAMI	Association for the Advancement of Medical Instrumentation
AAMSI	American Association for Medical Systems and Informatics
AAN	American Academy of Neurology
AAO	American Academy of Ophthalmology
AAOHNS	American Academy of Otolaryngology-Head and Neck Surgery
AAOS	American Academy of Orthopaedic Surgeons
AAP	American Academy of Pediatrics
AAPMR	American Academy of Physical Medicine and Rehabilitation
AATB	American Association of Tissue Banks
ACC	American College of Cardiology
ACEP	American College of Emergency Physicians
ACG	American College of Gastroenterology
ACNP	American College of Nuclear Physicians
ACOG	American College of Obstetricians and Gynecologists
ACP	American College of Physicians
ACPM	American College of Preventive Medicine
ACR	American College of Radiology
ACS	American Cancer Society or American College of Surgeons
ACT	American Council on Transplantation
ADA	American Dental Association or American Diabetes Association
ADAMHA	Alcohol, Drug Abuse, and Mental Health Administration
ADM	alcohol, drug abuse, and mental health
AEMB	Alliance for Engineering in Medicine and Biology
AGS	American Geriatrics Society
AHA	American Hospital Association or American Heart Association
AHCI	American Health Care Institute
AHSR	Association for Health Services Research
AIUM	American Institute of Ultrasound in Medicine
AMA	American Medical Association
AMCRA	American Medical Care and Review Association
AMPRA	American Medical Peer Review Association
AAMRC	American Medical Review Research Center
ANSI	American National Standards Institute
AP	Associated Press
APA	American Psychiatric Association
APHA	American Public Health Association
ARA	American Rheumatism Association
ASA	American Society of Anesthesiologists
ASCP	American Society of Clinical Pathologists
ASCPT	American Society for Clinical Pharmacology and Therapeutics

ASGE	American Society for Gastrointestinal Endoscopy
ASIM	American Society of Internal Medicine
ASPEN	American Society of Parenteral and Enteral Nutrition
ASTM	American Society of Testing and Materials
ASTP	American Society of Transplant Physicians
ASTS	American Society of Transplant Surgeons
AUA	American Urological Association
AZT	azidothymidine
BCBS	Blue Cross and Blue Shield
BCDSP	Boston Collaborative Drug Surveillance Program
BDDD	Division of Birth Defects and Developmental Disabilities (CDC)
BERC	Bureau Eligibility, Reimbursement and Coverage (HCFA)
BMEDSS	Biomedical Engineering Decision Support Services
BRS	Bibliographic Retrieval Service
CABG	coronary artery bypass grafting
CAMMD	Canadian Association of Manufacturers of Medical Devices
CAP	College of American Pathologists
CASSIS	Classification and Search Support Information System (Patent and Trademark Office)
CAT	computerized axial tomography
CBO	Centraal Begeleidingsorgaan voor de Intercollegiale Toetsing (The Netherlands)
CCC	Copenhagen Collaborating Center (WHO)
CDB	Center for Drugs and Biologics (FDA)
CDC	Centers for Disease Control
CDRH	Center for Devices and Radiological Health (FDA)
CEAP	Clinical Efficacy Assessment Project (ACP)
CFSAN	Center for Food Safety and Applied Nutrition (FDA)
CHA	Center for Health Affairs (Project HOPE)
CHAMPUS	Civilian Health and Medical Program of the Uniformed Services
CHID	Combined Health Information Database
CHPE	Center for Health Promotion and Education (CDC)
CHPRE	Center for Health Policy Research and Education (Duke University)
CMA	California Medical Association
CMSS	Council of Medical Specialty Societies
CMT	Center for Medical Technology Assessment (Linköping University)
COMPASS	Computerized On-Line Medicaid Pharmaceutical Analysis and Surveillance System (Health Information Designs, Inc.)
CPHA	Commission on Professional and Hospital Activities
CPT-4	Current Procedural Terminology, 4th Edition
CRISP	Computer Retrieval of Information on Scientific Projects (NIH)
CSDD	Center for the Study of Drug Development (Tufts University)
CSS	Council of Subspecialty Societies
CT	computed tomography
CVS	chorionic villi sampling
DATTA	Diagnostic and Therapeutic Technology Assessment Program (AMA)

DCCC	Duke Comprehensive Cancer Center Database
DEN	Device Experience Network (FDA)
DHHS	U.S. Department of Health and Human Services
DHSS	Department of Health and Social Security (United Kingdom)
DIMDI	Deutsches Institut für Medizinische Dokumentation und Information (Germany)
DIRLINE	Directory of Information Resources Online (NLM)
DOD	U.S. Department of Defense
DPPR	Drug Product Problem Reporting System (FDA, USP)
DRG	diagnosis-related group or Division of Research Grants (NIH)
DURbase	Drug Utilization Review base (Health Information Designs, Inc.)
EBRI	Employee Benefit Research Institute
ECRI	formerly Emergency Care Research Institute
ECRI/HDP	ECRI Health Devices Program
ECRI/TAP	ECRI Technology Assessment Program
EHLS	Division of Environmental Health Laboratory Sciences (CDC)
EMBASE	Excerpta Medica Database (Elsevier)
EPA	Environmental Protection Agency
ERIC	Educational Resources Information Center
ESRD	end stage renal disease
FAHS	Federation of American Health Systems
FDA	Food and Drug Administration
GHAA	Group Health Association of America
GHC	Group Health Cooperative of Puget Sound
GPIA	Generic Pharmaceutical Industry Association
GPO	U.S. Government Printing Office
GWUMC	George Washington University Medical Center
HANES	National Health and Nutrition Examination Survey (NCHS)
HBP	high blood pressure
HCFA	Health Care Financing Administration (DHHS)
HECLINET	Health Care Literature Information Network (DIMDI)
HHS	U.S. Department of Health and Human Services
HIAA	Health Insurance Association of America
HIMA	Health Industry Manufacturers Association
HMO	health maintenance organization
HRSA	Health Resources and Services Administration
HSR&D	Health Services Research and Development Service (VA)
IAF	Institute for Alternative Futures
ICD-9-CM	International Classification of Diseases, 9th Revision, Clinical Modification
IDE	investigational device exemption (FDA)
IEEE	Institute of Electrical and Electronics Engineers
IFMBE	International Federation for Medical and Biological Engineering
IFTF	Institute for the Future
IFVHSF	International Federation of Voluntary Health Service Funds

IHPS	Institute for Health Policy Studies (UCSF)
IMPAC	Information for Management Planning Analysis and Coordination (NIH)
IND	investigational new drug (FDA)
IOM	Institute of Medicine (NAS)
IRCS	International Research Communications System (Elsevier)
ISTAHC	International Society of Technology Assessment in Health Care
MDR	Medical Device Reporting regulation (FDA)
MEDITEC	Medizinische Technik
MEDLARS	Medical Literature Analysis and Retrieval System (NLM)
MEDLINE	MEDLARS online (NLM)
MeSH	Medical Subject Headings (NLM)
MHA	Maryland Hospital Association
MHRST	Medical and Health Related Sciences Thesaurus (NIH)
MRC	Medical Research Council (Canada)
MTPPI	Medical Technology and Practice Patterns Institute
NAHDO	National Association of Health Data Organizations
NAM	National Association of Manufacturers
NAS	National Academy of Sciences
NASA	National Aeronautics and Space Administration
NCEP	National Cholesterol Education Program
NCHS	National Center for Health Statistics
NCHSR/ HCTA	National Center for Health Services Research and Health Care Technology Assessment
NCI	National Cancer Institute
NCQHC	National Committee for Quality Health Care
NDA	new drug application (FDA)
Nd:YAG	Neodymium:yttrium aluminum garnet
NEMA	National Electrical Manufacturers Association
NEMT	Nordic Evaluation of Medical Technology
NHC	National Heart Council
NHLBI	National Heart, Lung, and Blood Institute
NHRDP	National Health Research and Development Program (Canada)
NHS	National Health Service (United Kingdom)
NHSPPS	National Health Services and Practice Patterns Survey
NIA	National Institute on Aging
NIAAA	National Institute on Alcohol Abuse and Alcoholism
NICHD	National Institute of Child Health and Human Development
NIDA	National Institute on Drug Abuse
NIH	National Institutes of Health (PHS, DHHS)
NIMH	National Institute of Mental Health
NINCDS	National Institute of Neurological and Communicative Disorders and Stroke
NIOSH	National Institute for Occupational Safety and Health
NLM	National Library of Medicine
NMR	nuclear magnetic resonance
NSEP	NHLBI Smoking and Education Program
NTIS	National Technical Information Service

OASH	Office of the Assistant Secretary for Health (DHHS)
ODPHP	Office of Disease Prevention and Health Promotion (DHHS)
OHTA	Office of Health Technology Assessment (NCHSR)
OMAR	Office of Medical Applications of Research (NIH)
ONHIC	ODPHP National Health Information Center
OPE	Office of Planning and Evaluation (NIH)
OPTN	Organ Procurement and Transplantation Network (UNOS)
ORD	Office of Research and Demonstrations (HCFA)
OSHA	Occupational Safety and Health Administration
OTA	Office of Technology Assessment (U.S. Congress)
PAHO	Pan American Health Organization
PDQ	Physician Data Query (NCI)
PHS	U.S. Public Health Service (DHHS)
PMA	Pharmaceutical Manufacturers Association
PPRC or PhysPRC	Physician Payment Review Commission
PPS	Medicare Prospective Payment System
PRO	professional review organization
ProPAC	Prospective Payment Assessment Commission
PRP	Medical Device and Laboratory Product Problem Reporting Program (FDA, USP)
PTO	U.S. Patent and Trademark Office
R&D	research and development
RESNA	Association for the Advancement of Rehabilitation Technology, formerly Rehabilitation Engineering Society of North America
RCT	randomized (controlled) clinical trial
RFA	request for application
RFP	request for proposal
RPA	Renal Physicians Association
RTECS	Registry of Toxic Effects of Chemical Substances (NIOSH, NLM)
SBA	Summary Basis of Approval (FDA)
SEER	Surveillance, Epidemiology, and End Results Program (NCI)
SIC	Standard Industrial Classification
SMD	Society for Medical Decision Making
SNM	Society of Nuclear Medicine
SNIVT	Society of Non-Invasive Vascular Technology
SPO	Special Projects Office (VA)
SPRI	Swedish Planning and Rationalization Institute of the Health Services
SPRILINE	Swedish Planning and Rationalization Institute of the Health Services line
SREPCIM	Society for Research and Education in Primary Care Internal Medicine
SSED	Summaries of Safety and Effectiveness Data (FDA)
TAF	Technology Assessment and Forecast Program (PTO)
TDC	Technical Data Center (OSHA)
TNO	Medical Technology Unit, Netherlands Organization for Applied Scientific Research
UCSF	University of California at San Francisco
UHC	University Hospital Consortium
UNOS	United Network for Organ Sharing
USDA	U.S. Department of Agriculture

USDHHS	U.S. Department of Health and Human Services
VA	Veterans Administration
WHO	World Health Organization
YAG	yttrium aluminum garnet

Part 1
Assessment Program Profiles and Report Citations

Part 1: Assessment Program Profiles and Report Citations

This part has two major sections. Beginning on page 3 are profiles of 68 medical technology assessment programs, with citations of their approximately 3,200 completed, ongoing, and planned assessments. The assessment program profiles are listed alphabetically by name of parent organization.

Following the profiles, beginning on page 254, is a subject index to report citations, to be used for locating citations on particular subjects among the profiles. The index has approximately 1,900 subject terms. These terms are listed alphabetically, each followed by one or more relevant assessment report codes. Each code has a two letter prefix indicating an assessment program and a number indicating the report's placement in the list of citations at the end of the program's profile earlier in Part 1. A list of prefixes and their respective programs is shown on page 252, immediately preceding the subject index.

American Academy of Neurology
Practice Committee
2221 University Avenue SE, Suite 335
Minneapolis, MN 55414
612-623-8115

Contact: Richard P. Hames, Director, Division of Medical Services and Communications; William H. Stuart M.D., 105 Collier Rd. NW, Suite 1030, Atlanta, GA 30309, 404-351-2270; or John P. Conomy M.D., Department of Neurology, Cleveland Clinic Foundation, 9500 Euclid Ave., Cleveland, OH 44106, 216-444-5555.

Overview: The American Academy of Neurology (AAN) is a 9,000-member medical specialty society founded in 1948. The Academy's major objectives are to stimulate the growth and development of the specialty of clinical neurology and clinical neurologists. The AAN Practice Committee assesses the clinical effectiveness of drugs, devices, and procedures involving the neurosciences.

Purpose: To review and evaluate clinical, procedural, and technological requests for opinion received by the Academy.

Primary intended users: Providers, generally; physicians; health/medical professional associations; third party payers; government regulators.

Technologies: *Medical or surgical procedure,* drug, device.

Intervention: *Treatment,* diagnosis, rehabilitation.

Stage: *New,* established or widespread practice, obsolete.

Properties: *Effectiveness;* safety; efficacy; cost; service requirements; acceptance/adoption level; ethical, legal, social implications.

Selection process: Individual practitioners in neurology and neurosurgery, medical organizations, and third party payers can request that an assessment be conducted. All requests must be in writing and sent to the Academy office. Requests are submitted to the Practice Committee for opinion and inclusion on the agenda. The Practice Committee does not set assessment topic priorities. The Committee, acting as a group, assesses all questions submitted to it, although the Committee has rejected such complicated topics as organ transplantation.

Methods: *Group judgment,* expert opinion.

The Practice Committee receives reports from several subcommittees that are, in most cases, chaired by a Practice Committee member. The subcommittees consider the procedure/treatment question and exercise one of two options: 1) develop recommendation for full committee as to whether the treatment/procedure is established, investigational, unacceptable, or indeterminate (as defined in accordance with the American Medical Association (AMA) Diagnostic and Therapeutic Technology Assessment plan); or 2) defer recommendation pending further research/study by subcommittee members. At each of the four regularly scheduled meetings per year the Practice Committee reviews and acts on the recommendations of the subcommittees. Practice Committee actions are then submitted to the Academy Executive Board as information items.

The following statement is incorporated into every response to a request for opinion: "This response is provided as a service of the American Academy of Neurology. It is based on current scientific and clinical information through (date of evaluation), and does not represent endorsement by the AAN of particular diagnostic and therapeutic procedures or treatment."

When major questions or issues confront the Committee, such as the use of magnetic resonance imaging as a diagnostic procedure, a wider consensus is sought. Working with the Council of Medical Specialty Societies (CMSS), the AMA, and other organizations, a consensus panel is convened and a position paper developed on the technology in question.

The turnaround time from selection of assessment topic to reporting of findings ranges from 1 week to 6 months.

Assessors: The Practice Committee is composed of 16 members from across the country who represent the interests and concerns of the practitioner.

Assessment reports include: Who sponsored/commissioned/ supported the assessment; stage of life-cycle of technology when assessed; recommendations for practice, future assessments, technology development, research.

Dissemination: Assessment results are disseminated through the minutes of the Practice Committee and through correspondence with other medical organizations and practitioners. The Academy office maintains a listing of Practice Committee decisions and responds to inquiries about procedures/treatment. The Council of Medical Specialty Societies also distributes Practice Committee assessments.

Budget: The assessment program is not budgeted as a separate activity. The approximate cost per assessment is not known.

Use: The Academy disseminates assessment results to its membership. Based on inquires received, third party payers rely on Practice Committee opinions in making reimbursement decisions.

Completed Reports

AA1 American Academy of Neurology, Practice Committee. Extracranial-intracranial bypass surgery for treatment or prevention of stroke. 1986 Feb. [Expert opinion, Group judgment]

AA2 ______. Hyperbaric oxygen therapy for treatment of senility, multiple sclerosis, and cerebral edema. 1986 Feb. [Expert opinion, Group judgment]

AA3 ______. Apheresis (therapeutic) in the treatment of Guillain-Barré Syndrome. 1985 Jun. [Expert opinion, Group judgment]

AA4 ______. Apheresis in treatment of systemic lupus erythematosus. 1985 Jun. [Expert opinion, Group judgment]

AA5 ______. Percutaneous transluminal angioplasty (PTA). 1985 Feb. [Expert opinion, Group judgment]

AA6 ______. Topographic mapping. 1985. Feb. [Expert opinion, Group judgment]

AA7 ______. Apheresis in treatment of chronic relapsing polyneuropathy. 1984 Feb. [Expert opinion, Group judgment]

AA8 ______. Autopsies on patients with slow virus diseases. 1984 Nov. [Expert opinion, Group judgment]

AA9 ______. EEG guidelines for epileptic mentally retarded. 1984 Nov. [Expert opinion, Group judgment]

AA10 ______. Electromyographic biofeedback in treatment of hyperactivity. 1984 Feb. [Expert opinion, Group judgment]

AA11 ______. Electronystagmography. 1984 Jun. [Expert opinion, Group judgment]

AA12 ______. Functional integration in the alleviation of chronic muscular pain and spasticity. 1984 Feb. [Expert opinion, Group judgment]

AA13 ______. Nuclear magnetic resonance. 1984 Feb. [Expert opinion, Group judgment]

AA14 ______. Sterotactic cingulatomy. 1984 Nov. [Expert opinion, Group judgment]

AA15 ______. Amyotrophic lateral sclerosis—injected modified neurotoxin for treatment. 1983 Feb. [Expert opinion, Group judgment]

AA16 ______. Edinburgh Masker for stuttering. 1983 Jun. [Expert opinion, Group judgment]

AA17 ______. Histamine desensitization for cluster headache. 1983 Jun. [Expert opinion, Group judgment]

AA18 ______. Melodic intonation therapy for aphasia. [Expert opinion, Group judgment]

AA19 ______. Modified neurotoxin in the treatment of ALS. 1983 Jun. [Expert opinion, Group judgment]

AA20 ______. Plasmapheresis in treatment of multiple sclerosis. 1983 Feb. [Expert opinion, Group judgment]

AA21 ______. Plasmapheresis in treatment of myasthenia gravis. 1983 Feb. [Expert opinion, Group judgment]

AA22 ______. Somatosensory evoked response. 1983 Nov. [Expert opinion, Group judgment]

AA23 ______. Trancutaneous electrical nerve stimulation for treatment of acute pain for ambulatory patients. 1983 Nov. [Expert opinion, Group judgment]

AA24 ______. Twenty-four hour EEG ambulatory monitoring. 1983 Jun. [Expert opinion, Group judgment]

AA25 ______. Biofeedback for headaches. 1982 Jun. [Expert opinion, Group judgment]

AA26 ______. Carotid infusion of BCNU for glioblastoma multiforme. 1982 Jun. [Expert opinion, Group judgment]

AA27 ______. Cerebellar stimulator implantation for cerebral palsy. 1982 Oct. [Expert opinion, Group judgment]

AA28 ______. Cerebellar stimulator implantation. 1982 Jun. [Expert opinion, Group judgment]

AA29 ______. Cochleostomy with neurovascular transplant in treatment of Ménière's Disease. 1982 Oct.[Expert opinion, Group judgment]

AA30 ______. EEG monitoring—ambulatory. 1982 Apr. [Expert opinion, Group judgment]

AA31 ______. EEG monitoring during open-heart surgery and immediate post-operative period. 1982 Oct. [Expert opinion, Group judgment]

AA32 ______. Negative pressure respirators for home use in chronic neuromuscular disease. 1982 Oct. [Expert opinion, Group judgment]

AA33 ______. Spinal cord stimulation for treatment of cerebral palsy. 1982 Jun. [Expert opinion, Group judgment]

AA34 ______. Taste and smell clinics. 1982 Jun. [Expert opinion, Group judgment]

AA35 ______. Acupuncture. 1981 Jul. [Expert opinion, Group judgment]

AA36 ______. Apheresis for multiple sclerosis. 1981 Jul. [Expert opinion, Group judgment]

AA37 ______. EEG interpretation and brain stem evoked response. 1981 Jul. [Expert opinion, Group judgment]

AA38 ______. Electrical nerve stimulation of post-surgical pain. 1981 Apr. [Expert opinion, Group judgment]

AA39 ______. Electrical stimulation for treatment of Bell's Palsy. 1981 Apr. [Expert opinion, Group judgment]

AA40 ______. Electrical stimulation for treatment of facial nerve palsy. 1981 May. [Expert opinion, Group judgment]

AA41 ______. Histamine therapy for Ménière's Disease. 1981 Jul. [Expert opinion, Group judgment]

AA42 ______. Prolotherapy. 1981 Jul. [Expert opinion, Group judgment]

AA43 ______. Visual evoked potentials. 1981 Jul. [Expert opinion, Group judgment]

AA44 ______. Biofeedback treatment for migraine headache. 1980 Apr. [Expert opinion, Group judgment]

AA45 ______. Continuous EEG monitoring during surgery. 1980 Apr. [Expert opinion, Group judgment]

AA46 ______. Intracranial pressure monitors. 1980 Oct. [Expert opinion, Group judgment]

AA47 ______. Neurosonology. 1980 Mar. [Expert opinion, Group judgment]

AA48 ______. Spinal stimulation for multiple sclerosis. 1980 May. [Expert opinion, Group judgment]

AA49 ______. Transfer factor treatment in multiple sclerosis. 1980 Apr. [Expert opinion, Group judgment]

AA50 ______. Ultrasonic arteriography. 1980 May. [Expert opinion, Group judgment]

American Academy of Ophthalmology

Ophthalmic Procedures Assessment Program
PO Box 7424
655 Beach Street
San Francisco, CA 94120-7424
415-561-8500

Contact: Lea Gamble, Director Health Policy Research; or David L. Guyton, M.D., Chairman, Committee on Ophthalmic Procedures Assessment, Wilmer Ophthalmological Institute, the Johns Hopkins Hospital, Baltimore, MD 21205, 301-955-8314.

Overview: The American Academy of Ophthalmology (AAO) is a professional association composed of over 14,000 physicians trained in the specialty of ophthalmology. It offers a wide range of membership services including continuing education programs, public and professional information materials, and scientific meetings. The Ophthalmic Procedures Assessment Program is the medical technology assessment program of the AAO.

Purpose: To present state-of-the-science information about ophthalmic technologies that will help Academy members make informed decisions about patient care.

Primary intended users: Physicians, third party payers, government regulators.

Technologies: *Medical or surgical procedure,* drug, device.

Ophthalmology-related orphan drugs and products, diagnostic and therapeutic devices, and medical and surgical procedures are assessed.

Intervention: *Treatment,* diagnosis.

Stage: *New,* emerging, established or widespread practice.

Sufficient information must be available in the scientific literature to develop assessments.

Properties: *Safety, effectiveness,* efficacy.

Comprehensive assessments usually follow this format: definition of terms, including development of technique or procedure, extent of current use; clinical implementation, including indications for use, comparison to conventional methods, advantages/disadvantages, patient population most likely to benefit, and effectiveness; safety; qualifications necessary to use technique; and current research and summary.

Selection process: Academy members, public and private third party payers, and government agencies can request that assessments be conducted. Requests will also be accepted from other sources. Usually requests for assessments are written inquiries asking the Academy's position/opinion on a certain technology. Inquiries from individuals and private third party payers are frequently received over the telephone, but the AAO requires that a written request be submitted. The Committee on Ophthalmic Procedures Assessment sets priorities. Technologies to be assessed must be within the scope of ophthalmology, and sufficient scientific information on which to base a decision must be available. If new information is available that substantially changes information contained in an assessment, a reassessment of the technology will be initiated.

Methods: *Information syntheses, group judgment,* expert opinion, epidemiological and other observational methods.

The scientific literature in refereed journals is reviewed and expert opinion and group judgment is sought in order to reach consensus. After a decision to evaluate a technology has been made, the following four steps are followed: 1) an expert is identified who develops a draft with references; 2) the draft is reviewed by other experts, generally AAO members, the Committee, staff, and legal counsel; 3) if substantial changes are needed, a revised draft is recirculated to all reviewers and, generally, a conference call is held to discuss differences in interpretation of findings in the literature; and 4) once a draft is acceptable to the reviewers, it is submitted to the Academy's Board of Directors for approval.

For noncontroversial technologies, the average turnaround time from selection of assessment topic to reporting of findings is 6 to 9 months. For controversial technologies the turnaround time can extend into years.

Assessors: The Committee is composed of three Academy members, staffed by the Academy's Office of Health Policy Research, and assisted by the membership of the Academy. Academy members participate as reviewers, as in-depth consultants, or by preparing the original draft assessment. A total of 400 Academy members, covering 40 technical areas, have agreed to participate, in some capacity, in the assessment effort. These members participate voluntarily and without remuneration. When appropriate, experts from related fields are consulted.

Assessment reports include: Who conducted the assessment; description of the technology; properties assessed; sources of data/information; findings or conclusions; recommendations for practice, future assessments, technology development, research; how the technology works, including theory, principles; development of the technology.

Dissemination: *Printed reports; journal articles;* press conferences/news releases, TV/radio broadcasts, video products.

The Academy prints the assessment reports, and notices of completed assessments appear in the AAO membership newsletter. The assessments are published in the AAO's scientific journal, displayed at the AAO annual meeting, and are mailed to specific organizations and interested individuals. The Academy's Order Department accepts telephone and written requests for assessment reports. Copies are provided free of charge.

Budget: $7,500. Funding source: 100 percent sponsors/members dues, contributions.

Use: Assessment reports are considered an educational service to the members and are provided in response to inquiries from the media, third party payers, and the public. Private and public third party payers use them to make policy decisions about coverage. Their purpose for requesting an assessment is generally stated.

Related activities: At the 1986 AAO annual meeting, the Committee on Ophthalmic Procedures Assessment sponsored a special scientific session entitled, "Radial Keratotomy in Perspective." The purpose of this session was to have opthalmologists representing a range of opinions address key questions about the procedure.

Completed Reports

AB1 American Academy of Ophthalmology. Epikeratophakia procedures for the correction of severe hyperopia, myopia, and keratoconus. San Francisco, CA: American Academy of Ophthalmology, expected completion October 1987. [Information syntheses, Expert opinion]

AB2 ______. Punctal occlusion for the dry eye. San Francisco, CA: American Academy of Ophthalmology, 1987. [Information syntheses, Expert opinion]

AB3 ______. Punctoplasty for siccakeratitis. San Francisco, CA: American Academy of Ophthalmology, expected completion June 1987. [Information syntheses, Expert opinion]

AB4 ______. Radial keratotomy for myopia. San Francisco, CA: American Academy of Ophthalmology, expected completion October, 1987. [Information syntheses, Expert opinion]

AB5 ______. Cataract surgery in the 1980's. San Francisco, CA: American Academy of Ophthalmology, 1987. [Information syntheses, Expert opinion]

AB6 ______. Keratophakia and keratomileusis: safety and effectiveness. San Francisco, CA: American Academy of Ophthalmology, 1986. [Information syntheses, Expert opinion]

AB7 ______. Thymoxamine: the need for orphan drug status. San Francisco, CA: American Academy of Ophthalmology, 1986. [Information syntheses, Expert opinion]

AB8 ______. Botulinum toxin therapy of eye muscle disorders: safety and effectiveness. San Francisco, CA: American Academy of Ophthalmology, 1984. [Information syntheses, Expert opinion]

AB9 Committee on Ophthalmic Procedures Assessment. [American Academy of Ophthalmology] Carbon dioxide laser surgery in head and neck surgery. San Francisco, CA: American Academy of Ophthalmology, 1984. [Information syntheses, Expert opinion]

AB10 ______. [American Academy of Ophthalmology] Cyanoacrylate tissue adhesive. San Francisco, CA: American Academy of Ophthalmology, 1984. [Information syntheses, Expert opinion]

AB11 ______. [American Academy of Ophthalmology] Therapeutic contact lenses for recurrent corneal erosion. San Francisco, CA: American Academy of Ophthalmology, 1984. [Information syntheses, Expert opinion]

AB12 Keltner JL. [American Academy of Ophthalmology] Academy recommendation: automated perimetry. Ophthalmology 1984;91:51-56. [Information syntheses, Expert opinion]

AB13 Trokel S. [American Academy of Ophthalmology] Academy recommendation: ophthalmic neodymium YAG lasers: safety and effectiveness. Ophthalmology 1984;91:539-42. [Information syntheses, Expert opinion]

AB14 American Academy of Ophthalmology. Laser trabecular surgery for open-angle glaucoma. San Francisco, CA: American Academy of Ophthalmology, 1983. [Information syntheses, Expert opinion]

American Academy of Pediatrics

141 Northwest Point Boulevard
PO Box 927
Elk Grove Village, IL 60009-0927
312-228-5005

Contact: Jean Lockhart, M.D.

Overview: The American Academy of Pediatrics (AAP) is a professional association composed of pediatricians and pediatric medical and surgical subspecialists. The Academy promotes optimal physical, mental, and social health for infants, children, adolescents, and young adults. It provides a range of services including advocacy for children and pediatrics, health systems delivery research, public information and education, continuing medical education, and analyses and review of child health policy issues. The Academy's technology assessment activities are an integral part of the information gathering and advisory functions of the numerous AAP Committees.

Purpose: The AAP Committees keep abreast of developments in the field and advise the membership and Executive Board on topics within the committees' areas of expertise.

Primary intended users: General public; physicians; health/medical professional associations; government regulators; public policy-makers, legislators; policy research organizations; liability, malpractice insurers.

Technologies: Drug, device, medical or surgical procedure, support system, organizational or administrative system.

Intervention: Prevention, diagnosis, treatment, rehabilitation.

Stage: Emerging, new, established or widespread practice.

Properties: Safety; efficacy; effectiveness; service requirements; system impact; ethical, legal, social implications.

Selection process: Topic suggestions can come from any source. Usually, assessment topics are suggested by committee members, AAP members, or through other organizational requests. The AAP accepts telephone and written requests and occasionally relies on formal contracts. For example, the Food and Drug Administration contracted with the AAP for advice relative to infant formulas and drugs. AAP staff screen the requests and then the appropriate committee considers the question. Assessment topic priorities are set by the individual committee and the Academy.

Methods: Information syntheses, expert opinion, group judgment.

The assessment method varies from committee to committee and by issue, although all committees generally rely on a type of group judgment. For statements, committees usually proceed in the following manner: 1) general discussion of issue; 2) preparation of first draft by committee member; 3) extensive review and preparation of bibliography by same member (in some cases, this information is reviewed by outside consultants); 4) presentation of second draft and discussion by committee; and, 5) revision of draft, if necessary. All reports must be approved by the Executive Board of the AAP.

The average turnaround time from selection of assessment topic to reporting of findings ranges from 4 months to 1 year.

Assessors: AAP has committees in such areas as adolescence, bioethics, drugs, fetus and newborn, hospital care, infectious diseases, nutrition, radiology, and surgery. Each committee consists of experts in the topic area. Committees can also bring in consultants for additional expertise on particular reports.

Dissemination: Printed reports; advisories to members/constituents; press conferences/news releases, TV/radio broadcasts.

Committees issue reports with the assessment findings. For smaller scale projects a note is made in the minutes or a recommendation given to the AAP Executive Board. AAP Committee statements are published in *Pediatrics* or information may appear in *AAP News.* Occasionally, letters are sent to government agencies such as the Environmental Protection Agency or the Consumer Product Safety Commission. Some reports are distributed directly to the AAP members, such as the *Report of the Committee on Infectious Diseases* (the "Red Book").

Budget: Not provided.

Related activities: The AAP publishes a quarterly newsletter, *Child Health Financing Report,* which contains the latest information about child health financing for privately insured children and those covered by Medicare. The Academy also sponsors an annual meeting, educational programs, and continuing education courses.

Completed Reports

AC1 American Academy of Pediatrics, Committee on Hospital Care. Emergency services. Pediatrics (To be published).

AC2 ______, Committee on Hospital Care. Guidelines for air and ground transportation. Pediatrics (To be published).

AC3 ______, Committee on Hospital Care. Quality assurance of hospital care of children. Pediatrics (To be published).

AC4 ______, Committee on Practice and Ambulatory Medicine. Screening for vision problems. Pediatrics (To be published).

AC5 ______, Committee on Accident and Poison Prevention. Revised first aid for the choking child. Pediatrics 1986 Jun.

AC6 ______, Committee on Child Health Financing. Medicaid policy statement. Pediatrics 1986 May.

AC7 ______, Committee on Disabilities. Screening for developmental disabilities. Pediatrics 1986 Sep.

AC8 ______, Committee on Disabilities. Transition of severely disabled children from hospital or chronic care facilities to the community. Pediatrics 1986 Sep.

AC9 ______, Committee on Early Childhood, Adoption, and Dependent Care. Oral and dental aspects of child abuse and neglect. Pediatrics 1986 Sep.

AC10 ______, Committee on Nutrition. Prudent lifestyle for children: dietary fat and cholesterol. Pediatrics 1986 Sep.

AC11 ______, Committee on Practice and Ambulatory Medicine. Vision screening and eye examination in children. Pediatrics 1986 Jun.

AC12 ______, Committee on Research. Guidelines for the Pediatric Cancer Center and the role of such centers in diagnosis and treatment. Pediatrics 1986 Jun.

AC13 ______, Committee on School Health. CPR training in the school. AAP News 1986 Jan.

AC14 ______, Committee on School Health. School attendance of children and adolescents with human T lymphotropic virus III/lymphadenopathy-associated virus infection. Pediatrics 1986 Mar.

AC15 ______, Committee on School Health. School health examinations. AAP News 1986 Feb.

AC16 ______, Committee on Infectious Diseases. Prevention of hepatitis B virus infections. Pediatrics 1985 Feb.

AC17 ______, Committee on Bioethics. Proposed guidelines on genetic engineering. Pediatrics 1985 Jun.

AC18 ______, Committee on Disabilities. Assisting disabled children. Pediatrics 1985 Jun.

AC19 ______, Committee on Disabilities. Provision of related services for children with chronic disabilities. Pediatrics 1985 Apr.

AC20 ______, Committee on Drugs. "Inactive" ingredients in pharmaceutical products. Pediatrics 1985 Oct.

AC21 ______, Committee on Drugs. Behavioral and cognitive effects of anticonvulsant therapy. Pediatrics 1985 Oct.

AC22 ______, Committee on Drugs. Guidelines for the elective use or conscious use of sedation, deep sedation, and general anesthesia in pediatric patients. Pediatrics 1985 Aug.

AC23 ______, Committee on Environmental Hazards. Smokeless tobacco—a carcinogenic hazard to children. Pediatrics 1985.

AC24 ______, Committee on Fetus and Newborn. High risk newborn care. Pediatrics 1985 Jul.

AC25 ______, Committee on Fetus and Newborn. Home phototherapy. Pediatrics 1985 Jul.

AC26 ______, Committee on Fetus and Newborn. Vitamin E and the prevention of retinopathy of prematurity. Pediatrics 1985 Aug.

AC27 ______, Committee on Hospital Care. Child life programs for hospitalized children. Pediatrics 1985 Sep.

AC28 ______, Committee on Hospital Care. Guidelines for pediatric intensive care units. Pediatrics 1983 Sep.

AC29 ______, Committee on Infectious Diseases. Hemophilus type b polysaccharide vaccine. Pediatrics 1985 Aug.

AC30 ______, Committee on Infectious Diseases. Recommendations for using pneumococcal vaccine in children. Pediatrics 1985 Jun.

AC31 ______, Committee on Infectious Diseases. Recommendations for using pneumococcal vaccine in children. Pediatrics 1985 Jun.

AC32 ______, Committee on Nutrition. Nutritional needs of low-birth-weight infants. Pediatrics 1985 May.

AC33 ______, Committee on Nutrition. Use of oral fluid therapy and posttreatment feeding following enteritis in children in a developed country. Pediatrics 1985 Feb.

AC34 ______, Committee on Practice and Ambulatory Medicine. Computers in your practice. Pediatrics 1985 Jul.

AC35 ______, Committee on Practice and Ambulatory Medicine. High risk newborn care. Pediatrics 1985 Jul.

AC36 ______, Committee on School Health. Health education and schools. Pediatrics 1985 Jun.

AC37 ______, Committee on Screening Genetics. Maternal phenylketonuria. Pediatrics 1985 Aug.

AC38 ______, Committee on Adolescence. A policy reference guide to the AAP's Council Committee and Executive Board statements. 1984.

AC39 ______, Committee on Drugs. Ethanol in liquid preparations intended for children. 1984.

AC40 ______, Committee on Drugs. Antimicrobial prophylaxis in pediatric surgical patients. Pediatrics 1984 Sep.

AC41 ______, Committee on Infectious Diseases. Antimicrobial prophylaxis in pediatric surgical patients. Pediatrics 1984 Sep.

AC42 ______, Committee on Infectious Diseases. Pertussis vaccine. Pediatrics 1984 Aug.

AC43 ______, Committee on Nutrition. Imitation and substitute milks. Pediatrics 1984 Jun.

AC44 ______, Committee on Research. Fetal research. Pediatrics 1984 Sep.

AC45 ______, Committee on School Health. Administration of medication in school. Pediatrics 1984 Sep.

AC46 ______, Committee on School Health. Alcohol abuse education in schools. Pediatrics 1984 Sep.

AC47 ______, Committee on School Health. Guidelines for urgent care in schools. Pediatrics 1984 Jul.

AC48 ______, Committee on School Health. Heat stress and school closings. Pediatrics 1984 Aug.

AC49 ______, Committee on Sports Medicine. Health appraisal guidelines for day camps and residence camps. Pediatrics 1984 Jun.

AC50 ______, Committee on Nutrition. The use of whole cow's milk in infancy. Pediatrics 1983 Aug.

AC51 ______, Committee on Adolescence. Rape and the adolescent. Pediatrics 1983 Nov.

AC52 ______, Committee on Adolescence. The role of the pediatrician in substance abuse counseling. Pediatrics 1983 Aug.

AC53 ______, Committee on Bioethics. Treatment of critically ill newborns. 1983.

AC54 ______, Committee on Drugs. Growth hormone in treatment of children with short stature. 1983.

AC55 ______, Committee on Drugs. "Look-alikes." Pediatrics 1983 Aug.

AC56 ______, Committee on Drugs. Benzyl alcohol: toxic agent in neonatal units. Pediatrics 1983 Sep.

AC57 ______, Committee on Drugs. Dimethyl sulfoxide (DMSO). Pediatrics 1983 Jan.

AC58 ______, Committee on Drugs. New therapy for severe cystic acne. Pediatrics 1983 Aug.

AC59 ______, Committee on Drugs. Valproate teratogenicity. Pediatrics 1983 Jun.

AC60 ______, Committee on Early Childhood, Adoption, and Dependent Care. Gonorrhea in prepubertal children. Pediatrics 1983 Apr.

AC61 ______, Committee on Fetus and Newborn. Benzyl alcohol: toxic agent in neonatal units. Pediatrics 1983 Sep.

AC62 ______, Committee on Nutrition. Soy-protein formulas: recommendations for use in infant feeding. [1983]

AC63 ______, Committee on Nutrition. Commentary on parenteral nutrition. Pediatrics 1983 Apr.

AC64 ______, Committee on Nutrition. Toward a prudent diet for children. Pediatrics 1983 Jan.

AC65 ______, Committee on Research. Reducing the toll of injuries in childhood requires support for a focused research effort. Pediatrics 1983 Nov.

AC66 ______, Committee on Sports Medicine. Sports and the child with epilepsy. Pediatrics 1983 Dec.

AC67 American Academy of Pediatrics, Committee on Fetus and Newborn. Criteria for early infant discharge and follow-up evaluation. Pediatrics 1982 Dec.

AC68 ______, Committee on Disabilities. The Doman-Delacato treatment of neurologically handicapped children. Pediatrics 1982 Nov.

AC69 ______, Committee on Drugs. Psychotropic drugs in pregnancy and lactation. Pediatrics 1982 Feb.

AC70 ______, Committee on Drugs. Valproic acid: benefits and risks. Pediatrics 1982 Aug.

AC71 ______, Committee on Hospital Care. Preoperative chest radiographs. Pediatrics 1983 May.

AC72 ______, Committee on Infectious Diseases. Aspirin and Reye syndrome. Pediatrics 1982 Jun.

AC73 ______, Committee on Nutrition. Promotion of breast feeding. 1982.

AC74 ______, Committee on Research. Guidelines for health supervision of pediatric visits as recommended by the American Academy of Pediatrics Committee on Practice and Ambulatory Medicine. News and Comment 1982 May.

AC75 ______, Committee on Screening Genetics. New issues in newborn screening for phenylketonuria and congenital hypothyroidism. Pediatrics 1982 Jan.

AC76 ______, Committee on Sports Medicine. Risks in long distance running for children. Pediatrics 1982 Jun.

AC77 ______, Committee on Nutrition. Nutritional aspects of obesity in infancy and childhood. Pediatrics 1981 Dec.

AC78 ______, Committee on Nutrition. Breast feeding and contraception. 1981

AC79 ______, Committee on Nutrition. Breast feeding and contraception. 1981.

AC80 ______, Committee on Nutrition. Plant fiber intake in pediatric diet. 1981.

AC81 ______, Committee on Nutrition. Sodium intake for infants in the U.S., 1981.

AC82 ______, Committee on Nutrition. Nutrition and lactation. Pediatrics 1981 Sep.

AC83 ______, Committee on Adolescence. Contraception for the adolescent. Pediatrics 1980 Mar.

AC84 ______, Committee on Drugs. Anticonvulsants and pregnancy. Pediatrics 1980 Feb.

AC85 ______, Committee on Drugs. Medroxyprogesterone acetate (Depo-Provcra). Pcdiatrics 1980 Mar.

AC86 ______, Committee on Drugs. Naloxone use in newborns. Pediatrics 1980 Mar.

AC87 ______, Committee on Nutrition. Vitamins and mineral supplement needs. 1980.

AC88 ______, Committee on Nutrition. Encouraging breast-feeding. Pediatrics 1980 Mar.

AC89 ______, Committee on Nutrition. Human milk banking. Pediatrics 1980 Apr.

AC90 ______, Committee on Nutrition. On the feeding of supplemental foods to infants. Pediatrics 1980 Jun.

AC91 ______, Committee on Radiology. Comparison radiographs of extremities in childhood: recommended usage. Pediatrics 1980 Mar.

AC92 ______, Committee on Radiology. Excretory urography for evaluation of enuresis. Pediatrics 1980 Mar.

AC93 ______, Committee on Screening Genetics. Prenatal diagnosis for pediatricians. Pediatrics 1980 Jun.

AC94 ______, Committee on Adolescence. Pregnancy and abortion counseling. Pediatrics 1979 Jun.

AC95 ______, Committee on Disabilities. Current approaches to evaluation and management of children with myelomeningocele. Pediatrics 1979 Apr.

AC96 ______, Committee on Sports Medicine. Accidental hypothermia. Pediatrics 1979 Jun.

AC97 ______,Committee on Drugs. Camphor: who needs it? Pediatrics 1978 Sep.

AC98 ______, Committee on Drugs. Commentary on anthelmintics. Pediatrics 1978 Aug.

AC99 ______, Committee on Drugs. Effect of medication during labor and delivery on infant outcome. Pediatrics 1978 Sep.

AC100 ______, Committee on Drugs. PUVA: a caution. Pediatrics 1978 Aug.

AC101 ______, Committee on Drugs. Treatment of congenital hypothyroidism. Pediatrics 1978 Sep.

AC102 ______, Committee on Drugs. Unapproved uses of approved drugs: the physician, the package insert, and the FDA. Pediatrics 1978 Aug.

AC103 ______, Committee on Drugs. Use of codeine- and dextromethorphan-containing cough syrups in pediatrics. Pediatrics 1978 Jul.

AC104 ______, Committee on Nutrition. Juice in ready-to-use bottles and nursing bottle caries. 1978.

AC105 ______, Committee on Nutrition. Breast-feeding. Pediatrics 1978 Oct.

AC106 ______, Committee on Radiology. Radiation of pregnant women. Pediatrics 1978 Jan.

AC107 ______, Committee on Radiology. Water-soluble contrast material. Pediatrics 1978 Jul.

AC108 ______, Committee on Nutrition. Nutritional aspects of vegetarianism, health foods and fad diets. Pediatrics 1977 Mar.

AC109 ______, Committee on Screening Genetics. Screening school children for urologic disease. Pediatrics 1977 Aug.

AC110 ______, Committee on Drugs. Adverse reactions to iodide therapy of asthma and other pulmonary diseases. Pediatrics 1976 Feb.

AC111 ______, Committee on Drugs. Generic prescribing. Pediatrics 1976 Feb.

AC112 ______, Committee on Nutrition. Commentary on breast-feeding and infant formulas, including proposed standards for formulas. Pediatrics 1976 Feb.

AC113 ______, Committee on Bioethics. AAP code of ethics for the use of fetuses and fetal material for research. 1975

AC114 ______, Committee on Fetus and Newborn. Report of the Ad Hoc Task Force on Circumcision. Pediatrics 1975 Oct.

AC115 ______, Committee on Disabilities. Early identification of children with learning disabilities: the preschool child. Pediatrics 1973 Nov.

American College of Cardiology/American Heart Association Task Force on Assessment of Diagnostic and Therapeutic Cardiovascular Procedures

American College of Cardiology
9111 Old Georgetown Road
Bethesda, MD 20814
301-897-5400

American Heart Association
National Center
7320 Greenville Avenue
Dallas, TX 75231
214-373-6300

Contact: Charles Fisch, M.D., Chairman ACC/AHA Task Force on Assessment of Diagnostic and Therapeutic Cardiovascular Procedures; David Feild, Associate Executive Vice President, American College of Cardiology; or Kathryn A. Taubert, Ph.D., Science Consultant, American Heart Association 214-706-1455.

Overview: The American College of Cardiology (ACC) is a professional medical society composed of physicians and scientists. Its mission is to ensure optimal care for persons with cardiovascular disease or the potential for developing cardiovascular disease and to contribute to the prevention of cardiovascular disease through educational and socio-economic activities. The American Heart Association (AHA) is a voluntary health agency supported by public contributions and the donated time of volunteers. Its mission is to reduce premature death and disability from cardiovascular disease and stroke. The Task Force on the Assessment of Diagnostic and Therapeutic Cardiovascular Procedures is a technology assessment program jointly sponsored by the AHA and the ACC.

Purpose: To define the role of noninvasive and invasive diagnostic and therapeutic procedures in the diagnosis and management of cardiovascular disease.

Primary intended users: Physicians.

Technologies: Medical or surgical procedure.

Specifically, diagnostic and therapeutic cardiovascular procedures are assessed.

Intervention: Diagnosis, treatment.

Stage: Established or widespread practice.

Properties: Effectiveness, indications/contraindications.

Selection process: Members of the American College of Cardiology or the American Heart Association can submit, in writing, requests for assessments to the Chairman of the ACC/AHA Task Force. The Task Force meets at least twice a year to discuss possible future assessments. Recommendations are forwarded to the officers of the

American College of Cardiology and the American Heart Association. The possibility of updating published assessment reports is currently under discussion.

Methods: Information syntheses, expert opinion, group judgment.

As part of the assessment process a series of committee meetings are held. As the assessment report develops, information is shared, via mail, between Task Force members. The approximate turnaround time from selection of assessment topic to reporting of findings is 18 months.

Assessors: Task Force members are physicians who specialize in cardiovascular medicine.

Assessment reports include: The purpose of the assessment, who sponsored/commissioned/supported the assessment, who conducted the assessment, description of the technology.

Dissemination: Journal articles.

Reports are published simultaneously in the *Journal of the American College of Cardiology* and *Circulation.* Copies of the assessment reports can be obtained by contacting the headquarters offices of the American College of Cardiology or the American Heart Association.

Budget: $25,000. The approximate direct costs per assessment ranges from $10,000 to $15,000. Volunteer time committed to this effort is significant and is not calculated in this amount. Funding source: 50 percent American College of Cardiology, 50 percent American Heart Association.

Use: The Task Force assessment activities are described in Institute of Medicine, Committee on Evaluating Medical Technologies in Clinical Use. *Assessing medical technologies.* Washington, DC: National Academy Press, 1985.

Related activities: Services available to ACC members include a government relations department that promotes cardiovascular issues, the *Cardiology* and *Affiliates in Training* newsletters, an endowments program, professional awards programs, and continuing education opportunities.

The 14 Scientific Councils of the AHA generate state-of-the-art and position papers concerning specific areas of cardiovascular disease such as arteriosclerosis, cardiovascular radiology, cardiovascular surgery, and thrombosis. The Association provides approximately $50 million annually for scientific research and additional support for public education programs. The AHA advocates legislation for research and education in the field.

Completed Reports

AD1 O'Rourke RA, Chatterjee K, Dodge HT, et al. [American College of Cardiology/American Heart Association Task Force on Assessment of Cardiovascular Procedures] Guidelines for clinical use of cardiac radionuclide imaging. J Am Coll Cardiol 1986 Dec;8:1471-83. [Group judgment]

AD2 Schlant RC, Blomqvist CG, Brandenburg RO, et al. [American College of Cardiology/American Heart Association Task Force on Assessment of Cardiovascular Procedures] Guidelines for exercise testing. J Am Coll Cardiol 1986;8:725-738. [Group judgment]

AD3 Frye RL, Collins JJ, DeSanctis RW, et al. [American College of Cardiology/American Heart Association Task Force on Assessment of Cardiovascular Procedures] Guidelines for permanent cardiac pacemaker implantation. J Am Coll Cardiol 1984;4:434-42. [Group judgment]

Ongoing Assessments

AD4 American College of Cardiology/American Heart Association Task Force on Assessment of Cardiovascular Procedures. Guidelines for ambulatory electrocardiographic monitoring. Ongoing. [Group judgment]

AD5 ______. Guidelines for clinical intracardiac electrophysiologic studies. Ongoing. [Group judgment]

AD6 ______. Guidelines for coronary angiography. Ongoing. [Group judgment]

AD7 ______. Guidelines for percutaneous transluminal coronary angioplasty (PTCA). Ongoing. [Group judgment]

American College of Obstetricians and Gynecologists Committee Opinions

600 Maryland Avenue SW
Washington, DC 20024
202-638-5577

Contact: Shirley A. Shelton, Associate Director, Division of Practice Activities; or the ACOG Resource Center.

Overview: The American College of Obstetricians and Gynecologists (ACOG) is a not-for-profit, professional organization comprised of more than 26,000 physicians trained in the specialty of obstetrics and gynecology. The purpose of the organization is to promote and maintain high standards for women's health care by providing quality continuing education for its members and establishing patient care standards. ACOG is governed by an Executive Board composed of seven selected officers from the membership and ten District representatives. The Committee Opinions program is one of two technology assessment programs sponsored by the College.

Purpose: To provide members and other interested parties with state-of-the-art information on the clinical application of new technologies.

Primary intended users: Physicians, third party payers, public policy-makers, legislators.

Technologies: *Medical or surgical procedure,* drug, device.

The committees assess new devices, equipment, and other therapeutic modalities for the treatment of reproductive disorders in women.

Intervention: *Treatment,* diagnosis.

Stage: *New,* emerging, established or widespread practice.

Technologies are assessed as they are being applied to clinical practice.

Properties: *Effectiveness,* safety, service requirements.

Selection process: Within the ACOG structure, the Executive Board, Health Care Commission, or individual members can request that an assessment be conducted. The College also receives requests from third party carriers and government agencies. Only written requests are accepted. Assessment topic priorities are set by the Executive Board, Health Care Commission, and the committee to whom the request is referred. All existing opinions/statements are reviewed within 18 to 24 months from date of publication for relevance and accuracy.

Methods: *Information syntheses,* expert opinion, group judgment.

A subject is selected and referred to a committee. The committee elects a member to review the literature and draft a preliminary report citing literature references. The committee discusses the preliminary draft, achieves consensus on areas of controversy, and submits a revised report to an expert panel for review and comment. Information from reviewers is synthesized and a final report prepared for review by the Health Care Commission and Executive Board prior to publication. At any step along the way, when agreement is in doubt, the advice of further technical experts may be sought.

The turnaround time from selection of the assessment topic to publication of the findings ranges from 18 to 24 months.

Assessors: Committee members represent the academic and the clinical practice communities, are geographically dispersed, and reflect a wide range of practice settings. Panel experts are chosen because of their recognized authority in the chosen subject. The Health Care Commission and the Executive Board members are academicians, clinical practice generalists, and subspecialists.

Assessment reports include: Description of the technology; sources of data/information; findings or conclusions; how the technology works, including theory, principles; whether the technology is experimental, investigational, or considered acceptable clinical practice.

Dissemination: *Advisories to members/constituents,* printed reports.

Assessments are published as committee opinions and are disseminated to the College membership as an insert in the monthly ACOG newsletter. The reports are available upon request to all other interested parties.

Budget: $15,000. Currently, the assessment activity is considered part of the charge of the obstetric and gynecologic standing committees and is not identified separately within the committee budget. Therefore, the approximate cost per assessment is not known. Approximately $15,000 is allocated for printing and distribution of the reports to the membership. Funding source: 100 percent parent organization.

Use: When appropriate, the report conclusions are conveyed in other documents prepared by the ACOG (such as educational resources) and used in responding to individuals and organizations requesting specific information. Third party carriers use the reports for insurance purposes and to determine if the technology is viewed as clinically applicable. Members use the reports to determine if the state-of-the-art of the technology is appropriate for application to their practices.

The publications *ACOG Standards for Obstetric-Gynecologic Services, Guidelines for Perinatal Care,* and *Precis,* a compendium of current information in the specialty, reflect committee opinions where applicable. New editions of these publications appear every 3 years.

Related activities: The College produces a scientific, refereed journal that primarily reports research and the results of controlled clinical studies. These reports, along with those published in similar journals, provide the data with which committees form their opinions. The College also issues *Technical Bulletins* (see separate profile on ACOG Committee on Technical Bulletins), conducts an annual scientific meeting with symposia on new information in the specialty, and offers free-standing postgraduate courses on a variety of topics, many of which convey information on technologic advances and, where applicable, committee opinions.

The College also provides a contraceptive slide rule for lay persons which spells out the risks/benefits, advantages/disadvantages, cost, and mortality rates for various forms of contraceptives.

Completed Reports

AE1 American College of Obstetricians and Gynecologists, Committee Opinion. Clinical use of bromocriptine. Pending. [Information syntheses]

AE2 ______. Teratogenicity of steroids. Pending. [Information syntheses]

AE3 ______. Ultrasonography in the monitoring of follicular growth. Pending. [Information syntheses]

AE4 ______. Hysteroscopy. Revised 1986 Jan. [Information syntheses]

AE5 ______. The use of cryosurgery in the treatment of CIN. Revised 1986 Nov. [Information syntheses]

AE6 ______. Contraception for women in their later reproductive years. 1985 Dec. [Information syntheses]

AE7 ______. Current role of electronic heart rate monitoring in labor. Revised 1985 Jul. [Information syntheses]

AE8 ______. Endometrial sampling. 1985 Jun. [Information syntheses]

AE9 ______. Prophylactic use of antibiotics with abdominal hysterectomy. [Information syntheses]

AE10 ______. Anticonvulsants and pregnancy. Revised 1984 Jul. [Information syntheses]

AE11 ______. Carbon dioxide laser. Revised 1984 Apr. [Information syntheses]

AE12 ______. Fetoscopy. Revised 1984 Jul. [Information syntheses]

AE13 ______. Human in vitro fertilization and embryo placement. 1984 Apr. [Information syntheses]

AE14 ______. Microsurgery. 1984 Apr. [Information syntheses]

AE15 ______. Needle aspiration cytology in the evaluation of breast lesions. 1984 Jun. [Information syntheses]

AE16 ______. Breast-feeding and contraception. 1981 May. [Information syntheses]

AE17 ______. ACOG statement on periodic cancer screening for women. 1980 Jun. [Information syntheses]

AE18 ______. ACOG statement on mammography. 1979 Sep. [Information syntheses]

American College of Obstetricians and Gynecologists Committee on Technical Bulletins

600 Maryland Avenue SW
Washington, DC 20024
202-638-5577

Contact: Rebecca Rinehart, Associate Director of Publications, Division of Education; or the ACOG Resource Center.

Overview: The American College of Obstetricians and Gynecologists (ACOG) is a not-for-profit, professional organization comprised of more than 26,000 physicians trained in the specialty of obstetrics and gynecology. The purpose of the organization is to promote and maintain high standards for women's health care by providing quality continuing education for its members and establishing patient care standards. ACOG is governed by an Executive Board composed of seven elected officers from the membership and ten District representatives. The Committee on Technical Bulletins is one of two technology assessment programs sponsored by the College.

Purpose: To provide practicing physicians with timely information on the latest proven techniques of clinical practice in the specialty.

Primary intended users: Physicians.

Technologies: *Medical or surgical procedure,* drug, device.

The Committee assesses the management of specific reproductive disorders, treatment therapies, and the application of new technologies.

Intervention: *Treatment,* prevention, diagnosis.

Stage: *Established or widespread practice,* new.

Technologies are assessed when they are determined to have widespread applicability in clinical practice.

Properties: *Effectiveness,* service requirements, acceptance/adoption level.

Selection process: The Committee on Technical Bulletins is responsible for surveying current clinical knowledge to determine the need to address new topics or to update existing *Bulletins.* Topics can also be suggested by the Learning Resources and the Health Care Commissions, other standing committees, the Executive Board, and individual members. Requests for assessments are made by Committee consensus and are submitted in writing. Assessment topic priorities are set by the Committee in consultation with the Learning Resources Commission.

Technical Bulletins generally are reviewed for relevance and accuracy within 3 years from date of publication unless new information requires earlier attention.

Methods: *Expert opinion,* group judgment.

Once a topic is selected by the Committee on Technical Bulletins, an expert on the topic is chosen to prepare a manuscript. The Committee reviews the author's draft and achieves consensus on areas of disagreement between members and the author. A revised draft is submitted to the Learning Resources Commission. Information from the reviewers is synthesized, consensus is reached regarding any further unresolved matters, and a final report is prepared for review by the Executive Board prior to publication.

The turnaround time from selection of the topic to the publication of findings averages between 18 to 24 months.

Assessors: Committee members are geographically dispersed and are representatives of the academic and clinical practice communities. Authors are recognized authorities in the topics selected. The Learning Resources Commission and the Executive Board members are academicians, clinical practice generalists and subspecialists.

Assessment reports include: Description of the technology; sources of data/information; findings or conclusions; how the technology works, including theory, principles.

Dissemination: *Printed reports,* advisories to members/constituents.

Assessments are published as *Technical Bulletins* and the results are disseminated to the College membership as an insert in the monthly ACOG newsletter. Requests for copies of the *Technical Bulletins* should be directed to the ACOG Distribution Center at the Washington, DC address.

Budget: $95,000. The approximate cost per assessment is $5,000 exclusive of Committee budget. Funding source: 100 percent parent organization.

Use: The College uses the *Technical Bulletins* to keep members informed regarding accepted clinical management techniques. Insurers report that they have introduced the *Bulletins* as evidence in malpractice suits, by both plaintiffs and defendants. Trial lawyers have also used the *Bulletins.*

The publications *ACOG Standards for Obstetric-Gynecologic Services, Guidelines for Perinatal Care,* and *Precis,* a compendium of current information in the specialty, reflect, where applicable, the findings of *Technical Bulletins.* New editions of these publications appear every 3-4 years.

Program evaluation: The ACOG Division of Education periodically asks participants and members attending courses and annual meetings to evaluate the usefulness of educational offerings. *Technical Bulletins* consistently have been rated high by respondents.

Related activities: ACOG produces a scientific, refereed journal that primarily reports research and the results of controlled clinical studies. The College also issues committee opinions (see separate profile on ACOG Committee Opinions), conducts an annual scientific meeting with symposia on new information in the specialty, and offers free-standing postgraduate courses on a variety of topics, many of which convey information on technologic advances.

The College also provides a contraceptive slide rule for lay persons that spells out the risks/benefits, advantages/disadvantages, cost, and mortality rates for various forms of contraceptives.

Completed Reports

AF1 American College of Obstetricians and Gynecologists, Committee on Technical Bulletins. Antimicrobial therapy for gynecologic infections. 1986 Oct. (Technical bulletin no. 97). [Expert opinion]

AF2 ______. Estrogen replacement therapy. 1986 Jun. (Technical bulletin no. 93). [Expert opinion]

AF3 ______. Management of diabetes mellitus in pregnancy. 1986 May. (Technical bulletin no. 92). [Expert opinion]

AF4 ______. Management of isoimmunization in pregnancy. 1986 Jan. (Technical bulletin no. 90). [Expert opinion]

AF5 ______. Management of preeclampsia. 1986 Mar. (Technical Bulletin no. 91). [Expert opinion]

AF6 ______. Management of the breech presentation. 1986 Aug. (Technical bulletin no. 95). [Expert opinion]

AF7 ______. Genitourinary fistula. 1985 Jan. (Technical bulletin no 83). [Expert opinion]

AF8 ______. Gonorrhea and chlamydia infections. 1985 Nov. (Technical bulletin no. 89). [Expert opinion]

AF9 ______. Management of endometriosis. 1985 Mar. (Technical bulletin no. 85). [Expert opinion]

AF10 ______. Blood component therapy. 1984 Jul. (Technical bulletin no. 78). [Expert opinion]

AF11 ______. Carcinoma of the endometrium. 1984 Mar. (Technical bulletin no. 75). [Expert opinion]

AF12 ______. Carcinoma of the vulva. 1984 Jun. (Technical Bulletin no. 77). [Expert opinion]

AF13 ______. Cervical cytology: evaluation and management of abnormalities. 1984 Oct. (Technical bulletin no. 81). [Expert opinion]

AF14 ______. Prevention of Rho(D) isoimmunization. 1984 Aug. (Technical bulletin no. 79). [Expert opinion]

AF15 ______. Septic shock. 1984 Mar. (Technical bulletin no. 75). [Expert opinion]

AF16 ______. Hemorrhagic shock. 1984 Dec. (Technical bulletin no. 82). [Expert opinion]

AF17 ______. Automobile passenger restraints for children and pregnant women. 1983 Dec. (Technical bulletin no. 74). [Expert opinion]

AF18 ______. Cancer of the ovary. 1983 Oct. (Technical bulletin no. 73). [Expert opinion]

AF19 ______. Diagnosis and management of invasive cervical carcinomas. 1983 May. (Technical bulletin no. 69). [Expert opinion]

AF20 ______. Dysmenorrhea. 1983 Mar. (Technical bulletin no. 68). [Expert opinion]

AF21 ______. Epidemiology and diagnosis of breast disease. 1983 Sep. (Technical bulletin no. 71). [Expert opinion]

AF22 ______. Osteoporosis. 1983 Oct. (Technical bulletin no. 72). [Expert oppinion]

AF23 ______. Anesthesia for cesarean section. 1982 May. (Technical bulletin no. 65). [Expert opinion]

AF24 ______. Dysfunctional uterine bleeding. 1982 Sep. (Technical bulletin no. 66). [Expert opinion]

AF25 ______. Immunization during pregnancy. 1982 May. (Technical bulletin no. 64). [Expert opinion]

AF26 ______. Prenatal detection of neural tube defects. 1982 Oct. (Technical bulletin no. 67). [Expert opinion]

AF27 ______. Diagnostic ultrasound in obstetrics and gynecology. 1981 Oct. (Technical bulletin no. 63). [Expert opinion]

AF28 ______. Neonatal metabolic diseases. 1981 Jan. (Technical bulletin no. 60). [Expert opinion]

AF29 ______. Rubella—a clinical update. 1981 Jul. (Technical bulletin no. 62). [Expert opinion]

AF30 ______. Management of gestational trophoblastic neoplasia. 1980 Dec. (Technical bulleltin no. 59). [Expert opinion]

AF31 ______. Pregnancy, work, and disability. 1980 May. (Technical bulletin no. 58). [Expert opinion]

AF32 ______. Cigarette smoking and pregnancy. 1979 Sep. (Technical bulletin no. 53). [Expert opinion]

AF33 ______. Diagnosis and management of missed abortion and antepartum fetal death. 1979 Nov. (Technical bulletin no. 55). [Expert opinion]

AF34 ______. Methods of midtrimester abortion. 1979 Dec. (Technical bulletin no. 56). [Expert opinion]

AF35 ______. Induction of labor. 1978 May. (Technical bulletin no. 49). [Expert opinion]

AF36 ______. Sexually transmitted diseases (STD): other than gonorrhea and syphilis. (Technical bulletin no. 51). 1978 Jul. [Expert opinion]

AF37 ______. Classification and staging of malignant tumors in the female pelvis. 1977 Jun. (Technical bulletin no. 47). [Expert opinion]

AF38 ______. Communication of sexual problems in office gynecology. 1977 Apr. (Technical bulletin no. 45). [Expert opinion]

AF39 ______. Intrapartum fetal monitoring. 1977 Jan. (Technical bulletin no. 44). [Expert opinion]

AF40 ______. Prevention of hospital-acquired urinary tract infections in gynecology patients. 1977 May. (Technical bulletin no. 46). [Expert opinion]

AF41 ______. Fetal blood sampling. 1976 Oct. (Technical bulletin no. 42). [Expert opinion]

AF42 ______. Oral contraception 1976 Jul. (Technical bulletin no. 41). [Expert opinion]

AF43 ______. Prevention of Tay-Sachs disease: carrier identification and genetic counseling. 1976 Jan. (Technical bulletin no. 34). [Expert opinion]

AF44 ______. Urinary incontinence in the female. 1979 Feb. (Technical bulletin no. 36). [Expert opinion]

AF45 ______. Fetal heart rate monitoring. 1975 Jun. (Technical bulletin no. 32). [Expert opinion]

American College of Physicians

Clinical Efficacy Assessment Project
4200 Pine Street
Philadelphia, PA 19104
215-243-1200; 800-523-1546

Contact: Linda Johnson White, Director; or John R. Ball, M.D.

Overview: The American College of Physicians (ACP) is a national medical society with a membership of over 63,000 internists and related subspecialists. It works to uphold health care standards through its activities in continuing education, health policy analysis, quality assurance, and medical technology assessment. The Clinical Efficacy Assessment Project (CEAP) is an expansion of the College's participation in the Blue Cross and Blue Shield Association's Medical Necessity Project beginning in 1976, which identified outmoded tests in order to curtail reimbursement for unnecessary medical procedures. Recognizing the need for complete and accurate technology assessment on a continuing basis, the ACP expanded the program in 1981 with a 3-year grant from the John A. Hartford Foundation of New York City. In 1984, the CEAP became a fully funded activity of the College. Beginning in 1986, ACP has accepted contributions to the CEAP from interested individuals and organizations.

Purpose: To help physicians practice high-quality, more efficient, and cost-effective medicine. CEAP recommendations are intended to provide physicians with current information and guidelines regarding the use of tests, procedures, and therapies and the rationale for such recommendations founded on both the literature and broad-based expert opinion.

Primary intended users: Providers, generally; physicians; other care givers; health/medical professional associations; third party payers; government regulators; public policy-makers, legislators; policy research organizations.

Technologies: *Medical or surgical procedure,* drug, device, organizational or administrative system.

Intervention: *Diagnosis,* prevention, treatment, rehabilitation.

Stage: *Established or widespread practice,* new, obsolete.

Properties: *Efficacy,* safety, effectiveness, cost, service requirements.

Selection process: The Clinical Efficacy Assessment Subcommittee identifies potential technologies for CEAP evaluations by reviewing policy needs, practitioner opinion, academic opinion, recent journal articles, and professional meetings focusing on emerging technologies. Recommendations and requests also are received from other ACP committees as well as outside organizations. In selecting technologies to be evaluated, the Clinical Efficacy Assessment Subcommittee examines the following attributes:

1) degree of interest to practitioners of internal medicine, whether or not internists are directly responsible for its application; 2) potential for wide application, or prevalence of current usage; 3) potential for significant benefit if widely applied; and 4) potential for risk if widely applied, particularly in relation to potential benefit.

The Subcommittee will consider requests from College members and others for reevaluation of a statement if the request contains compelling documentation. Staff also solicit advice from the Council of Subspecialty Societies, the Council of Medical Societies, and other experts as to the availability of new information on a technology. If substantive, new information is available, the Subcommittee will consider reassessment.

Methods: *Information syntheses,* expert opinion, group judgment, cost analyses.

Notice of a pending CEAP evaluation is published in *Annals of Internal Medicine, ACP Observer, New England Journal of Medicine,* and the *International Journal of Technology Assessment in Health Care.* The notices invite comments from interested parties. For special or major evaluations, other specialty journals may be asked to publish notices of CEAP evaluations.

ACP staff, in consultation with the CEA Subcommittee, select the appropriate member societies of the Council of Subspecialty Societies (CSS) and Council of Medical Societies (CMS) to review the technology in question. These societies are asked to provide opinion and data on the safety, efficacy, effectiveness, and cost of the technology, as well as to identify other experts (proponents, opponents, and those who are neutral on the topic) to provide information on the technology.

Consultants undertake a comprehensive review of the scientific literature. Assessments of other organizations are reviewed and, when possible and necessary, information regarding ongoing clinical trials is obtained. A synthesis of this information, the comments from persons responding to the published notices, and the opinions of the CSS/CMS members and other experts form the scientific base of the CEAP evaluation.

Consultants assess a technology by the method best suited to the topic. The methods include, but are not limited to, data synthesis, meta-analysis, clinical decision analysis, and consensus development. At times, a combination of methods is used. When possible, risk-benefit and cost-effectiveness analyses are performed.

The approximate turnaround time from selection of assessment topic to reporting of findings is 9 months to 1 year.

Assessors: Physicians trained in clinical epidemiology, statistics, economics, decision analysis, and technology assessment are commissioned to conduct CEAP evaluations. These physicians are selected from candidates suggested by the CEAP Subcommittee, members of the Technology Assessment Committee of the Society for Research and Education in Primary Care Internal Medicine (SREPCIM), and others. When the evaluation of a specific topic requires special expertise, the principal consultant is asked to collaborate with a qualified content expert in the assessment of the topic.

Assessment reports include: Abstract; who sponsored/commissioned/supported the assessment; who conducted the assessment; description of the technology; stage of life-cycle of technology when assessed; properties assessed; procedure used for the assessment; sources of data/information; methods for collecting data/information; methods for analyzing/synthesizing data/information; results; findings or conclusions; limitations of findings; implications of findings for practice; recommendations for practice, future assessments, technology development, research; how the technology works, including theory, principles.

CEAP statements have five components: 1) a general description of the technology, its uses, potential uses, and rationale; 2) an overview of the safety of the technology; 3) a review of the technology's efficacy; 4) information on its cost; and 5) appropriate conclusions and recommendations. Areas requiring further research also are summarized. Key points in the statement refer to the appropriate published literature and the effective date of the literature review is noted. A detailed and referenced background paper that supports and provides the rationale for the CEAP statement and recommendations also is developed. Whereas the CEAP statement follows a standard format, the background paper may be prepared in the style best suited to the analysis of the subject.

Dissemination: CEAP statements become position papers of the American College of Physicians upon approval by the Board of Regents. The position and background papers are submitted to *ACP Observer* and to *Annals of Internal Medicine* for publication. If the *Annals* declines to publish the position paper, it is published in full in *ACP Observer*. If the *Annals* accepts the position paper for publication, an abstract will be published in *ACP Observer*. Thus, all College members and many others receive all CEAP statements through these publications. Background papers that are not published in *Annals* remain the property of their authors and may be submitted to other journals for publication. In addition, the *International Journal for Technology Assessment in Health Care* has been given permission to republish abstracts of all ACP position papers.

Single copies of CEAP statements are available free of charge from the College. A three-ring binder *Clinical Efficacy Reports*, containing the full collection of CEAP statements is available from ACP.

In 1987, ACP published the manual *Common Diagnostic Tests: Use and Interpretation*, available from the ACP publications department. The purpose of this manual is to help physicians determine when diagnostic tests are likely to make desirable differences in patient care. Based on a critical review of published articles, the manual provides recommendations for using selected tests in cardiopulmonary medicine, hematology, infectious diseases, oncology, and other diagnostic applications. The manual calls for additional research for tests for which the published literature is insufficient for making well founded recommendations. The manual chapters are derived from papers commissioned by the Blue Cross and Blue Shield Association for its Medical Necessity Project. These were reviewed through the CEAP process, approved by the ACP, and published in the *Annals of Internal Medicine*. The appendices are texts of the Blue Cross and Blue Shield Medical Necessity guidelines.

Budget: $150,000. If the total program budget is divided by the number of assessments per year, the cost is $10,000.

Approximate consultant cost per assessment is $3,500. Funding sources: 95 percent parent organization; 5 percent foundations, other private grants.

Use: CEAP statements are used by third party payers, training directors in residency programs, and as an educational service to college members as evidence of its commitment to quality care.

The establishment of the Association of Ambulatory Cardiac Catheters (AACC) was a direct result of a CEAP paper. The AACC is now organizing quality assurance activities with the objective of receiving JCAH accreditation for freestanding units. The CEAP endoscopy papers were cited in the 1985 presidential address to the American Gastroenterology Association.

CEAP is described in Institute of Medicine, Committee on Evaluating Medical Technologies in Clinical Use. *Assessing medical technologies.* Washington, DC: National Academy Press, 1985.

Program evaluation: As part of its grant award, the John A. Hartford Foundation stipulated and funded an evaluation of the CEAP. In 1983, the Blue Cross and Blue Shield Association conducted the evaluation which included a questionnaire that was sent to all major third party payers and government agencies. Recipients were asked about their knowledge of the CEAP, if the reports were relevant, and if the CEAP reports were used for educational and policy-setting purposes. Findings indicated that CEAP reports were used for educational and policy-setting purposes. The program was not modified as a result of the evaluation, but the mailing list was expanded.

Completed Reports

AG1 American College of Physicians, Clinical Efficacy Assessment Project. A comparative assessment of coronary artery bypass surgery and percutaneous transluminal coronary angioplasty. Expected completion 1988. [Information syntheses]

AG2 ______. Allergy testing. Expected completion 1988. [Information syntheses]

AG3 ______. Chemical aversion therapy in the treatment of alcoholism, expected completion 1988. [Information syntheses]

AG4 ______. Clinical ecology, expected completion 1988. [Information syntheses]

AG5 ______. Exercise thallium scanning, expected completion 1988. [Information syntheses]

AG6 ______. How to study the carotid arteries, expected completion 1988. [Information syntheses]

AG7 ______. How to study the gallbladder, expected completion 1988. [Information syntheses]

AG8 ______. Intravenous pyelography, expected completion 1988. [Information syntheses]

AG9 ______. Laboratory evaluation of the patient after myocardial infarction, expected completion 1988. [Information syntheses]

AG10 ______. Preoperative pulmonary function tests, expected completion 1988. [Information syntheses]

AG11 ______. Rehabilitation of the myocardial infarction patient, expected completion 1988. [Information syntheses]

AG12 ______. Bone mineral densitometry, 1987. [Information syntheses]

AG13 ______. Magnetic resonance imaging of the brain and spine, 1987. [Information syntheses]

AG14 ______. Methotrexate for rheumatoid arthritis, 1987. [Information syntheses]

AG15 ______. Parenteral nutrition, 1987. [Information syntheses]

AG16 ______. A comparative assessment of standard and computed tomography in the evaluation of neoplasms of the chest. 1986. [Information syntheses]

AG17 ______. Automated ambulatory blood pressure monitoring. Ann Intern Med 1986;104:275-8. [Information syntheses]

AG18 ______. Cardiokymography. ACP Observer 1986 Jan:8,10. [Information syntheses]

AG19 ______. Congestive heart failure and thoracentesis, 1986. [Information syntheses]

AG20 ______. Pneumococcal vaccine. Ann Intern Med 1986;104:118-120

AG21 ______. The diagnostic spinal tap. Ann Intern Med 1986;104:880-5,840-8. [Information syntheses]

AG22 ______. Apheresis in chronic inflammatory demyelinating polyneuropathy and in renal transplantation. Ann Inter Med 1985;103:630-3. [Information syntheses]

AG23 ______. Biofeedback for gastrointestinal disorders. Ann Intern Med 1985;103:291-3,240-44. [Information syntheses]

AG24 ______. Biofeedback for headaches. Ann Intern Med 1985;102:128-31. [Information syntheses]

AG25 ______. Biofeedback for hypertension. Ann Intern Med 1985;102:709-15. [Information syntheses]

AG26 ______. Biofeedback for neuromuscular disorders. Ann Intern Med 1985;102:854-8. [Information syntheses]

AG27 ______. Colonoscopy: management of colorectal neoplasia. 1985. [Information syntheses]

AG28 ______. Diagnostic thoracentesis and pleural biopsy. Ann Intern Med 1985;103:799-802. [Information syntheses]

AG29 ______. Esophagogastroduodenoscopy (EGD). [Information syntheses]

AG30 ______. Lithotripsy. Ann Intern Med 1985;103:626-9. [Information syntheses]

AG31 ______. Screening for breast cancer. Ann Intern Med 1985;103:143-6,79-85. [Information syntheses]

AG32 ______. The safety and efficacy of ambulatory cardiac catheterization in the hospital and free standing setting. Ann Intern Med 1985:103;294-8. [Information syntheses]

AG33 ______. Thrombolysis for evolving myocardial infarction. Ann Intern Med 1985;103:463-9. [Information syntheses]

AG34 ______. Apheresis in chronic severe rheumatoid arthritis. 1984. [Information syntheses]

AG35 ______. Clinical usefulness of hemoglobin A1C measurements. Ann Intern Med 1984;101:710-3. [Information syntheses]

AG36 ______. Efficacy of endoscopic retrograde cholangiopancreatography (ERCP) and endoscopic retrograde sphincterotomy (ERS). 1984. [Information syntheses]

AG37 ______. Endocardial electrical stimulation. Ann Intern Med 1984;100:452-4. [Information syntheses]

AG38 ______. Endoscopic injection sclerotherapy. Ann Intern Med 1984;100:608-10. [Information syntheses]

AG39 ______. Ergonovine provocative testing. Ann Intern Med 1984;100:152-2. [Information syntheses]

AG40 ______. Heparin infusion pumps. Ann Intern Med 1984;100:305-6. [Information syntheses]

AG41 ______. Hepatitis B vaccine. Ann Intern Med 1984;100:149-50. [Information syntheses]

AG42 ______. Radiologic methods to evaluate bone mineral content. Ann Intern Med 1984;100:108-11. [Information syntheses]

AG43 ______. 13C and 14C glycocholate tests. 1983. [Information syntheses]

AG44 ______. 13C and 14C glycocholate, H2 breath, 13C trioctanoin, and 14C triolein breath tests. 1983. [Information syntheses]

AG45 ______. 14C xylose breath test. 1983. [Information syntheses]

AG46 ______. Home blood glucose monitoring. Ann Intern Med 1983;99:272-4. [Information syntheses]

AG47 ______. Hyperbaric oxygen therapy: acute, traumatic peripheral ischemia. 1983. [Information syntheses]

AG48 ______. Hyperbaric oxygen therapy: chronic vascular insufficiency. 1983. [Information syntheses]

AG49 ______. Hyperbaric oxygen therapy: decubitus ulcers. 1983. [Information syntheses]

AG50 ______. Hyperbaric oxygen therapy: senility. [Information syntheses]

AG51 ______. Lactulose H2 breath test. 1983. [Information syntheses]

AG52 ______. Management of diabetes mellitus: computerized insulin infusion pumps. Ann Intern Med 1983;99::272-4. [Information syntheses]

AG53 ______. Management of diabetes mellitus: external infusion pumps. Ann Intern Med 1983;99:272-4. [Information syntheses]

AG54 ______. Management of diabetes mellitus: pancreatic transplants. Ann Intern Med 1983;99:272-4. [Information syntheses]

AG55 ______. Percutaneous transluminal angioplasty: carotid, vertebral, and subclavian arteries. Ann Intern Med 1983;99:864-9. [Information syntheses]

AG56 ______. Percutaneous transluminal angioplasty: coronary arteries. Ann Intern Med 1983;99:864-9. [Information syntheses]

AG57 ______. Percutaneous transluminal angioplasty: iliac, femoral, and popliteal arteries. Ann Intern Med 1983;99:864-9. [Information syntheses]

AG58 ______. Percutaneous transluminal angioplasty: renal arteries. Ann Intern Med 1983;99:864-9. [Information syntheses]

AG59 ______. The dexamethasone suppression test. Ann Intern Med 1983;100:307-8. [Information syntheses]

AG60 ______. The H2 breath test. 1983. [Information syntheses]

AG61 ______. Antilymphocyte (ALG) and antithymocyte (ATG) globulin in renal transplantation. 1982. [Information syntheses.

AG62 ______. Bentonite flocculation test. 1982. [Information syntheses]

AG63 ______. DNA antibody test. 1982. [Information syntheses]

AG64 ______. Immunotherapy of cancer. 1982. [Information syntheses]

AG65 ______. Kunkel test (total serum gammaglobulin). 1982. [Information syntheses]

AG66 ______. Phonocardiography. 1982. [Information syntheses]

AG67 ______. 24-hour sphygmomanometry. 1981. [Information syntheses]

AG68 ______. 25 hydroxyvitamin D level. 1981. [Information syntheses]

AG69 ______. Cytotoxic food testing. 1981. [Information syntheses]

AG70 ______. Gastric analysis by the capsule method (Heidelberg). 1981. [Information syntheses]

AG71 ______. Human tumor cell drug sensitivity assay in the treatment of solid tumors. 1981. [Information syntheses]

AG72 ______. Hyperbaric oxygen therapy: actinomycosis. 1981. [Information syntheses]

AG73 ______. Hyperbaric oxygen therapy: arthritis. 1981. [Information syntheses]

AG74 ______. Hyperbaric oxygen therapy: osteomyelitis. 1981. [Information syntheses]

AG75 ______. Intracutaneous titration. 1981. [Information syntheses]

AG76 ______. Intravenous histamine therapy. 1981. [Information syntheses]

AG77 ______. Management of histapenia. 1981. [Information syntheses]

AG78 ______. Radioallergosorbent technique (RAST). 1981. [Information syntheses]

AG79 ______. Ultrasonic arteriography, B mode. 1981. [Information syntheses]

AG80 ______. Ultrasonic arteriography, B-scan and Doppler ultrasound. 1981. [Information syntheses]

AG81 ______. Hemodialysis for the treatment of schizophrenia. 1980. [Information syntheses]

AG82 ______. Urine autoinjection. 1980. [Information syntheses]

AG83 ______. Whole body hyperthermia for cancer patients. 1980. [Information syntheses]

American College of Radiology

Task Force on Breast Cancer
1891 Preston White Drive
Reston, VA 22091
703-648-8925

Contact: Marie Zinninger, M.S.N., Coordinator; Gerald Dodd, M.D., Chairman, Task Force on Breast Cancer.

Overview: The American College of Radiology (ACR) serves radiologists with programs addressing the practice of radiology and the delivery of comprehensive radiological health services. The purposes of the ACR are to advance the science of radiology, improve radiologic service to the patient, study the economic aspects of the practice of radiology, and encourage improved and continuing education for radiologists and allied professional fields.

The ACR has more than 20,000 members and fellows in diagnostic and therapeutic radiology, radiologic physics, and related disciplines. ACR members participate in commissions and committees that prepare publications and conduct programs directed to meeting member needs. These include quality assurance, practice and accreditation, management consulting, professional placement, self-evaluation, continuing education, manpower, practice management, and the development and conduct of special scientific courses needed in the field. The subject of this profile is the ACR Task Force on Breast Cancer.

Purpose: To coordinate the activities of various ACR committees concerned with mammography and breast cancer. These include the Committee on Breast Cancer, Committee on Breast Imaging, Committee on Mammography Equipment, the Committee on Mammography Accreditation of the Commission on Radiologic Practice, and the ACR/American Cancer Society Joint Committee on Mammography. Issues addressed by the Task Force include education of radiologists and referring physicians, mammography policy statements and guidelines, mammography quality assurance, and liaison with other national medical organizations such as the American Cancer Society.

Primary intended users: Physicians; patients; health/medical professional associations; voluntary associations, organizations.

Technologies: *Medical or surgical procedure,* device.

Intervention: *Diagnosis,* prevention.

The major emphasis of the program is on early detection of breast cancer.

Stage: Established or widespread practice.

Properties: *Safety; effectiveness;* cost; ethical, legal, social implications.

Selection process: ACR assessments are requested by such outside organizations as the Office of Health Technology Assessment, American Cancer Society (ACS), Blue Cross and Blue Shield Association, the Conference of Radiation Control Programs Directors, Inc., and other sources. In addition, they may be requested by ACR members and other physicians, and by the ACR committees cited above that work with the Task Force. Assessment priorities are normally set by the Task Force.

Methods: *Group judgment,* information syntheses, expert opinion, cost analyses, epidemiological and other observational methods.

Assessments are generally initiated by the Committee on Breast Cancer, Committee on Breast Imaging, Committee on Mammography Equipment, Committee on Mammography Accreditation, or ACR/ACS Joint Committee on Mammography, as appropriate. Reports are often drafted jointly by committee members and staff.

When a consensus is reached at the committee level, it is forwarded to the Task Force for review and approval. The Task Force normally meets twice a year, though it may meet more often as needed. Upon Task Force approval, reports are submitted to the ACR Board of Chancellors for acceptance. The final endorsement comes at the ACR annual meeting where the ACR Council of approximately 175 physicians acts upon a resolution. Average turnaround time for assessments is approximately one year.

As guidelines are based on current available information, they are to be revised as more is learned about the control of breast cancer. Thus, in 1986 the Task Force issued supplementary statements to the 1982 policy statement on mammography; these supplementary statements addressed the capabilities and limitations of mammography in the detection and diagnosis of breast cancer and performance guidelines for mammography.

Assessors: The Task Force on Breast Cancer has 14 members. Of these, 12 are physicians and 2 are radiological physicists. There are 10-12 members on each of the committees; members are gynecologists, surgeons, radiation oncologists, internists, pathologists, family practitioners, and members of other organizations such as the American Cancer Society and National Cancer Institute.

Assessment reports include: Purpose of the assessment; relationship of the assessment to prior or concurrent assessments of the technology or other technologies intended for similar purposes; who sponsored/commissioned/supported the assessment; description of the technology; stage of life-cycle of technology when assessed; properties assessed; sources of data/information; findings or conclusions; limitations of findings; implications of findings for practice; recommendations for practice, future assessments, technology development, research; how the technology works, including theory, principles.

Dissemination: *Printed reports;* advisories to members/constituents; press conference/news releases, TV radio broadcasts, video products; clearinghouses.

Individual Task Force policy statements are available from the ACR at no charge. Policy statements also appear in the newsletter *ACR Bulletin*. The ACR *Mammography Resource Kit* includes the policy statements on mammography, as well as reprints of other organizations' statements on mammography, order forms for public service announcements, information about mammography training programs, mammography bibliography, audiovisual materials on mammography, protocol information for patients, and related educational and reference materials. The kit is available upon written request to ACR members at no charge and to others for $25.

Use: Portions of ACR policy statements on mammography appear in publications of the National Cancer Institute, American Cancer Society, and other organizations. ACR policy statements on mammography help form the basis for recommended mammography guidelines issued by medical specialty organizations such as the American College of Obstetricians and Gynecologists and the American Academy of Family Physicians. ACR mammography guidelines are also cited in guidelines and suggested state regulations offered by the Conference of Radiation Control Program Directors, used by many state radiation control programs.

ACR policy statements have been cited in assessments by the Blue Cross and Blue Shield Association, the Office of Health Technology Assessment, and other agencies. For example, ACR opinions have been used in the Blue Cross and Blue Shield Association Medical Necessity guidelines on bronchoscopy (1977), angiocardiography (1977), angiography (1977), diagnostic imaging (1984), and routine preoperative and general hospital admission chest x-rays (1987).

ACR opinions have also been cited in the National Council on Radiation Protection and Measurements Report No. 85, *Mammography: A User's Guide* (1986); State of New York Department of Health memorandum *Quality Assurance Programs for Providers of Mammography Services* (1987); and the Food and Drug Administration Center for Devices and Radiological Health *Mammographic Phantom Evaluation Project Report* (1983).

Articles written by Task Force members on topics related to mammography policy statements appear in the published periodical literature and in texts. Examples are the following:

McClelland, R, Feig SA. Guidelines for mammography. In Feig SA, McClelland R, eds. *Breast carcinoma: current diagnosis and treatment.* New York: ACR and Masson, 1983:365-69.

Bird RE, McClelland R. How to initiate and operate a low-cost screening mammography center. *Radiology* 1986;161(2):43-47.

Budget: The Task Force operations budget is approximately $26,000. This amount does not include the value of the time volunteered to the Task Force by the member radiologists, physicists, and other professionals; it also does not include costs for the other committees involved in generating statements.

Related activities: The Task Force on Breast Cancer coordinates and cosponsors with the American College of Pathologists, ACS, and American Society for Therapeutic Radiology and Oncology a biennial National Conference on Breast Cancer. The ACR and the ACS have a liaison committee to support the ACS Breast Cancer Detection Awareness Program to educate asymptomatic women and their physicians in the importance of breast cancer detection, including screening mammography.

The ACR Mammography Accreditation Program, directed by the ACR Committee on Practice Accreditation and assisted by the Task Force on Breast Cancer, provides voluntary peer review and evaluation services of mammography facility staff qualifications, equipment, quality control and quality assurance programs, image quality and breast dose. Facilities meeting the criteria of the Mammography Accreditation Program are given a 3-year accreditation, a certificate for each approved mammography unit, and a listing on the ACS referral list of approved mammographic centers.

The Patterns of Care Study of cancer treatment, which has been supported by the National Cancer Institute and conducted by ACR since 1971, has conducted surveys of structure, process, and outcomes for a national sample of radiation treatment facilities. As part of the study, ACR assembled review committees of radiation therapists to reach consensus in the form of decision trees for the management of ten disease types in which radiation therapy is involved. The ACR Practice Accreditation Program in Radiation Oncology, which evolved from the Patterns of Care Study, provides a voluntary quality assurance service for radiation therapy facilities. This program involves individual facility visits modeled in order to provide feedback to radiation therapists on their practice relative to regional and national norms established through the Patterns of Care Study.

Based on site visits by teams of selected ACR member surveyors, the ACR Practice Survey Program is a voluntary review and evaluation service offered to diagnostic radiologists in a variety of practice settings. Both accreditation and consultative surveys are available.

Additional ACR publications related to technology assessment include the following.

ACR policy statements on computed tomography, imaging center guidelines, magnetic resonance, and obstetrical/ultrasound examination guidelines.

Acceptance testing protocols: a systematic approach to evaluation of radiology equipment. 1983.

Imaging equipment compendium: a comparative reference of equipment characteristics. 1983. 1985 update, supplement.

List of MR sites.

Planning guides for radiologic installations.

Proceedings of the Eighth Conference on Computer Applications in Radiology. 1984.

Completed Reports

AH1 American College of Radiology, Task Force on Breast Cancer. Policy statement on oscillating grids for mammography equipment. Expected 1987. [Group judgment]

AH2 ______. Resolution no. 1: supplementary mammography statement. 1986 Sep. [Group judgment]

AH3 ______. Resolution no. 2: mammography performance guidelines. 1986 Sep. [Group judgment]

AH4 ______. Policy statement: breast cancer screening centers. 1985. [Group judgment]

AH5 ______. Policy statement on sonography for the detection and diagnosis of breast disease. 1984. [Group judgment]

AH6 ______. Policy statement on thermography for the detection of breast cancer. 1983 Sep 28. [Group judgment]

AH7 ______. Statement of the preservation of mammograms. 1983. [Group judgment]

AH8 ______. Policy statement: guidelines for mammography. 1982 Sep 22. [Group judgment]

American Dental Association
Council on Dental Materials, Instruments, and Equipment

211 East Chicago Avenue
Chicago, IL 60611
312-440-2507

Contact: Dr. P.L. Fan, Associate Secretary.

Overview: The American Dental Association (ADA) is a professional association that provides a variety of services to assist its members practice dentistry and deliver health care to the public. The ADA's objectives include encouraging the improvement of the public's health, promoting the art and science of dentistry, and representing the interests of the dental profession and the public that it serves. The Council on Dental Materials, Instruments, and Equipment is one of two technology assessment programs sponsored by the ADA; the other being the Council on Dental Therapeutics. The Council was established in 1966 to centralize the ADA's activities in the standardization and evaluation of dental materials, instruments, and equipment. This activity had been initiated by the Association in 1928 at the National Bureau of Standards.

The Council performs its duties through its Specification Program, Evaluation Programs (which include the Certification Program, the Acceptance Program and the Recognition Program), Complaint Report Program, and Status Report Program. This profile focuses on the Acceptance Program component. Additional information on other Council activities can be found in the Council's textbook, *Dentists' Desk Reference: Materials, Instruments and Equipment.*

Purpose: To evaluate materials, instruments, and equipment for which evidence of safety and usefulness has been established by biological, laboratory, or clinical evaluations and for which physical standards or specifications do not exist.

Primary intended users: General public, patients, health product manufacturers, dentists.

Technologies: Device.

The following are examples of product areas presently covered by the Council's Acceptance Program: alloys for cast dental restorative and prosthetic devices, autoclave sterilizers, composite resin materials for occlusal restorations, crown and bridge resins, electrosurgical devices; x-ray equipment, denture adherents, denture cleansers, endosseous implants, glass ionomer cements, denture cleaning devices, nitrous oxide/oxygen sedation machines and devices, oral irrigating devices, orthodontic bracket attachment materials, powered oral hygiene devices, precision attachments, processing devices for radiographic film; scaling/stain removal devices, and visible radiation emitting devices.

Intervention: *Treatment,* prevention, diagnosis.

Stage: *New,* emerging, established or widespread practice.

Properties: *Effectiveness,* safety, efficacy.

Selection process: Commercial products are evaluated at the request of the manufacturer or distributor, or at the Council's initiative. All submissions and other information are sent in writing to the Council. Only complete submissions will be accepted; partial submissions will be returned. Each submission must include a summary report covering all information on safety and efficacy of the material, instrument, or item of equipment.

Submissions normally include the following: name and use of item; patent number relating to product; composition, physical, and chemical properties of dental materials; materials used in construction and method of operation of a device; and evidence of safety and usefulness of the product based on in vitro, biological, and clinical evaluations. Evidence of safety and usefulness of the product may be in the form of published reports or unpublished information obtained from appropriate scientific studies using in vitro, biological, and clinical observations.

Methods: Information syntheses, expert opinion, group judgment, bench testing.

The Council evaluates the information available and arrives at a decision, classifying the product as "acceptable," "provisionally acceptable," or "unacceptable." Products classified as "acceptable" usually retain that status for 3 years. Acceptance is renewable and may be reconsidered at any time. If there is a change in manufacturer or distributor of the product, the acceptance automatically expires.

"Acceptable" products are listed in *Dentists' Desk Reference: Materials, Instruments and Equipment.* The manufacturer or distributor may use the Seal of Acceptance and the Council's authorized statement.

"Provisionally acceptable" products consist of those that lack sufficient evidence to justify classification as "acceptable," but for which there is reasonable evidence of safety and usefulness including clinical feasibility. The Council may authorize the use of a suitable statement to specifically define the area of usefulness. Products in this classification category are reviewed each year and ordinarily are not continued for more than 3 years.

"Unacceptable" products are those that are obsolete, markedly inferior, useless, or dangerous to the health of the user.

Dissemination: Acceptable products are listed in the ADA publication *Dentists' Desk Reference: Materials, Instruments and Equipment* and in the *Journal of the American Dental Association.* See for example, Product listing: classified dental materials, instruments, and equipment. *J Am Dent Assoc* 1986 Dec;113:1013-1015.

Budget: Not available. Funding source: 100 percent parent organization. Evaluators and consultants donate their time.

Use: The information is used by the ADA membership and the public.

Related Activities: The Council's Certification Program evaluates products and classifies them as "certified" when they meet formal certification requirements. The results of the Certification Program are also published in the *Journal of the American Dental Association.*

Completed Reports

AJ1 American Dental Association, Council on Dental Materials, Instruments and Equipment. Dentin bonding systems: an update. J Am Dent Assoc 1987;114:91-95.

AJ2 ______. Dental endosseous implants. J Am Dent Assoc 1986;113:949-950.

AJ3 ______. Posterior composite resins. J Am Dent Assoc 1986;112:717-709.

AJ4 ______. Posterior composite resins: an update. J Am Dent Assoc 1986;113:950-952.

AJ5 ______. The effects of blue light on the retina and the use of protective filtering glasses. J Am Dent Assoc 1986;112:533-535.

AJ6 ______. Recent developments in materials and process for ceramic crowns. J Am Dent Assoc 1985;110:548-549.

AJ7 ______. Report on base metal alloys for crown and bridge applications: benefits and risks. J Am Dent Assoc 1985;111:479-483.

AJ8 ______. Status report on professional scaling and stain-removal devices. J Am Dent Assoc 1985;111:801-802.

AJ9 ______. Visible light-cured composites and activating units. J Am Dent Assoc 1985;110:100-103

AJ10 ______, Council on Dental Research, and Council on Dental Therapeutics. Hydroxylapatite, beta tricalcium phosphate, and autogenous and allogenic bone for filling periodontal defects, alveolar ridge augmentation, and pulp capping. J Am Dent Assoc 1984;108:822-831.

AJ11 ______, Council on Dental Therapeutics. Patch tests for sensitivity to mercury or nickel. J Am Dent Assoc 1984;108:381.

AJ12 ______. Classification system for cast alloys. J Am Dent Assoc 1984;109:766.

AJ13 ______. Mouth protectors and sports team dentists. J Am Dent Assoc 1984;109:84-87.

AJ14 ______. Recommendations in dental mercury hygiene, 1984. J Am Dent Assoc 1984;109:617-619.

AJ15 ______. Recommendations in radiographic practices, 1984. J Am Dent Assoc 1984;109:764-765.

AJ16 ______. Reported sensitivity to glass ionomer luting cements. J Am Dent Assoc 1984;109:617-619.

AJ17 ______. Resin dental bonding systems. J Am Dent Assoc 1984;108:240-241.

AJ18 ______. Status report on enamel bonding of composites, preformed laminate, and laboratory fabricated resin veneers. J Am Dent Assoc 1984;109:762-764.

AJ19 ______. Denture cleansers. J Am Dent Assoc 1983;106:77-79.

AJ20 ______. Pit and fissure sealants. J Am Dent Assoc 1983;107:465.

AJ21 ______. Safety of dental amalgam. J Am Dent Assoc 1983;106:519-520.

AJ22 ______. Status report on amalgamators. J Am Dent Assoc 1983;107:639-640.

AJ23 ______. Status report on posterior composites. J Am Dent Asso 1983;107:71-75.

AJ24 ______. Status report: the periodontal ligament injection. J Am Dent Assoc 1983;106:222-224.

AJ25 ______. Biological effects of nickel-containing dental alloys. J Am Dent Assoc 1982;104:501-505.

AJ26 ______. Biological effects of radiation from dental radiography. J Am Dent Assoc 1982;105:275-281.

AJ27 ______. High copper-content amalgam alloys. J Am Dent Assoc 1982;105:1077-1080.

AJ28 ______. Recommendations for radiographic darkrooms and darkroom practices. J Am Dent Assoc 1982;104:636-637.

AJ29 ______. State of the art and science of bonding in orthodontic treatment. J Am Dent Assoc 1982;105:844-850.

AJ30 ______. Status report on beta titanium orthodontic wire. J Am Dent Assoc 1982;105:684-685.

AJ31 ______. Status report on microfilled composite restorative resins. J Am Dent Assoc 1982-105:488-492.

AJ32 ______. Status report on precious metal scrap. J Am Dent Assoc 1982;105:1080-1081.

AJ33 ______. Status report: dental visible light-curing units. J Am Dent Assoc 1982;104:505.

AJ34 ______. A status report on resilient denture base materials. J Am Dent Assoc 1981;103:450-451.

AJ35 ______. ADA Council issues updated mercury hygiene measures recommended. ADA News 1981 Sep 7.

AJ36 ______. Classification and definition of alloys used for casting substrates for porcelain veneering. J Am Dent Assoc 1981;103:755-757.

AJ37 ______. Council update on "adhesion" and "adhesive" materials. J Am Dent Assoc 1981;103:252-253.

AJ38 ______. Current status of sterilization instruments, devices, and methods for the dental office. J Am Dent Assoc 1981;102:683-689.

AJ39 ______. How to improve shade matching in the dental operatory. J Am Dent Assoc 1981;102:209-210.

AJ40 ______. Porcelain-metal alloy compatibility: criteria and test methods. J Am Dent Assoc 1981;102:71-72.

AJ41 ______. Recommendations in radiographic practices. J Am Dent Assoc 1981;103:103-104

AJ42 ______. The desirability of using radiopaque plastics in dentistry: a status report. J Am Dent Assoc 1981;102:347-349.

AJ43 ______. Council position on nitrous oxide scavenging and monitoring devices. J Am Dent Assoc 1980;101:62.

AJ44 ______. Council reevaluates position on dental endosseous implants. J Am Dent Assoc 1980;100:247.

AJ45 ______. Prevention of problems with removable partial dentures. J Am Dent Assoc 1980;100:919-921.

AJ46 ______. Status report on low-gold-content alloys for fixed prostheses. J Am Dent Assoc 1980;100:237-240.

American Dental Association
Council on Dental Therapeutics

211 East Chicago Avenue
Chicago, IL 60611
312-440-2523

Contact: Kenneth H. Burrell, Secretary.

Overview: The American Dental Association (ADA) is a professional association that provides a variety of services to assist the profession in delivering health care to the public. The ADA's objectives include encouraging the improvements of the public's health, promoting the art and science of dentistry, and representing the interests of the members of the dental profession and the public that it serves. The Council on Dental Therapeutics is one of two technology assessment programs sponsored by the ADA; the other being the Council on Dental Materials, Instruments, and Equipment. The Council supplies reliable information and confers a seal of acceptance, provisional acceptance, and unacceptance on recently developed dental products.

Purpose: To study, evaluate, and disseminate information on 1) the proper use of dental therapeutics, their adjuncts, and dental cosmetic agents offered to the public or profession; and 2) aspects of the dental practice environment related to the health of dentists, dental auxiliaries, and the public.

Primary intended users: General public, patients, dentists.

Technologies: Drug, medical or surgical procedure.

Examples of technologies evaluated by the Council are: topical fluoride preparations, analgesics, antianxiety agents, anticholinergic drugs, antihistamines for control of allergic reactions, artificial salivas, astringents for gingival retraction, chemical disinfecting/sterilizing agents, corticosteroids, fluoride dentrifices, fluoride mouthrinses, formocresol preparations, hand antiseptics, hemostatic agents, hypochlorite substances, inhalation anesthetics, local anesthetics, muscle relaxants, nutritional supplements, oral antiseptics, periodontal dressings, pharmaceutical aids, phenolic compounds, respiratory stimulants, root canal calcium chelating agents, sedatives and hypnotics, sterilizing agents, topical protectants, vasoconstrictors, and zinc oxide preparations.

Intervention: Prevention, diagnosis, and treatment.

Stages: *New,* emerging, established or widespread practice.

Properties: Safety, efficacy, effectiveness.

The Council also considers if the products meet standards of acceptance with respect to composition, advertising, and labeling.

Selection process: Commercial products are evaluated at the request of a manufacturer or distributor, or at the Council's initiative. Any firm may submit appropriate products to the Council for the consideration of acceptance. Communications must be submitted in writing through the Secretary of the Council.

The Manufacturers normally submit the following types of information: product name, composition, physical and chemical properties of product; evidence of safety and effectiveness; government regulations related to the product; and promotional materials.

Methods: Information syntheses, expert opinion, group judgment, bench testing.

The steps required for the review of products in the Council's acceptance program depend on several factors. For example, if a product is essentially the same as an existing accepted product and does not require chemical analysis by the Council's laboratory or review by consultants, the process will require fewer steps.

After consideration of a product has been completed, the Council classifies the product as "accepted," "provisionally accepted," or "unaccepted." Products are generally accepted for three years. Acceptance is renewable and may be reconsidered at any time. If there is a change in the product's manufacturer or distributor, the acceptance automatically expires.

"Accepted" products include those for which there is adequate evidence of safety and effectiveness. They may use the Council's "Seal of Acceptance" and/or an authorized statement, unless otherwise provided. "Provisionally accepted" products include those for which there is reasonable evidence of safety and effectiveness, but which lack sufficient evidence of dental effectiveness to justify being accepted. These products meet other qualifications and standards established by the Council. "Unaccepted" products include those for which the Council has determined that there is no substantial evidence of effectiveness, or that a question of safety exists.

Dissemination: Accepted products are listed in *Accepted Dental Therapeutics* and may be described in suitable reports in the *Journal of the American Dental Association* See for example, Product listing: accepted therapeutic products. *J Am Dent Assoc* 1986 Dec;113:1018-1023. When it is in the best interest of the public or the profession, the Council may submit reports on unaccepted products for publication in the *Journal of the American Dental Association.*

Budget: Not available. Funding source: 100 percent parent organization. Evaluators and consultants donate their time.

Use: The information is used by the ADA membership and the public.

Completed Reports

AK1 American Dental Association, Council on Dental Therapeutics, Council on Dental Materials, Instruments, and Equipment. The use of root canal filling materials containing paraformaldehyde: a status report. J Am Dent Assoc 1987 Jan;114:95.

AK2 ______. American Dental Association, Council on Dental Therapeutics. Acceptance of Promise with Fluoride and Sensodyne-F toothpastes for sensitive teeth.] Am Dent Assoc 1986;113:673-5.

AK3 ______. Guidelines for acceptance of chemotherapeutic products for the control of supragingival dental plaque and gingivitis. J Am Dent Assoc 1986;112:529-32.

AK4 ______. Recommendations for evaluating agents for the reduction of dentinal hypersensitivity. J Am Dent Assoc 1986;112:709-10.

AK5 ______, Council on Prosthetic Services and Dental Laboratory Relations. Guidelines for infection control in the dental office and the commercial dental laboratory. J Am Dent Assoc 1985;110:969-72.

AK6 ______. Acceptance of OMNI-II disinfectant for instruments and equipment. J Am Dent Assoc 1985;110.

AK7 ______. Acceptance of Sensodyne toothpaste for sensitive teeth. J Am Dent Assoc 1985;110.

AK8 ______. Prevention of bacterial endocarditis: a committee report of the American Heart Association. J Am Dent Assoc 1985;110.

AK9 ______. Herpes simplex virus disease: implications for dental personnel. J Am Dent Assoc 1984;108:381-2.

AK10 ______, Council on Dental Research and Council on Dental Therapeutics. Report of symposium: root surface caries. J Am Dent Assoc 1983;106.

AK11 American Dental Association. Report of the President's Conference on the examination, diagnosis, and management of temporomandibular disorders. J Am Dent Assoc 1983;106:75-7.

AK12 American Dental Association, Council on Dental Therapeutics. Evaluation of Denquel Sensitive Teeth toothpaste. J Am Dent Assoc 1982;105.

AK13 ______. Council accepts Aim with sodium monofluorophosphate. J Am Dent Assoc 1980;101:822.

AK14 ______. Council accepts dilution claims for Sporicidin. J Am Dent Assoc 1980;100:918.

AK15 ______. Office emergencies and emergency kits. J Am Dent Assoc 1980;101.

American Diabetes Association

1660 Duke Street
Alexandria, VA 22314
703-549-1500

Contact: Richard Kahn, Ph.D., Assistant Executive Vice President.

Overview: The American Diabetes Association (ADA) is a not-for-profit membership association that promotes efforts to prevent and cure diabetes and works to improve the well-being of people with diabetes and their families. It provides professional education programs, patient information materials/programs, research grant awards, and public awareness about diabetes. ADA's technology assessment activities include sponsoring consensus conferences, developing position papers, and publishing review articles.

Purpose: To provide health professionals and the public with accurate and comprehensive information about technologies relevant to diabetes.

Primary intended users: General public; people concerned about their health; patients; providers, generally; physicians; other care givers; health product manufacturers; health/medical professional associations; health industry associations; consumer associations; employers; unions and other employee organizations; third party payers; government regulators; voluntary associations, organizations; biomedical researchers; reporters, writers, news media; information/computer industry; labs, blood banks; public policy-makers, legislators; policy research organizations.

Technologies: Drug, device, medical or surgical procedure, support system, organizational or administrative system.

Intervention: Diagnosis, treatment, rehabilitation.

Stage: New, established or widespread practice.

Properties: Safety; efficacy; effectiveness; cost; cost-benefit; cost-effectiveness; service requirements; acceptance/adoption level; system impact; economic implications; ethical, legal, social implications.

Selection process: ADA board members and officers, professional members, and other agencies and institutions can request that an assessment be conducted. Written requests are submitted to the volunteer leadership or senior staff. The volunteer leadership sets the assessment topic priorities.

Methods: Information syntheses, expert opinion, group judgment, cost analyses.

The assessment process is conducted in committee meetings, symposia, and conferences. The approximate turnaround time from selection of assessment topic to reporting of findings is 6 months.

Assessors: The assessors have expertise in a wide variety of areas related to diabetes including medicine, nutrition, exercise, law, and public health.

Assessment reports include: The purpose of the assessment; relationship of this assessment to prior or concurrent assessments of the technology or other technologies intended for similar purposes; who conducted the assessment; description of the technology; properties assessed; procedure used for the assessment; sources of data/information; methods for collecting data/information; methods for analyzing/synthesizing data/information; results; findings or conclusions; limitations of findings; implications of findings for practice; recommendations for practice, future assessments, technology development, research; how the technology works, including theory, principles; development of the technology; coverage/reimbursement status of the technology.

Dissemination: Printed reports; journal articles; advisories to members/constituents; press conferences/news releases; TV/radio broadcasts, video products.

The ADA accepts telephone and written requests for copies of assessment reports.

Budget: $100,000. The approximate cost per assessment ranges from $1,000 to $50,000. Funding sources: 5 percent government grants/contracts; 15 percent foundations, other private grants; 80 percent sponsors/members dues, contributions.

Use: The ADA uses the assessment reports and position statements as a guide for new program development and as an authoritative source of information. Reports are cited in government documents, newspaper articles, lay public magazines, and other publications.

Related activities: The ADA conducts an annual scientific session at which hundreds of original research reports are presented. The Association sponsors an annual postgraduate course, a research symposium, and other conferences intended to disseminate new information or to provide a forum for discussing important topics related to diabetes.

Completed Reports

AL1 American Diabetes Association, Consensus Development Panel. Consensus statement on self-monitoring of blood glucose. Diabetes Care 1987;10:95-99. [Expert opinion, Group judgment]

AL2 American Diabetes Association, Task Force of the Council on Nutrition Sciences and Metabolism. Position statment on use of noncaloric sweeteners. 1987. [Expert opinion, Group judgment]

AL3 American Diabetes Association. Nutritional recommendations and principles for individuals with diabetes mellitus. Diabetes Care 1987;10:126-132. [Expert opinion, Group judgment]

AL4 American Diabetes Association and the Centers for Disease Control, Task Force on Financing Quality Health Care for Persons with Diabetes. Third-party reimbursement for diabetes outpatient education. 1986. [Expert opinion, Group judgment]

AL5 American Diabetes Association. Position statment on polydextrose. 1986. [Expert opinion, Group judgment]

AL6 ———. Bedside blood glucose monitoring in hospitals. Diabetes Care 1986;9:89. [Expert opinion, Group judgment]

AL7 ______. Gestational diabetes mellitus. Diabetes Care 1986;9:430-431. [Expert opinion, Group judgment]

AL8 ______. Continuous subcutaneous insulin infusion. Diabetes 1985;34:946. [Expert opinion, Group judgment]

AL9 ______. Office guide to diagnosis and classification of diabetes mellitus and other categories of glucose intolerance. Diabetes Care 1981;4:335. [Expert opinion, Group judgment]

AL10 Olefsky JM, Crapo P. [American Diabetes Association] Fructose, xylitol, and sorbitol. Diabetes Care 1980;3:390-393. [Expert opinion, Group judgment]

American Gastroenterological Association

Patient Care Committee
c/o John Balint, M.D.
Chairman, Department of Medicine
Albany Medical College
47 New Scotland Avenue
Albany, NY 12208
518-445-5376

Contact: John Balint, M.D.

Overview: The American Gastroenterological Association (AGA) is a professional society for gastroenterologists concerned with patient care education, research, and public policy.

Purpose: To evaluate the safety and efficacy of new diagnostic and treatment modalities in digestive diseases and to develop effective and affordable methodologies for data collection.

Primary intended users: Patients; physicians; acute facility administrators; health product manufacturers; health/medical professional associations; third party payers; government regulators; biomedical researchers; public policy-makers, legislators.

Technologies: *Device,* drug, medical or surgical procedure.

Specifically, endoscopic instrumentation for diagnosis and treatment, new imaging technology, and nutritional support systems are assessed.

Intervention: *Treatment,* diagnosis.

Stage: *New,* emerging, established or widespread practice.

Properties: *Effectiveness,* safety, cost-benefit, cost-effectiveness, acceptance/adoption level.

Selection process: Anyone can request that an assessment be conducted. Generally, Committee members initiate a request, although the Committee will respond to requests from any organization. The Committee sets assessment topic priorities and decides on the most appropriate response to a request.

Methods: *Information syntheses,* expert opinion, group judgment, epidemiological and other observational methods.

Committee members conduct the assessment process and are assigned specific tasks to complete. Assessments are based largely on literature reviews, although, the Committee wants to develop questionnaire methods for prospective evaluations. The turnaround time from selection of assessment topic to reporting of findings ranges from 6 months to 2 years.

Assessors: The Patient Care Committee consists of practicing gastroenterologists, surgeons, endoscopists, and pediatric gastroenterologists.

Assessment reports include: The purpose of the assessment; stage of life-cycle of technology when assessed; properties assessed; procedure used for the assessment; sources of data/information; methods for collecting data/information; results; findings or conclusions; limitations of findings; implications of findings for practice; and recommendations for practice, future assessments, technology development, research.

Dissemination: Printed reports, journal articles.

Assessment results are published in the journal *Gastroenterology* and are presented at AGA meetings. Copies of the assessments can be requested from the Patient Care Committee.

Budget: Not available. The approximate cost per assessment is not known. In general, Committee members donate their time. Funding source: 100 percent parent organization.

Related activities: The Patient Care Committee sponsors symposia at their annual meeting that are designed to help the practicing gastroenterologist evaluate and properly use diagnostic and treatment modalities.

Completed Reports

AM1 Sitzman JV, Pitt HA. [American Gastroenterological Association, Patient Care Committee] Guidelines for total parenteral nutrition. Gastroenterology 1987 (in press).

AM2 Kreek MJ, Balint JA. [American Gastroenterological Association, Patient Care Committee] "Skinny needle" cholangiography: results of a pilot study of a voluntary prospective method for gathering risk data on new procedures. Gastroenterology 1980;78:598-604. [Information syntheses]

Ongoing Assessments

AM3 American Gastroenterological Association, Patient Care Committee. Diagnostic procedures in jaundice. Ongoing.

AM4 American Gastroenterological Association, Patient Care Committee. Diagnostic procedures in noncardiac chest pain. Ongoing.

American Hospital Association

Hospital Technology Series Program
Division of Clinical Services and Technology
840 North Lake Shore Drive
Chicago, IL 60611
312-280-6084

Contact: Henry C. Alder, Director; Suzanna Pribyl, Manager, Technology Policy and Planning; or Susan A. Frankel, Manager, Marketing and Publications.

Overview: The American Hospital Association (AHA) is a trade association that represents member hospitals, providing advocacy, policy development, publications, data services, educational programs, and special projects. Its Hospital Technology Series Program, initiated in 1982, is a health care technology evaluation and information dissemination program for hospital administrators.

Purpose: To assist hospital administrators in making prudent and informed management decisions regarding new and existing technologies to support clinical services planning activities.

Primary intended users: Providers, generally; acute facility administrators; long-term care facility administrators.

Technologies: Device, support system.

The Program deals primarily with service implications of technological advances on the planning and delivery of clinical services from the hospital perspective. The Program generally does not evaluate procedures, although they are discussed insofar as they bear upon strategic equipment and service choices.

Intervention: Diagnosis, treatment.

Properties: *Service requirements, system impact,* efficacy, effectiveness, cost, cost-benefit, cost-effectiveness, acceptance/adoption level, economic implications.

Evaluations also consider manufacturer issues, such as vendor stability, the capacity for technologies to be upgraded, and other compared attributes of competing technologies. Although evaluations do not include brand name ratings, they sometimes provide brand-specific information, such as cost and installation information and service support arrangements. Specifically, evaluations are most concerned with the following: 1) cost and organizational implications, 2) installation costs, 3) staffing and training requirements, 4) probable number of patients affected, 5) effects on other hospital resources, and 6) effectiveness (not patient outcomes, but effects on the use of hospital resources, such as inpatient versus outpatient stay and average length of stay).

Selection process: Program staff select subjects for assessment after reviewing their importance to hospital management, especially their impact on costs. Technologies are reassessed based on new information and the perceived needs of hospitals. Reassessments follow the same format as the original assessments.

Methods: Information syntheses, expert opinion, cost analyses.

Evaluations consist of syntheses of the literature, focused interviews with manufacturers and users, and compilations of reported experience by users in such areas as negotiating purchase contracts and common mistakes made in implementation.

The approximate turnaround time from selection of assessment topic to reporting of findings is 6 months.

Assessors: The evaluations are conducted or directed by staff of the Division of Clinical Services and Technology who have expertise in hospital and business administration, health care administration, and clinical engineering. Outside consultants with medical and scientific expertise are also employed.

Assessment reports include: Who conducted the assessment; description of the technology; properties assessed; results; findings or conclusions; implications of findings for practice; recommendations for practice, future assessments, technology development, research; how the technology works, including theory, principles; development of the technology; procurement/deployment information; regulatory agency approval status; coverage/reimbursement status of the technology.

Dissemination: *Printed reports,* journal articles, advisories to members/constituents.

Evaluation findings are reported in *Guideline Reports* issued approximately 4 times a year and disseminated to member hospitals. Selected *Guideline Reports* are summarized in *Hospitals* magazine. They may be obtained as part of a subscription to the *AHA Hospital Technology Series* or ordered separately for a nominal fee.

In addition to *Guideline Reports* the *AHA Hospital Technology Series* includes the following:

Executive Briefing; an overview of major developments affecting hospitals' use of technology in the delivery of patient care; directed to hospitals' chief executive officers and distributed monthly.

Technology Scanner; a collection of categorized summaries of articles relevant to hospital technology, drawn from more than 80 medical and technical journals. Directed to hospital administrators and distributed monthly.

Special Reports; brief updates on current technological issues.

Budget: $368,000. Funding sources: 100 percent sales of subscriptions and reports.

Use: Approximately 1,700 hospitals subscribe to the *Hospital Technology Series.*

Related activities: The AHA's Division of Clinical Services and Technology also produces *MediTrends,* an environmental assessment of clinical services focusing on medical technology.

Completed Reports

AN1 American Hospital Association, Hospital Technology Series Program. Positron emission tomography. 1987. (Guideline report) [Information syntheses, Expert opinion, Cost analyses]

AN2 ———. Radiation therapy planning. 1987. (Guideline report) [Information syntheses, Expert opinion, Cost analyses]

AN3 ______. Topographic brain mapping. 1987. (Guideline report) [Information syntheses, Expert opinion, Cost analyses]

AN4 ______. Cine-CT: progress and opportunities. 1986. (Guideline report) [Information syntheses, Expert opinion, Cost analyses]

AN5 ______. Implementing laser technology in the community hospital. 1986. (Guideline report) [Information syntheses, Expert opinion, Cost analyses]

AN6 ______. Purchasing a satellite receiving earth terminal. 1986. (Guideline report) [Information syntheses, Expert opinion, Cost analyses]

AN7 ______. Lithotripters. 1985. (Guideline report) [Information syntheses, Expert opinion, Cost analyses]

AN8 ______. NMR—issues for 1985 and beyond. 1985. (Guideline report) [Information syntheses, Expert opinion, Cost analyses]

AN9 ______. Picture archiving and communication systems. 1985. (Guideline report) [Information syntheses, Expert opinion, Cost analyses]

AN10 ______. A medical device recall and reporting system. 1984. (Guideline report) [Information syntheses, Expert opinion, Cost analyses]

AN11 ______. Adult volume ventilators. 1984. (Guideline report) [Information syntheses, Expert opinion, Cost analyses]

AN12 ______. Bar coding technology—applications in health care. 1984. (Guideline report)

AN13 ______. Computerized tomographic scanners. 1984. (Guideline report) [Information syntheses, Expert opinion, Cost analyses]

AN14 ______. Echocardiography. 1984. (Guideline report) [Information syntheses, Expert opinion, Cost analyses]

AN15 ______. Equipment acquisition under prospective payment. 1984. (Guideline report) [Information syntheses, Expert opinion, Cost analyses]

AN16 ______. Microcomputers in hospitals. 1984. (Guideline report) [Information syntheses, Expert opinion, Cost analyses]

AN17 ______. Trends in nuclear medicine. 1984. (Guideline report) [Information syntheses, Expert opinion, Cost analyses]

AN18 ______. Materials management information systems. 1983. (Guideline report) [Information syntheses, Expert opinion, Cost analyses]

AN19 ______. Medicare technology assessment. 1983. (Guideline report) [Information syntheses, Expert opinion, Cost analyses]

AN20 ______. Nuclear magnetic resonance (NMR). 1983. (Guideline report) [Information syntheses, Expert opinion, Cost analyses]

AN21 ______. Automated indirect blood pressure measurement devices. 1982. (Guideline report) [Information syntheses, Expert opinion, Cost analyses]

AN22 ______. Automated infusion devices. 1982. (Guideline report) [Information syntheses, Expert opinion, Cost analyses]

AN23 ______. Autotransfusion units. 1982. (Guideline report) [Information syntheses, Expert opinion, Cost analyses]

AN24 ______. Buying and selling used medical equipment. 1982. (Guideline report) [Information syntheses, Expert opinion, Cost analyses]

AN25 ______. Clinical laboratory information systems. 1982. (Guideline report) [Informaton syntheses, Expert opinion, Cost analyses]

AN26 ______. Computerized arrhythmia monitoring systems. 1982. (Guideline report) [Information syntheses, Expert opinion, Cost analyses]

AN27 ______. Digital subtraction angiography. 1982. (Guideline report) [Information syntheses, Expert opinion, Cost analyses]

AN28 ______. Ethylene oxide sterilization. 1982. (Guideline report) [Information synthesis, expert opinion, Cost analyses]

AN29 ______. Evaluation methods for intensive care units. 1982. (Guideline report) [Information syntheses, Expert opinion, Cost analyses]

AN30 ______. Medicare technology assessment. 1982. (Guideline report) [Information syntheses, Expert opinion, Cost analyses]

AN31 ______. Medicare technology assessment. 1981. (Guideline report) [Information syntheses, Expert opinion, Cost analyses]

American Medical Association Council on Scientific Affairs

535 North Dearborn Street
Chicago, IL 60610
312-645-5335

Contact: William R. Hendee, Ph,D., Secretary; or Vicki Grosso, Council and Committee Coordinator.

Overview: The American Medical Association (AMA) is a professional association that provides a wide range of services and products to advance the field of medicine. The Council on Scientific Affairs was formed in 1976 by the AMA.

Purpose: To provide accurate, balanced, and up-to-date information on medical technology to the practicing medical community and to communicate the concerns and opinions of physicians to the health care community.

Primary intended users: General public; people concerned about their health; patients; providers, generally; physicians; acute facility administrators; long-term care facility administrators; other care givers; health product manufacturers; health/medical professional associations; health industry associations; consumer associations; employers; unions and other employee organizations; third party payers; government regulators; voluntary associations, organizations; biomedical researchers; public policymakers, legislators.

Technologies: *Medical or surgical procedure,* drug, device.

Intervention: *Diagnosis, treatment,* prevention, rehabilitation.

Stage: Emerging, new, established or widespread practice, obsolete.

Properties: *Safety, effectiveness,* efficacy.

Selection process: Any responsible party may request an assessment. Requests are made to the Secretary or Council members. The members of the Council then set the priorities for assessment.

Methods: *Group judgment,* information syntheses, expert opinion.

Issues of importance to the practicing medical community are identified. Often expert panels are organized and charged with addressing pertinent issues. Reports are developed by the panel and submitted to the Council for approval. In other cases, issues are analyzed by staff. Reports are developed and reviewed by three or four consultants. They are then submitted to the Council for approval. The approximate turnaround time from selection of assessment topic to reporting of findings is 6 to 12 months.

Assessors: The Council has access to experts in all areas of medicine.

Assessment reports include: Abstract; the purpose of the assessment; description of the technology; stage of life-cycle of technology when assessed; properties assessed; sources of data/information; results; findings or conclusions; limitations of findings;

implications of findings for practice; recommendations for practice, future assessments, technology development, research; how the technology works, including theory, principles; development of the technology.

Dissemination: Printed reports; journal articles; advisories to members/constituents; press conferences/news releases, TV/radio broadcasts, video products.

The reports are 20-25 pages in length with an initial synopsis. The results are disseminated through the *Journal of the American Medical Association (JAMA)* or the popular press. Copies of the assessment reports may be obtained from *JAMA* or by requesting reprints.

Budget: $613,782. The cost per assessment varies. Funding source: 100 percent parent organization.

Use: The AMA uses the assessment reports as a source of information for physicians to incorporate in their decision-making processes.

Completed Reports

AO1 American Medical Association, Council on Scientific Affairs. Drugs and athletes—Progress Report. 1986. [Group judgment]

AO2 ______. Glucocorticoid-induced osteonecrosis. 1986. [Group judgment]

AO3 ______. Herpes simplex and school children. 1986. [Group judgment]

AO4 ______. Lasers in medicine and surgery. JAMA 1986 Aug 15;256(7):900-907. [Group judgment]

AO5 ______. OTC diet preparations containing phenylpropanolamine (Resolution 100, I-85). 1986. [Group judgment]

AO6 ______. Preventing death and disability from fires by the new rapid response automatic sprinklers and smoke detectors (Resolution 2, A-85). 1986. [Group judgment]

AO7 ______. Safe use of radioactive materials in medical practice (Resolution 66, A-85). 1986. [Group judgment]

AO8 ______. Statement on liver transplantation. 1986. [Group judgment]

AO9 ______. The Heimlich maneuver—interim report (Resolution 52, I-85). 1986. [Group judgment]

AO10 ______. Use of immunosuppressants in organ transplantation. 1986. [Group judgment]

AO11 ______. AMA diagnostic and treatment guidelines concerning child abuse and neglect. JAMA 1985 Aug 9;254(6):796-800. [Group judgment]

AO12 ______. Aspartame: review of safety issues. JAMA 1985 Jul 18;254:400-402. [Group judgment]

AO13 ______. Autopsies: interim report (Substitute Resolution 11, A-84). 1985. [Group judgment]

AO14 ______. Current status of therapeutic plasmapheresis and related techniques. JAMA 1985 Feb 8;253:819-825. [Group judgment]

AO15 ______. Dementia. 1985 [Group judgment]

AO16 ______. Drugs and athletes—interim report. 1985. [Group judgment]

AO17 ______. Guidelines for handling parenteral antineoplastics. JAMA 1985 Mar 15;253:1590-1592. [Group judgment]

AO18 ______. Guidelines for reporting estimates of probability of paternity. JAMA 1985 Jun 14;253:3298. [Group judgment]

AO19 ______. Harmful effects of UVA and UVB light. 1985. [Group judgment]

AO20 ______. SI units for clinical laboratory data. JAMA 1985 May 3;253:2553-2554. [Group judgment]

AO21 ______. Saccharin: review of safety issues. JAMA 1985 Nov 8;254(18):2622-2624. [Group judgment]

AO22 ______. Scientific status of refreshing recollection by the use of hypnosis. JAMA 1985 Apr 5;253:1918-1923. [Group judgment]

AO23 ______. The use of cardiac pacemakers in medical practice. JAMA 1985 Oct 11;254 (14) 1952-1954. [Group judgment]

AO24 ______. Vitamin preparations as dietary supplements and as therapeutic agents. 1985. [Group judgment]

AO25 ______. Xenografts: Review of the literature and current status. JAMA 1985 Dec 20;254(23):3353. [Group judgment; Information syntheses]

AO26 ______. Caffeine labeling. JAMA 1984 Aug 10;252:803-806. [Group judgment]

AO27 ______. Chelation therapy. 1984. [Group judgment]

AO28 ______. Combined modality approaches to cancer therapy. JAMA 1984 May 11;251:2398-2407. [Group judgment]

AO29 ______. Early detection of breast cancer. JAMA 1984 Dec 7;252:3008-3011. [Group judgment]

AO30 ______. Nicotine chewing gum for cessation of smoking. 1984. [Group judgment]

AO31 ______. Percutaneous transluminal angioplasty. JAMA 1984 Feb 10;251:764-768. [Group judgment]

AO32 ______. Prescription Abuse Data Synthesis (PADS) Project and the AMA prescription drug abuse activity. 1984. [Group judgment]

AO33 ______. The acquired immunodeficiency syndrome. JAMA 1984 Oct 19;252:2037-2043. [Group judgment]

AO34 ______. A guide to the hospital management of injuries arising from exposure to or involving ionizing radiation. 1983. [Group judgment]

AO35 ______. AMA's role in technology assessment (Resolution 131 (A-83). 1983. [Group judgment]

AO36 ______. Calcium channel blocking agents. JAMA 1983 Nov 11;250:2522-2524. [Group judgment]

AO37 ______. Choking: the Heimlich maneuver (abdominal thrust) vs. back blows. 1983. [Group judgment]

AO38 ______. Cochlear implants. JAMA 1983 Jul 15;250:391-392. [Group judgment]

AO39 ______. Dietary and pharmacologic therapy for the lipid risk factors. JAMA 1983 Oct 14;250:1873-1879. [Group judgment]

AO40 ______. Effects of competition in medicine. JAMA 1983 Apr 8;249:1864-1868. [Group judgment]

AO41 ______. Estrogen replacement in the menopause. JAMA 1983 Jan 21;249:359. [Group judgment]

AO42 ______. Exercise programs for the elderly. 1983. [Group judgment]

AO43 ______. In-utero fetal surgery: (Resolution 73 (I-81). JAMA 1983 Sep 16;250:1443-1444. [Group judgment]

AO44 ______. Maternal alcohol use. JAMA 1983 May 13;249:2517-2521. [Group judgment]

AO45 ______. Medical evaluations of healthy persons. JAMA 1983 Mar 25;249:1626-1633. [Group judgment]

AO46 ______. Methaqualone, abuse limits its usefulness. JAMA 1983 Dec 9;250:3052. [Group judgment]

AO47 ______. Nonsmoking in hospitals. 1983. [Group judgment]

AO48 ______. Pharmaceutical dissolution of gallstones. JAMA 1983 Nov 4;250:2373-2374. [Group judgment]

AO49 ______. Update on venereal disease. 1983. [Group judgment]

AO50 ______. AMA involvement in prevention and treatment of child abuse and neglect (Substitute Resolution 75, A-81). 1982. [Group judgment]

AO51 ______. Addition of thiamine to alcoholic beverages (Resolution 140, A-81). 1982. [Group judgment]

AO52 ______. Continuous ambulatory peritoneal dialysis. JAMA 1982 Nov 12;248:2340. [Group judgment]

AO53 ______. Dimethyl sulfoxide. JAMA 1982 Sep 17;248:1369. [Group judgment]

AO54 ______. Drug abuse related to prescribing practices. JAMA 1982 Feb 12;247:864. [Group judgment]

AO55 ______. Genetic counseling and prevention of birth defects. JAMA 1982 Jul 9;248:221. [Group judgment]

AO56 ______. Health care needs of a homosexual population. JAMA 1982 Aug 13;248:736. [Group judgment]

AO57 ______. Infant formula marketing (Resolution 155, A-81). 1982. [Group judgment]

AO58 ______. Maternal serum a-fetoprotein monitoring. JAMA 1982 Mar 12;247:1478. [Group judgment]

AO59 ______. Pneumococcal, influenza and hepatitis-B vaccine (Resolution 75, A-82). 1982. [Group judgment]

AO60 ______. Acupuncture. 1981. [Group judgment]

AO61 ______. Electronic fetal monitoring. JAMA 1981 Nov 20;246:2370. [Group judgment]

AO62 ______. Evalution of iridology. 1981. [Group judgment]

AO63 ______. Hypnotic drugs and treatment of insomnia. JAMA 1981 Feb 20;245:749. [Group judgment]

AO64 ______. Indications and contraindications for exercise testing. JAMA 1981 Aug 28;246:1015. [Group judgment]

AO65 ______. Marijuana, its health hazards and therapeutic potentials. JAMA 1981 Oct 16;246:1823. [Group judgment]

AO66 ______. Medical care for indigent and culturally displaced obstetrical patients and their newborns. Committee on Maternal and Child Health. JAMA 1981 Mar 20;245:1159. [Group judgment]

AO67 ______. Organ donor recruitment. JAMA 1981 Nov 13;246:2157. [Group judgment]

AO68 ______. Physician-supervised exercise programs in rehabilitation of patients with coronary heart disease. JAMA 1981 Apr 10;245:1463. [Group judgment]

AO69 ______. Prescription of tranquilizers and antidepressants for women (Board of Trustees report X, I-80). 1981. [Group judgment]

AO70 ______. Health care technology assessment—1980. 1980. [Group judgment]

AO71 ______. Hypoglycemic treatment, guidelines for the non-insulin-dependent diabetic. JAMA 1980 May 23-30;243:2078. [Group judgment]

AO72 ______. Importance of diagnostic computerized tomographic scanning. 1980. [Group judgment]

AO73 ______. Infant nutrition (Resolution III, I-78.) 1980. [Group judgment]

AO74 ______. Marijuana in the 80's. 1980. [Group judgment]

AO75 ______. Progress in adoption of SI units. 1980. [Group judgment]

AO76 ______. The nutritive quality of processed foods: general policies for nutrient additions. 1980. [Group judgment]

American Medical Association
Diagnostic and Therapeutic Technology Assessment

535 North Dearborn Street
Chicago, IL 60610
312-645-4530

Contact: William T. McGivney, Ph.D., Director; or Andrea L. Schneider, Program Administrator. Telex 910-221-0300.

Overview: The American Medical Association (AMA) is a professional association that provides a wide range of services and products to advance the field of medicine. The Diagnostic and Therapeutic Technology Assessment program (DATTA) was established by the AMA in 1982.

Purpose: To provide accurate, balanced, and up-to-date information on medical technology to the practicing medical community; and to communicate the concerns and opinions of physicians to other constituents of the health care community.

Primary intended users: General public; people concerned about their health; patients; providers, generally; physicians; acute facility administrators; long-term care facility administrators; other care givers; health product manufacturers; health/medical professional associations; health industry associations; consumer associations; employers; unions and other employee organizations; third party payers; government regulators; voluntary associations, organizations; biomedical researchers; public policymakers; legislators.

Technologies: *Medical or surgical procedure,* drug, device.

Intervention: *Diagnosis, treatment,* prevention, rehabilitation.

Stage: *New,* emerging, established or widespread practice, obsolete.

Properties: *Safety, effectiveness,* efficacy.

Selection process: Any responsible party may request that an assessment be conducted. Written requests should be submitted to the Director. The DATTA Subcommittee, Director, and AMA Executive staff set assessment topic priorities. The need to reassess the technologies is considered periodically.

Methods: *Expert opinion,* information syntheses.

DATTA formulates questions to examine the safety and effectiveness of a technology when applied for very specific indications. Individuals with expertise in the topic are selected from a reference panel and asked (by mail) to rate the safety and effectiveness of the technology as established, investigational, or unacceptable. Panelists are encouraged to provide supporting data and relevant considerations. The evaluations of the panelists are collated, compiled, and synthesized with an extensive analysis of the biomedical literature. The approximate turnaround time from selection of topic to reporting of findings is 120 days.

Assessors: DATTA is operated by AMA staff under direction of a subcommittee of the AMA Council on Scientific Affairs. Staff selects panelists for each assessment from a reference panel of 1,000 physicians appointed by the Council on Scientific Affairs. Panelists represent a broad spectrum of specialties and subspecialties.

Assessment reports include: Description of the technology; stage of life-cycle of technology when assessed; properties assessed; sources of data/information; results; findings or conclusions; limitations of findings; implications of findings for practice; recommendations for practice, future assessments, technology development, research; how the technology works, including theory, principles.

Dissemination: Printed reports; journal articles; advisories to members/constituents; press conferences/news releases, TV/radio broadcasts, video products.

The assessment reports contain an initial synopsis and are usually 8 to 10 pages in length. DATTA results are usually published in the *Journal of the American Medical Association,* disseminated in the popular press, and are distributed to certain individuals and organizations on a mailing list. Individual copies of DATTA reports may be obtained from the AMA. Subscriptions to the DATTA series, including new and past reports and the newsletter *AMA Tech,* are available from the AMA.

Budget: $380,000. The approximate cost per assessment is $15,000. Funding source: 100 percent parent organization.

Use: The AMA uses the assessment reports as a source of information for physicians to use for decision-making purposes. They are also used by third party payers, group practices, specialty societies, individual patients, public policy-makers. Articles describing the program include the following citations:

Institute of Medicine, Committee on Evaluating Medical Technologies in Clinical Use. *Assessing medical technologies*. Washington, DC: National Academy Press, 1985.

Monaco GP, Burke RL. Insurance as gatekeeper—part two: policy obstacles in unproven methods litigation. *Forum* 1985;spring.

Petitti DB. Competing technologies, implications for the cost and complexity of medical care. *New Engl J Med* 1986 Dec 4.

Rose M, Leibenluft RF. Antitrust implications of medical technology assessment. *New Engl J Med* 1986 Jun 5.

The following assessment reports of the Office of Health Technology Assessment (National Center for Health Services Research and Health Care Technology Assessment) reference DATTA statements:

1983

Anti-gastroesophageal reflux implantation
Diathermy as a physical therapy modality
Fully automated ambulatory blood pressure monitoring of hypertension

1984

Ambulatory electroencephalographic (EEG) monitoring
External open-loop pump for the subcutaneous infusion of insulin in diabetes
Implantable pump for chronic heparin therapy Streptokinase infusion for acute myocardial infarction
Transplantation of the pancreas

1985

Apheresis in the treatment of guillian-barre syndrome
Extracorporeal shock wave lithotripsy (ESWL) procedure for treatment of kidney stones
Patient selection criteria for percutaneous transluminal coronary angioplasty of a stenotic lesion in a single coronary artery
Percutaneous ultrasound procedures for the treatment of kidney stones
Reassessment of cardiokymography (No longer valid)
Transurethral ureteroscopic lithotripsy procedures for the treatment of kidney stones

Completed Reports

AP1 American Medical Association, Diagnostic and Therapeutic Technology Assessment. Ablation of accessory pathways in Wolff-Parkinson-White Syndrome. Mar 31, 1986. [Expert opinion, Information syntheses]

AP2 ______. Angelchik antireflux prosthesis treatment of gastroesophageal reflux. JAMA 1986 Sep 12. [Expert opinion, Information syntheses]

AP3 ______. Autologous bone marrow transplantation. JAMA 1986 Jul 4. [Expert opinion, Information syntheses]

AP4 ______. BCG immunotherapy in bladder cancer. Mar 31, 1986. [Expert opinion, Information syntheses]

AP5 ______. Cardiac rehabilitation services. Jul 16, 1986. [Expert opinion, Information syntheses]

AP6 ______. Garren gastric bubble for morbid obesity. JAMA 1986 Dec 19. [Expert opinion, Information syntheses]

AP7 ______. Mammographic screening for breast cancer. Oct 19, 1986. [Expert opinion, Information syntheses]

AP8 ______. Microsurgical reconstruction for brachial plexus injury. Jul 16, 1986. [Expert opinion, Information syntheses]

AP9 ______. Continuous arteriovenous hemofiltration (CAVH) for fluid removal. JAMA 1985 Mar 1. [Expert opinion, Information syntheses]

AP10 ______. Diagnostic intraoperative ultrasound. JAMA 1985 Jul 12. [Expert opinion, Information syntheses]

AP11 ______. Endoscopic electrocoagulation for gastrointestinal hemorrhage. JAMA 1985 May 11. [Expert opinion, Information syntheses]

AP12 ______. Endoscopic laser photocoagulation for gastrointestinal hemorrhage. JAMA 1985 May 11. [Expert opinion, Information syntheses]

AP13 ______. Endoscopic thermal coagulation for gastrointestinal hemorrhage. JAMA 1985 May 11. [Expert opinion, Information syntheses]

AP14 ______. Endoscopic topical therapy for gastrointestinal hemorrhage. JAMA 1985 May 11. [Expert opinion, Information syntheses]

AP15 ______. Enhanced computed tomography in head trauma. JAMA 1985 Dec 20. [Expert opinion, Information syntheses]

AP16 ______. Non-invasive extracorporeal lithotripsy for disruption of kidney stones—Update. Feb 15, 1985. [Expert opinion, Information syntheses]

AP17 ______. Sperm penetration assay in identifying male infertility. JAMA 1985 Oct 11. [Expert opinion, Information syntheses]

AP18 ______. Sterotactic cingulatomy treatment for psychiatric disorders. JAMA 1985 Nov 15. [Expert opinion, Information syntheses]

AP19 ______. Apnea monitoring for 24-hour surveillance of newborns at risk for sudden infant death syndrome. JAMA 1984 Jan 27. [Expert opinion, Information syntheses]

AP20 ______. Bone marrow transplantation in childhood leukemia. JAMA 1984 Apr 27. [Expert opinion, Information syntheses]

AP21 ______. Cardiokymography for (non-invasive) cardiological diagnosis. JAMA 1984 Feb 24. [Expert opinion, Information syntheses]

AP22 ______. Diaphanography (transillumination of the the breast) for cancer screening. JAMA 1984 Apr 18. [Expert opinion, Information syntheses]

AP23 ______. Endoscopic transurethral nephrolithotomy for disruption of kidney stones. JAMA 1984 Dec 21. [Expert opinion, Information syntheses]

AP24 ______. Gastric restrictive surgery for morbid obesity. JAMA 1984 Jun 8. [Expert opinion, Information syntheses]

AP25 ______. Hyperthermia treatment for cancer—Update. Sep 17, 1984. [Expert opinion, Information syntheses]

AP26 ______. Implanted electrospinal stimulator for scoliosis. JAMA 1984 May 25. [Expert opinion, Information syntheses]

AP27 ______. Percutaneous nephrolithotomy for kidney stone removal. JAMA 1984 Dec 2. [Expert opinion, Information syntheses]

AP28 ______. 24-hour ambulatory EEG monitoring for diagnosing seizure disorders. JAMA 1983 Dec 23. [Expert opinion, Information syntheses]

AP29 ______. Biofeedback for managing vascular and tension headaches. JAMA 1983 Nov 14. [Expert opinion, Information syntheses]

AP30 ______. CO2 laser for the treatment of gynecologic malignancies. JAMA 1983 Aug 5. [Expert opinion, Information systheses]

AP31 ______. Chelation therapy (with EDTA) for atherosclerosis. JAMA 1983 Aug 5. [Expert opinion, Information syntheses]

AP32 ______. Cranial electrostimulation for treatment of anxiety and/or depression. JAMA 1984 Feb 24. [Expert opinion, Information syntheses]

AP33 ______. Diathermy for treating musculoskeletal conditions. JAMA 1983 Jul 22-29. [Expert opinion, Information syntheses]

AP34 ______. Implantable infusion pump for continuous drug therapy. JAMA 1983 Oct 14. [Expert opinion, Information syntheses]

AP35 ______. Mandatory EKG prior to elective surgery. JAMA 1983 Jul 29. [Expert opinion, Information syntheses]

AP36 ______. Quantitative EEG (fast Fourier transform analysis) operative monitoring of cerebrovascular status. JAMA 1983 Jul 15. [Expert opinion, Information syntheses]

AP37 ______. Radial keratotomy for the treatment of myopia. JAMA 1983 Jul 15. [Expert opinon, Information syntheses]

AP38 ______. Thermography (electronic and liquid crystal) for diagnosing low-back pain. Ongoing. [Expert opinion, Information syntheses]

American Medical Association Drug Evaluations

535 North Dearborn Street
Chicago, IL 60610
312-645-4560

Contact: Donald R. Bennett, M.D., Ph.D., Director; or Marilyn A. Mayo, Assistant to the Director. Telex 910-221-0300.

Overview: The American Medical Association (AMA) is a professional association that provides many services and products to advance the field of medicine. The AMA Drug Evaluations section was established in 1971, however, the Department of Drugs has been a part of the AMA for 75 years. Every 2 to 3 years it publishes the reference book *Drug Evaluations*; the sixth edition was published in 1986.

Purpose: To provide physicians and other health care professionals with up-to-date, objective information on the clinical use of drugs and to serve as a reference source for practical, comparative, evaluative information on drug therapy.

Primary intended users: Providers, generally; physicians; health product manufacturers; health/medical professional associations; public policy-makers, legislators.

Technologies: Drug.

Intervention: Treatment.

Stage: Emerging, new, established or widespread practice, obsolete.

Properties: Safety, efficacy, effectiveness.

Selection process: Assessment topics are identified primarily by AMA scientific staff review of current drug utilization. Occasionally, requests are received from physicians. The requests are submitted to the Director who sets priorities in consultation with the Drug Evaluations editor and scientific staff.

Methods: Information syntheses, expert opinion.

The staff of the AMA Department of Drugs prepares chapters based on the current scientific literature. The chapters are reviewed by consultants and the medical staffs of the appropriate pharmaceutical manufacturers. Following consensus revision, the chapters are reviewed by designees or members of the American Society for Clinical Pharmacology and Therapeutics (ASCPT). For the sixth edition, more than 500 distinguished consultants contributed their comments to the draft versions. Thus, this publication is a joint scientific contribution to the field of applied therapeutics by the AMA, a large consultant body, and the ASCPT. The consultants have expertise in pharmacology and therapeutics. A new edition of *Drug Evaluations* is produced every 2 to 3 years.

Assessors: AMA professional staff, medical staff of pharmaceutical manufacturers, and expert consultants in pharmacology and therapeutics participate in the assessments.

Assessment reports include: Description of the technology; stage of life-cycle of technology when assessed; properties assessed; sources of data/information; results; findings or conclusions; limitations of findings; implications of findings for practice; recommendations for practice, future assessments, technology development, research; how the technology works, including theory, principles. The text describes approximately 2,000 drugs.

Dissemination: The text is sold by the AMA directly and by a commercial publisher.

Budget: The cost of producing each text is $1,500,000; this averages $500 for each drug evaluation. Funding source: 100 percent parent organization.

Use: *Drug Evaluations* provides physicians information on comparative drug therapy to improve their prescribing practices. There are numerous citations in the biomedical literature to this text.

Completed Reports

AQ1 American Medical Association. Drug evaluations. Philadelphia:Saunders, 1986. [Information syntheses, Expert opinion]

American Society for Gastrointestinal Endoscopy

Committee on Technology Assessment
13 Elm Street
Manchester, MA 01944
617-927-8330

Contact: William T. Maloney, Executive Director; or John H. Bond Jr., M.D., Chairman, Veterans Administration Hospital, 54th St. and 48th Ave. South, Minneapolis, MN 55417,612-725-6767.

Overview: The purposes of the American Society for Gastrointestinal Endoscopy (ASGE) are 1) to further knowledge of gastrointestinal disease through the use of endoscopic techniques in clinical practice and research; 2) to establish and maintain the highest standards of practices for the diagnostic and therapeutic use of gastrointestinal endoscopic methods; 3) to provide guidelines for training programs and to further the teaching of gastrointestinal endoscopy; 4) to assist all those involved with health care as it relates to gastrointestinal endoscopy; and 5) to facilitate development of improved instruments of gastrointestinal endoscopy.

The Society has 3,840 members. Its activities include educational, audiovisual, scientific, and research programs, as well as publication of a bimonthly journal *Gastrointestinal Endoscopy* and guidelines and statements on training and practice.

Various activities relating to technology assessment were organized under the direction of a five-member Committee on Technology Assessment in May 1986. The Society functions as an information source, and is capable of offering expert and consensus opinions and other assistance in matters that relate to gastrointestinal endoscopic technology.

Purpose: To explore and define technology issues that apply to gastrointestinal endoscopy.

Primary intended users: Providers, generally; physicians.

Technologies: Device, medical or surgical procedure.

Interest is focused primarily on the use in clinical practice of emerging and established gastrointestinal endoscopic procedures and other technical procedures that relate to endoscopy. The Society is also concerned with the development and assessment of new instruments and techniques as well as innovative uses of existing methods and instruments.

Intervention: *Diagnosis, treatment.*

Stage: Emerging, new, established or widespread practice, obsolete.

Existing and established endoscopic methods and related instruments are assessed. Emerging procedures and instruments are also assessed, especially those that appear likely to be adopted by large numbers of physicians who use endoscopy.

Properties: *Safety, efficacy, effectiveness,* cost-effectiveness.

Emphasis is on the correct use of endoscopic instruments and techniques with respect to accepted indications and contraindications, safety considerations, effectiveness, and cost-effectiveness, and on training in endoscopic procedures.

Selection process: The ASGE Governing Board directs the activities of the Technology Assessment Committee. In some instances the Board directs that specific questions be reviewed while in other cases, committees may recommend areas for study that they consider important or controversial. The Society solicits the views of its members, usually by means of questionnaires and surveys, to identify problem areas.

All ASGE statements on the use of endoscopic procedures are updated periodically, and out-of-date statements are withdrawn.

Methods: *Group judgment,* information syntheses, expert opinion, cost analyses.

The Society has several assessment procedures, including information gathering and syntheses. In this process, published information is reviewed, the opinions of expert consultants are solicited, and conclusions are formulated by a panel of experienced endoscopists.

The ASGE conducts prospective studies of various problems pertaining to the use of endoscopy in which members submit data according to a protocol. One of the most useful has been the National ASGE Survey on Upper Gastrointestinal Bleeding (Silverstein FE, et al. *Gastrointest Endosc* 1981;27:73-103) which included the participation of 277 members.

A comprehensive review of a specific technology requires about 9 to 12 months, although this is highly variable and depends on the complexity of the problem.

Assessors: Society members who participate in technology assessment have extensive clinical experience in endoscopy. They are usually acknowledged experts in specific areas of endoscopy as well as established investigators who have made significant contributions to the field in its technical and clinical aspects.

Assessment reports include: Description of the technology; properties assessed; procedure used for the assessment; sources of data/information; methods for collecting data/information; methods for analyzing/synthesizing data/information; results; findings or conclusions; limitations of findings; implications of findings for practice; recommendations for practice, future assessments, technology development, research.

Dissemination: Printed reports, journal articles.

The conclusions that result from a review process may be formulated as a guideline statement with recommendations directed to Society members and the medical community at large. Statements, recommendations, and reviews are usually published as pamphlets or monographs, which are available free from the Manchester office.

Budget: Not provided. The approximate cost of an assessment, based on the number of meetings to generate a report, is $5,000 to $25,000. A complex review of a broad area or an intricate problem that requires considerable discussion might require greater funding.

Use: The ASGE uses the assessments to promote high standards of practice, patient care, and training in matters that pertain to endoscopy. Although the work of the ASGE as a professional society is primarily directed toward practicing physicians, it is also available to health care institutions, government agencies, certifying bodies, organizations that regulate health care delivery, and virtually any organization with legitimate interests in health care. It is also available to the general public. It is the ASGE's impression that some of these groups have used its reports, but this usage is not tracked.

Related activities: The results and conclusions of investigative work sponsored by the ASGE and relating, at times, to technology assessment are usually presented in open forums such as the plenary session of the Society and in the Society's journal, *Gastrointestinal Endoscopy*.

Completed Reports

AS1 Boyce HW. Treatment of esophageal stenosis. In: American Society for Gastrointestinal Endoscopy, Committee on Technology Assessment. Therapeutic gastrointestinal endoscopy: an information resource manual. 1987. [Information syntheses, Expert opinion, Group judgment, Cost analyses]

AS2 Fleischer DE. Esophageal cancer: laser treatment. In: American Society for Gastrointestinal Endoscopy, Committee on Technology Assessment. Therapeutic gastrointestinal endoscopy: an information resource manual. 1987. [Information syntheses, Expert opinion, Group judgment, Cost analyses]

AS3 Jensen DM. Gastrointestinal angiomata: current diagnosis and treatment. In: American society for Gastrointestinal Endoscopy, Committee on Technology Assessment. Therapeutic gastrointestinal endoscopy: an information resource manual. 1987. [Information syntheses, Expert opinion, Group judgment, Cost analyses]

AS4 Johnston JH. Ulcer hemorrhage—heater probe treatment. In: American Society for Gastrointestinal Endoscopy, Committee on Technology Assessment. Therapeutic gastrointestinal endoscopy: an information resource manual. 1987. [Information syntheses, Expert opinion, Group judgment, Cost analyses]

AS5 Kozarek RA. Balloon dilation. In: American Society for Gastrointestinal Endoscopy, Committee on Technology Assessment. Therapeutic gastrointestinal endoscopy: an information resource manual. 1987. [Information synthesis, Expert opinion, Group judgment, Cost analyses]

AS6 Mellow MH. Endoscopic laser treatment of colon cancer. In: American Society for Gastrointestinal Endoscopy, Committee on Technology Assessment. Therapeutic gastrointestinal endoscopy: an information resource manual. 1987. [Information syntheses, Expert opinion, Group judgment, Cost analyses]

AS7 Overholt BF. Ulcer hemorrhage—laser treatment. In: American Society for Gastrointestinal Endoscopy, Committee on Technology Assessment. Therapeutic gastrointestinal endoscopy: an information resource manual. 1987. [Information syntheses, Expert opinion, Group judgment, Cost analyses]

AS8 Papp JP. Control of upper gastrointestinal bleeding by monopolar electrocoagulation. In: American Society for Gastrointestinal Endoscopy, Committee on Technology Assessment. Therapeutic gastrointestinal endoscopy: an information resource manual. 1987. [Information syntheses, Expert opinion, Group judgment, Cost analyses]

AS9 Ponsky JL. Percutaneous endoscopic gastrostomy and jejunostomy. In: American Society for Gastrointestinal Endoscopy, Committee on Technology Assessment. Therapeutic gastrointestinal endoscopy: an information resource manual. 1987. [Information synthesis, Expert opinion, Group judgment, Cost analyses]

AS10 Protell RL. Ulcer hemorrhage—bicap probe treatment. In: American Society for Gastrointestinal Endoscopy, Committee on Technology Assessment. Therapeutic gastrointestinal endoscopy: an information resource manual. 1987. [Information sytheses, Expert opinion, Group judgment, Cost analyses]

AS11 Silvis SE. Endoscopic retrograde sphincterotomy (ERS). In: American Society for Gastrointestinal Endoscopy, Committee on Technology Assessment. Therapeutic gastrointestinal endoscopy: an information resource manual. 1987. [Information syntheses;Expert opinion, Group judgment, Cost analyses]

AS12 Sivak MV. Sclerotherapy of esophageal varices. In: American Society for Gastrointestinal Endoscopy, Committee on Technology Assessment. Therapeutic gastrointestinal endoscopy: an information resource manual. 1987. [Information syntheses, Expert opinion, Group judgment, Cost analyses]

AS13 Wayne JD. Colonoscopic polypectomy. In: American Society for Gastrointestinal Endoscopy, Committee on Technology Assessment. Therapeutic gastrointestinal endoscopy: an information resource manual. 1987. [Information syntheses, Expert opinion, Group judgment, Cost analyses]

AS14 Webb WA. Esophageal and gastric foreign bodies: endoscopic removal. In: American Society for Gastrointestinal Endoscopy, Committee on Technology Assessment. Therapeutic gastrointestinal endoscopy: an information resource manual. 1987. [Information syntheses, Expert opinion, Group judgment, Cost analyses]

AS15 American Society for Gastrointestinal Endoscopy. Appropriate use of gastrointestinal endoscopy. 1986 Jun.

AS16 ______. Flexible sigmoidoscopy. Revised 1986 Mar.

AS17 ______. Standards of practice for gastrointestinal endoscopy. Revised 1986 Mar.

AS18 ______. Statement of endoscopic training. Revised 1986 Mar.

AS19 ______. The role of colonoscopy in the management of patients with colonic polyps. Revised 1986 May.

AS20 ______. The role of colonoscopy in the patients with inflammatory bowel diseases. Revised 1986 May.

AS21 ______. The role of endoscopy in the management of esophagitis. Revised 1986 Mar.

AS22 ______. The role of endoscopy in the management of the patient with peptic ulcer disease. Revised 1986 Mar.

AS23 ______. The role of endoscopy in the management of upper gastrointestinal hemorrhage. Revised 1986 Mar.

AS24 ______. The role of endoscopy in the patient with lower gastrointestinal bleeding. 1986 May.

AS25 ______. The role of endoscopy in the surveillance of premalignant conditions of the upper gastrointestinal tract. Revised 1986 Mar.

Battelle Memorial Institute

Battelle Human Affairs Research Centers
4000 NE 41st Street
Seattle, WA 98105
206-525-3130

Battelle Medical Technology Assessment Program
2030 M Street NW
Washington, DC 20036
202-785-8400

Contact: Roger W. Evans, Ph.D., Senior Research Scientist, Human Affairs Research Centers; Bryan R. Luce, Ph.D., Director, Medical Technology Assessment Program.

Overview: The Battelle Memorial Institute is a nonprofit organization devoted to the advancement and use of science and technology. The Battelle Human Affairs Research Centers is a component of the Pacific Northwest Division of Battelle Memorial Institute. Assessments of health care technologies are undertaken by the Health and Population Study Center in Seattle, and by the Medical Technoloy Assessment Program (MEDTAP) in Washington, DC.

Purpose: To assess medical technologies.

Primary intended uses: General public; patients; providers, generally; physicians; acute facility administrators; health product manufacturers; health/medical professional associations; health industry associations; employers; third party payers; government regulators; reporters, writers, news media; public policy-makers, legislators.

Technologies: *Drug, device,* medical or surgical procedure, support system, organizational or administrative system.

Intervention: *Treatment,* prevention, diagnosis, rehabilitation.

Stage: *New,* emerging, established or widespread practice.

Properties: *Cost-effectiveness;* effectiveness; cost; service requirements; acceptance/ adoption level; economic implications; ethical, legal, social implications; health status effects; reimbursement implications.

Selection process: Anyone can request that an assessment be conducted; requests do not follow a specific format. All assessments are done through either a contract or grant. Generally the sponsor, whether it is industry or government, sets assessment topic priorities.

Methods: *Cost analyses,* information syntheses, expert opinion, group judgment, modeling, epidemiological or other observational methods, prospective economic clinical trials/studies, retrospective cost-effectiveness studies, quality of life questionnaires, cost of illness simulation techniques.

The assessment process varies depending upon the issue addressed. The turnaround time from selection of assessment topic to reporting of findings averages 1 year but ranges from 4 months to 3 years.

Assessors: The assessors have expertise in conducting cost effectiveness research, quality of life/health status measurement, and prospective economic clinical studies.

Assessment reports include: Abstract; the assessment's intended audience; the purpose of the assessment; relationship of this assessment to prior or concurrent assessments of the technology or other technologies intended for similar purposes; who sponsored/commissioned/supported the assessment; who conducted the assessment; description of the technology; stage of life-cycle of technology when assessed; properties assessed; procedure used for the assessment; sources of data/information; methods for collecting data/information; methods for analyzing/synthesizing data/information; results; findings or conclusions; limitations of findings; implications of findings for practice; recommendations for practice, future assessments, technology development, research; how the technology works, including theory, principles; where technology is in use; regulatory agency approval status; coverage/reimbursement status of the technology.

Dissemination: Printed reports, journal articles.

Copies of assessments may be obtained by writing to: Battelle Human Affairs Research Centers or to Battelle MEDTAP. For the National Heart Transplantation Study and the National Kidney Dialysis and Kidney Transplantation Study, Battelle printed a total of some 80 Update Series reports on various aspects of these major studies. All are available from Battelle; some have been published in journals. Due to agreements with its clients, Battelle MEDTAP is unable to provide a complete list of ongoing assessments.

Budget: $200,000. The cost per assessment ranges from $40,000 to $3,000,000. Funding source: 100 percent private industry contracts.

Use: Most assessments are used for health policy and reimbursement decisions or marketing purposes. The Battelle National Heart Transplant Study was particularly important in assisting the Health Care Financing Administration and the Secretary of the U.S. Department of Health and Human Services in formulating Medicare reimbursement policy.

Battelle's assessment activities are described in Institute of Medicine, Committee on Evaluating Medical Technologies in Clinical Use. *Assessing medical technologies.* Washington, DC: National Academy Press, 1985.

Completed Reports

BA1 Luce BR, Ellrodt AG, Camaeron JM, Reidinger M. [Battelle Medical Technology Assessment Program] Managing acute hypertension: cost considerations. Am J Emer Med 1986;6(supplement):31-34. [Cost analyses]

BA2 Health Industry Manufacturers Association. [Battelle Medical Technology Assessment Program] A guide to cost-effectiveness analysis for medical device and diagnostic manufacturers. Washington, D.C.: Health Industry Manufacturers Association, 1985. (HIMA Report Number B5-2, HIMA Research Report Series Number 3). [Cost analyses]

BA3 Battelle Human Affairs Research Centers. National Heart Transplantation Study, Final Report to the Health Care Financing Administration. 1984.

BA4 Battelle Human Affairs Research Centers. National Kidney Dialysis and Kidney Transplantation Study, Final Report submitted to the Health Care Financing Administration. 1984.

Ongoing Assessments

BA5 Battelle Human Affairs Research Centers. Cost-effectiveness of cyclosporine as primary immunosuppressive therapy for kidney transplantation recipients, sponsored by the Health Care Financing Administration. Ongoing.

BA6 Battelle Medical Technology Assessment Program. Cost-effectiveness of the implantable cardiac defibrillator. Ongoing.

Blue Cross and Blue Shield Association Medical Necessity Program

676 North St. Clair Street, 11th Floor
Chicago, IL 60611
312-440-5577

Contact: Susan Gleeson, Executive Director, Technology Management Department; David Tennenbaum, Manager, Medical Necessity Program 312-440-6155.

Overview: The Blue Cross and Blue Shield Association represents member Blue Cross and Blue Shield plans and advises them on health care insurance issues. As an association, it provides medical, financial, and administrative consultation and technical assistance to member plans.

The identification of obsolete procedures by Blue Cross and Blue Shield plans began in 1975 with the California Blue Shield Medical Policy Committee. The Medical Necessity Program was begun in 1976 under the National Association of Blue Shield Plans (which merged in 1978 with the Blue Cross Association to form the Blue Cross and Blue Shield Association), representing one of the first national private initiatives to assess medical technology for coverage purposes. Since its inception, the Program has worked in cooperation with such organizations as the American College of Physicians, the American College of Radiology, and the American College of Surgeons. As a result of its participation in the Medical Necessity Program, the American College of Physicians established the Clinical Efficacy Assessment Project.

Purpose: To provide advice to member Blue Cross and Blue Shield plans on the clinically appropriate uses of existing medical technologies.

Primary intended users: Physicians, medical policy staff, Blue Cross and Blue Shield plans.

Technologies: *Medical or surgical procedure,* device.

Intervention: *Diagnosis,* treatment, rehabilitation.

Stage: *Established or widespread practice,* obsolete.

Properties: *Effectiveness,* efficacy, medical necessity.

Selection process: Blue Cross and Blue Shield plans submit requests for assessments to Program staff. The staff sets assessment topic priorities in consultation with a Medical Advisory Panel comprised of medical directors from selected Blue Cross and Blue Shield plans. Technologies are reassessed when an ongoing review of new clinical evidence suggests this is warranted.

Methods: *Information syntheses,* expert opinion.

The Program commissions experts on the respective assessment topics to develop comprehensive literature review articles. A Medical Necessity Program conference may be held where national medical organization representatives review the commissioned articles. Draft clinical guidelines based on the articles are also reviewed. Final guidelines are then developed by Program staff in consultation with the commissioned experts. Recently, several medical necessity topics have been assessed by the Clinical Efficacy Assessment Subcommittee of the American College of Physicians.

The approximate turnaround time from selection of assessment topic to reporting of findings is 1 year.

Assessors: Both external consultants and internal staff have medical, clinical, and research expertise including data analysis and interpretation.

Assessment reports include: Who conducted the assessment; description of the technology; properties assessed; results; findings or conclusions; recommendations for practice, future assessments, technology development, research.

Dissemination: *Advisories to members/constituents;* printed reports; journal articles; press conferences/news releases, TV/radio broadcasts.

The Association distributes *Medical Necessity Program Guidelines* to Blue Cross and Blue Shield plans. The plans generally publicize the *Guidelines* and distribute them to providers in their service area. *Guidelines* can be obtained from the Association upon request. The literature review articles are published by the authors in medical peer-reviewed journals.

Budget: $350,000. Funding source: 100 percent parent organization.

Use: The literature review articles and *Medical Necessity Guidelines* constitute clinical advice to the plans, which use them in establishing their medical policies. Organizations such as the American College of Physicians have endorsed many Medical Necessity Program products. *Guidelines* are often used by health care institutions' utilization review and quality assurance programs.

The Program is cited in the following documents:

Government Accounting Office. *OPM should promote medical necessity programs for federal employees' health insurance.* 1980 Jul 29.

Greenberg G and Derzon RA. Determining health insurance coverage of technology: problems and options. *Med Care* 1981;19(10):967-78.

Institute of Medicine, Committee for Evaluating Medical Technologies in Clinical Use. *Assessing medical technologies.* Washington, DC: National Academy Press, 1985.

Lewin and Associates. *A forward plan for Medicare coverage and technology assessment.* 1986 Dec.

Completed Reports

BC1 Blue Cross and Blue Shield, Medical Necessity Program. Activated partial thromboplastin time and prothrombin time. 1987. [Information syntheses]

BC2 ______. Arterial blood gas analysis. 1987. [Information syntheses]

BC3 ______. Biochemical profiles in ambulatory screening and preadmission testing of adults. 1987. [Information syntheses]

BC4 ______. Blood cultures. 1987. [Information syntheses]

BC5 ______. Blood urea nitrogen concentration and serum creatinine concentration. 1987. [Information syntheses]

BC6 ______. Carcinoembryonic antigen. 1987. [Information syntheses]

BC7 ______. Cardiac enzyme assays in the diagnosis of myocardial infarction. 1987. [Information syntheses]

BC8 ______. Complete blood count and leukocyte differential count. 1987. [Information syntheses]

BC9 ______. Erythrocyte sedimentation rate. 1987. [Information syntheses]

BC10 ______. Routine preoperative and general hospital admission chest x-rays. 1987. [Information syntheses]

BC11 ______. Routine preoperative and general hospital admission electrocardiograms. 1987. [Information syntheses]

BC12 ______. Serum electrolytes and serum osmolality. 1987. [Information syntheses]

BC13 ______. Syphilis tests. 1987. [Information syntheses]

BC14 ______. Throat cultures and rapid test for diagnosing group A streptococcal pharyngitis. 1987. [Information syntheses]

BC15 ______. Urinalysis, urine culture, and other tests in the diagnosis of women with acute dysuria. 1987. [Information syntheses]

BC16 ______. Anticoagulant therapy in the myocardial infarction patient. 1985. [Information syntheses]

BC17 ______. Cardiac exercise stress test. 1985. [Information syntheses]

BC18 ______. Cardiokymography. 1985. [Information syntheses]

BC19 ______. Coronary angiography and cardiac catheterization. 1985. [Information syntheses]

BC20 ______. Doppler flow velocity study. 1985. [Information syntheses]

BC21 ______. Echocardiogram. 1985. [Information syntheses]

BC22 ______. Electrocardiogram. 1985. [Information syntheses]

BC23 ______. Intensive cardiac care unit. 1985. [Information syntheses]

BC24 ______. Outpatient cardiac rehabilitation. 1985. [Information syntheses]

BC25 ______. Permanent cardiac pacemakers. 1985. [Information syntheses]

BC26 ______. Serum lipoprotein evaluation. 1985. [Information syntheses]

BC27 ______. Vectorcardiogram. 1985. [Information syntheses]

BC28 ______. CT scan in the evaluation of headaches, cerebrovascular disease and dementia. 1984. [Information syntheses]

BC29 ______. Chest x-ray examinations. 1984. [Information syntheses]

BC30 ______. Diagnostic imaging in the evaluation of breast disease. 1984. [Information syntheses]

BC31 ______. Head CT scan and ultrasound in the pediatric patient. 1984. [Information syntheses]

BC32 ______. Outmoded radionuclide imaging procedures. 1984. [Information syntheses]

BC33 ______. Radionuclide bone scan and x-ray of bones in the evaluation of bone metastases. 1984. [Information syntheses]

BC34 ______. Radionuclide brain scan in the evaluation of adult intracranial disease. [Information syntheses]

BC35 ______. Ultrasound and x-ray pelvimetry in maternity care. 1984. [Information syntheses]

BC36 ______. Upper gastrointestinal fluoroscopic study. 1984. [Information syntheses]

BC37 ______. Routine admission testing—medical admissions. 1983. [Information syntheses]

BC38 ______. Routine admission testing—surgical admissions. 1983. [Information syntheses]

BC39 ______. Diagnostic studies for respiratory patients: arterial blood gas analysis. 1982. [Information syntheses]

BC40 ______. Diagnostic studies for respiratory patients: pulmonary function tests. 1982. [Information syntheses]

BC41 ______. Oxygen therapy. 1982. [Information syntheses]

BC42 ______. Respiratory therapy: aerosol therapy. 1982. [Information syntheses]

BC43 ______. Respiratory therapy: incentive spirometry. 1982. [Information syntheses]

BC44 ______. Respiratory therapy: intermittent positive pressure breathing. 1982. [Information syntheses]

BC45 ______. Respiratory therapy: postural drainage. 1982. [Information syntheses]

Blue Cross and Blue Shield Association
Technology Evaluation and Coverage Program

676 North St. Clair, 11th Floor
Chicago, IL 60611
312-440-5577

Contact: Susan Gleeson, Executive Director, Technology Management Department.

Overview: The Blue Cross and Blue Shield Association represents member Blue Cross and Blue Shield plans and advises them on health care insurance issues. As a trade association, it provides medical, financial, and administrative consultation and technical assistance publications. Its Technology Evaluation and Coverage (TEC) Program was formally established in 1985, having evolved from activities originally begun under the National Association of Blue Shield Plans in the late 1960s.

Purpose: To provide advice to member Blue Cross and Blue Shield plans to assist them in determining the eligibility for coverage of new and emerging technologies.

Primary intended users: Blue Cross and Blue Shield plans.

Technologies: Device, medical or surgical procedure, support system.

Intervention: *Treatment,* diagnosis.

Stage: *New,* emerging.

Properties: *Effectiveness,* safety, efficacy, cost, cost-effectiveness, service requirements.

In order to be recommended as eligible for coverage: (1) a technology must have final approval from the appropriate government regulatory agency, e.g., Food and Drug Administration; (2) scientific evidence must permit conclusions concerning the effect of the technology on health outcomes; (3) the technology must improve the net health outcome; (4) the technology must be as beneficial as any established alternative; and (5) the improvement must be attainable outside the investigational settings.

Methods: *Information syntheses,* expert opinion, group judgment, cost analyses.

TEC staff or commissioned experts review and synthesize the published literature. Responses to specific assessment criteria underlie and define the process. A Medical Advisory Panel appointed by the Association monitors the validity of the process and outcome.

Approximate turnaround time from selection of assessment topic to reporting of findings is 3 to 6 months.

Assessors: The Medical Advisory Panel includes seven physicians who are medical directors of Blue Cross and Blue Shield plans, as well as non-voting outside experts. Assessors have expertise in the medical, clinical, ethics, and research fields, including data analysis and interpretation.

Assessment reports include: The purpose of the assessment; relationship of this assessment to prior or concurrent assessments of the technology or other technologies intended for similar purposes; description of the technology; properties assessed;

procedure used for the assessment; sources of data/information; findings or conclusions; limitations of findings; implications of findings for practice; recommendations for practice, future assessments, technology development, research; how the technology works, including theory, principles.

Dissemination: *Advisories to members/constituents,* printed reports.

Advisory bulletins, newsletters, and reports are distributed to member plans. TEC evaluations are available only from the Blue Cross and Blue Shield Association and are normally made available only to member Blue Cross and Blue Shield plans.

Budget: $600,000. Funding source: 100 percent parent organization.

Use: The Association uses the reports only to provide advice to member plans. The coverage recommendations associated with each report, however, appear to be rapidly communicated among affected providers and other health insurance carriers.

One example of outside use is the citation of the Association's document, *Extracorporeal shock wave lithotripsy: clinical assessments, utilization and cost projects,* May 1985 in a publication issued by the Congressional Office of Technology Assessment: *Effects of federal policies on extracorporeal shock wave lithotripsy,* 1985.

The Program is cited in the following documents:

Greenberg G and Derzon RA. Determining health insurance coverage of technology: problems and options. *Med Care* 1981;19(10):967-78.

Institute of Medicine, Committee for Evaluating Medical Technologies in Clinical Use. *Assessing medical technologies.* Washington, DC: National Academy Press, 1985.

Lewin and Associates. *A forward plan for Medicare coverage and technology assessment.* 1986 Dec.

Completed Reports

BS1 Blue Cross and Blue Shield Association, Technology Evaluation and Coverage Program. Absorptiometry, dual photon for osteoporosis monitoring. 1986. [Information syntheses]

BS2 ______. Absorptiometry, single and dual photon. 1986. [Information syntheses]

BS3 ______. Ambulatory uterine monitoring. 1986. [Information syntheses]

BS4 ______. Angelchik antireflux prosthesis. 1986. [Information syntheses]

BS5 ______. Automated and semi-automated ambulatory blood pressure monitoring. 1986. [Information syntheses]

BS6 ______. Automatic implantable cardioverter defibrillator. 1986. [Information syntheses]

BS7 ______. Bone marrow transplantation, allogeneic. 1986. [Information syntheses]

BS8 ______. Bone marrow transplantation, autologous. 1986. [Information syntheses]

BS9 ______. Chorionic villi sampling. 1986. [Information syntheses]

BS10 ______. Collagen implants. 1986. [Information syntheses]

BS11 ______. Continuous arteriovenous hemofiltration. 1986. [Information syntheses]

BS12 ______. Continuous passive motion device. 1986.

BS13 ______. Corneal endothelial cell microscopy. 1986. [Informatiaon syntheses]

BS14 ______. Electrical bone growth stimulation. 1986. [Information syntheses]

BS15 ______. Electrical nerve stimulation (implantable spinal cord stimulator). 1986. [Information syntheses]

BS16 ______. Electrical nerve stimulation of the ear. 1986. [Information syntheses]

BS17 ______. Epidural analgesia therapy. 1986. [Information syntheses]

BS18 ______. Epikeratophakia. 1986. [Information syntheses]

BS19 ______. Extracranial-intracranial artery bypass surgery. 1986. [Information syntheses]

BS20 ______. Gastric bubble. 1986. [Information syntheses]

BS21 ______. Home phototherapy for neonatal jaundice. 1986. [Information syntheses]

BS22 ______. Hyperthermia, local. 1986. [Information syntheses]

BS23 ______. Implantable infusion pump. 1986. [Information syntheses]

BS24 ______. In vitro fertilization. 1986. [Information syntheses]

BS25 ______. Iontophoresis. 1986. [Information syntheses]

BS26 ______. Isolated limb perfusion. 1986. [Information syntheses]

BS27 ______. Lacate infusion for panic disorder. 1986. [Information syntheses]

BS28 ______. Nasal continuous positive airway pressure. 1986. [Information syntheses]

BS29 ______. Nd:YAG laser—gastrointestinal bleeding. 1986. [Information syntheses]

BS30 ______. Nd:YAG laser—posterior capsulotomy. 1986. [Information syntheses]

BS31 ______. Nd:YAG laser—tracheo-bronchial obstruction. 1986. [Information syntheses]

BS32 ______. Psoralens and ultraviolet A (PUVA). 1986. [Information syntheses]

BS33 ______. SIDS (home apnea monitoring of siblings). 1986. [Information syntheses]

BS34 ______. Signal averaged ECG. 1986. [Information syntheses]

BS35 ______. Sperm penetration assay. 1986. [Information syntheses]

BS36 ______. Videofluoroscopic evaluation in speech pathology. 1986. [Information syntheses]

Brandeis University Health Policy Center

Organ Procurement Project
415 South Street
Waltham, MA 02254
617-736-3900

Contact: Jeffrey Prottas, Senior Research Associate; or Helen Levine Batten, Research Associate.

Overview: The Brandeis University Health Policy Center studies, develops, and demonstrates aspects of national health policy. The Organ Procurement Project first conducted an evaluation of the organ procurement system in 1983. Surveys of key medical professionals, donor families, and the general public were undertaken in 1984-1986. Currently, a study of the causes of failure to transplant organs and a reevaluation of the organ procurement system are in progress.

Purpose: To improve the supply and distribution of cadaveric organs.

Primary intended users: General public; health/medical professional associations; government regulators; public policy-makers, legislators.

Technologies: *Organizational or administrative system,* support system.

Intervention: Administration.

Stage: *Established or widespread practice,* emerging, new.

Properties: *Service requirements;* cost-effectiveness; economic implications; ethical, legal, social implications.

Methods: Epidemiological and other observational methods.

Case studies, survey research, and cost-data analysis are the methods used to conduct assessments. The turnaround time from selection of assessment topic to reporting of findings varies.

Assessors: The assessors have extensive experience and expertise in organ procurement and medical sociology.

Assessment reports include: Abstract; the assessment's intended audience; the purpose of the assessment; relationship of this assessment to prior or concurrent assessments of the technology or other technologies intended for similar purposes; who sponsored/commissioned/supported the assessment; who conducted the assessment; description of the technology; stage of life-cycle of technology when assessed; properties assessed; procedure used for the assessment; sources of data/information; methods for collecting data/information; methods for analyzing/synthesizing data/information; results; findings or conclusions; limitations of findings; implications of findings for practice; recommendations for practice, future assessments, technology development, research.

Dissemination: *Printed reports,* journal articles.

Copies of assessment reports are available upon request.

Budget: The budget and cost per assessment varies. Funding source: 100 percent parent organization.

Use: The assessment reports are used to further the development of national health policy.

Completed Reports

BU1 Batten HL, Prottas JM. [Brandeis University, Health Policy Center, Organ Procurement Project] Kind strangers: families of organ donors. Health Affairs, forthcoming. [Epidemiological and other observational methods]

BU2 Prottas JM, Batten HL. [Brandeis University, Health Policy Center, Organ Procurement Project] Attitudes and incentives in organ procurement: report to the Health Care Financing Administration. 1986 Apr. [Epidemiological and other observational methods]

BU3 Prottas JM. [Brandeis University, Health Policy Center, Organ Procurement Project] Organ procurement in Europe and the United States. Millbank Mem Fund Q 1985;63(1):94-126. [Epidemiological and other observational methods]

BU4 Prottas JM. [Brandeis University, Health Policy Center, Organ Procurement Project] The structure and effectiveness of the U.S. procurement system. Inquiry 1985;22(4)365-376. [Epidemiological and other observational methods]

BU5 Prottas JM. [Brandeis University, Health Policy Center, Organ Procurement Project] Encouraging altruisms: public attitudes and the marketing of organ donation. Milbank Mem Fund Q 1983;61:278-306. [Epidemiological and other observational methods]

BU6 Prottas JM. [Brandeis University, Health Policy Center, Organ Procurment Project] Obtaining replacements: the organizational framework of organ procurement. J Health Polit Policy Law 1983;8(2):235-250. [Epidemiological and other observational methods]

California Medical Association

Medical Practice Opinion Program
PO Box 7690
San Francisco, CA 94120-7690
415-863-5522

Contact: Robert Sparacino, Manager, Department of Specialty Sections and Scientific Programs.

Overview: The California Medical Association (CMA) is a not-for-profit, voluntary professional medical association whose members number almost 34,000. Its principal services include legislative advocacy, insurance programs, peer review, financial management, continuing medical education, socio-economic research and reports, and administration of accreditation and licensing programs for hospitals. The Medical Practice Opinion Program began in 1972 and since its inception, approximately 350 opinions have been issued.

Purpose: To provide CMA's members, its component medical societies, and other interested organizations with objective, authoritative, scientific opinion on questions of medical practice in California. The opinions offered are based on training, experience, and literature reviewed by specialists. The opinions are advisory only and are not intended to be interpreted as directives, instructions, or policy statements. Opinions are always subject to revision as dictated by new information.

Primary intended users: General public; physicians; health/medical professional associations; health industry associations; unions and other employee organizations; third party payers; government regulators; voluntary associations, organizations.

Technologies: Drug, device, medical or surgical procedure.

Intervention: Diagnosis, treatment.

Stage: *New,* emerging, established or widespread practice, obsolete.

Properties: Acceptance/adoption level, safety, effectiveness, limitations of use.

Selection process: CMA members, component medical societies, voluntary/professional medical associations, government agencies, third party payers or any other organization with a vital interest in a subject may pose a question for review. Requests must be submitted in writing and include background material that describes the technology in question.

Staff, in collaboration with the chairmen of CMA's 24 advisory panels and the chairman of the Commission on Quality Care Review, set the assessment topic priorities. Topics are generally addressed in the order received. An issue that demands immediate attention is processed promptly.

All opinions are reviewed annually by the appropriate advisory panels and the Commission on Quality Care Review. Some subjects warrant review within that annual interval.

Methods: *Group judgment,* expert opinion, information syntheses.

Following approval of the question by the appropriate advisory panel chairman, staff prepares a questionnaire with background material that typically includes policy or position statements from state/national organizations; testimonials from physicians who are known to be expert in the field; and a selection of recent, pertinent journal articles.

Advisory panel members review the material and submit their opinions individually; these opinions are the foundation of the consensus opinion. Some questions involve more than one panel. Staff prepare the consensus opinion which is subject to the review and approval of the panel chairmen, the panel members and, finally, the Commission on Quality Care Review. Once approved, the opinion is sent to the original inquirer and then published in *The Western Journal of Medicine,* the official scientific publication of California and eight other western state medical associations and five research societies.

The approximate turnaround time from selection of assessment topic to reporting of findings is 4 months. Complex questions involving multiple panels usually take longer.

Assessors: Officers of the state's principal specialty societies, California medical school department chairmen, and representatives of CMA's 24 specialty sections comprise the membership of each advisory panel, which includes an equal number of private practicing physicians and full-time medical school faculty physicians.

Assessment reports include: The purpose of the assessment; who conducted the assessment; description of the technology; stage of life-cycle of technology when assessed; properties assessed; implications of findings for practice; how the technology works, including theory, principles; regulatory agency approval status.

Dissemination: Printed reports; journal articles; advisories to members/constituents.

Copies of medical practice opinions can be obtained by calling or writing the CMA Department of Specialty Sections and Scientific Programs, in the Division of Scientific and Educational Activities.

Budget: $15,000. Funding source: 100 percent sponsors/members dues, contributions.

Use: The CMA provides the opinions to its members and component medical societies as a member service and will share them with persons or organizations outside its immediate membership as a public service.

Generally, health associations, government agencies, and insurance companies most frequently initiate CMA's review of new technologies. The opinions assist these organizations in formulating their own views on the scientific standing of new medical or surgical procedures.

Program evaluation: Internal monitoring of the program is performed by the Commission on Quality Care Review and the Scientific Board's 24 advisory panels. However, no formal evaluation of the program has been conducted.

Completed Reports

CA1 California Medical Association, Medical Practice Opinion Program. Arthroscopic stapling of an unstable shoulder. 1985 Sep. (Medical Practice Opinion #335) [Group judgment]

CA2 ———. Diagnosis of obstructive sleep apnea in children. 1987 Feb. (Medical Practice Opinion #346) [Group judgment]

CA3 ______. Hubbard method of detoxification. 1987 Apr. (Medical Practice Opinion #347) [Group judgment]

CA4 ______. Topographic brain mapping. 1987 Mar. (Medical Practice Opinion #345) [Group judgment]

CA5 ______. Ambulatory monitoring of uterine activity. 1986 Jul. (Medical Practice Opinion #342) [Group judgment]

CA6 ______. Contralateral breast surgery following mastectomy. 1986 Feb. (Medical Practice Opinion #338) [Group judgment]

CA7 ______. Epikeratophakia in children.. 1986 Dec. (Medical Practice Opinion #344) [Group judgment]

CA8 ______. Gastric bubble for treatment of obesity. 1986 Aug. (Medical Practice Opinion #343) [Group judgment]

CA9 ______. Hospital admission following rigid esophagoscopy. 1986 Jul. (Medical Practice Opinion #339) [Group judgment]

CA10 ______. Sleep studies for obstructive sleep apnea. 1986 Feb. (Medical Practice Opinion #340) [Group judgment]

CA11 ______. Vertebral artery surgery. 1986 Sep. (Medical Practice Opinion #341) [Group judgment]

CA12 ______. Acoustic impedance testing in school screening. 1985 Sep. (Medical Practice Opinion #325) [Group judgment]

CA13 ______. Anticholinergic drugs for nicotine addiction. 1985 May. (Medical Practice Opinion #322) [Group judgment]

CA14 ______. Assistant surgeon at cataract surgery. 1985 May. (Medical Practice Opinion #324) [Group judgment]

CA15 ______. Assistant surgeon at elective abdominal tubal ligation. 1985 Nov. (Medical Practice Opinion #333) [Group judgment]

CA16 ______. Chorionic villus biopsy. 1985 Sep. (Medical Practice Opinion #328) [Group judgment]

CA17 ______. Cytoxan therapy for multiple sclerosis. 1985 Oct. (Medical Practice Opinion #329) [Group judgment]

CA18 ______. Discography for cervical and lumbar disorders. 1985 Feb. (Medical Practice Opinion #317) [Group judgment]

CA19 ______. Early detection of lung cancer. 1985 Dec. (Medical Practice Opinion #337) [Group judgment]

CA20 ______. Echocine for diagnosis of sinusitis. 1985 Jun. (Medical Practice Opinion #318) [Group judgment]

CA21 ______. Extracorporeal shock-wave lithotripsy. 1985 Sep. (Medical Practice Opinion #32) [Group judgment]

CA22 ______. In vitro fertilization. 1985 Jun. (Medical Practice Opinion #278) [Group judgment]

CA23 ______. Indications for tonsillectomy. 1985 Dec. (Medical Practice Opinion #326) [Group judgment]

CA24 ______. Intraosseous pressure measurement. 1985 Oct. (Medical Practice Opinion #334) [Group judgment]

CA25 ______. Laser irradiation for pain of Charcot-Marie-Tooth disease. 1985 May. (Medical Practice Opinion #321) [Group judgment]

CA26 ______. Laser therapy for plantar warts. 1985 May. (Medical Practice Opinion #320) [Group judgment]

CA27 ______. Magnetic resonance imaging. 1985 Sep. (Medical Practice Opinion #277) [Group judgment]

CA28 ______. Microsurgery in the treatment of infertility. 1985 Aug. (Medical Practice Opinion #308) [Group judgment]

CA29 ______. Neurostimulation for urethral sphincter spasticity. 1985 Dec. (Medical Practice Opinion #336) [Group judgment]

CA30 ______. Permanent eyeliner. 1985 Nov. (Medical Practice Opinion #332) [Group judgment]

CA31 ______. Radial keratotomy for myopia. 1985 Apr. (Medical Practice Opinion #244) [Group judgment]

CA32 ______. Reconsideration of percutaneous and transluminal coronary angioplasty. 1985 Feb. [Group judgment]

CA33 ______. Stereotactic heavy-ion irradiation for arteriovenous malformations. 1985 Sep. (Medical Practice Opinion #316) [Group judgment]

CA34 ______. Suction lipectomy. 1985 Dec. (Medical Practice Opinion #286) [Group judgment]

CA35 ______. Transmission of disease via mouth to mouth resuscitation. 1985 June. (Medical Practice Opinion #323) [Group judgment]

CA36 ______. Treatment of rheumatoid arthritis with flagyl. 1985 Oct. (Medical Practice Opinion #330) [Group judgment]

CA37 ______. Treatment of rheumatoid arthritis with sex hormones. 1985 Oct. (Medical Practice Opinion #331) [Group judgment]

CA38 ______. YAG laser for posterior lens capsules. 1985 Apr. (Medical Practice Opinion #319) [Group judgment]

CA39 ______. Assistant surgeon for arthroscopic procedures. 1984 Apr. (Medical Practice Opinion #239) [Group judgment]

CA40 ______. Assistant surgeon for septorhinoplasty. 1984 Jan. (Medical Practice Opinion #307) [Group judgment]

CA41 ______. Aversion therapy for alcoholism. 1984 Feb. (Medical Practice Opinion #311) [Group judgment]

CA42 ______. Biochemical biopsy. 1984 Nov. (Medical Practice Opinion #285) [Group judgment]

CA43 ______. Cardiac pacemakers. 1984 Mar. (Medical Practice Opinion #291) [Group judgment]

CA44 ______. Computed tomography—multiplanar reconstruction. 1984 Nov. (Medical Practice Opinion #310) [Group judgment]

CA45 ______. Cranial electrotherapy stimulation. 1984 Nov. (Medical Practice Opinion #315) [Group judgment]

CA46 ______. Cytotoxic testing for food allergy. 1984 Feb. (Medical Practice Opinion #265) [Group judgment]

CA47 ______. Heart-lung transplantation. 1984 Sep. (Medical Practice Opinion #309) [Group judgment]

CA48 ______. Immunotherapy for melanoma. 1984 Feb. (Medical Practice Opinion #305) [Group judgment]

CA49 ______. Immunotherapy for treatment of cancer. 1984 Jul. (Medical Practice Opinion #204) [Group judgment]

CA50 ______. Intradermal provocative titration/diagnosis of food allergy. 1984 Feb. (Medical Practice Opinion #293) [Group judgment]

CA51 ______. Kinetic therapy for lumbago. 1984 Nov. (Medical Practice Opinion #312) [Group judgment]

CA52 ______. Radioallergosorbent test (RAST) 1984 Dec. (Medical Practice Opinion #255) [Group judgment]

CA53 ______. Rinkel serial intracutaneous titration/diagnosis. 1984 Feb. (Medical Practice Opinion #295) [Group judgment]

CA54 ______. Sublingual challenge technique/diagnosis of food allergy. 1984 Feb. (Medical Practice Opinion #294) [Group judgment]

CA55 ______. Temporomandibular joint procedure. 1984 Feb. (Medical Practice Opinion #270) [Group judgment]

CA56 ______. Tuberculosis surveillance program for hospital employees. 1984 Oct. (Medical Practice Opinion #304) [Group judgment]

CA57 ______. Use of sclerosant injections for neck, back and lower extremity pain. (Medical Practice Opinion #313) [Group judgment]

CA58 ______. Video electroencephalographic monitoring. 1984 Nov. (Medical Practice Opinion #314) [Group judgment]

CA59 ______. Barbiturate coma. 1983 Feb. (Medical Practice Opinion #280) [Group judgment]

CA60 ______. Bilio-pancreatic bypass surgery for obesity. 1983 Mar. (Medical Practice Opinion #284) [Group judgment]

CA61 ______. Biofeedback. 1983 Aug. (Medical Practice Opinion #240) [Group judgment]

CA62 ______. Collagen implant. 1983 Apr. (Medical Practice Opinion #283) [Group judgment]

CA63 ______. Computerized tomography for lumbar spine. Feb 1983. (Medical Practice Opinion #282) [Group judgment]

CA64 ______. Continuous passive motion for stiffening conditions. 1983 Mar. (Medical Practice Opinion #306) [Group judgment]

CA65 ______. Endothelial cell counts. 1983 Sep. (Medical Practice Opinion #303) [Group judgment]

CA66 ______. Ericsson sex selection method. 1983 Sep. (Medical Practice Opinion #298) [Group judgment]

CA67 ______. Hyperbaric oxygen therapy. 1983 Sep. (Medical Practice Opinion #243) [Group judgment]

CA68 ______. Hyperthermia treatment for cancer. 1983 Oct. (Medical Practice Opinion #296) [Group judgment]

CA69 ______. Interferon for the treatment of cancer. 1983 Sep. (Medical Practice Opinion #299) [Group judgment]

CA70 ______. Interferon for the treatment of infectious diseases. 1983 Sep. (Medical Practice Opinion #300) [Group judgment]

CA71 ______. Intravenous streptokinase after myocardial infarction. 1983 June. (Medical Practice Opinion #287) [Group judgment]

CA72 ______. Laser photoradiation therapy for carcinoma. 1983 Feb. (Medical Practice Opinion #279) [Group judgment]

CA73 ______. Liver transplantation. 1983 Sep. (Medical Practice Opinion #297) [Group judgment]

CA74 ______. Nissen's fundoplication—gastric reservoir reduction for morbid obesity. 1983 May. (Medical Practice Opinion #290) [Group judgment]

CA75 ______. Noninvasive muscle stimulators for prevention of muscle atrophy. 1983 Jul. (Medical Practice Opinion #292) [Group judgment]

CA76 ______. Palatopharyngoplasty for the treatment of snoring. 1983 Dec. (Medical Practice Opinion #301) [Group judgment]

CA77 ______. Rectal mucosal replacement. 1983 Nov. (Medical Practice Opinion #288) [Group judgment]

CA78 ______. Stapedectomy for otosclerosis. 1983 Sep. (Medical Practice Opinion #302) [Group judgment]

CA79 ______. Thrombolytic therapy for pulmonary embolism. 1983 Feb. (Medical Practice Opinion #281) [Group judgment]

CA80 ______. Assistant surgeon for laser iridotomy. 1982 Jul. (Medical Practice Opinion #272) [Group judgment]

CA81 ______. Bone densitometry. 1982 Nov. (Medical Practice Opinion #254) [Group judgment]

CA82 ______. Challenge food testing for depression. 1982 Feb. (Medical Practice Opinion #257b) [Group judgment]

CA83 ______. Challenge food testing for respiratory disorders. 1982 Feb. (Medical Practice Opinion #257c) [Group judgment]

CA84 ______. Challenge food testing for rheumatoid arthritis. 1982 Feb. (Medical Practice Opinion #257a) [Group judgment]

CA85 ______. Constant blood pressure monitoring. 1982 Aug. (Medical Practice Opinion #275) [Group judgment]

CA86 ______. Human tumor stem cell assay. 1982 Jul. (Medical Practice Opinion #273) [Group judgment]

CA87 ______. Intraarterial BCNU chemotherapy. 1982 Oct. (Medical Practice Opinion #276) [Group judgment]

CA88 ______. Methylethylketone damage of the immune system. 1982 Nov. (Medical Practice Opinion #261) [Group judgment]

CA89 ______. Needleless insulin injection. 1982 Dec. (Medical Practice Opinion #274) [Group judgment]

CA90 ______. Plasmapheresis for rheumatoid arthritis. 1982 Aug. (Medical Practice Opinion #263) [Group judgment]

CA91 ______. Plasmapheresis for six conditions. 1982 Sep. (Medical Practice Opinion #249) [Group judgment]

CA92 ______. Sleep disorder therapy. 1982 Dec. (Medical Practice Opinion #271) [Group judgment]

CA93 ______. Thermography for spinal problems. 1982 Jul. (Medical Practice Opinion #269) [Group judgment]

CA94 ______. Transcutaneous electrical nerve stimulation. 1982 Jul. (Medical Practice Opinion #82) [Group judgment]

CA95 ______. Viral and bacterial vaccines for arthritis. 1982 Jun. (Medical Practice Opinion #268) [Group judgment]

CA96 ______. Anesthesia by hypnosis. 1981 Aug. (Medical Practice Opinion #250) [Group judgment]

CA97 ______. Cochlear implant for deafness. 1981 Aug. (Medical Practice Opinion #178) [Group judgment]

CA98 ______. DMSO. 1981 Jan. (Medical Practice Opinion #248) [Group judgment]

CA99 ______. Esterine for treatment of rheumatoid arthritis. 1981 Dec. (Medical Practice Opinion #253) [Group judgment]

CA100 ______. Heart transplants. 1981 Dec. (Medical Practice Opinion #252) [Group judgment]

CA101 ______. High gastric bypass for morbid obesity. 1981 Feb. (Medical Practice Opinion #246) [Group judgment]

CA102 ______. Intermittent positive pressure breathing. 1981 Aug. (Medical Practice Opinion #259) [Group judgment]

CA103 ______. Paper radioallergosorbent test (PRAST) 1981 Aug. (Medical Practice Opinion #256) [Group judgment]

CA104 ______. Plasmapheresis treatment of multiple sclerosis. 1981 Dec. (Medical Practice Opinion #212) [Group judgment]

CA105 ______. Singer-Blom valve operation. 1981 Jul. (Medical Practice Opinion #262) [Group judgment]

CA106 ______. Stat-tek glucose analyzer for diabetes. 1981 Aug. (Medical Practice Opinion #260) [Group judgment]

CA107 ______. Clinical ecology. 1980 Dec. (Medical Practice Opinion #264) [Group judgment]

CA108 ______. Injections of universal bacterial antigen. 1980 Jan. (Medical Practice Opinion #210) [Group judgment]

CA109 ______. Microsurgical lumbar discectomy. 1980 Feb. (Medical Practice Opinion #238) [Group judgment]

CBO (Centraal Begeleidingsorgaan voor de Intercollegiale Toetsing)

National Organization for Quality Assurance in Hospitals
Consensus Development Program
PO Box 20064, Churchilllaan 11
3502 LB Utrecht, The Netherlands
(31-30) 96-06-47

Contact: Evert Reerink, M.D., Ph.D., Executive Director.

Overview: CBO is an independent foundation established in 1979 by the National Specialists Organization in the Netherlands and the Dutch Association of Medical Directors of Hospitals. The Board of Trustees consists of representatives of those organizations, the National Hospital Association, the Society of Dutch Sick Funds, the Society of Private Insurance Companies, the Royal Netherlands Medical Association, and the Ministry of Welfare, Health and Culture. CBO is a World Health Organization Collaborating Center for Quality Assurance in Health Care. This profile describes the CBO consensus development program.

Purpose: To develop statements that facilitate a uniform approach among hospital clinicians in dealing with patient problems of national concern.

Primary intended users: Providers, generally; physicians; acute facility administrators; long-term care facility administrators.

Technologies: *Medical or surgical procedure.*

Intervention: *Diagnosis, treatment,* prevention, rehabilitation.

Stage: *Established or widespread practice.*

Properties: *Safety, effectiveness,* service requirements, acceptance/adoption level.

Selection process: CBO selects the assessment topics from suggestions made by the hospitals. Topics may be reassessed when consensus statements are out of date, e.g., are 5 or more years old, or when the findings of consensus efforts are inconclusive. Blood transfusion therapy is the first topic to be reassessed.

Methods: *Group judgment, expert opinion.*

Panels consisting of 6 to 20 experts are given 6 to 18 months to produce a draft consensus report. The draft report contains 2- to 4-page papers individually authored by the panelists and a draft consensus statement consisting of as many as 30 numbered statements on the topic generated by the panelists. The report is put into a booklet and circulated to a larger group of health care workers interested in the topic. This larger group—usually between 100 to 150 people, but sometimes more—convenes for a 1-day meeting to review the draft report with the panelists. Following this meeting, the panel completes a final consensus statement in narrative form.

Assessors: Consensus panels are usually composed of physician specialists relevant to the topic (e.g., neurosurgeons, radiologists, and dermatologists); a few panels have included other types of personnel (e.g., laboratory technicians for blood transfusion therapy panel, nurses for treatment of bedsores panel, and epidemiologists for follow-up colorectal cancer panel).

Assessment reports include: The first five assessment reports appeared in narrative form only. All subsequent statements have appeared first as draft statements in booklet form that include table of contents, list of participants, introductory paragraph, the short papers individually authored by the panelists, and the draft numbered consensus statements. The final statements are narratives distilled from the draft booklets. Final statements may reflect disagreements among panel members.

Dissemination: The draft consensus statements in booklet form and the final statements are available from the CBO. The final statements are also published approximately 1 year following their release in the *Nederlands Tydschrift voor Geneeskunde* (Dutch Journal of Medicine). Only one report, on melanoma of the skin (1984) has been translated into English; all others are in Dutch.

Budget: The entire CBO budget is approximately $900,000, some $135,000 of which is devoted to consensus activities. CBO is funded from levies applied to Dutch hospitals based on their number of beds.

Use: CBO has attempted to gauge the impact of some consensus statements. CBO staff have worked with hospital quality assurance committees to determine whether consensus guidelines on melanoma of the skin and blood transfusion therapy have been incorporated into quality assurance criteria and practices.

Related activities: CBO is devoted to enhancing quality assurance in Dutch hospitals. It assesses and works to improve the quality of procedures in specific hospitals, assists in setting criteria for quality assurance, and provides a second-opinion service. CBO also offers assistance to other organizations in assessing new technologies, developing information systems, and developing clinical protocols. Because of statutory limitations, CBO is not engaged in research.

Completed Reports

CB1 CBO (Centraal Begeleidingsorgaan voor de Intercollegiale Toetsing) Consensus Development Program. Diagnosis of atopic syndrome. 1987. [Dutch language only] [Group judgment, Expert opinion]

CB2 ______. Follow-up colorectal cancer. 1987. [Dutch language only] [Group judgment, Expert opinion]

CB3 ______. Hemophilia. 1987. [Dutch language only] [Group judgment, Expert opinion]

CB4 ______. Hypercholesterolemia. 1987. [Dutch language only] [Group judgment, Expert opinion]

CB5 ______. Prevention of herpes neonatorum. 1987. [Dutch language only] [Group judgment, Expert opinion]

CB6 ______. Suspect lymph nodules in the neck. 1987. [Dutch language only] [Group judgment, Expert opinion]

CB7 ______. Total hip prostheses. 1987. [Dutch language only] [Group judgment, Expert opinion]

CB8 ______. Diagnosis of deep venous thrombosis. 1986. [Dutch language only] [Group judgment, Expert opinion]

CB9 ______. Non-scrotal testis. 1986. [Dutch language only] [Group judgment, Expert opinion]

CB10 ______. Treatment of bedsores. 1986. [Dutch language only] [Group judgment, Expert opinion]

CB11 ______. Foot problems of diabetic patients. 1985. [Dutch language only] [Group judgment, Expert opinion]

CB12 ______. Osteoporosis. 1985. [Dutch language only] [Group judgment, Expert opinion]

CB13 ______. Prevention of bedsores. 1985. [Dutch language only] [Group judgment, Expert opinion]

CB14 ______. Solid solitary thyroid nodule. 1985. [Dutch language only] [Group judgment, Expert opinion]

CB15 ______. Melanoma of the skin. 1984. [Group judgment, Expert opinon]

CB16 ______. Severe brain damage. 1984. [Dutch language only] [Group judgment, Expert opinion]

CB17 ______. Thrombocytes transfusion policy. 1984. [Dutch language only] [Group judgment, Expert opinion]

CB18 ______. Mammography policy. 1983. [Dutch language only] [Group judgment, Expert opinion]

CB19 ______. Traumatic lesions of the back. 1983. [Dutch language only] [Group judgment, Expert opinion]

CB20 ______. Blood transfusion therapy. 1982. [Dutch language only] [Group judgment, Expert opinion]

College of American Pathologists

Surveys Program
5202 Old Orchard Road
Skokie, IL 60077-1034
312-966-5700

Contact: William E. Williamson, Director Laboratory Improvement Programs.

Overview: The College of American Pathologists is a professional association dedicated to serving the needs of its members in the fields of pathology, medicine, and patient care. With over 10,000 members, its services include periodicals, educational programs, Professional Affairs Assistance, and other programs.

The College's Surveys Program is an ongoing assessment of laboratory technology that provides subscribing laboratories with an evaluation of their own accuracy and precision. This Program began with circulation of samples to assess the technology in limited areas of clinical chemistry and hematology. Over the past 25 years the program has grown to over 50 surveys, assessing the technology of virtually all areas of laboratory medicine. The program currently provides technology assessment information to over 12,000 participating laboratories in the United States and several foreign countries.

Purpose: To assess laboratory technology and to provide individual subscribing laboratories with these assessments as well as evaluations of their own accuracy and precision.

Primary intended users: Labs, blood banks.

Technologies: *Device*, medical or surgical procedure, support system.

Laboratory methods, systems, and instrument performance are assessed.

Intervention: *Diagnosis*, treatment.

Stage: *Established or widespread practice,* new, obsolete.

Properties: Safety, effectiveness, acceptance/adoption level.

The Program assesses the laboratories for safety and effectiveness with respect to accuracy and precision of results. Based on performance, assessments provide mechanisms for determining acceptance and level of technology.

Selection process: Any medical laboratory may request that an assessment of its performance be conducted and compared with its peers. Since this is a voluntary program, laboratories need only to subscribe to the surveys in which they wish to participate. Assessment topics are determined and prioritized by CAP committees of experts in the laboratory discipline involved in the technology assessment.

Methods: Bench testing.

Unknown simulated patient samples (e.g., blood products, spinal fluid, urine) are sent quarterly to participating laboratories. Laboratories are given a certain amount of time to analyze samples for specified constituents and return data for computer analysis of performance.

Selection of assessment topics (simulated patient sample content) is determined 18 months prior to the surveys. However, the actual turnaround time for the assessment process, from the standpoint of the participant, is approximately 8 weeks from receipt of samples for analysis to reporting of findings.

Assessors: The expert committees that operate the various assessment programs are made up of pathologists and doctoral scientists with expertise in the given area of technology assessment.

Assessment reports include: The assessment's intended audience; relationship of this assessment to prior or concurrent assessments of the technology or other technologies intended for similar purposes; sources of data/information; methods for collecting data/information; methods for analyzing/synthesizing data/information; results; findings or conclusions; limitations of findings; where technology is in use.

Dissemination: *Printed reports,* journal articles, advisories to members/constituents.

Assessment products include CAP Surveys Program quarterly summary reports, CAP conference proceedings, articles in *Archives of Pathology and Laboratory Medicine* and the quarterly CAP newsletter, *Summing Up.* The summary reports are mailed to participating laboratories listing their own results and summarizing the results of all participants.

Generally, summary reports are available only to participants. Conference proceedings and *Summing Up* can be purchased from CAP. Selected studies are published in the scientific literature.

Budget: $15,000,000. Funding source: 85 percent sponsors/members dues, contributions; 15 percent parent organization.

Use: The CAP uses the assessments to monitor the state of the art. Members of the expert committees also use the assessments as the basis for articles in professional journals.

Scientific professionals may use the reports for the noncommercial purpose of scientific or educational advancement as defined in the CAP copyright. Generally permission is requested prior to publication. Government and regulatory agencies also use the results to establish compliance and regulatory requirements.

Program evaluation: Various Federal agencies assess the Program to determine compliance with Federal Equivalency Requirements.

The CAP evaluated the Surveys Program in 1981 as the result of a database conference it sponsored that was attended by representatives of clinical laboratories, the diagnostic industry, and government. The conference participants requested the evaluation because they regarded the CAP database as an important resource for the advancement of technology in the clinical laboratory field.

The College funded the evaluation, which consisted of compiling data from its clinical laboratory improvement programs for the years 1970 to 1980. The resulting compendium, *Data ReCap 1970-1980: A Compilation of Data from the College of American Pathologists Clinical Laboratory Improvement Program,* was published in 1981 and documented laboratory performance over the decade and the state of the art in 1980.

Related activities: The quarterly newsletter *Summing Up* highlights various areas of technology assessment based upon the surveys performance. Annual conferences are sponsored by the various expert committees of the Surveys Program which, based upon the technology assessments, focus on the relevance of clinical laboratory testing to patient care. These conferences periodically review and redefine analytical goals based upon the performance assessments of the Surveys Program. As new specialized technologies emerge, new committees are formed to monitor and assess performance.

Completed Reports

CP1 Howanitz PJ, ed. Quality assurance in physician office, bedside, and home testing. Skokie, IL: College of American Pathologists. Expected 1987. [Expert opinion, Bench testing]

CP2 Triplett DA, ed. Advances in coagulation testing: interpretation and application. Skokie, IL: College of American Pathologists. Expected 1987. [Expert opinion, Bench testing]

CP3 Smith JW, ed. The role of clinical microbiology in cost-effective health care. CAP Conference/1984. Skokie, IL: College of American Pathologists, 1985. [Expert opinion, Bench testing]

CP4 Rippey JH, Nakamura RM, eds. Diagnostic immunology: technology assessment and quality assurance. CAP Conference/1983. Skokie, IL: College of American Pathologists, 1984. [Expert opinion, Bench testing]

CP5 Homburger HA, ed. Clinical and analytical concepts in enzymology. CAP Conference/1982. Skokie, IL: College of American Pathologists, 1983. [Expert opinion, Bench testing]

CP6 Polesky HF, Walker RH, eds. Safety in transfusion practices. CAP Conference/Aspen 1980. Skokie, IL: College of American Pathologists, 1981. [Expert opinion, Bench testing]

CP7 Sommers HM, ed. Clinical relevance in microbiology. CAP Conference/Aspen 1979. Skokie, IL: College of American Pathologists, 1981. [Expert opinion, Bench testing]

CP8 Triplett DA, ed. Standardization of coagulation assays: an overview. CAP Conference/Aspen 1980. Skokie, IL: College of American Pathologists, 1981. [Expert opinion, Bench testing]

CP9 Keitagaes PW, Nakamura RM, eds. Diagnostic immunology: current and future trends. CAP Conference/Aspen 1978. Skokie, IL: College of American Pathologists, 1980. [Expert opinion, Bench testing]

CP10 Koepke JA, ed. Differential leukocyte counting. CAP Conference/Aspen 1977. Skokie, IL: College of American Pathologists, 1978. [Expert opinion, Bench testing]

Congress of the United States
Office of Technology Assessment Health Program
Washington, D.C. 20510
202-228-6590

Contact: Clyde J. Behney, Program Manager for Health.

Overview: The Office of Technology Assessment (OTA) is a nonpartisan analytical support agency that serves the U.S. Congress. The Office was authorized in 1972, funded in late 1973, and began full operations in 1974. The Health Program was established in 1975.

OTA has three operating divisions: the Energy, Materials, and International Security Division; the Science, Information and Natural Resources Division; and the Health and Life Sciences Division. Within the Health and Life Sciences Division are three programs: the Food and Renewable Resources Program; the Biological Applications Program; and the Health Program. This profile deals primarily with assessment activities of the Health Program.

OTA is governed by a 12-member bipartisan Congressional board of six senators and six representatives. The board is advised by an Advisory Council of 10 public members eminent in science, technology, and education, appointed by the board. The Comptroller General of the United States and the director of the Congressional Research Service of the Library of Congress are also members. The OTA director is appointed by the board and serves as a nonvoting member.

Purpose: To help Congress anticipate and plan for the consequences of technological applications, and to examine the ways, expected and unexpected, in which technology affects people's lives. The OTA clarifies for Congress both the range of policy options and the potential impacts of adopting each option, but it makes no formal recommendations. The OTA also provides advice to Congressional committee members and staff, presents testimony at hearings, and conducts workshops with committees. Although the OTA is responsible to the needs of the Congress and its products are designed for use by the Congress, they have a wider applicability as well.

Primary intended users: Legislators, government regulators, public policy-makers.

Technologies: Drug, device, medical or surgical procedure, support system, organizational or administrative system, personnel.

The OTA focuses its evaluation efforts on broad policy technological issues or on case studies from which further research questions or generalizable lessons can be gained.

Intervention: Prevention, diagnosis, treatment, rehabilitation.

Stage: *New, established or widespread practice,* emerging, obsolete.

Properties: *Safety; efficacy; cost-effectiveness;* effectiveness; cost; acceptance/adoption level; system impact; economic implications; ethical, legal, social implications.

The scope of OTA assessments is quite broad, reflecting the extent to which legislative policy issues are influenced by technological developments.

Selection process: Under OTA statute, studies may be initiated by a request from a Congressional committee chairman. The OTA will also respond formally to requests for information from any member of Congress or any Congressional committee. OTA staff members screen the proposed study to determine what resources and time it might require and what modifications it might need to suit the OTA's resources and Congressional needs. The staff then presents a formal study proposal to the OTA Board, which makes the final decision on whether to undertake it.

Methods: *Information syntheses,* expert opinion, modeling, cost analysis.

The OTA generally does not support original research, but synthesizes existing knowledge from the medical and health policy literature with the help of expert advisors.

The OTA staff develops an initial draft with advice from an expert advisory panel appointed for each main report. The draft is then circulated for review and comment to groups and experts both in the government and in the private sector. Advisory panel assistance includes review and comment, although its consensus is not sought for report content or findings and reports are not formally approved by the panel. OTA staff are responsible for drafting the final report. Case studies of specific technologies have been used often in conjunction with reports dealing with broad issues such as studies of cost-effectiveness and cost-benefit analyses of technologies. Such case studies usually are prepared by experts under commissions from the OTA and occasionally by OTA staff.

The bulk of OTA's work involves comprehensive, in-depth assessments that may take 18 months or more to complete. It is also provides shorter responses to meet Congressional needs, largely based on information in past and current assessments. OTA can structure longer-range assessments so that the results, in various stages, can be sent to Congress in the form of interim reports.

Assessors: OTA multidisciplinary staff teams plan, direct, and draft all assessments. Staff members have expertise in such areas as medicine, law, sociology, epidemiology, statistics, public health, public policy, and biology. The Health Program has about 13 permanent staff and 12 to 14 other in-house staff on temporary appointments. Outside contract work is usually for special material to be included in OTA reports. OTA uses expert advisory panels as a way of ensuring that reports are objective, fair, and authoritative. The Health Program is advised regarding overall planning by a standing 15-member Health Program Advisory Committee composed of experts in a variety of fields relevant to health care technology assessment. This committee generally is not involved directly in specific studies. The staff rely extensively on the broad technical and professional resources of the private sector, including universities, research organizations, industry, and public interest groups.

Assessment reports include: Abstract; the purpose of the assessment; relationship of this assessment to prior or concurrent assessments of the technology or other technologies intended for similar purposes; who sponsored/commissioned/supported the assessment; who conducted the assessment; description of the technology; stage of life-cycle of technology when assessed; properties assessed; procedure used for the assessment; sources of data/information; methods for collecting data/information; results; findings or conclusions; limitations of findings; implications of findings for practice; recommendations for practice, future assessments, technology development, research; how the technology works, including theory, principles; development of the technology; where technology is in use.

Dissemination: *Printed reports;* journal articles; press conferences/news releases; TV/radio broadcasts, video products; briefings to Congressional committees and staff.

Reports approved by the OTA Director are sent to the Technology Assessment Board and to the requesting Congressional committee(s). Summaries are also sent to all members of Congress and then the report and summary are released to the public. Summaries of all OTA reports are available free of charge from the OTA. OTA studies are also available from the U.S. Government Printing Office or the National Technical Information Service.

Budget: $1.6 million (fiscal year 1987). The approximate cost per assessment is $400,000 to $700,000. Funding source: 100 percent parent organization.

Use: OTA reports have generally been well-received by Congress and the various sectors of the health care industry. Because of the nature of congressional decisions, it is difficult to attribute legislative change or other congressional actions to any one factor. However, in several instances Congress has based funding and policy decisions on OTA report findings.

The OTA Health Program is described in: Institute of Medicine, Committee on Evaluating Medical Technologies in Clinical Use. *Assessing medical technologies.* Washington, DC: National Academy Press, 1985.

Related activities: The OTA was mandated by Congress to select and appoint the members of the Prospective Payment Assessment Commission (ProPAC), which advises the Secretary of DHHS regarding the hospital prospective payment system used for Medicare. The OTA acts as an observer and evaluator of ProPAC, reports annually to Congress on the functioning of the Commission, and appoints replacement commissioners each year. The OTA has similar responsibilities for the Physician Payment Review Commission.

Completed Reports

CU1 Congress of the United States, Office of Technology Assessment. Assessing the quality of medical care. Washington, D.C.: U.S. Government Printing Office. To be completed in Spring 1988.

CU2 ______. Diagnostic and predictive medical tests. Washington, D.C.: U.S. Government Printing Office. To be completed in Spring 1988.

CU3 ______. Drug labeling in developing countries. Washington, D.C.: U.S. Government Printing Office. To be completed in Winter 1988/89.

CU4 ______. Nontraditional methods of cancer management. Washington, D.C.: U.S. Government Printing Office. To be completed in Summer 1988.

CU5 ______. Carcinogen regulatory policy. Washington, D.C.: U.S. Government Printing Office. To be completed Spring 1987.

CU6 ______. Clinical staffing issues in the Indian Health Service. Washington, D.C.: Office of Technology Assessment. Special report. To be released in Spring 1987.

CU7 ______. Effectiveness and costs of ambulatory tocodynamometry. Washington, D.C.: U.S. Government Printing Office. To be completed in Spring 1987.

CU8 ______. Immuno-augmentative therapy. Washington, D.C.: U.S. Government Printing Office. To be completed in Winter 1987/1988.

CU9 ______. Mammography screening for the Medicare population. Washington, D.C.: Office of Technology Assessment. To be completed in Summer 1987.

CU10 ______. Mental health services for children. Washington, D.C.: U.S. Government Printing Office, January 1987.

CU11 ______. Review of study comparing inpatient hospital costs in the Veterans Administration to those in non-VA facilities. Washington, D.C.: Office of Technology Assessment. To be completed in February 1987.

CU12 ______. Technology and child health. Washington, D.C.: U.S. Government Printing Office. To be completed in Spring 1987.

CU13 ______. Extracorporeal shock-wave lithotripsy. Washington, D.C.: U.S. Government Printing Office, May 1986. (Health technology case study series #36)

CU14 ______. Indian health care. Washington, D.C.: U.S. Government Printing Office, April 1986.

CU15 ______. Nurse practitioners, certified nurse-midwives, and assistants: a policy analysis. Washington, D.C.: U.S. Government Printing Office, December 1986. (Health technology case study series #37)

CU16 ______. OTA's second report on the Prospective Payment Assessment Commission (special report). Washington, D.C.: Office of Technology Assessment, March 1986.

CU17 ______. Passive smoking in the workplace: selected issues. Washington, D.C.: Office of Technology Assessment, May 1986.

CU18 ______. Payment for physician services: strategies for Medicare. Washington, D.C.: U.S. Government Printing Office, February 1986.

CU19 ______. Technologies for detecting heritable mutations in human beings. Washington, D.C.: U.S. Government Printing Office, September 1986.

CU20 ______. Blood policy and technology. Washington, D.C.: U.S. Government Printing Office, January 1985.

CU21 ______. Evaluation of HCFA's Part A data base. Washington, D.C.: Office of Technology Assessment, July 1985.

CU22 ______. Medical devices and the Veterans Administration. Washington, D.C.: U.S. Government Printing Office, February 1985.

CU23 ______. Medicare's prospective payment system: strategies for evaluating cost, quality, and medical technology. Washington, D.C.: U.S. Government Printing Office, October 1985.

CU24 ______. OTA's first report on the Prospective Payment Assessment Commission (special report). Washington, D.C.: Office of Technology Assessment, March 1985.

CU25 ______. Preventing illness and injury in the workplace. Washington, D.C.: U.S. Government Printing Office, April 1985.

CU26 ______. Replacing the Rosebud Sioux Hospital: number of beds and whether a surgical suite is needed. Washington, D.C.: Office of Technology Assessment , August 1985.

CU27 ______. Review of the Public Health Service's response to AIDS. Washington, D.C.: U.S. Government Printing Office, February 1985.

CU28 ______. Status of biomedical research and related technology for tropical diseases. Washington, D.C.: U.S. Government Printing Office, September 1985.

CU29 ______. Technologies for managing urinary incontinence. Washington, D.C.: U.S. Government Printing Office, July 1985. (Health technology case study series #33)

CU30 ______. The cost effectiveness of digital subtraction angiography in the detection of cerebrovascular disease. Washington, D.C.: U.S. Government Printing Office, May 1985. (Health technology case study series #34)

CU31 ______. The effectiveness and costs of continuous ambulatory peritoneal dialysis. Washington, D.C.: U.S. Government Printing Office, September 1985. (Health technology case study series #35)

CU32 ______ The hemodialysis equipment and disposables industry. Washington, D.C.: U.S. Government Printing Office, December 1984. (Health technology case study series #32)

CU33 ______. Federal policies and the medical devices industry. Washington, D.C.: U.S. Goverment Printing Office, October 1984.

CU34 ______. Intensive care units: costs, outcome, and decisionmaking. Washington, D.C.: U.S. Government Printing Office, October 1984. (Health technology case study series #28)

CU35 ______. Medical technology and costs of the Medicare program. Washington, D.C.: U.S. Government Printing Office, July 1984.

CU36 ______. Nuclear magnetic resonance imaging technology: a clinical, industrial, and policy analysis. Washington, D.C.: U.S. Government Printing Office, September 1984. (Health technology case study series #27)

CU37 ______. The Boston elbow. Washington, D.C.: U.S. Government Printing Office, November 1984. (Health technology case study series #29)

CU38 ______. The contact lens industry. Washington, D.C.: U.S. Government Printing Office, December 1984 (Health technology case study series #31)

CU39 ______. The health effects of fish oil. Washington, D.C.: Office of Technology Assessment, February 1984.

CU40 ______. The market for wheelchairs: innovations and public policy. Washington, D.C.: U.S. Government Printing Office, November 1984. (Health technology case study series #30)

CU41 ______. The use of immunosuppressive drugs in kidney transplantation. Washington, D.C.: Office of Technology Assessment, March 1984.

CU42 ______. Update of Federal activities regarding the use of pneumococcal vaccine. Washington, D.C.: U.S. Government Printing Office, May 1984.

CU43 ______. Assistive devices for severe speech impairments. Washington, D.C.: U.S. Government Printing Office, December 1983. (Health technology case study series #26)

CU44 ______. Diagnosis-related groups (DRGs) and the Medicare program: implications for medical technology, Washington, D.C.: U.S. Government Printing Office, July 1983.

CU45 ______. Quality and relevance of research and related activities at the Gorgas Memorial Laboratory. Washington, D.C.: U.S. Government Printing Office, August 1983.

CU46 ______. Technology and learning disabilities. Washington, D.C.: U.S. Government Printing Office, December 1983. (Health technology case study series #25)

CU47 ______. The effectiveness and costs of alcoholism treatment. Washington, D.C.: U.S. Government Printing Office, March 1983. (Health technology case study series #22)

CU48 ______. The impact of randomized clinical trials on health policy and medical practice. Washington, D.C.: U.S. Government Printing Office, August 1983.

CU49 ______. The safety, efficacy, and cost effectiveness of therapeutic apheresis. Washington, D.C.: U.S. Government Printing Office, July 1983. (Health technology case study series #23)

CU50 ______. Variations in hospital length of stay: their relationships to health outcomes. Washington, D.C.: U.S. Government Printing Office, August 1983. (Health technology case study series #24)

CU51 ______. Assessment of four common X-ray procedures. Washington, D.C.: U.S. Government Printing Office, April 1982. (Health technology case study series #19)

CU52 ______. Cardiac radionuclide imaging and cost-effectiveness. Washington, D.C.: U.S. Government Printing Office, May 1982. (Health technology case study series #13)

CU53 ______. MEDLARS and health information policy. Washington, D.C.: U.S. Government Printing Office, September 1982.

CU54 ______. Mandatory passive restraint systems in automobiles. Washington, D.C.: U.S. Government Printing Office, September 1982. (Health technology case study series #20)

CU55 ______. Medical technology under proposals to increase competition in health care. Washington, D.C.: U.S. Government Printing Office, October 1982.

CU56 ______. Postmarketing surveillance of prescription drugs. Washington, D.C.: U.S. Government Printing Office, November 1982.

CU57 ______. Selected telecommunications devices for hearing-impaired persons. Washington, D.C.: U.S. Government Printing Office, December 1982. (Health technology case study series #21)

CU58 ______. Strategies for medical technology assessment. Washington, D.C.: U.S. Government Printing Office, September 1982.

CU59 ______. Technology and handicapped people. Washington, D.C.: U.S. Government Printing Office, May 1982.

CU60 ______. Technology transfer at the National Institutes of Health. Washington, D.C.: U.S. Government Printing Office, March 1982.

CU61 ______. The artificial heart: cost, risks, and benefits. Washington, D.C.: U.S. Government Printing Office, May 1982. (Health technology case study series #9)

CU62 ______. Allocating costs and benefits in disease prevention: an application to cervical cancer screening. Washington, D.C.: U.S. Government Printing Office, May 1981. (Health technology case study series #7)

CU63 ______. Assessing selected respiratory therapy modalities: trends and relative costs in the Washington, D.C. area. Washington, D.C.: U.S. Government Printing Office, July 1981. (Health technology case study series #12)

CU64 ______. Benefit and cost analysis of medical interventions: the case of cimetidine and peptic ulcer disease. Washington, D.C.: U.S. Government Printing Office, September 1981. (Health technology case study series #11)

CU65 ______. Cost-benefit/cost-effectiveness of medical technologies: a case study of orthopedic joint implants. Washington, D.C.: U.S. Government Printing Office, September 1981. (Health technology case study series #14)

CU66 ______. Cost-effectiveness of automated multichannel chemistry analyzers. Washington, D.C.: U.S. Government Printing Office, April 1981. (Health technology case study series #4)

CU67 ______. Cost-effectiveness of influenza vaccination. Washington, D.C.: U.S. Government Printing Office, December 1981.

CU68 ______. Elective hysterectomy: costs, risks and benefits. Washington, D.C.: U.S. Government Printing Office, October 1981. (Health technology case study series #15)

CU69 ______. Formal analysis, policy formulation, and end-stage renal disease. Washington, D.C.: U.S. Government Printing Office, April 1981. (Health technology case study series #1)

CU70 ______. Periodontal disease: assessing the effectiveness and costs of the Keyes technique. Washington, D.C.: U.S. Government Printing Office, May 1981. (Health technology case study series #5)

CU71 ______. Policy implications of computed tomography (CT) scanners: an update. Washington, D.C.: U.S. Government Printing Office, January 1981.

CU72 ______. Screening for colon cancer. Washington, D.C.: U.S. Government Printing Office, April 1981. (Health technology case study series #3)

CU73 ______. Surgery for breast cancer. Washington, D.C.: U.S. Government Printing Office, October 1981. (Health technology case study series #17)

CU74 ______. Technologies for determining cancer risks from the environment. Washington, D.C.: U.S. Government Printing Office, June 1981.

CU75 ______. The cost-effectiveness of bone marrow transplant therapy and its policy implications. Washington, D.C.: U.S. Government Printing Office, May 1981. (Health technology case study series #6)

CU76 ______. The cost-effectiveness of upper gastrointestinal endoscopy. Washington, D.C.: U.S. Government Printing Office, May 1981. (Health technology case study series #8)

CU77 ______. The costs and effectiveness of neonatal intensive care. Washington, D.C.: U.S. Government Printing Office, August 1981. (Health technology case study series #10)

CU78 ______. The costs and effectiveness of nurse practitioners. Washington, D.C.: U.S. Government Printing Office, July 1981. (Health technology case study series #16)

CU79 ______. The feasibility of economic evaluation of diagnostic procedures: the case of CT scanning. Washington, D.C.: U.S. Government Printing Office, April 1981. (Health technology case study series #2)

CU80 ______. Compensation for vaccine-related injuries. Washington, D.C.: U.S. Government Printing Office, November, 1980.

CU81 ______. Methodological issues and literature review. Washington, D.C.: U.S. Government Printing Office, September 1980. (Background paper #1 of the Series on implications of cost-effectiveness analysis of medical technology)

CU82 ______. The efficacy and cost effectiveness of psychotherapy. Washington, D.C.: U.S. Government Printing Office, October 1980. (Health technology case study series #18)

CU83 ______. The implications of cost-effectiveness analysis of medical technology. Washington, D.C.: U.S. Government Printing Office, August 1980.

CU84 ______. The management of health care technology in ten countries. Washington, D.C.: U.S. Government Printing Office, October 1980. (Background paper #4 of the Series on implications of cost-effectiveness analysis of medical technology)

CU85 ______. A review of selected federal vaccine and immunization policies. Washington, D.C.: U.S. Government Printing Office, September 1979.

CU86 ______. Computer technology in medical education and assessment. Washington, D.C.: U.S. Government Printing Office, September 1979.

CU87 ______. Assessing the efficacy and safety of medical technologies. Washington, D.C.: U.S. Government Printing Office, September 1978.

CU88 ______. Policy implications of computed tomography (CT) scanners. Washington, D.C.: U.S. Government Printing Office, August 1978.

CU89 ______. Cancer testing technology and saccharin. Washington, D.C.: U.S. Government Printing Office, October 1977.

CU90 ______. Policy implications of medical information systems. Washington, D.C.: U.S. Government Printing Office, November 1977.

CU91 ______. Development of medical technology: opportunities for assessment. Washington, D.C.: U.S. Government Printing Office, August 1976.

CU92 ______. Drug bioequivalence. Washington, D.C.: U.S. Government Printing Office, July 1974.

Duke University

Center for Health Policy Research and Education
Box GM, Duke Station
Durham, NC 27706
919-684-3023

Contact: David M. Eddy, M.D., Ph.D., Director. Telex 802829 DUKTELCOM DURM.

Overview: The Center for Health Policy Research and Education (CHPRE) was created in 1980 with a core grant from the Duke Endowment. From the start, it has focused on the development and application of methods to assess health technologies. It also works to analyze particular health practices and to educate policy makers. Its products are technology assessment methods, assessments, and educational programs.

Purpose: To develop methods of technology assessment, to improve health by evaluation of particular health practices, and to educate policy makers.

Primary intended users: Providers, generally; physicians; acute facility administrators; health product manufacturers; health/medical professional associations; health industry associations; employers; third party payers; government regulators; voluntary associations, organizations; public policy-makers, legislators.

Technologies: Drug, device, medical or surgical procedure.

Assessments have focused on the impact of technologies on individuals as well as on populations.

Intervention: *Prevention, treatment,* diagnosis, rehabilitation.

Stage: Emerging, new, established or widespread practice, obsolete.

The program is concerned with controversial technologies at any stage.

Properties: *Efficacy, cost-effectiveness,* safety, effectiveness, cost, system impact, economic implications.

Selection process: Any organization may request that an assessment be conducted, including third party payers; state, federal, and international governments; hospitals; health maintenance organizations; professional societies; health industries; trade associations; and venture capitalists.

Assessment topic priorities are set by the Center staff. Major criteria are: 1) a request from a major organization currently facing a decision about the technology; 2) the importance (magnitude of the health and economic impact) of the health problem and the expected difference made by the technology; 3) the degree of uncertainty or controversy about the technology; and 4) the existence of methodological issues (anticipated difficulty and novelty of the analysis).

Reassessments are performed at the request of an organization or when new information becomes available that could modify the results of an active assessment (an assessment still being used for decisions).

Methods: *Information syntheses;* expert opinion; group judgment; modeling; cost analyses.

Existing information is analyzed to estimate the effect of the technology on important health and economic outcomes. Typically, quantitative methods are used to interpret and synthesize the information, and to estimate effects that have not been or can not be observed experimentally (e.g., life expectancy and population effects). To the greatest extent possible, analyses rest on empirical observations. When unavoidable, expert judgments are formally incorporated into the assessment.

Assessments are typically performed in eight steps: 1) problem formulation (performed in conjunction with the requesting organization); 2) information gathering; 3) model development; 4) analysis; 5) preparation of drafts; 6) cycles of external review and revision; 7) approval; and 8) final report.

Turnaround time from selection of assessment topic to reporting of findings depends on the time constraints of the requesting organization, prior familiarity with the assessment problem, and the review process. The time ranges from 1 week to 2 years; the average is 6 months.

Assessors: Assessors are experts in medicine, statistics, mathematics, operations research, computer science, and law.

Assessment reports include: Abstract; the purpose of the assessment; relationship of this assessment to prior or concurrent assessments of the technology or other technologies intended for similar purposes; who sponsored/commissioned/supported the assessment; who conducted the assessment; description of the technology; properties assessed; procedure used for the assessment; sources of data/information; methods for collecting data/information; methods for analyzing/synthesizing data/information; results; findings or conclusions; limitations of findings; implications of findings for practice; recommendations for practice, future assessments, technology development, research.

Dissemination: Printed reports, journal articles, advisories to members/constituents.

Assessment results are also disseminated by the requesting organizations through their own channels. Copies of assessment reports are available upon request or in the open scientific literature.

Budget: $1,000,000. Assessments cost CHPRE from $3,000 to $60,000; charges have ranged from no charge to $45,000. Funding sources: 10 percent parent organization; 30 percent government grants/contracts; 60 percent foundations, other private grants.

Use: Duke University does not formally use the assessment reports. The requesting organizations have used the results to help set third party coverage policies, to design practice standards, to draft legislation, to develop recommendations for national policy, and to design national health programs. The use of assessments is usually known because CHPRE staff works with the requesting organization through the implementation stage. In addition, assessment authors are frequently invited to speak on their topics.

Examples of use include the following: 1) publication by the American Cancer Society of the *ACS Guidelines on the Cancer-Related Health Checkup;* 2) publication by the World Health Organization of *Control of Oral Cancer in Developing Countries;* 3) adoption by the National Cancer Institute of a computer program for *Setting National Cancer Control Priorities for the Year 2000* and 4) acceptance by the Minister of Health, Chile, of recommendations for cancer control priorities.

Program evaluation: In 1986, the Hartford Foundation evaluated CHPRE at the end of a 3-year grant that funded the development and application of a new set of assessment methods. An independent consultant to the Foundation read project reports and background material and visited the Center for 1 day. The evaluation's findings were positive. Following the evaluation, the Center received a second grant from the Foundation to continue development of the assessment method.

Related activities: Computer software is being prepared to enable others to use some of the quantitative technology assessment methods developed at the Center. CHPRE plans to offer several 1-day seminars to acquaint researchers and policy-makers with technology assessment methods developed by the Center.

Completed Reports

DC1 Adar R, Critchfield GC, Eddy DM. [Duke University, Center for Health Policy and Education] A confidence profile analysis of the results of percutaneous transluminal angioplasty in the treatment of ischemic femoropopliteal artery disease, expected publication 1988. [Information syntheses]

DC2 Critchfield GC, Eddy DM. [______] A confidence profile analysis of the effectiveness of disulfiram in the treatment of chronic alcoholism. Med Care, submitted for publication. [Information syntheses]

DC3 Critchfield GC, Eddy DM. [______] Screening for osteoporosis, expected publication 1988. [Information syntheses]

DC4 Eddy DM, Hasselblad V, McGivney W, Hendee W. [______] The value of mammography screening for women age 40-49, submitted for publication. [Information syntheses]

DC5 Eddy DM. [______] Screening by mammography for women over age 65, reassessment, expected publication 1988. [Information syntheses]

DC6 ______. [______] Screening for breast cancer, reassessment, expected publication 1988. [Information syntheses]

DC7 ______. [______] Screening for cervical cancer, reassessment, expected publication 1988. [Information syntheses]

DC8 ______. [______] Screening for colorectal cancer, reassessment, expected publication 1988. [Information syntheses]

DC9 ______. [______] Screening for glaucoma, reassessment, expected publication 1988. [Information syntheses]

DC10 ______. [______] Screening for lung cancer, reassessment, expected publication, 1988. [Information syntheses]

DC11 Gavin NI, Hasselblad V, Eddy DM. [______] The role of adjuvant tamoxifen treatment of postmenopausal women with stage II breast cancer, expected publication 1988. [Information syntheses]

DC12 Hasselblad V. [______] Analysis of the prevention of mental retardation by screening for maple syrup urine disease, expected publication 1988. [Information syntheses]

DC13 Brandeau ML, Eddy DM. [______] The workup of the asymptomatic patient with a positive fecal occult blood test. Med Decis Making 1987;7:32-46. [Information syntheses]

DC14 Eddy DM, Wolpert RL, Rosenberg ML. [______] Estimating the effectiveness of interventions to prevent youth suicides: a report to the Secretary's Task Force on Youth Suicide. 1987. [Information syntheses]

DC15 Eddy DM, Nugent FW, Eddy JF, et al. [______] Screening for colorectal cancer in a high-risk population: results of a mathematical model. Gastroenterology 1987;92:682-692. [Information syntheses]

DC16 Eddy DM. [______] The use of confidence profiles to assess tissue-type plasminogen activator. In: Califf RM, Wanger GS, eds. Acute coronary care. Boston: Martinus Nijhoff Publishing, 1987. [Information syntheses]

DC17 ______. [______] Priorities for cancer control in Chile. Report prepared for the World Health Organization. 1986. [Information syntheses]

DC18 ______. [______] Priorities for cancer control in India. Report prepared for the World Health Organization. 1986. [Information syntheses]

DC19 ______. [______] The effectiveness, cost, & cost-effectiveness of breast cancer screening with annual mammography & breast physical exam. for women over 65. Report prepared for Committee on Ways & Means, Subcommittee on Health, U.S. House of Representatives. 1986 Jan 7. [Information syntheses]

DC20 Eddy JF, Eddy, DM. [______] The value of corneal endothelial cell microscopy for cataract surgery. Report prepared for the Blue Cross and Blue Shield Association. 1986. [Information syntheses]

DC21 Eddy DM. [______] Priorities for cancer control in Chile. Report prepared for the World Health Organization. 1985. [Information syntheses]

DC22 ______. [______] Priorities for cancer control in India. Report prepared for the World Health Organization. 1985. [Information syntheses]

DC23 A WHO Meeting [______] Control of oral cancer in developing countries. Bull WHO 1984;62:817-830. [Information syntheses]

DC24 ______. [______] The economic impact of cancer and cancer prevention in private industry. Report prepared for the American Cancer Society. 1984. [Information syntheses]

DC25 Eddy DM, Eddy JF, Sanders LE. [______] Surgical treatment of obesity. Evidence of effectiveness and risks. Report prepared for the North Carolina Blue Cross and Blue Shield Asociation. 1983. [Information syntheses]

DC26 Eddy DM, Sanders L, Eddy J. [______] The value of screening for glaucoma with tonometry. Surv Ophthalmol 1983;28:194-205. [Information syntheses]

DC27 Eddy DM. [______] Appropriateness of cervical cancer screening. Gynecol Oncol 1981;12:S168-187. [Information syntheses]

DC28 ______. [______] Screening for colon cancer: a technology assessment. 1981. (Office of Technology Assessment background paper #2: case studies of medical technologies) [Information syntheses]

DC29 ______. [______] Guidelines for the cancer-related checkup: recommendations and rationale. CA-A Cancer J Clin 1980;30:193-240. [Information syntheses]

ECRI Health Devices Program

5200 Butler Pike
Plymouth Meeting, PA 19462
215-825-6000

Contact: Robert Mosenkis, Vice President of Publications. Telex 510-660-8023. Telefax 215-834-1275.

Overview: ECRI, formerly the Emergency Care Research Institute, is an independent not-for-profit corporation that works to improve the quality of patient care. It provides a wide range of services dealing with health care technology including research, evaluation, assessment, consulting, environmental testing, and publications development. The Health Devices Program (HDP) was established by ECRI in 1971.

Purpose: To conduct assessments that provide independent, objective judgment for selection, purchase, and use of medical instruments, equipment, and systems; to function as a clearinghouse for investigating and resolving hazards and deficiencies in medical devices; and to encourage the improvement of medical devices through an informed marketplace.

Primary intended users: Providers, generally; physicians; acute facility administrators; biomedical researchers.

Technologies: *Device,* support system, organizational or administrative system.

All types of diagnostic and therapeutic medical devices, equipment, and support systems, as well as some preventive and rehabilitative technologies are assessed. Examples range from disposables, such as incontinent pads and suction canisters, to electric beds, patient monitoring systems, anesthesia machines, infusion and imaging technologies, and clinical laboratory instruments. Comparative evaluations are usually conducted within a product category.

Intervention: *Treatment,* prevention, diagnosis, rehabilitation.

Stage: *Established or widespread practice,* new.

Properties: *Effectiveness,* safety, efficacy, cost, cost-effectiveness, service requirements, acceptance/adoption level, performance, ease of use, reliability, and appropriateness of use.

Selection process: Hospital members of the Health Devices Program may request that an assessment be conducted. ECRI/HDP may also determine the need for an evaluation based on inquiries received from member hospitals. Requests for assessments are made either informally by telephone conversation with staff members, by written correspondence, or by responding to periodic HDP member surveys. Topic selection is based on the volume of inquiries received from ECRI/HDP member hospitals; the ECRI's senior staff's experience regarding a product's importance to hospitals and to safe, efficacious, and cost-effective patient care; and the results of membership questionnaires.

Device categories are reassessed when member hospitals request more current information than is available from previous evaluations. This normally occurs when a significant number of new product models appear on the market in a given category.

Methods: *Bench testing,* information syntheses, expert opinion, group judgment, cost analyses, clinical trials.

The ECRI/HDP comparative evaluations are based on ECRI laboratory and clinical evaluations. Laboratory evaluations are conducted in ECRI's facility, and clinical studies (in vivo evaluations of device performance) are conducted in selected member hospitals. Evaluations follow appropriately reviewed medical/scientific protocols developed by ECRI. There is an extensive review process that involves both in-house and independent reviewers, typically including clinicians with special expertise in the subject area.

The approximate turnaround time from selection of assessment topic to reporting of findings is 6 to 9 months.

Assessors: Evaluations are conducted primarily by engineers, physicians, and chemists. As needed, ECRI's interdisciplinary staff collaborate on evaluations. ECRI employs more than 120 full-time staff with expertise in medical, engineering, and analytical sciences.

Assessment reports include: Abstract; the purpose of the assessment; relationship of this assessment to prior or concurrent assessments of the technology or other technologies intended for similar purposes; description of the technology; stage of life-cycle of technology when assessed; properties assessed; procedure used for the assessment; sources of data/information; methods for collecting data/information; methods for analyzing/synthesizing data/information; results; findings or conclusions; limitations of findings; implications of findings for practice; recommendations for practice, future assessments, technology development, research; how the technology works, including theory, principles; development of the technology; procurement/deployment information; product recall history, liability actions.

Dissemination: *Journal articles;* advisories to members/constituents; clearinghouses, data/citation bases, on-line services. Specifically, abstracts are published in *Health Devices Alerts* and are available in an online database.

For each evaluation, a comprehensive report is published containing tables that show the product's characteristics and performance on each evaluation criterion. Model-specific listings of advantages and disadvantages and ratings (e.g., recommended, not recommended) are also included. All reports are published in ECRI's monthly journal, *Health Devices* which began publication in 1971. *Health Devices* also contains reports of hazards with medical devices, as reported by ECRI/HDP member hospitals and investigated by ECRI engineers.

Copies of individual issues of *Health Devices* may be purchased from ECRI's Circulation Department. Hospitals and others may become members of the Health Devices Program and receive subscriptions to the weekly *Health Devices Alerts*, the bimonthly journal, *Health Technology: Critical Issues for Decision Makers*, and telephone consultation privileges. Individual subscriptions to *Health Devices* alone are not available. Summaries of relevant evaluations are also published in the *Technology for Health Care* family of seven specialized monthly newsletters. *Health Devices* is not indexed by the National Library of Medicine for the MEDLARS system. However, indexes and database searches are available directly from ECRI.

Budget: $2,000,000. Based on the type of device being evaluated, the cost per assessment ranges from $40,000 to $100,000. Funding source: 100 percent sponsors/members dues, contributions.

Use: Assessments reports are used by ECRI to serve the health care community and patients in the nation's hospitals. These reports are also used by members of the Health Devices Program (which includes hospitals representing about 70 percent of all acute-care beds in the U.S.) in a variety of ways involving selection, acquisition, and use of medical devices.

Regular surveys of ECRI/HDP members and an annual membership renewal rate exceeding 95 percent provide indications of the value of these evaluations to member hospitals. Numerous specific product improvements have been directly attributed to ECRI/HDP evaluations. For instance, following an extensive 1973 study of electrosurgical machines, most manufacturers undertook major redesign to improve safety. Over the past decade 90 percent of the nation's inventory of these devices has been replaced. The impact has been significant; fewer electrosurgical burns are reported to ECRI.

ECRI estimates that cost savings in the hundreds of millions of dollars can be attributed to ECRI evaluations and other technology-related efforts on behalf of member hospitals. One example is the National Electrical Code controversy over isolated power in anesthetizing locations.

ECRI assessment activities are described in Institute of Medicine, Committee on Evaluating Medical Technologies in Clinical Use. *Assessing medical technologies.* Washington, DC: National Academy Press, 1985.

Related activities: The Health Devices Program is closely related to other ECRI activities including: the Technology Assessment Program; a technology risk management program that produces the four-volume *Hospital Risk Control* information service; accident investigation, forensic engineering, engineering and management consultation; and field technical services for hospitals.

Completed Reports

EH1 ECRI Health Devices Program. Carbon dioxide monitors. Health Devices 1986;15:255-85.

EH2 ______. Continuous passive motion (CPM) leg exercisers. Health Devices 1986;15:3-22.

EH3 ______. EEG monitors. Health Devices 1986;15:71-95.

EH4 ______. Electric beds. Health Devices 1986;15-299-316.

EH5 ______. Electrosurgical active electrode pencils, hand controlled. Health Devices 1986;15:151-77.

EH6 ______. Neonatal ventilators. Health Devices 1986;15:219-46.

EH7 ______. Patient care management system, Space-Labs. Health Devices 1986;15:286-94.

EH8 ______. Peritoneal dialysis cyclers. Health Devices 1986;15:31-61.

EH9 ______. Sphygmomanometers, automatic. Health Devices 1986;15:187-208.

EH10 ______. Surgical drapes. Health Devices 1986;15:111-40.

EH11 ______. Arrhythmia monitoring systems, computerized. Health Devices 1985;14:287-319.

EH12 ______. Batteries, zinc air. Health Devices 1985;14:209-211.

EH13 ______. Electrode monitoring systems, electrosurgical. Health Devices 1985;14:115-31.

EH14 ______. Infusion controllers. Health Devices 1985;14:219-256.

EH15 ______. Oxygen-air proportioners. Health Devices 1985;14:263-76.

EH16 ______. Physiologic monitoring systems. Health Devices 1985;14:143-182.

EH17 ______. Positive end expiratory pressure (PEEP) valves. Health Devices 1985;14:379-99.

EH18 ______. Suction canisters (aspirator collection bottles). Health Devices 1985;14:411-34.

EH19 ______. Suction regulators. Health Devices 1985;14:191-209.

EH20 ______. Blood warmers. Health Devices 1984;13:191-219.

EH21 ______. Disposable pressure transducers. Health Devices 1984;13:268-90.

EH22 ______. Electrocardiographs, three-channel. Health Devices 1984;13:235-59.

EH23 ______. Enteral feeding pumps. Health Devices 1984;14:9-30.

EH24 ______. Infant radiant warmers. Health Devices 1984;13:119-45.

EH25 ______. Infusion pumps. Health Devices 1983-84;13:31-62.

EH26 ______. Patient bed scales. Health Devices 1984;13:75-91.

EH27 ______. Pneumatic tourniquets. Health Devices 1984;13:299-316.

EH28 ______. Anesthesia unit gas scavengers. Health Devices 1983;12:267-286.

EH29 ______. Blood gas/pH analyzers. Health Devices 1983;12:59-78.

EH30 ______. Defibrillators, line-powered. Health Devices 1983;12:291-314.

EH31 ______. External transcutanaeous pacemakers, Pace*Aid Model 50C. Health Devices 1983;13:3-13.

EH32 ______. Heat and moisture exchange humidifiers. Health Devices 1983;12:155-67.

EH33 ______. Incontinent pads. Health Devices 1983;12:108-18.

EH34 ______. Oxygen analyzers. Health Devices 1983;12:183-97.

EH35 ______. Oxygen monitors, transcutaneous. Health Devices 1983;12:213-51.

EH36 ______. Suction canisters (aspirator collection bottles). Health Devices 1983;12:127-49.

EH37 ______. Surgical gloves, latex. Health Devices 1983;12:83-98.

EH38 ______. Arrhythmia monitoring systems, computerized. Health Devices 1982;11:211-247.

EH39 ______. Electronic intermittent thermometers. Health Devices 1982;12:3-20.

EH40 ______. Ethylene oxide sterilizers. Health Devices 1982;11:287-301.

EH41 ______. Fetal monitors. Health Devices 1982;11:123-44.

EH42 ______. Infant incubators. Health Devices 1982;11:191-9.

EH43 ______. Infant transport incubators. Health Devices 1982;11:179-91.

EH44 ______. Infusion controllers. Health Devices 1982;11:75-96.

EH45 ______. Operating room ECG monitors. Health Devices 1982;11:155-74.

EH46 ______. Physiologic monitoring systems. Health Devices 1982;11:211-47.

EH47 ______. Surgical case carts. Health Devices 1982;11:311-24.

EH48 ______. Surgical case carts. Health Devices 1982;12:33-9.

EH49 ______. Volume ventilators. Health Devices 1982;11:264-83.

EH50 ______. X-ray film processors. Health Devices 1982;11:99-115.

ECRI Technology Assessment Program

5200 Butler Pike
Plymouth Meeting, PA 19462
215-825-6000

Contact: Malin VanAntwerp, Director of Policy Analysis. Telex 510-660-8023. Telefax 215-834-1275.

Overview: ECRI, formerly the Emergency Care Research Institute, is an independent, not-for-profit corporation that works to improve the quality of patient care. It provides a wide range of services dealing with health care technology including research, evaluation, assessment, consulting, environmental testing, and publications development. The Technology Assessment Program (ECRI/TAP) was established by ECRI in 1981.

Purpose: To provide to interested parties assessments of emerging and regularly used health care technologies.

Primary intended users: Providers, generally; physicians; acute facility administrators; other care givers; health product manufacturers; health/medical professional associations; health industry associations; consumer associations; employers; third party payers; government regulators; voluntary associations, organizations; financial analysts, consultants; reporters, writers, news media; information/computer industry; labs, blood banks; public policy-makers, legislators; policy research organizations; lawyers; liability, malpractice insurers.

Technologies: *Device,* medical or surgical procedure, support system.

Primarily diagnostic and therapeutic equipment are assessed. Occasionally, surgical procedures and clinical laboratory diagnostics are assessed.

Intervention: *Treatment,* diagnosis, rehabilitation.

Stage: *New,* emerging, established or widespread practice, obsolete.

Technologies are generally assessed when it is appropriate for a "typical" hospital (i.e., smaller than a tertiary care/medical center hospital but at least a 200-bed facility) to consider acquiring the technology, and sometimes when a technology may be unsafe or obsolete.

Properties: *Effectiveness;* safety; efficacy; cost; cost-effectiveness; service requirements; acceptance/adoption level; system impact; economic implications; ethical, legal, social implications.

Selection process: Assessment topics and priorities are set by ECRI/TAP staff. Decisions are based on their review of clinical journals, manufacturing/industry trade literature, and input from other ECRI staff (clinical/biomedical engineers, hospital consultants, etc.) who have contact with hospitals. A technology is reassessed when the previously published material becomes significantly outdated by more recent developments.

Methods: *Information syntheses,* expert opinion, group judgment, cost analyses.

A comprehensive review, evaluation, and synthesis of the published literature is at the core of the assessment process. ECRI in-house experts, nationally prominent clinicians, and others familiar with the technology conduct a thorough three-step review of draft assessment reports.

The average turnaround time from selection of assessment topic to reporting of findings is 2 to 3 months.

Assessors: The primary assessors are members of ECRI's interdisciplinary policy analysis staff which includes attorneys and experts in health care administration and planning. As needed, additional assessors are selected from ECRI's 120-member, full-time staff, or from among outside clinicians. The staff have expertise in medicine, engineering, and other relevant disciplines.

Assessment reports include: Abstract; the assessment's intended audience; the purpose of the assessment; relationship of this assessment to prior or concurrent assessments of the technology or other technologies intended for similar purposes; who sponsored/commissioned/supported the assessment; who conducted the assessment; description of the technology; stage of life-cycle of technology when assessed; properties assessed; procedure used for the assessment; sources of data/information; methods for collecting data/information; methods for analyzing/synthesizing data/information; results; findings or conclusions; limitations of findings; implications of findings for practice; recommendations for practice, future assessments, technology development, research; how the technology works, including theory, principles; development of the technology; procurement/deployment information; where technology is in use; regulatory agency approval status; coverage/reimbursement status of the technology.

Dissemination: Journal articles.

The assessment products are comprehensive assessment reports and *New Technology Briefs.* Both comprehensive technology assessment reports and *New Technology Briefs* are published, beginning with the January/February 1987 issue, in ECRI's new *Health Technology: Critical Issues for Decision Makers.* This journal combines two previous ECRI publications, the *Journal of Health Care Technology* and *Issues in Health Care Technology,* which had been published since 1984 and 1981, respectively. Copies of the assessments can be acquired by subscribing to *Health Technology* (either independently or by membership in the Health Devices Program) or purchasing single copies; reports are not available separately. Individual copies of back issues of the *Journal of Health Care Technology* may also be purchased from ECRI's Circulation Department.

Budget: $300,000. The approximate cost of an assessment ranges from $3,000 to $15,000 depending on the report's length and comprehensiveness. Funding sources: 67 percent sponsors/members dues, contributions; 33 percent subscriptions to *Health Technology*.

Use: Reports are used to support consulting and technical advice provided by ECRI personnel to hospitals. Based on responses from reader surveys, reports receive wide circulation in hospitals and are used for a variety of purposes, such as equipment acquisition and replacement decisions. Perhaps the most-cited of any assessment report is "Deaths during General Anesthesia," published in the *Journal of Health Care Technology* 1985;1:55-75, which was reprinted in full in the *Newsletter of the American Society of Anesthesiologists*.

ECRI assessment activities are described in Institute of Medicine, Committee on Evaluating Medical Technologies in Clinical Use. *Assessing medical technologies*. Washington, DC: National Academy Press, 1985.

Program evaluation: The only evaluations of the program have been reader surveys conducted on 3 occasions by the two ECRI predecessor publications.

Related activities: The Technology Assessment Program is closely related to ECRI's Health Devices Program (HDP); all HDP members receive *Health Technology* as one of their membership benefits. The ECRI/TAP staff also work closely with other ECRI activities. These include a technology risk management program that produces the four-volume *Hospital Risk Control* information service; accident investigation, forensic engineering, engineering, and management consultation; and field technical services for hospitals.

Completed Reports

ET1 ECRI Technology Assessment Program. Artificial urinary sphincters. Issues Health Care Technol 1986;sec.5.U.1. [Information syntheses]

ET2 ______. Automatic implantable cardioverter/defibrillator. Issues Health Care Technol 1986;sec.5.D.3. [Information syntheses]

ET3 ______. Bone mineral assessment, noninvasive (dual photon absorptiometry and quantitative computed tomography). J Health Care Technol 1986;2:183-200. [Information syntheses]

ET4 ______. Cardiokymography. Issues Health Care Technol 1986;sec.5.C.8. [Information syntheses]

ET5 ______. Chorionic villus sampling (CVS). Issues Health Care Technol 1986;sec.5.C.6. [Information syntheses]

ET6 ______. Clinical use of mass spectrometers. Issues Health Care Technol 1986;sec.5.M.2. [Information syntheses]

ET7 ______. Computer-processed EEG monitoring during surgery. Issues Health Care Technol 1986;sec.5.E.4. [Information syntheses]

ET8 ______. Extracorporeal membrane oxygenation (ECMO) for newborn respiratory failure. Issues Health Care Technol 1986;5.E.6. [Information syntheses]

ET9 ______. Gastric bubble. Issues Health Care Technol 1986;sec.5.G.1. [Information syntheses]

ET10 ______. Image transmission and data compression. J Health Care Technol 1986;3:83-93. [Information syntheses]

ET11 ______. Interpretive reporting of clinical laboratory test results. J Health Care Technol 1986;2:269-82. [Information syntheses]

ET12 ______. Legal system, insurance, and health care: the liability problem. J Health Care Technol 1986;2:247-68. [Information syntheses]

ET13 ______. Low-osmolality radiographic contrast agents. Issues Health Care Technol 1986;sec.5.L.4. [Information syntheses]

ET14 ______. Medicare payment for new technologies. J Health Care Technol 1986;3:13-32. [Information syntheses]

ET15 ______. Multichannel cochlear implants for profound deafness. Issues Health Care Technol 1986;sec.5.C.7. [Information syntheses]

ET16 ______. Percutaneous balloon valvuloplasty. Issues Health Care Technol 1986;sec.5.P.9. [Information syntheses]

ET17 ______. Percutaneous transluminal coronary angioplasty (PTCA). Issues Health Care Technol 1986;sec.5.P.2. [Information syntheses]

ET18 ______. Personal emergency response system (PERS). Issues Health Care Technol 1986;sec. 5.P.10. [Information syntheses]

ET19 ______. Physician office laboratories. J Health Care Technol 1986;3:95-115. [Information syntheses]

ET20 ______. Pulse oximeters. Issues Health Care Technol 1986;sec.5.O.1. [Information syntheses]

ET21 ______. SPECT imaging. J Health Care Technol 1986;3:33-62. [Information syntheses]

ET22 ______. Temporary external noninvasive pacemakers. Issues Health Care Technol 1986;sec.5.P.11. [Information syntheses]

ET23 ______. Three-dimensional computed tomography. Issues Health Care Technol 1986;sec.5.T.6. [Information syntheses]

ET24 ______. Two-dimensional Doppler echocardiography. Issues Health Care Technol 1986;sec.5.E.5. [Information syntheses]

ET25 ______. Urinalysis, automated. J Health Care Technol 1986;2:201-10. [Information syntheses]

ET26 ______. Angelchik gastroesophageal antireflux prosthesis. Issues Health Care Technol 1985;sec.5.A.4. [Information syntheses]

ET27 ______. Automated microbiology systems. Issues Health Care Technol 1985;sec.5.M.5. [Information syntheses]

ET28 ______. Automated microbiology systems. J Health Care Technol 1985;1:213-30. [Information syntheses]

ET29 ______. Bone marrow transplantation. Issues Health Care Technol 1985;sec.5.B.5. [Information syntheses]

ET30 ______. CT-assisted stereotactic neurosurgery. Issues Health Care Technol 1985;sec.5.S.3. [Information syntheses]

ET31 ______. Continuous passive motion (CPM) devices. Issues Health Care Technol 1985;sec.5.C.4. [Information syntheses]

ET32 ______. Deaths during general anesthesia. J Health Care Technol 1985;1:155-75. [Information syntheses]

ET33 ______. Digital subtraction angiography (DSA). J Health Care Technol 1985;1:177-212. [Information syntheses]

ET34 ______. Freestanding imaging centers. J Health Care Technol 1985;1:257-278. [Information syntheses]

ET35 ______. Hyperthermia treatment of tumors. Issues Health Care Technol 1985;sec.5.H.2. [Information syntheses]

ET36 ______. Imatron high-speed CT scanner. Issues Health Care Technol 1985;sec.5.C.5. [Information synthesis]

ET37 ______. Implantable vascular access ports. Issues Health Care Technology 1985;sec.5.V.2. [Information syntheses]

ET38 ______. Laser angioplasty for atherosclerosis. Issues Health Care Technol 1985;sec.5.L.3. [Information syntheses]

ET39 ______. Leukocyte differential counters, automated. J Health Care Technol 1985;2:51-72. [Information syntheses]

ET40 ______. Magnetic resonance imaging (MRI). J Health Care Technol 1985;2:23-50. [Information syntheses]

ET41 ______. Monitoring of exhaled CO2 levels during anesthesia. Issues Health Care Technol 1985;sec.5.M.4. [Information syntheses]

ET42 ______. Patient-controlled analgesia. Issues Health Care Technol 1985;sec.5.P.8. [Information syntheses]

ET43 ______. Streptokinase thrombolysis of coronary arteries. Issues Health Care Technol 1985;sec.5.T.1. [Information syntheses]

ET44 ______. Therapeutic apheresis. J Health Care Technol 1985;1:279-98. [Information syntheses]

ET45 ______. Thermography for breast cancer prescreening. Issues Health Care Technol 1985;sec.5.T.5. [Information syntheses]

ET46 ______. Tumor markers. J Health Care Technol 1985;2:105-28. [Information syntheses]

ET47 ______. Two-dimensional Doppler echocardiography. J Health Care Technol 1985;2:129-50. [Information syntheses]

ET48 ______. Cementless hip prosthesis. Issues Health Care Technol 1984;sec.5.H.3. [Information syntheses]

ET49 ______. Digital imaging storage and retrieval. J Health Care Technol 1984;1:13-38. [Information syntheses]

ET50 ______. Dual-photon absorptiometry for bone mineral content. Issues Health Care Technol 1984;sec.5.A.3. [Information syntheses]

ET51 ______. Extracorporeal shock-wave lithotripsy (ESWL). Issues Health Care Technol 1984;sec.5.L.2. [Information syntheses]

ET52 ______. Percutaneous nephrostomy. Issues Health Care Technol 1984;sec.5.N.1. [Information syntheses]

ET53 ______. Photoradiation therapy (PRT) of tumors. Issues Health Care Technol 1984;sec.5.P.6. [Information syntheses]

ET54 ______. Plasminogen activator thrombolysis of coronary arteries. Issues Health Care Technol 1984;sec.5.T.4. [Information syntheses]

ET55 ______. Plethysmography for diagnosing deep vein thrombosis. Issues Health Care Technol 1984;sec.5.P.7. [Information syntheses]

ET56 ______. Prenatal alpha-fetoprotein (AFP) testing. Issues Health Care Technol 1984;sec.5.A.2. [Information syntheses]

ET57 ______. Surgery for morbid obesity. Issues Health Care Technol 1984;sec.5.S.2. [Information syntheses]

ET58 ______. Therapeutic drug monitoring (TDM). J Health Care Technol 1984;1:39-61. [Information syntheses]

ET59 ______. Transcatheter therapeutic embolization. Issues Health Care Technol 1984;sec.5.E.3. [Information syntheses]

ET60 ______. X-ray image digitizing systems. Issues Health Care Technol 1984;sec.5.D.4. [Information syntheses]

ET61 ______. Chemonucleolysis of herniated lumbar disks. Issues Health Care Technol 1983;sec.5.C.3. [Information syntheses]

ET62 ______. Collagen implants for smoothing skin. Issues Health Care Technol 1983;sec.5.C.2. [Information syntheses]

ET63 ______. Digital radiography and fluoroscopy. Issues Health Care Technol 1983;sec.5.D.2. [Information syntheses]

ET64 ______. Mobile computerized ECG interpretive systems. Issues Health Care Technol 1983;sec.5.E.2. [Information syntheses]

ET65 ______. Noninvasive bilirubinometers. Issues Health Care Technol 1983;sec.5.B.4. [Information syntheses]

ET66 ______. Penile prostheses. Issues Health Care Technol 1983;sec.5.P.5. [Information syntheses]

ET67 ______. Percutaneous lithotripsy of kidney stones. Issues Health Care Technol 1983;sec.5.L.1. [Information syntheses]

ET68 ______. Percutaneous transluminal angioplasty (PTA) of peripheral arteries. Issues Health Care Technol 1983;sec.5.P.4. [Information syntheses]

ET69 ______. Single-channel cochlear implants for profound deafness. Issues Health Care Technol 1983;sec.5.C.1. [Information syntheses]

ET70 ______. Transcutaneous CO2 monitors. Issues Health Care Technol 1983;sec.5.M.3. [Information syntheses]

ET71 ______. Transdermal delivery of nitroglycerin. Issues Health Care Technol 1983;sec.5.T.2. [Information syntheses]

ET72 ______. Transrectal ultrasound of the prostate. Issues Health Care Technol 1983;sec.5.T.3. [Information syntheses]

ET73 ______. Automatic indirect blood pressure monitors. Issues Health Care Technol 1982;sec.5.B.2. [Information syntheses]

ET74 ______. Blood substitute. Issues Health Care Technol 1982;sec.5.B.3. [Information syntheses]

ET75 ______. Diagnostic and operative arthroscopy. Issues Health Care Technol 1982;sec.5.A.1. [Information syntheses]

ET76 ______. Dual-energy scanned projection radiography. Issues Health Care Technol 1982;sec.5.D.1. [Information syntheses]

ET77 ______. Hyperbaric oxygen (HBO) therapy. Issues Health Care Technol 1982;sec.5.H.1. [Information syntheses]

ET78 ______. Implantable drug infusion pumps. Issues Health Care Technol 1982;sec.5.I.4. [Information syntheses]

ET79 ______. Intra-aortic balloon pumps. Issues Health Care Technol 1982;sec.5.I.3. [Information syntheses]

ET80 ______. Multiprogrammable pacemakers. Issues Health Care Technol 1982;sec.5.P.3. [Information syntheses]

ET81 ______. Multiprogrammable pacemakers. Issues Health Care Technol 1982;sec.5.P.3. [Information syntheses]

ET82 ______. Radial keratotomy. Issues Health Care Technol 1982;sec.5.R.1. [Information syntheses]

ET83 ______. Bone growth stimulators. Issues Health Care Technol 1981;sec.5.B.1. [Information syntheses]

ET84 ______. Evoked potential (EP) response measurement. Issues Health Care Technol 1981;sec.5.E.1. [Information syntheses]

ET85 ______. High-frequency ventilators. Issues Health Care Technol 1981;sec.5.V.1. [Information syntheses]

ET86 ______. Insulin delivery devices. Issues Health Care Technol 1981;sec.5.I.2. [Information syntheses]

ET87 ______. Insulin infusion systems (controlled). Issues Health Care Technol 1981;sec.5.I.1. [Information syntheses]

ET88 ______. Noninvasive blood gas oxygen monitors. Issues Health Care Technol 1981;sec.5.M.1. [Information syntheses]

ET89 ______. Remote control fluoroscopy units. Issues Health Care Technol 1981;sec.5.F.1. [Information syntheses]

ET90 ______. Therapeutic plasmapheresis. Issues Health Care Technol 1981;sec.5.P.1. [Information syntheses]

Food and Drug Administration

5600 Fishers Lane
Rockville, MD 20857
301-443-5470

Individual profiles on the Food and Drug Administration's Center for Devices and Radiological Health, Center for Drugs and Biologics, and the Center for Food Safety and Applied Nutrition follow this overview of the agency.

The Food and Drug Administration (FDA) is a component of the Public Health Service (PHS) within the U.S. Department of Health and Human Services (DHHS). Its purpose is to ensure that: (1) food is safe and wholesome; (2) drugs (both human and veterinary), biological products, such as vaccines and blood for transfusion, and medical devices are safe and effective; (3) cosmetics are safe; (4) the use of radiological products does not result in unnecessary exposure to radiation; and (5) all of these products are honestly and informatively labeled.

The FDA accomplishes its mission through premarket clearance; monitoring, using inspections, investigations, and surveillance; compliance activities involving corrections and penalties; promulgation of regulations; and bioresearch monitoring and good laboratory practices.

The body of law defining FDA's authority is comprehensive, providing a variety of controls required by the nature of the market, the products, and potential risks.

Statutes include: the Food, Drug, and Cosmetic Act (FD&C Act); the Public Health Service Act (PHS Act of 1944); the Fair Packaging and Labeling Act of 1966; and the Orphan Drug Act of 1983.

Federal laws define the requirements applicable to firms dealing in interstate commerce, as well as the authority of the agency that will administer and enforce each law. The FDA must make regulations telling how the law is to be applied. Regulations also describe the approval processes for many individual products and set forth required standards of product composition or performance. All FDA regulations, amendments, and other notices are published in the *Federal Register,* issued daily by the Federal Government.

The FDA's principal components include: the Commissioner, Deputy Commissioner, and the staff and line organizations. The line organizations concerned with technology assessment are the four product-oriented centers: Center for Devices and Radiological Health, Center for Drugs and Biologics, Center for Food Safety and Applied Nutrition, and the Center for Veterinary Medicine. The first three are described separately in this directory. The National Center for Toxicological Research is a part of FDA's science foundation.

The Center for Devices and Radiological Health is responsible for ensuring the safety and effectiveness (efficacy) of medical devices, as provided for by the 1976 Medical Device Amendments to the Food, Drug, and Cosmetic Act; and eliminating unnecessary human exposure to man-made radiation from medical, occupational, and consumer products, as provided for by the Radiation Control for Health and Safety Act of 1968.

The Center for Drugs and Biologics (CDB) is responsible for ensuring that all human-use drugs and biologics manufactured for interstate sale are safe and effective (efficacious) and that product labeling is truthful and informative.

The Center for Food Safety and Applied Nutrition (CFSAN) regulates foods and cosmetics to ensure that foods are pure and wholesome, safe to eat, and produced under sanitary conditions; that cosmetics are safe and made from appropriate ingredients; and that the labeling of foods and cosmetics is truthful and informative.

General information on the FDA's other functions may be obtained from the Associate Commissioner for Consumer Affairs at the above address. News of FDA activities is also available through the *FDA Consumer,* a magazine issued 10 times a year by the U.S. Government Printing Office, Washington, DC 20402; stock no. 717-009-00000-2; $17 per year.

Food and Drug Administration
Center for Devices and Radiological Health

12720 Twinbrook Parkway
Rockville, MD 20857
301-443-5807

Contact: Bobbi Dresser, Program Analyst, (for general information).

Overview: The FDA Center for Devices and Radiological Health (CDRH) is responsible for ensuring the safety and effectiveness (efficacy) of medical devices, as provided for by the 1976 Medical Device Amendments to the Food, Drug, and Cosmetic Act; and eliminating unnecessary human exposure to man-made radiation from medical, occupational, and consumer products, as provided for by the Radiation Control for Health and Safety (RCHS) Act of 1968.

CDRH classifies each type of device into the appropriate regulatory control category (Class I, devices requiring only general controls; Class II, devices requiring standards; and Class III, devices requiring premarket approval). CDRH applies general controls, such as labeling, registration, listing, Good Manufacturing Practices, and repair/replace/refund requirements. It develops performance standards for Class II devices; conducts premarket review of new devices through the premarket notification, premarket approval, and product development protocol provisions of the Amendments; and encourages the discovery and development of useful new devices, while protecting the rights and safety of human subjects in testing of devices.

In the area of radiological health, CDRH conducts epidemiological and experimental research to assess the risk from various forms and sources of radiation; develops radiation measurement instruments and methods useful in evaluating radiation-emitting devices and products; develops performance standards for radiation-emitting devices and products; develops guidelines for the use of radiation-emitting devices and products to prevent unnecessary radiation exposure; and implements survey programs to determine trends in, and the current state of the use of radiation-emitting devices and products.

The CDRH review and approval process generates Premarket Approval Applications (PMAs), Summaries of Safety and Effectiveness Data (SSED), and other reports.

Purpose: To ensure the safety and effectiveness of medical devices; to eliminate unnecessary human exposure to man-made radiation from medical, occupational, and consumer products; and to educate consumers, industry, and health professionals to enable them to make more informed judgments.

(Note: CDRH assessment activities primarily address *efficacy* as the term is used in this Directory, especially with regard to premarket approval of new devices. The agency uses the term *effectiveness* in characterizing its activities because this term is used in the agency's legislative language.)

Primary intended users: General public; people concerned about their health; patients; providers, generally; health product manufacturers.

Technologies: *Devices,* medical or surgical procedure, support system.

Intervention: *Diagnosis, treatment,* prevention.

Stage: *Emerging, new,* established or widespread practice, obsolete.

Emerging and new technologies are assessed to prevent problems; mature technologies are assessed to solve problems.

Properties: *Safety; efficacy;* effectiveness.

Medical devices are assessed for safety and effectiveness (efficacy) in their broadest sense; certain radiological screening procedures are also assessed for medical productivity.

Selection process: Manufacturers submit an application to initiate PMAs. Other topics are selected internally and assessment of topic priorities are established as part of the program planning process. New information, particularly awareness of an unforeseen problem, can lead to reassessment.

Methods: *Information syntheses, group judgment,* expert opinion for device premarketing approval; also, epidemiological and other observational methods for postmarketing surveillance of devices and for radiological health.

The assessment process is usually conducted by panels who base their assessments on information synthesized by CDRH staff. Some assessments are prepared internally by the scientific staff.

PMAs have a statutory turnaround time of 180 days; other projects may average 2 to 3 years, with a range from 1 to 5 years.

Assessors: The panel members are usually clinicians who are experts in the field and may be experienced in the use of similar technologies.

Assessment reports include: Abstract; the assessment's intended audience; the purpose of the assessment; relationship of this assessment to prior or concurrent assessments of the technology or other technologies intended for similar purposes; who sponsored/commissioned/supported the assessment; who conducted the assessment; description of the technology; stage of life-cycle of technology when assessed; properties assessed; procedure used for the assessment; sources of data/information; methods for collecting data/information; methods for analyzing/synthesizing data/information; results; findings or conclusions; limitations of findings; implications of findings for practice; recommendations for practice, future assessments, technology development, research; development of the technology; regulatory agency approval status; summary of pre-clinical and clinical data.

Dissemination: Printed reports, journal articles.

Reports are available from either the National Technical Information Service, 5285 Port Royal Rd., Springfield, VA 22161 or the Superintendent of Documents, U.S. Government Printing Office, Washington, DC 20402. Assessment results may also be published in the *Federal Register.*

Budget: Not provided. The approximate cost for a PMA is $24,000 and for x-ray criteria, $270,000. Funding source: 100 percent parent organization.

Use: SSEDs, by statute, are required for the information of parties outside the organization. Other types of assessments are used to develop educational or regulatory strategies. Based on requests for copies and references in other documents, the assessments are used by manufacturers, other government agencies, and foreign governments. Modifications of medical practice indicate that physicians also use the assessments.

Related activities: CDRH coordinates several postmarketing surveillance activities for medical devices and in vitro diagnostic (laboratory) products. The Device Experience Network (DEN) is a computer database system that collects, stores, and retrieves problem reports for these products submitted voluntarily by health professionals. The Medical Device and Laboratory Product Problem Reporting Program (PRP) provides DEN with its primary source of device experience information. PRP is funded by FDA, and is conducted by the United States Pharmacopeia. The Medical Device Reporting (MDR) database, established following enactment of the 1984 MDR regulations, contains mandatory reports from manufacturers and importers pertaining to device performance failures and malfunctions that have resulted in injury, death, or any hazard to safety.

Completed Reports

FA1 Alcon Laboratories, Inc. [Food and Drug Administration, Center for Devices and Radiological Health] Scanlens (Scafilcon A contact lens): summary of safety and effectiveness. 1987 Jan 16. (PMA no. P850033-000).

FA2 Paragon Optical Inc. [______] Paraperm E.W. blue rigid gas permeable contact len: summary of safety and effectiveness. 1987 Feb 18. (PMA no. P850038-000).

FA3 Precision-Cosmet., Inc. [______] Kelman (TM) omnifit II model 2100: summary of safety and effectiveness. 1987 Feb 2. (PMA no. P850059-000).

FA4 Scimed Life Systems, Inc. [______] Scimed PTCA dilatation catheter: summary of safety and effectiveness. 1987 Jan 16. (PMA no. P860019-000).

FA5 Stericon Laboratories. [______] Stericon saline solution: summary of safety and effectiveness. 1987 Jan 16. (PMA no. P850070-000).

FA6 Abbott Laboratories. [______] Abbott anti-delta diagnostic kit (RIA): summary of safety and effectiveness. 1986 Aug 7. (PMA no. P850062-000).

FA7 Advanced Biosearch Assn. [______] Orthopak (R) bone growth stimulator: summary of safety and effectiveness. 1986 Apr 9. (PMA no. P850022-000).

FA8 Akorn, Inc. [______] Sodium chloride tablets, USP: summary of safety and effectiveness. 1986 Mar 14. (PMA no. 850037-000).

FA9 Allergan Pharmaceuticals, Inc. [______] Oxysept system: summary of safety and effectiveness. 1986 Nov 20. (PMA no. P850088-000).

FA10 American Edwards Division of American Supply Corporation. [______] Duromedics bileaflet heart valve: summary of safety and effectiveness. 1986 Sep 26. (PMA no. P850006-000).

FA11 American Edwards Laboratories. [______] Amer. Ed. Labs. PTCA: summary of safety and effectiveness. 1986 Jul 9. (PMA no. P850021-000).

FA12 American Medical Electronics, Inc. [______] Physio-stim (TM) I & II Model 6000 & 7000: summary of safety and effectiveness. 1986 Apr 18. (PMA no. P850007-000).

FA13 Barnes-Hind Inc. [______] Softmate (R) hydrogen peroxide disinfection system: summary of safety and effectiveness. 1986 Oct 6. (PMA no. P840066-000).

FA14 Bausch & Lomb (R). [______] B & L (R) (Amefocon A) oxygen permeable lens: summary of safety and effectiveness. 1986 Aug 7. (PMA no. P830050-000).

FA15 Bausch & Lomb (R). [______] B & L sterile all purpose solution & contact cleaner: summary of safety and effectiveness. 1986 Dec 16. (PMA no. P830002-000).

FA16 Bausch & Lomb. [______] B & L Sensitive Eyes (TM) saline/cleaning solution: summary of safety and effectiveness. 1986 Jul 7. (PMA no. 850036-000).

FA17 Bausch & Lomb. [______] B & L Therma-zyne, Fizziclean: summary of safety and effectiveness. 1986 Nov 5. (PMA no. P850093-000).

FA18 Bausch & Lomb. [______] Sensitive eyes chemical disinfectant: summary of safety and effectiveness. 1986 Jan 2. (PMA no. P840020-000).

FA19 Bausch & Lomb. [______] Silsoft (Elastofilcon A) contact lenses: summary of safety and effectiveness. 1986 Feb 2. (PMA no. P850068-000).

FA20 Blairex Laboratories, Inc. [______] Blairex sterile saline solution: summary of safety and effectiveness. 1986 Mar 6. (PMA no. P850045-000).

FA21 Briggs Ophthalmics Corp. [______] Sunsoft (Methafilcon A) hydrophilic contact lens: summary of safety and effectiveness. 1986 Aug 7. (PMA no. P850077-001).

FA22 Briggs Ophthalmics Corporation. [______] Sunsoft (Methafilcon A) hydrophilic contact lens: summary of safety and effectiveness. 1986 Mar 28. (PMA no. P850077-000).

FA23 CTL, Inc. [______] Customeyes (TM) 45L & 55L (Bufilcon A): summary of safety and effectiveness. 1986 Jul 1. (PMA no. P850057-000).

FA24 CTL, Inc. [______] Customeyes 70L & 79L (Lidofilcon A & B): summary of safety and efectiveness. 1986 Jul 1. (PMA no. P850058-000).

FA25 Cardiac Pacemakers, Inc. [______] Models 925, 2040, 2041, 6564: summary of safety and effectiveness. 1986 Jan 24. (PMA no. P840068-000).

FA26 Carl Zeiss, Inc. [______] Visulas Nd:Yag laser: summary of safety and effectiveness. 1986 Aug 7. (PMA no. P850083-000).

FA27 Cilco, Inc. [______] Sodium chrondroitin sulfate: summary of safety and effectiveness. 1986 Nov 5. (PMA no. P820079-000).

FA28 Cilco. [______] Viscoat (TM): summary of safety and effectiveness. 1986 Jun 6. (PMA no.P840064-000).

FA29 Coast Contact Lens, Inc. [______] Hydra (Methafilcon A) contact lens: summary of safety and effectiveness. 1986 Aug 7. (PMA no. P850079-001).

FA30 Coast Contact Lens, Inc. [______] Hydrasoft (Methafilcon A) contact lens: summary of safety and effectiveness. 1986 Mar 28. (PMA no. P850079-000).

FA31 Coburn Optical Industries. [______] Intraocular lens: summary of safety and effectiveness. 1986 Dec 16. (PMA no. P860002-000).

FA32 Coburn Optical. [______] J loop posterior chamber type II 0 & I0: summary of safety and effectiveness. 1986 Jul 1. (PMA no. P840039-000).

FA33 Coherent Medical Division. [______] Neodymium:Yag ophthalmic laser system 9900: summary of safety and effectiveness. 1986 Dec 31. (PMA no. P830054-000).

FA34 Coopervision Cilco. [______] Optiflex anterior chamber lenses (L1-L5): summary of safety and effectiveness. 1986 Jun 18. (PMA no. P8200035-000).

FA35 Coopervision Cilco. [______] SM-1, CR-1, & GR-1 IOLS: summary of safety and effectiveness. 1986 Jun 11. (PMA no. P840060-000).

FA36 Coopervision, Inc. [______] Coopervision peroxide system: summary of safety and effectiveness. 1986 Mar 12. (PMA no. P830023-000).

FA37 Coopervision, Inc. [______] Mirasoak (TM) rinsing, disinfecting & storage solution: summary of safety and effectiveness. 1986 Aug 18. (PMA no. P810038-000).

FA38 Coopervision. [______] Miraflow extra strength cleaner: summary of safety and effectiveness. 1986 Nov 5. (PMA no. P850055-000).

FA39 Corometrics Medical Systems, Inc. [______] Model 515 neonatal monitor: summary of safety and effectiveness. 1986 Jan 31. (PMA no. P840037-000).

FA40 Custom Tint Lab., Inc. [______] Permatint (R): summary of safety and effectiveness. 1986 Mar 14. (PMA no. P820059-000).

FA41 Custom Tint Lab., Inc. [______] Permatint (R): summary of safety and effectiveness. 1986 Mar 26. (PMA no. P820059-000).

FA42 Datoscope Corporation. [______] Novacol (TM) textured collagen hemostatic agent: summary of safety and effectiveness. 1986 Jul 7. (PMA no. P850023-000).

FA43 Dey Laboratories, Inc. [______] Dey-vial (R): summary of safety and effectiveness. 1986 Apr 1. (PMA no.P840061-000).

FA44 Elscint, Inc. [______] Gyrex, models S3500 & S5000: summary of safety and effectiveness. 1986 Sep 9. (PMA no. P840007-000).

FA45 Ethicon, Inc. [______] PDS suture (dyed): summary of safety and effectiveness. 1986 Jul 22. (PMA no. N18331-016).

FA46 Food and Drug Administration, Center for Devices and Radiological Health. A practioner's guide to the ultrasonic therapy equipment standard. 1986. (NTIS Order No. PB86-113933/AS).

FA47 ______. Basic concepts in the selection of patients for dental x-ray examinations. 1986. (GPO Stock No. 017-015-00230-6, NTIS Order No. PB86-126067/AS).

FA48 ______. Computer program for absorbed dose to the breast in mammography. 1986. (GPO Stock No. 017-015-00228-4, NTIS Order No. PB86-114774/AS).

FA49 ______. Embryo, fetus, infant . . . recommendations to minimize diagnostic nuclear medicine exposure. 1986. (FDA Pub No. FDA86-8254).

FA50 ______. Evaluation of radiation exposure from diagnostic radiology examinations—technique/exposure guides for the craniocaudal projection in mammography. 1986. (NTIS Order No. PB86-126075/AS).

FA51 ______. Evaluation of radiation exposure from diagnostic radiology examinations: general recommendations. 1986. (NTIS Order No. PB86-125903/AS).

FA52 ______. Problem definition study: rubella antibody testing. 1986. (NTIS Order No. PB86-131935).

FA53 ______. Recommendations for evaluation of radiation exposure from diagnostic radiology examinations. 1986. (NTIS Order No. PB86-125846/AS).

FA54 ______. To cement or not to cement? or has the FDA approved the use of this device? 1986. (FDA Pub No. FDA86-4202).

FA55 Gambro, Inc. [______] Gambro fiber plasmafilter: summary of safety and effectiveness. 1986 Jul 7. (PMA no. P83006-000).

FA56 Gish Biomedical, Inc. [______] Micro Yag Nd:Yag laser system: summary of safety and effectiveness. 1986 May 30. (PMA no. P850063-000).

FA57 Gynotech, Inc. [______] Dilapan (TM): summary of safety and effectiveness. 1986 Jun 11. (PMA no. P840045-000).

FA58 Helitrex, Inc. [______] Collacote (TM): summary of safety and effectiveness. 1986 Jan 2. (PMA no. P840062-000).

FA59 Hilitrex, Inc. [______] Helistat (TM) absorbable collagen hemostatic sponge: summary of safety and effectiveness. 1986 Jan 2. (PMA no. P850010-000).

FA60 Hybritech Inc. [______] Tandem (R)-R carcinoembryonic antigen assay: summary of safety and effectiveness. 1986 Jul 1. (PMA no. P840019-000).

FA61 Hybritech Inc. [______] Tandem-R PSA immunoradiometric assay: summary of safety and effectiveness. 1986 Apr 9. (PMA no. P850048-000).

FA62 Iolab Corp. [______] Model 91-50 IOL: summary of safety and effectiveness. 1986 Feb 14. (PMA no. P820044-000).

FA63 Iolab. [______] Microruptor MR-2 Nd:Yag laser system: summary of safety and effectiveness. 1986 Mar 28 (PMA no. P840012-000).

FA64 Kontur Kontact Lens Co. Inc. [______] Kontur soft (Methafilcon A) contact lens: summary of safety and effectiveness. 1986 Aug 7. (PMA no. P850078-000).

FA65 Kontur Kontact Lens Co. Inc. [______] Kontur soft (Methafilcon A) contact lens: summary of safety and effectiveness. 1986 Mar 28. (PMA no. P850078-000).

FA66 Litton Datamedix. [______] Litton transcutaneous C02 system: summary of safety and effectiveness. 1986 Sep 26. (PMA no. P850087-000).

FA67 Medi-tech. [______] Med-tech coronary balloon dilatation catheter system: summary of safety and effectiveness. 1986 Feb 10. (PMA no. P840040-000).

FA68 Medtronic, Inc. [______] Activitrax models 8400, 8402, 8403: summary of safety and effectiveness. 1986 Jul 11. (PMA no. P850051-000).

FA69 Medtronic, Inc. [______] Medtronic (R) scoliosis system, model 3100-2: summary of safety and effectiveness. 1986 Jan 2. (PMA no. P840022-000).

FA70 Medtronic, Inc. [______] Steroid tip (TM) model 4503 & 4003 transvenous pacing: summary of safety and effectiveness. 1986 Aug 22. (PMA no. P830061-000).

FA71 Medtronic. [______] Model 5525 transvenous atrial & Model 5025 ventrical: summary of safety and effectiveness. 1986 Aug 22. (PMA no. P850089-000).

FA72 N & N Menicon Inc. [______] (Mafilcon) soft contact lenses: summary of safety and effectiveness. 1986 Dec 17. (PMA no. PB00031-000).

FA73 National Patent Development Corp. [______] GE-101E caries removal agent/system: summary of safety and effectiveness. 1986 May 2. (PMA no. P830035-000).

FA74 Oculua Contact Lens Company. [______] Ocusil (TM) contact lens: summary of safety and effectiveness. 1986 Jan2. (PMA no. P840050-000).

FA75 Ocumed Inc. [______] Sodium chloride tablets 250 MG: summary of safety and effectiveness. 1986 Mar 12. (PMA no. P850016-000).

FA76 Optical Radiation Corporation. [______] Styles 31-34 posterior IOLS: summary of safety and effectiveness. 1986 Jun 18. (PMA no. P830056-000).

FA77 Organon Teknika Corp. [______] Hepanostika (TM) HBEAG/anti HBE microelisa (TM) system: summary of safety and effectiveness. 1986 Jul 1. (PMA no. P840070-000).

FA78 Pacemaker Systems, Inc. a Siemens Co. [______] DDD pulse generator 674: summary of safety and effectiveness. 1986 Sep 8. (PMA no. P840014-000).

FA79 Paco Pharmaceutical Services, Inc. [______] Nonpreserved saline solution: summary of safety and effectiveness. 1986 Sep 23. (PMA no. P850025-000).

FA80 Paco Pharmaceutical Services, Inc. [______] Sorbic acid preserved daily cleaner: summary of safety and effectiveness. 1986 Nov 10. (PMA no. P850076-000).

FA81 Paco Pharmaceutical Services, Inc. [______] Sorbic acid preserved lens lubricant: summary of safety and effectiveness. 1986 Oct 9. (PMA no. P850075-000).

FA82 Paco Research Corp. [______] Charter Labs saline solution: summary of safety and effectiveness. 1986 Dec 17. (PMA no. P840069-000).

FA83 Permeable Contact Lenses, Inc. [______] SGP lens (TM): summary of safety and effectiveness. 1986 Jan 21. (PMA no. P840055-000).

FA84 Phillips Medical Systems, Inc. [______] Gyroscan (TM): summary of safety and effectiveness. 1986 Sep 16. (PMA no. P840063-000).

FA85 Roche Diagnostic Systems. [______] Cobas bact: summary of safety and effectiveness. 1986 Jul 7. (PMA no. P840065-000).

FA86 Sarn, Inc. [______] Therapore (TM) system: summary of safety and effectiveness. 1986 Dec 24. (PMA no. 850092-000).

FA87 Seecor, Inc. [______] Stat-Pace II: summary of safety and effectiveness. 1986 Jul 1. (PMA no.P840002-000).

FA88 Sharplan Lasers Inc. [______] Model 702: summary of safety and effectiveness. 1986 May 8. (PMA no. P850060-000).

FA89 Sorin Biomedica, Fiat, USA Inc. [______] AB-Core K hepatitis B core antigen 1251: summary of safety and effectiveness. 1986 Apr 10. (PMA no. P850044-000).

FA90 Stericon Laboratories. [______] Crystalens saline spray: summary of safety and effectiveness. 1986 Mar 24. (PMA no. P850065-000).

FA91 Syntex Opthalmics Inc. [______] Polycon contact lens: summary of safety and effectiveness. 1986 Feb 10.(PMA no. N18120-015).

FA92 Telectronics LTD. [______] Telectronics pasar model 4171 PG: summary of safety and effectiveness. 1986 Nov 10. (PMA no. P850027-000).

FA93 Thompson CGR Medical Corp. [______] Magniscan 5000 MRI System: summary of safety and effectiveness. 1986 Oct 6. (PMA no. 850043-000).

FA94 Toray Industries Inc. [______] Toray soft contact lenses: summary of safety and effectiveness. 1986 Mar 5. (PMA no. P840044-000).

FA95 Travenol Labs, Inc. [______] Gamma dab (1251) AFP RIA kit: summary of safety and effectiveness. 1986 Jun 17. (PMA no. P790032-000).

FA96 UCO Optics, Inc. [______] Aquasept II: summary of safety and effectiveness. 1986 Feb 14. (PMA no. N17679-008).

FA97 University Optical Products Co. [______] The Boston lens II Alges (R) bifocal contact lens: summary of safety and effectiveness. 1986 Jan 24. (PMA no. P850008-000).

FA98 University Optical Products Company. [______] Alges (TM) (Hefilcon A) contact lens: summary of safety and effectiveness. 1986 Apr 28. (PMA no. P850002-000).

FA99 W.L. Gore & Assoc., Inc. [______] Gore-Tex (R) expanded PTFE suture: summary of safety and effectiveness.1986 Feb 28. (PMA no. P820083-000).

FA100 W.L. Gore & Associates, Inc. [______] Gore-tex expanded PTFE prosthetic ligament: summary of safety and effectiveness. 1986 Nov 18. (PMA no. P850074-000).

FA101 Wesley-Jessen. [______] Durasoft 4 (ofilcon A) spherical hydrophilic lens: summary of safety and effectiveness. 1986 Aug 14. (PMA no. P85).

FA102 Alcon Labs., Inc. [______] Polquat disinfection system: summary of safety and effectiveness. 1985 Sep 18. (PMA no. P830034-000).

FA103 Allergan. [______] Model no. ALS-IV heat disinfection unit: summary of safety and effectiveness. 1985 May 20. (PMA no. P840054-000).

FA104 Bausch & Lomb. [______] B & L 58 (TM) (Etafilcona) contact lens: summary of safety and effectiveness. 1985 Sep 23. (PMA no. P850039-000).

FA105 Bausch & Lomb. [______] B & L Sensitive Eyes (TM) daily cleaner: summary of safety and effectiveness. 1985 Jul 9. (PMA no. P830013-000).

FA106 Cardiac Pacemakers, Inc. [______] AID-B automatic implantable cardiovertor defibrillator: summary of safety and effectiveness. 1985 Nov 15. (PMA no. P830060-000).

FA107 Centers for Disease Control. [______] AFP mid-pregnancy reference preparation: summary of safety and effectiveness. 1985 Jan 3 (PMA no. P820077-000).

FA108 Cilco. [______] Cilco Nd:Yag laser: summary of safety and effectiveness. 1985 Sep 11. (PMA no. P840047-000).

FA109 Clin-Therm Corporation. [______] Clini-Therm Mark I/IV: summary of safety and effectiveness. 1985 Sep 11. (PMA no. P840015-000).

FA110 Coopervision Inc. [______] Horizon (TM) Yag laser model 2000: summary of safety and effectiveness. 1985 Aug 15. (PMA no. P850001-000).

FA111 Davis & Geck. [______] Novafil (TM): summary of safety and effectiveness. 1985 Nov 18. (PMA no. P840041-000).

FA112 Depuy, Inc. [______] New Jersey integrated knee replacement system: summary of safety and effectiveness. 1985 May 20. (PMA no. P830055-000).

FA113 Depuy, Inc. [______] New Jersey integrated knee replacement system: summary of safety and effectiveness. 1985 May 20. (PMA no. P830055-002).

FA114 Dornier System GMBH. [______] Dornier lithotripter, model HM3: summary of safety and effectiveness. 1985 Jan 16. (PMA no. P840008-000).

FA115 Drs. Lloyd and Mary Garren. [______] Garren gastric bubble: summary of safety and efectiveness. 1985 Oct 29.(PMA no. P840025-000).

FA116 Food and Drug Administration, Center for Devices and Radiological Health. Assessment and modification of clinical utility in diagnostic radiology: the oral cholecystogram and the upper gastrointestinal examinations. 1985. (NTIS order no. PB-85-246916/AS).

FA117 ______. Evaluation of radiation exposure from diagnostic radiology examinations (technique/exposure guides for the dental bitewing projection). 1985. (FDA pub no. 85-8245).

FA118 ______. Extremity radiography following trauma: an overview. 1985. (GPO Stock No. 017-015-00224-1, NTIS order no. PB85-115053).

FA119 ______. Handbook of glandular tissue doses in mammography. 1985. (NTIS order no. PB85-209914/AS).

FA120 ______. Patient exposure reduction during scoliosis radiography. 1985. (GPO stock no. 017-015-00227-6).

FA121 ______. Quality control guide for sunlamp products. 1985. (NTIS order no. PB85-124808).

FA122 ______. Recommendations for quality assurance programs in nuclear medicine facilities. (GPO stock no. 017-015-00225-0, NTIS order no. 85-145720/AS).

FA123 ______. Reducing patient exposure during scoliosis radiography. 1985. (FDA pub no. FDA 85-8252).

FA124 ______. Surface cracking of polyurethane tubing resulting from subcutaneous implantation in dogs. 1985. (NTIS order no. PB85-171619/AS).

FA125 ______. Therapeutic microwave and shortwave diathermy: a review of thermal effectiveness, safe use, and state of the art: 1984. 1985. (GPO stock no. 017-015-00226-8, NTIS order no. PB85-170165/AS).

FA126 Frigitronics, Inc. [______] Saturn II (TM) (Synergicon A) contact lens: summary of safety and effectiveness. 1985 Mar 22 (PMA no. P840004-000).

FA127 General Electric, Co. [______] GE signa magnetic resonance diagnostic imaging system: summary of safety and effectiveness. 1985 Jun 5. (PMA no. P830074-000)/

FA128 Heyer Schulte Corp. [______] Sauflon (R) PW (Lidofilcon B): summary of safety and effectiveness. 1985 May 10. (PMA no. P790020-008).

FA129 Heyer Schulte Corp. [______] Sauflon (r) 70 (Lidofilcon A): summary of safety and effectiveness. 1985 May 10 (PMA no. P790020-002).

FA130 Hoffman-La Roche Inc. [______] CEA-Rooche (R) EIA: summary of safety and effectiveness. 1985 Jun 12. (PMA no. P840027-000).

FA131 Hybritech, Inc. [______] Tandem (R)-E AFP: summary of safety and effectiveness. 1985 May 23. (PMA no. P840035-000).

FA132 Hydracon. [______] Hydracon (R) contact lenses: summary of safety and effectiveness. 1985 Nov 19. (PMA no. P820017-001).

FA133 International Hydron Corp. [______] X-70 soft contact lens: summary of safety and effectiveness. 1985 May 10. (PMA no. P830047-000).

FA134 Johnson & Johnson. [______] 3-Coll (TM) collagen absorbable hemostat: summary of safety and effectiveness. 1985 Nov 15. (PMA no. 830079-000).

FA135 Kallestad Labs, Inc. [______] Quantitope 1251 AFP kit and control serum: summary of safety and effectiveness. 1985 Feb 17. (PMA no. PB00025-000).

FA136 Lasers for Medicine, Inc. [______] Phototome (TM) system 2700: summary of safety and effectiveness. 1985 Sep 18. (PMA no. P850019-000).

FA137 McGhan/3M. [______] Styles 30 & 31 posterior chamber IOLS: summary of safety and effectiveness. 1985 Oct 17. (PMA no. P830040-000).

FA138 Medical Inc. [______] Omniscience prosthetic cardiac valve: summary of safety and effectiveness. 1985 Sep 11. (PMA no. P830039-000).

FA139 Medical Lasers, Inc. [______] Meditec OPL3 Nd:Yag laser: summary of safety and effectiveness. 1985 Feb 21. (PMA no. P830025-000).

FA140 Medtronic, Inc. [______] Itrel (R) totally implantable spinal cord stimulation system: summary of safety and effectiveness. 1985 Jan 2. (PMA no. P840001-000).

FA141 National Patent Development Corporation. [______] Hydron hydrophilic contact lens: summary of safety and effectiveness. 1985 Nov 18. (PMA no. P78007-016).

FA142 Nucleus LTD. [______] Nucleus multichannel implantable hearing prosthesis: summary of safety and effectiveness. 1985 Dec 9. (PMA no. P840024-000).

FA143 Optical Plastic Research. [______] Softview spherical & toric contact lens: summary of safety and effectiveness. 1985 Feb 20. (PMA no. P830003-000).

FA144 Paris Contact Lens Lab. [______] Softsite (Hefilcon A) contact lens: summary of safety and effectiveness. 1985 Nov 21. (PMA no. N17793-006).

FA145 Pharmafair, Inc. [______] Saltair tablets (250MG): summary of safety and effectiveness. 1985 Jun 5. (PMA no. P840034-000).

FA146 Product Development Corp. [______] Soft hydrophilic contact lens: summary of safety and effectiveness. 1985 Nov 21. (PMA no. P850041-000).

FA147 Repro-Med System, Inc. [______] Repro-Med-THD: summary of safety and effectiveness. 1985 Jan 25. (PMA no. P820034-000).

FA148 Salvatori Ophthalmics, Inc. [______] Synsoft (TM) (polymacon) bifocal contact lens: summary of safety and effectiveness. 1985 Mar 22. (PMA no. P840006-000).

FA149 Siemans Medical Systems, Inc. [______] Magnetom: summary of safety and effectiveness. 1985 Jan 2. (PMA no. P830081-000).

FA150 Soft Lense Inc. [______] Hydrocurve II bifocal lens: summary of safety and effectiveness. 1985 Mar 22. (PMA no. N17752-016).

FA151 Surgidev Corp. [______] Style 17 & 17A posterior chamber IOLS: summary of safety and effectiveness. 1985 Oct 17. (PMA no. P830033-000).

FA152 University Optical Products Company. [______] Alges (TM) (Hefilcon A) contact lens: summary of safety and effectiveness. 1985 Dec 4. (PMA no. 850002-000).

FA153 Visiontech, Inc. [______] Sauflon PW-70 A & B: summary of safety and effectiveness. 1985 Jun 19. (PMA no. P840031-000).

FA154 Wesley Jessen. [______] Airlens (R) (Airfocon A) lens blue & clear: summary of safety and effectiveness. 1985 Jan 18. (PMA no. P830070-000).

FA155 Wesley-Jessen. [______] Durasoft (R) 3 for extended wear: summary of safety and effectiveness. 1985 Sep 11. (PMA no. P830039-000).

FA156 3M. [______] 3M brand cochlear implant system/house design: summary of safety and effectiveness. 1984 Dec 24. (PMA no. P830069-000).

FA157 Abbott Laboratories. [______] Abbott CEA-EIA kit: summary of safety and effectiveness. 1984 Aug 21. (PMA no. P830066-000).

FA158 Abbott Labs. [______] Corzyme (TM)-M diagnostic kit: summary of safety and effectiveness. 1984 Jan 26. (PMA no. P830014-000).

FA159 Abbott. [______] Abbott AFP: summary of safety and effectiveness. 1984 Jul 25. (PMA no. P780005-000).

FA160 Advanced Optical Inc. [______] Softics (TM) (polymacon): summary of safety and effectiveness. 1984 Jul3. (PMA no. P830012-000).

FA161 Alden Optical Labs., Inc. [______] AL-47 soft contact lens: summary of safety and effectiveness. 1984 Mar 9. (PMA no. P820078-000).

FA162 Allergan Optical. [______] The soft lens thermal disinfecting unit: summary of safety and effectiveness. 1984 Jan 4. (PMA no. P820082-000).

FA163 Allergan Pharmaceuticals, Inc. [______] ND:Yag posterior capsulotomy model 100: summary of safety and effectiveness. 1984 Nov 26. (PMA no. P830062-000).

FA164 Amersham Corporation. [______] Amersham AFP: summary of safety and effectiveness. 1984 Jul 6 (PMA no. P78006-000).

FA165 Analytab Products, Inc. [______] Uniscept (TM): summary of safety and effectiveness. 1984 Apr 25. (PMA no. P830028-000).

FA166 BSD Medical Corp. [______] BSD 1000 hyperthermia system: summary of safety and effectiveness. 1984 Aug 27. (PMA no. P820088-002).

FA167 BSD Medical Corporation. [______] BSD 1000 hyperthermia system: summary of safety and effectiveness. 1984 Jan 25. (PMA no. P820088-000).

FA168 Barnes-Hind Pharmaceuticals. [______] Gas permeable regimen: summary of safety and effectiveness. 1984 Apr 25. (PMA no. P820053-000).

FA169 Biotronik Sales, Inc. [______] Diplos model 03: summary of safety and effectiveness. 1984 Apr 6. (PMA no. P820076-000).

FA170 CIBA Vision Care Corporation. [______] Cibatint (TM) tinting process: summary of safety and effectiveness. 1984 Apr 10. (PMA no. P820086-000).

FA171 Coburn Optical Industries, Inc. [______] Neodymium-Yag op laser OPL-3: summary of safety and effectiveness. 1984Sep 7. (PMA no. P830064-000).

FA172 Coherent Medical Division. [______] Neodymium:Yag ophthalmic laser system 9900.: summary of safety and effectiveness. 1984 Jul 30. (PMA no. P830054-000).

FA173 Comfort Flex Hydrophilics Inc. [______] TRI POL 43 contact lens: summary of safety and effectiveness. 1984 Apr 17. (PMA no. P780013-004).

FA174 Diasonics, Inc. [______] Diasonics NMR imaging system: summary of safety and effectiveness. 1984 Apr 25. (PMA no. P830053-000).

FA175 Dow Corning Wright [______] CMW bone cement: summary of safety and effectiveness. 1984 Apr 24. (PMA no. N18466-000).

FA176 EM Labs. [______] Palacos R bone cement: summary of safety and effectiveness. 1984 Feb 28. (PMA no. P810020-000).

FA177 Fonar Corp. [______] Fonar NMR whole body scanner beta 3000: summary of safety and effectiveness. 1984 Nov 13. (PMA no. P830076).

FA178 Food and Drug Administration, Center for Devices and Radiological Health. A basic quality assurance program for small diagnostic radiology facilities. 1984. (NTIS order no. PB84-119098).

FA179 ______. A study of DC defibrillator safety and performance—performance and safety standard—volume II. 1984. (NTIS order no. PB84-188838).

FA180 ______. A study of the common characteristics, hazards, and performance problems of endoscopes and endoscopic accessories. 1984. (NTIS order no. PB84-187202).

FA181 ______. An investigation of cerebrospinal fluid shunt valves—test results for twenty-five valves: final report—Phase III.

FA182 ______. Computerized treatment planning systems—proceedings of a symposium held at Henry Ford Hospital, Detroit, Michigan. 1984. (NTIS order no. 84-155118).

FA183 ______. Development of test methods and draft standard for cardiac monitors. 1984. (NTIS order no. PB84-187756).

FA184 ______. Development of test methods for disposable ECG electrodes—Volume I. 1984. (NTIS order no. PB84-193960).

FA185 ______. Evaluation of automated differential cell counting devices—Volume I: review of literature and labeling. 1984. (NTIS order no. PB84-189356).

FA186 ______. Hypodermic thermocouple tissue cryometers. 1984. (NTIS order no. PB84-190776).

FA187 ______. Instrumentation for nonionizing radiation measurement. 1984. (NTIS order no. 84-180603).

FA188 ______. Investigation and studies in electrosurgery. 1984. (NTIS order no. PB84-191634).

FA189 ______. Problem definition study in liquid crystal forehead temperature strips. 1984. (NTIS order no. PB84-187483).

FA190 ______. Prosthetic heart valves: a study of in vitro performance, phase II final report part II. 1984. (NTIS order no. PB84-162387).

FA191 ______. Prosthetic heart valves: a study of in vitro performance, phase II final report part III. 1984. (NTIS order no. PB84-162395).

FA192 ______. Prosthetic heart valves: a study of in vitro performance, phase II final report part I. 1984. (NTIS order no. PB84-162379).

FA193 ______. Safety and performance of angiographic and lymphographic injectors. 1984. (NTIS order no. PB84-195544).

FA194 ______. Safety and performance of resuscitators. 1984. (NTIS order no. PB84-195635).

FA195 ______. Safety and performance of ventilators. 1984.(NTIS Order no. PB84-188721).

FA196 ______. Standard for cardiac monitors, heart rate meters, and alarms. 1984. (NTIS Order no. PB84-188812).

FA197 Frontier Contact Lense. [______] Hydro marc lenses (hydrophilic): summary of safety and effectiveness. 1984 Sep 17. (PMA no. N18033-006).

FA198 Hydracon. [______] Hydracon (R) contact lenses: summary of safety and effectiveness. 1984 Aug 7. (PMA no. P820017-002).

FA199 Intermedics Inc. [______] Cosmos (TM) system: summary of safety and effectiveness. 1984 Apr 25. (PMA no. P830026-000).

FA200 Intermedics, Inc. [______] Cybertach (TM) 60 pulse generator & programmer: summary of safety and effectiveness. 1984 Dec 12. (PMA no. P820022-000).

FA201 Medtronic, Inc. [______] Isomed (R) electrospinal orthosis single channel S: summary of safety and effectiveness. 1984 Jan 25. (PMA no. P810062-000).

FA202 Metrosoft, Inc. [______] Metro 55 (Methafilcon A): summary of safety and effectiveness. 1984 Jul 3. (PMA no. P830077-000).

FA203 Ocu-Ease Optical Products, Inc. [______] Ocuflex: summary of safety and effectiveness. 1984 Apr 25. (PMA no. P820051-000).

FA204 Organon Teknika Corp. [______] Curesis plasma separator: summary of safety and effectiveness. 1984 Nov 9. (PMA no. P830010-000).

FA205 Pacesetter Systems Inc. [______] Model 283 pulse generator & model 370/375 supports: summary of safety and effectiveness. 1984 Apr 20. (PMA no. P830045-000).

FA206 Picker International. [______] Nuclear magnetic resonance scanner models NMR 1000: summary of safety and effectiveness. 1984 Jun 8. (PMA no. P830052-000).

FA207 Polymer Technology Corporation. [______] Boston lens (R) lens-clear: summary of safety and effectiveness. 1984 Jan 27. (PMA no. P820065-000).

FA208 Radiometer! America. [______] Radiometer TCM-10 transcutaneous carbon dioxide monitor: summary of safety and effectiveness. 1984 Apr 13. (PMA no. P800043-002).

FA209 Radionics, Inc. [______] Cosman ICP tele-sensor (R): summary of safety and effectiveness. 1984 Nov 21. (PMA no. P820012-000).

FA210 Salvatori Ophthalmics, Inc. [______] Paraperm 02 clear & blue lens: summary of safety and effectiveness. 1984 Apr 25. (PMA no. 820062-000).

FA211 Syntex Ophthalmics Inc. [______] Soft contact lens: summary of safety and effectiveness. 1984 Jan 17. (PMA no. N17987-007).

FA212 Technicare Corporation. [______] Teslacon (TM) NMR imaging system: summary of safety and effectiveness. 1984 Apr 25. (PMA no. P830051-000).

FA213 Vision Ease Contact Lens Co. [______] VE soft hydrophilic contact lens: summary of safety and effectiveness. 1984 Mar 9. (PMA no. P830049-000).

FA214 Wampole Labs. [______] AFP RIA kit: summary of safety and effectiveness. 1984 Feb 17. (PMA no.P76001-000).

FA215 Abbott Labs. [______] Abbott AFP-EIA diagnostic kit for cancer: summary of safety and effectiveness. 1983 Jul 19. (PMA no. P820060).

FA216 Alcon Laboratories, Inc. [______] Micro-therm disinfectant unit: summary of safety and effectiveness. 1983 Jan 25. (PMA no. P820041-000).

FA217 Alcon Laboratories, Inc. [______] Opti-clean (TM) LC 1323: summary of safety and effectiveness. 1983 May 13. (PMA no. P820036-000).

FA218 Alcon Labs, Inc. [______] Alcon enzyme cleaner: summary of safety and effectiveness. 1983 Jan 25.(PMA no. P820001-000).

FA219 Allergan Medical Optics. [______] Model AC10 & AC20 I0LS: summary of safety and effectiveness. 1983 Aug 16. (PMA no. P810056-000).

FA220 Allergan Medical Optics. [______] Models PC10 & PC21: summary of safety and effectiveness. 1983 Jun 17. (PMA no. P820049-000).

FA221 Allergan Pharmaceuticals, Inc. [______] Lens Plus (TM): summary of safety and effectiveness. 1983 Jul 19. (PMA no. P820050-000).

FA222 Amcon Inc. [______] The Amcon Way Plus: summary of safety and effectiveness. 1983 Feb 22. (PMA no. P800069-002).

FA223 Apothecary Products, Inc. [______] The normaline kit: summary of safety and effectiveness. 1983 Jun 17. (PMA no. P800055-002).

FA224 Asahi Chemical Industry America, Inc. [______] Plasmaflo AP-O5H Asahi plasma separator: summary of safety and effectiveness. 1983 Aug 12. (PMA no. P820033-000).

FA225 Avicon, Inc. [______] Microfibrillar collagen hemostat non-woven web: summary of safety and effectiveness. 1983 Feb 15. (PMA no. P800002-000).

FA226 Barnes-Hind/Hydrocurve, Inc. [______] Soft lens salt tablets: summary of safety and effectiveness. 1983 Jul 29. (PMA no. P800067-000).

FA227 Bausch & Lomb Optics Center. [______] Sensitive Eyes (TM) saline & cleaning solution: summary of safety and effectiveness. 1983 Sep 16. (PMA no. P820031-000).

FA228 Bausch and Lomb. [———Devics and Radiological Health] 03/04 (TM) lens series: summary of safety and effectiveness. 1983 Aug 16. (PMA no. N16895-025).

FA229 Blairex Laboratories, Inc. [______] The Blairex system: summary of safety and effectiveness. 1983 Feb 18. (PMA no. PB00028-003).

FA230 Boehringer Mannheim Diagnostics Inc. [______] Micur-mic systems: summary of safety and effectiveness. 1983 Jul 19. (PMA no. P820073-000).

FA231 C.C. Kelly Enterprises. [______] Eyerisol (R): summary of safety and effectiveness. 1983 May 31. (PMA no. P810034-000).

FA232 CIBA Vision Care [______] Salt tablets: summary of safety and effectiveness. 1983 Feb 18. (PMA no. P810015-001).

FA233 CIBA Vision Care Corporation. [______] Septicon (TM) disinfection regimen for use with . . . : summary of safety and effectiveness. 1983 Apr 8. (PMA no. P820040-000).

FA234 CIBA Vision Care Corporation. [______] Softcon (Vifilcon A) soft contact extended wear lens: summary of safety and effectiveness. 1983 Apr 29. (PMA no. P820021-000).

FA235 Cabot Medical Corp. [______] Lamicel (TM): summary of safety and effectiveness. 1983 Jul 19. (PMA no. P820075-000).

FA236 Cilco, Inc. [______] Models IS & IP: summary of safety and effectiveness. 1983 Apr 26. (PMA no. P800049-000).

FA237 Cilco, Inc. [______] Posterior chamber intraocular lenses: summary of safety and effectiveness. 1983 Apr 1. (PMA no. P810018-001).

FA238 Con-cise. [______] Paraperm O2 contact lens clear & blue: summary of safety and effectiveness. 1983 Dec 8. (PMA no. P820061-000).

FA239 Contact Lens Corporation of America. [______] Softact II (polymacon): summary of safety and effectiveness. 1983 Aug 5. (PMA no. P830006-000).

FA240 Coopervision Cilco. [______] Model AC (ACI-AC5): summary of safety and effectiveness. 1983 Apr 12. (PMA no. P810001-000).

FA241 Coopervision, Inc. [______] Heatcase (TM): summary of safety and effectiveness. 1983 Jul 19. (PMA no. P830001-000).

FA242 Cordis Corp. [______] Gemini (R) theta model 415A cardiac pacer: summary of safety and effectiveness. 1983 Dec 7. (PMA no. P830007-000).

FA243 Custom Tint Lab., Inc. [______] Permatint (R): summary of safety and effectiveness. 1983 Nov 9. (PMA no. P820059-000).

FA244 Depuy (R). [______] Prosthesis, hip, hemi-femoral, metal: summary of safety and effectiveness. 1983 Sep 16. (PMA no. P820024-000).

FA245 Dow Corning Corporation. [______] Silicon(R) (silafilcon A) contact lens daily wear: summary of safety and effectiveness. 1983 Dec 12. (PMA no. P800054-004).

FA246 Eaton Medical Corporation. [______] Easy Eyes (TM): summary of safety and effectiveness. 1983 Jul 19. (PMA no. P830009-000).

FA247 Electro-Biology, Inc. [______] Scolitron (TM) stimulator: summary of safety and effectiveness. 1983 Feb 25. (PMA no. P820008-000).

FA248 Food and Drug Administration, Center for Devices and Radiological Health. Investigation of the risks & hazards with devices associated with peritoneal dialysis (including intermittent dialysis & continuous ambulatory peritoneal dialysis) & sorbent regenerated dialysate delivery systems. 1983. (NTIS order no. PB83-175984).

FA249 ______. Vascular catheter devices: a study of safety and performance—volume 1. 1983. (NTIS order no. PB83-144659).

FA250 ______. Vascular catheter devices: a study of safety and performance—volume 2. 1983. (NTIS order no. 83-144667).

FA251 Frigitronics, Inc. [______] Opus-III contact lenses: summary of safety and effectiveness. 1983 Sep 2. (PMA no. P820074-000).

FA252 Frigitronics, Inc. [______] Softmark: summary of safety and effectiveness. 1983 Jul 19. (PMA no. P820027-000).

FA253 Horizon Pharmacal, Inc. [______] The Horizon system: summary of safety and effectiveness. 1983 Feb 18. (PMA no. P810009-002).

FA254 Hydracon. [______] Hydracon (R) contact lenses: summary of safety and effectiveness. 1983 Mar 25. (PMA no. P820017-000).

FA255 Intermedics Intraocular Inc. [______] Models 011 & 011B iridocapsular IOLS: summary of safety and effectiveness. 1983 Jan 25. (PMA no. P810042-000).

FA256 Intermedics Intraocular Inc. [______] Models 019B, 019C, 019E, 019F, 019J, 019K: summary of safety and effectiveness. 1983 Feb 25. (PMA no. P810055-000).

FA257 Kestrel. [______] Kestrel no. 695 heater: summary of safety and effectiveness. 1983 Jun 10. (PMA no. P820087-000).

FA258 Marlin Industries. [______] Marlin squeeze bottle & Marlin salt tablets: summary of safety and effectiveness. 1983 Feb 18. (PMA no. P800038-001).

FA259 Medtronic, Inc. [______] Versatrax model 7000 universal A-V pulse generator: summary of safety and effectiveness. 1983 Jan 7. (PMA no. P820003-000).

FA260 Narco Scientific. [______] Monitoring system TCPC02: summary of safety and effectiveness. 1983 Feb 15. (PMA no. P820025-000).

FA261 National Patent Development Corporation. [______] Hydron (TM) saline system (135 & 250 mg): summary of safety and effectiveness. 1983 Feb 25. (PMA no. P810047-002).

FA262 New England Nuclear. [______] Rianen (TM) (3H) progestin receptor assay kit: summary of safety and effectiveness. 1983 Oct 12. (PMA no. P820052-000).

FA263 Optacryl Inc. [______] Optacryl 60-clear: summary of safety and effectiveness. 1983 Dec 8. (PMA no. P820056-000).

FA264 Optech, Inc, [______] Optech fre-flex soft contact lens: summary of safety and effectiveness.1983 Feb 15. (PMA no. P810050-000).

FA265 Osmed, Inc. [______] Drilac cubes (TM): summary of safety and effectiveness. 1983 Feb 25. (PMA no. P800012-000).

FA266 Pacesetter Systems, Inc. [______] Programalith (TM) model 223 pulse generator 398 P: summary of safety and effectiveness. 1983 Feb 25. (PMA no. P820023-000).

FA267 Paragon Optical Inc. [______] Paraperm O2 contact lens: summary of safety and effectiveness. 1983 Dec 8. (PMA no. P820063-000).

FA268 Parker Hannifin Corporation. [______] Cryomax (TM): summary of safety and effectiveness. 1983 Feb 18. (PMA no. P820002-000).

FA269 Pharmacia Diagnostics. [______] Healon: summary of safety and effectiveness. 1983 Feb 8. (PMA no. P810031-000).

FA270 Precision-Cosmet Co., Inc. [______] Circular open loop posterior IOLS & Kratz elliptic: summary of safety and effectiveness. 1983 Aug 9 (PMA no. P820072-000).

FA271 Precision-Cosmet, Co. [______] AMVISC (R): summary of safety and effectiveness. 1983 Nov 28. (PMA no. P810025-000).

FA272 Professional Supplies. [______] The soft rinse system: summary of safety and effectiveness. 1983 Feb 18. (PMA no. P800060-003).

FA273 Sensormedics. [______] Cutaneous gas monitor: summary of safety and effectiveness. 1983 Sep 16. (PMA no. P830008-000).

FA274 St. Jude Medical Inc. [______] Bileaflet-center opening cardiac valve: summary of safety and effectiveness. 1983 Mar 1. (PMA no. P810002-000).

FA275 Storz Instrument Co. [______] Lincoff-design scleral buckling balloon catheter: summary of safety and effectiveness. 1983 Nov 21. (PMA no. P820009-000).

FA276 Telectronics, Inc. [______] Autima (TM) model 2251 & model 2600: summary of safety and effectiveness. 1983 Mar 11. (PMA no. P820018-000).

FA277 Travenol Laboratories. [______] Plasma separation system: summary of safety and effectiveness. 1983 Nov 3. (PMA no. P820032-000).

FA278 Upjohn. [______] Gelfoam: summary of safety and effectiveness. 1983 Aug 29. (PMA no. N18286-000).

FA279 Wesley Jesson Inc. [______] Durasoft (R) Trufocal (TM): summary of safety and effectiveness. 1983 Jun 3. (PMA no. N17852-008).

FA280 Advanced Catheter Systems. [______] Simpson-Robert coronary balloon dilatation catheter: summary of safety and effectiveness. 1982 Mar 26. (PMA no. P810046-000).

FA281 Allergan Pharmaceuticals. [______] Lens-wet (TM): summary of safety and effectiveness. 1982 May 14. (PMA no. P800065-000).

FA282 Amcon Inc. [______] Nor-Sa-Tab: summary of safety and effectiveness. 1982 Feb 19. (PMA no. P800069-000).

FA283 American Medical Products Corporation. [______] Collastat: summary of safety and effectiveness. 1982 Jan 5. (PMA no. P810006-000).

FA284 Apothecary Products, Inc. [______] The normaline kit: summary of safety and effectiveness. 1982 Jan 12. (PMA no. P800055-000).

FA285 Avery Labs, Inc. [______] Spinal epidural electrode for P.E.N.S. models E-355: summary of safety and effectiveness. 1982 Mar 2. (PMA no. P810033-000).

FA286 Barnes-Hind Pharmaceuticals, Inc. [______] Softmate weekly cleaning solution: summary of safety and effectiveness. 1982 Mar 26. (PMA no. P810017-000).

FA287 Bausch & Lomb. [______] Sensitive eyes (TM) saline solution: summary of safety and effectiveness. 1982 Nov 11. (PMA no. P810039-000).

FA288 Bausch and Lomb. [______] Soflens (r) polymacon P.A.1 series: summary of safety and effectiveness. 1982 Dec 17. (PMA no. N16895 019).

FA289 Biochem International Inc. [______] Lifespan (TM) 100 TCPC02 monitor: summary of safety and effectiveness. 1982 Oct 1. (PMA no. P820019-000).

FA290 CIBA Vision Care. [______] Weicon (R) (Tefilicon) hydrophilic contact lens: summary of safety and effectiveness. 1982 Jul 27. (PMA no. P810005-002).

FA291 Central Pharmaceuticals, Inc. [______] Central's pharm. salt tablets for disinfection: summary of safety and effectiveness. 1982 Jan 15. (PMA no. P810030-000).

FA292 Cobe Laboratories, Inc. [______] Cobe century (R) TPE system: summary of safety and effectiveness. 1982 Mar 9. (PMA no. P810023-000).

FA293 Coburn Optical Industries, Inc. [______] Binkhorst & Fedorov I iris clip IOLS: summary of safety and effectiveness. 1982 Aug 31. (PMA no. P800027-000).

FA294 Cooper Labs, Inc. [______] Clerz lubricating & rewetting eye drops: summary of safety and effectiveness. 1982 Jul 13. (PMA no. PB00034-000).

FA295 Coopervision Cilco. [______] Posterior chamber intraocular lenses: summary of safety and effectiveness. 1982 Aug 31. (PMA no. P810018-000).

FA296 Coopervision, Inc. [______] Cooper (TM) 38 (polymacon) hydrophilic contact lens: summary of safety and effectiveness. 1982 May 21. (PMA no. P810057-000).

FA297 Coopervision, Inc. [______] Mirasol (TM): summary of safety and effectiveness. 1982 Jan 12. (PMA no. P810008-000).

FA298 Coopervision, Inc. [______] Models B-13F (P-10) & B-1H (P-11): summary of safety and effectiveness. 1982 May 25. (PMA no. P810032-000).

FA299 Cordis Corp. [______] Cordis sequicor theta models 233D & 233E: summary of safety and effectiveness. 1982 Dec 10. (PMA no. P820014-000).

FA300 Danker and Wohlk, Inc. [______] Danker silicone lens (Dimefocon-A): summary of safety and effectiveness. 1982 Jun 13. (PMA no. P790010-000).

FA301 ______. Quality assurance in nuclear medicine—proceedings of an international symposium and workshop, held in Washington, D.C., April 27-29. 1981. 1982. (GPO Stock No. 017-015-00221-7, NTIS Order No. PB84-199306).

FA302 Genetics Lab. [______] Bioflow (TM): summary of safety and effectiveness. 1982 Jul 20. (PMA no. P800064-000).

FA303 Hewlett-Packard Co. [______] H-P capnometer model 47210A, option A10 cutaneous: summary of safety and effectiveness. 1982 Apr 13. (PMA no. P810043-000).

FA304 Horizon Pharmacal, Inc. [______] The Horizon system: summary of safety and effectiveness. 1982 Jan 12. (PMA no. P810009-000).

FA305 Howmedica, Inc. [______] Deklene (TM): summary of safety and effectiveness. 1982 Jun 4. (PMA no. P810028-000).

FA306 Interface Biomedical Labs., Inc. [______] Superstat: summary of safety and effectiveness. 1982 Jun 25. (PMA no. P810040-000).

FA307 Intermedics Infusaid, Inc. [______] Infusaid implantable infusion pump model 100, 200, 4: summary of safety and effectiveness. 1982 Mar 26. (PMA no. P800036-000).

FA308 International Hydron Corporation. [______ Hydron (TM) saline system (135 & 250 mg): summary of safety and effectiveness. 1982 Apr 9. (PMA no. P810047-000).

FA309 International Hydron Corporation. [______] Hydron (R) lens care unit: summary of safety and effectiveness. 1982 Oct 9. (PMA no. P820007-000).

FA310 Johnson and Johnson Co. [______] Chamber lens models 101, 101B, 101T: summary of safety and effectiveness. 1982 Mar 26. (PMA no. P790027-000).

FA311 Kontron Cardiovascular Inc. [______] Kontron cutaneous PC02 monitor: summary of safety and effectiveness. 1982 Jun 18. (PMA no. P810037-000).

FA312 Medtronic, Inc. [______] Medtronic (r) Hall prosthetic heart valve: summary of safety and effectiveness. 1982 Jan 29. (PMA no. P790018-000).

FA313 Metrosoft, Inc. [______] Metrosoft (TM) II (polymacon) hydrophilic contact: summary of safety and effectiveness. 1982 Sep 24. (PMA no. P820026-000).

FA314 Orange Medical Instruments. [______] Transconjunctival oxygen monitor: summary of safety and effectiveness. 1982 Nov 19. (PMA no. P820011-000).

FA315 Pharmacia, Inc. [______] Medallion (R): summary of safety and effectiveness. 1982 Jan 1. (PMA no. P810060-000).

FA316 Precision-Cosmet. [______] Tennant (TM) & Kelman (TM) type II: summary of safety and effectiveness. 1982 Apr 20. (PMA no. PB00016-000).

FA317 Professional Pharmaceal Co. [______] Salt tablets: summary of safety and effectiveness. 1982 Jan 5. (PMA no.P810003-000).

FA318 Professional Supplies. [______] The soft rinse system: summary of safety and effectiveness. 1982 Jan 1. (PMA no. P800060-000).

FA319 Radionics, Inc. [______] Cosman ICP Tele-sensor (R): summary of safety and effectiveness. 1982 Oct 1. (PMA no. P820012-000).

FA320 Richards Medical Co. [______] Osteo ceramic hip: summary of safety and effectiveness. 1982 Dec 10. (PMA no. P810048-000).

FA321 Salvatori Ophthalmics, Inc. [______] (Polymacon) contact lenses: summary of safety and effectiveness. 1982 Sep 17. (PMA no. P820005-000).

FA322 Sherman Labs, Inc. [______] Sof! Pro-clean contact lens cleaner: summary of safety and effectivness. 1982 Jul 23. (PMA no. P810041-000).

FA323 Siemens-Elema Pacmaker Div. [______] Endocardial pacemaker lead w/carbon tip: summary of safety and effectiveness. 1982 Sep 24. (PMA no. P800041-000).

FA324 Standard Pharmacal Corp. [______] Lens-sol: summary of safety and effectiveness. 1982 Mar 26. (PMA no. P810012-000).

FA325 Syntex Ophthalmics Inc. [______] Polycon contact lens: summary of safety and effectiveness. 1982 Sep 21 (PMA no. N18120-008).

FA326 Teledyne, Inc. [______] Sleep sentry (TM): summary of safety and effectiveness. 1982 Sep 17. (PMA no. P81004-000).

FA327 Unilab, Inc. [______] Kiel Surgibone: summary of safety and effectiveness. 1982 Jun 18. (PMA no. P800044-000).

FA328 Warner Lambert. [______] Autobac MTS plus test system: summary of safety and effectiveness. 1982 Mar 26. (PMA no. P810024-000).

FA329 Soft Lense Inc. [______] Hydrocurve: summary of safety and effectiveness. 1980 Jan 11. (PMA no. N17752-000).

FA330 Soft Lense Inc. [______] Hydrocurve: summary of safety and effectiveness. 1980 Mar 14. (PMA no. N17752-001).

Food and Drug Administration
Center for Drugs and Biologics

5600 Fishers Lane
Rockville, MD 20857
301-443-2894

Contact: Don McLearn (for general information); Linda Carter (for information on new SBAs) 301-443-4330; or FOI staff (Freedom of Information inquiries) 301-443-6310.

Overview: The FDA Center for Drugs and Biologics (CDB) is responsible for ensuring that all human drugs and biologics manufactured for interstate sale are safe and effective and that product labeling is truthful and informative. Drugs and biologics are evaluated to prevent potentially dangerous or ineffective drugs, vaccines, toxoids, immune sera, antigens and allergenic products, and blood and blood products from entering the nation's health care system. For many newly approved drugs, CDB prepares a Summary Basis of Approval (SBA).

Purpose: To evaluate and approve new drugs for marketing on the basis of safety and effectiveness (efficacy), to assure that these drugs are properly labeled, and to share with the public the key facts on which approval is based.

Primary intended users: General public; people concerned about their health; patients; providers, generally; health product manufacturers.

Technologies: *Drug.*

Human-use drugs for therapeutic use are assessed.

Intervention: *Treatment,* prevention, diagnosis.

Stage: *New.*

SBAs are prepared when the drug is released for use in the practice of medicine.

Properties: *Safety, efficacy,* effectiveness.

Selection process: The CDB has criteria that determine which drugs justify an SBA. No one can request that an assessment be done beyond the intended target group of a given drug.

Methods: *Information syntheses, expert opinion,* for premarketing approval; epidemiological and other observational methods for postmarketing surveillance.

Preparations of the SBA is based on information generated by the New Drug Application process, through which manufacturers submit information for new drug approval. The approval process actually involves two stages, called the Investigational New Drug (IND) and the New Drug Application (NDA). Before CDB will permit a new drug to be tested on humans, the drug's sponsor must file an IND. The IND contains the drug's structural formula, the results of animal testing, the proposed protocol for clinical testing on humans, and other data. The CDB reviews the IND to determine whether the data are complete and sufficient to initiate clinical trials.

After the trials, but before marketing, the manufacturer files an NDA, which must contain full information about the proposed product, including the results of the clinical testing. When the claims for safety, efficacy, and labeling have been approved, the drug may go on the market, but the manufacturer must continue to send periodic reports on adverse reactions and other aspects of drug experience. The CDB may require changes of labeling or take other actions because of dangers that are revealed in this way. If a manufacturer wants to change a drug with an approved NDA—for example, to claim a new use for it—a supplemental NDA may have to be filed and approved.

The average total approval time for an NDA, i.e., from receipt by the CDB of the application to the approval date, is approximately 2 years. This includes time required by the manufacturer to provide information in response to agency actions, which average 6 months.

Assessors: Each IND and NDA is reviewed by a team of FDA scientists—a physician, pharmacologist, a chemist, a pharmacokineticist, and a biometrician (usually, a biologist, and a microbiologist. The Center may also present important NDAs to advisory committees, whose recommendations are valued but are not binding.

The Summary Basis of Approval is generally developed collaboratively by the CDB and the NDA sponsor, with experts on medicine, biostatistics, chemistry, pharmacology, and toxicology. On occasion, the sponsor may develop a draft and submit it to the CDB.

Assessment reports include: Results, findings or conclusions, regulatory agency approval status.

Dissemination: *Printed reports;* clearinghouses, data/citation bases, on-line services.

SBAs are available through the FDA's Freedom of Information Office, 301-443-6310, and from the National Technical Information Service, 5285 Port Royal Rd., Springfield, VA 22161.

Budget: $250,000. The approximate cost per assessment is under $5,000. Funding source: 100 percent parent organization.

Use: Pharmaceutical firms use the SBAs as a source of information on the industry. They are also reviewed by consumer advocates, health professionals in universities, and others.

Related activities: The CDB issues an annual list of *Approved Drug Products* with monthly updates. Subscriptions are available for $103 per year through the U.S. Government Printing Office, Washington, DC 20204; stock no. 917-001-00000-6.

CDB coordinates a number of postmarketing surveillance programs, including spontaneous reaction reporting programs, adverse reaction registries, and research programs. Manufacturers are required to send problem reports to CDB; many health professionals and hospitals send them voluntarily. The Drug Product Problem Reporting Program (DPPR), maintained by the United States Pharmacopeia, is a computer database containing voluntary reports from providers on problems experienced when pharmaceutical products are received, used, or dispensed. These might include unsatisfactory packaging, labeling, or insert information; poor pharmaceutical quality, stability; therapeutic effectiveness, or related characteristics.

Completed Reports

FD1 Food and Drug Administration, Center for Drugs and Biologics. Acetohydroxamic acid. 1987. (Summary basis of approval, NDA # 18-749). [Information syntheses, Expert opinion, Epidemiological and other observational methods, Clinical trials, Bench testing]

FD2 ______. Allopurinol 100 mg. 1987. (Summary basis of approval, NDA # 18-832). [Information syntheses, Expert opinion, Epidemiological and other observational methods, Clinical trials, Bench testing]

FD3 ______. Allopurinol 300 mg. 1987. (Summary basis of approval, NDA # 18-832). [Information syntheses, Expert opinion, Epidemiological and other observational methods, Clinical trials, Bench testing]

FD4 ______. Betamethasone dipropionate. 1987. (Summary basis of approval, NDA #19-136). [Information syntheses, Expert opinion, Epidemiological and other observational methods, Clinical trials, Bench testing]

FD5 ______. Betamethasone dipropionate. 1987. (Summary basis of approval, NDA #19-137). [Information syntheses, Expert opinion, Epidemiological and other observational methods, Clinical trials, Bench testing]

FD6 ______. Betamethasone dipropionate. 1987. (Summary basis of approval, NDA #19-138). [Information syntheses, Expert opinion, Epidemiological and other observational methods, Clinical trials, Bench testing]

FD7 ______. Bronalide inhaler system. 1987. (Summary basis of approval, NDA #18-340). [Information syntheses, Expert opinion, Epidemiological and other observational methods, Clinical trials, Bench testing]

FD8 ______. Bumetanide injectable. 1987. (Summary basis of approval, NDA #18-226). [Information syntheses, Expert opinion, Epidemiological and other observational methods, Clinical trials, Bench testing]

FD9 ______. Bumetanide tablets. 1987. (Summary basis of approval, NDA #18-225). [Information syntheses, Expert opinion, Epidemiological and other observational methods, Clinical trials, Bench testing]

FD10 ______. Clonidine. 1987. (Summary basis of approval, NDA # 18-891). [Information syntheses, Expert opinion, Epidemiological and other observational methods, Clincial trials, Bench testing]

FD11 ______. Clotrimazole. 1987. (Summary basis of approval, NDA #18-827). [Information syntheses, Expert opinion, Epidemiological and other observational methods, Clinical trials, Bench testing]

FD12 ______. Dopamine HCl. 1987. (Summary basis of approval substitute, NDA # 19-099) [Information syntheses, Expert opinion, Epidemiological and other observational methods, Clinical trials, Bench testing]

FD13 ______. Dopamine HCl. 1987. (Summary basis of approval substitute, NDA # 19-099). [Information syntheses, Expert opinion, Epidemiological and other observational methods, Clinical trials, Bench testing]

FD14 ______. Enalapril maleate/hydro-chlorothiazide. 1987. (Summary basis of approval substitute, NDA # 19-221). [Information syntheses, Expert opinion, Epidemiological and other observational methods, Clinical trials, Bench testing]

FD15 ______. Hydromorphone HC1. 1987. (Summary basis of approval, NDA # 19-034). [Information syntheses, Expert opinion, Epidemiological and other observational methods, Clinical trials, Bench testing]

FD16 ______. Ibuprofen. 1987. (Summary basis of approval, NDA #18-989). [Information syntheses, Expert opinion, Epidemiological and other observational methods, Clinical trials, Bench testing]

FD17 ______. Ibuprofen. 1987. (Summary basis of approval, NDA #19-012). [Information syntheses, Expert opinion, Epidemiological and other observational methods, Clinical trials, Bench testing]

FD18 ______. Potassium chloride. 1987. (Summary basis of approval substitute, NDA # 19-123). [Information syntheses, Expert opinion, Epidemiological and other observational methods, Clinical trials, Bench testing]

FD19 ______. Potassium chloride. 1987. (Summary basis of approval, NDA # 19-439). [Information syntheses, Expert opinion, Epidemiological and other observational methods, Clinical trials, Bench testing]

FD20 ______. Potassium chloride. 1987. (Summary basis of approval, NDA# 19-123). [Information syntheses, Expert opinion, Epidemiological and other observational methods, Clinical trials, Bench testing]

FD21 ______. Potassium citrate. 1987. (Summary basis of approval, NDA #19-071). [Information syntheses, Expert opinion, Epidemiological and other observational methods, Clinical trials, Bench testing]

FD22 ______. Propranolol HCl liquid. 1987. (Summary basis of approval substitute, NDA# 19-536). [Information syntheses, Expert opinion, Epidemiological and other observational methods, Clinical trials, Bench testing]

FD23 ______. Propranolol SR/hydrochlorothiazide. 1987. (Summary basis of approval, NDA # 19-059). [Information syntheses, Expert opinion, Epidemiological and other observational methods, Clinical trials, Bench testing]

FD24 ______. Propranolol hydrochloride. 1987. (Summary basis of approval, NDA #18-553). [Information syntheses, Expert opinion, Epidemiological and other observational methods, Clinical trials, Bench testing]

FD25 ______. Ranitidine HCl. 1987. (Summary basis of approval NDA # 18-703). [Information syntheses, Expert opinion, Epidemiological and other observational methods, Clinical trials, Bench testing]

FD26 ______. Ranitidine HCl. 1987. (Summary basis of approval substitute, NDA # 19-593). [Information syntheses, Expert opinion, Epidemiological and other observational methods, Clinical trials, Bench testing]

FD27 ______. Sodium cellulose phosphate. 1987. (Summary basis of approval, NDA #18-757). [Information syntheses, Expert opinion, Epidemiological and other observational methods, Clinical trials, Bench testing]

FD28 ______. Triamterene and hydrochlorothiazide. 1987. (Summary basis of approval, NDA # 19-129). [Information syntheses, Expert opinion, Epidemiological and other observational methods, Clinical trials, Bench testing]

FD29 ______. Verapamil HCl. 1987. (Summary basis of approval substitute, NDA # 19-152). [Information syntheses, Expert opinion, Epidemiological and other observational methods, Clinical trials, Bench testing]

FD30 ______. Verapamil. 1987. (Summary basis of approval substitute, NDA # 18-817/S-003). [Information syntheses, Expert opinion, Epidemiological and other observational methods, Clinical trials, Bench testing]

FD31 ______. Alclometasone dipropionate. 1983. (NTIS order no. PB83-915901). [Information syntheses, Expert opinion, Epidemiological and other observational methods, Clinical trials, Bench testing]

FD32 ______. Aminocaproic acid injection. 1983. (NTIS order no. PB83-915901). [Information syntheses, Expert opinion, Epidemiological and other observational methods, Clinical trials, Bench testing]

FD33 ______. Betamethasone valerate. 1983. (NTIS order no. PB83-915902). [Information syntheses, Expert opinion, Epidemiological and other observational methods, Clinical trials, Bench testing]

FD34 ______. Chymopapain. 1983. (NTIS order no. PB83-915901). [Information syntheses, Expert opinion, Epidemiological and other observational methods, Clinical trials, Bench testing]

FD35 ______. Ciclopirox olamine. 1983. (NTIS order no. PB83-915901). [Information syntheses, Expert opinion, Epidemiological and other observational methods, Clinical trials, Bench testing]

FD36 ______. Dextromethorphan resin complex. 1983. (NTIS order no. PB83-915901. [Information syntheses, Expert opinion, Epidemiological and other observational methods, Clinical trials, Bench testing]

FD37 ______. Diethylpropion hydrochloride. 1983. (NTIS order no. PB83-915901). [Information syntheses, Expert opinion, Epidemiological and other observational methods, Clinical trials, Bench testing]

FD38 ______. Diltiazem hydrochloride. 1983. (NTIS order no. PB83-915901). [Information syntheses, Expert opinion, Epidemiological and other observational methods, Clinical trials, Bench testing]

FD39 ______. Econazole nitrate. 1983. (NTIS order no. PB83-915901). [Information syntheses, Expert opinion, Epidemiological and other observational methods, Clinical trials, Bench testin]

FD40 ______. Etomidate. 1983. (NTIS order no. PB83-91590). [Information syntheses, Expert opinion, Epidemiological and other observational methods, Clinical trials, Bench testing]

FD41 ______. Guanabenz acetate. 1983. (NTIS order no. PB83-915903). [Information syntheses, Expert opinion, Epidemiological and other observational methods, Clinical trials, Bench testing]

FD42 ______. Guanadrel sulfate. 1983. (NTIS order no. PB 83-915901). [Information syntehese, Expert opinion, Epidemiological and other observational methods, Clinical trials, Bench testing]

FD43 ______. Human insulin (recombinant DNA orgin) isophane suspension. 1983. (NTIS order no. PB83-915901). [Information syntheses, Expert opinion, Epidemiological and other observational methods, Clinical trials, Bench testing]

FD44 ______. Hydrocortisone butyrate. 1983. (NTIS order no. PB83-915901). [Information syntheses, Expert opinion, Epidemiological and other observational methods, Clinical trials, Bench testing]

FD45 ______. Nadolol-bendroflumethiazide. 1983. (NTIS order no. PB 83-915903). [Information syntheses, Expert opinion, Epidemiological and other observational methods, Clinical trials, Bench testing]

FD46 ______. Pentazocine HCl and naloxone HCl. 1983. (NTIS order no. PB83-915901). [Information syntheses, Expert opinion, Epidemiological and other observational methods, Clinical trials, Bench testing]

FD47 ______. Praziquantel, 1983. (NTIS order No. PB83-915901). [Information syntheses, Expert opinion, Epidemiological and other observational methods, Clinical trials, Bench testing]

FD48 ______. Regular human insulin (recombinant DNA origin) injection. 1983. (NTIS order no. PB83-915901). [Information syntheses, Expert opinion, Epidemiological and other observational methods, Clinical trails, Bench testing]

FD49 ______. Selenium sulfide. 1983. (NTIS order no. PB83-915902). [Information syntheses, Expert opinion, Epidemiological and other observational methods, Clinical trials, Bench testing]

FD50 ______. Technetium Tc 99m albumin colloid kit. 1983. (NTIS order no. PB83-915902). [Information syntheses, Expert opinion, Epidemiological and other observational methods, Clinical trials, Bench testing]

FD51 ______. Tioconazole. 1983. (NTIS order no. PB83-915902). [Information syntheses, Expert opinion, Epidemiological and other observational methods, Clinical trials, Bench testing]

FD52 ______. Triazolam. 1983. (NTIS order no. PB83-915901). [Information syntheses, Expert opinion, Epidemiological and other observational methods, Clinical trials, Bench testing]

FD53 ______. Vidarabine. 1983. (NTIS order no. PB83-915903). [Information syntheses, Expert opinion, Epidemiological and other observational methods, Clinical trials, Bench testing]

FD54 ______. Xenon Xe 127 gas. 1983 (NTIS order no. PB83-915901). [Information syntheses, Expert opinion, Epidemiological and other observational methods, Clinical trials, Bench testing]

FD55 ______. 8% amino acid injection. 1982. (NTIS order no. PB82-915904). [Information syntheses, Expert opinion, Epidemiological and other observational methods, Clinical trials, Bench testing]

FD56 ______. Acyclovir. 1982. (NTIS order no. PB82-915902). [Information syntheses, Expert opinion, Epidemiological and other observational methods, Clinical trials, Bench testing]

FD57 ______. Albuterol sulfate. 1982. (NTIS order no. PB82-915903). [Information syntheses, Expert opinion, Epidemiological and other observational methods, Clinical trials, Bench testing]

FD58 ______. Alprazolam. 1982. (NTIS order no. PB82-915901). [Information syntheses, Expert opinion, Epidemiological and other observational methods, Clinical trials, Bench testing]

FD59 ______. Alprostadil (PGE1). 1982. (NTIS order no. PB82-915901). [Information syntheses, Expert opinion, Epidemiological and other observational methods, Clinical trials, Bench testing]

FD60 ______. Amcinonide. 1982. (NTIS order no. PB82-915901). [Information syntheses, Expert opinion, Epidemiological and other observational methods, Clinical trials, Bench testing]

FD61 ______. Amiloride HCl. 1982. (NTIS order no. PB82-915901). [Information syntheses, Expert opinion, Epidemiological and other observational methods, Clinical trials, Bench testing]

FD62 ______. Amiloride HCl/hydrochlorothiazide. 1982. (NTIS order no. PB82-915901). [Information syntheses, Expert opinion, Epidemiological and other observational methods, Clinical trials, Bench testing]

FD63 ______. Aminophylline, USP. 1982/ (NTIS order no. PB82-915903). [Information syntheses, Expert opinion, Epidemiological and other observational methods, Clinical trials, Bench testing]

FD64 ______. Azatadine maleate & pseud. sulfate. 1982. (NTIS order no. PB82-915902). [Information syntheses, Expert opinion, Epidemiological and other observational methods, Clinical trials, Bench testing]

FD65 ______. Azlocillin sodium. 1982. (NTIS order no. PB82-915904). [Information syntheses, Expert opinion, Epidemiological and other observational methods, Clinical trials, Bench testing]

FD66 ______. Bacampicillin hydrochloride. 1982. (NTIS order no. PB82-915902). [Information syntheses, Expert opinion, Epidemiological and other observational methods, Clinical trials, Bench testing]

FD67 ______. Benoxaprofen. 1982. (NTIS order no. PB82-915903). [Information syntheses, Expert opinion, Epidemiological and other observational methods, Clinical trials, Bench testing]

FD68 ______. Bupivacaine hydrochloride. 1982. (NTIS order no. PB82-915901). [Information syntheses, Expert opinion, Epidemiological and other observational methods, Clinical trials, Bench testing]

FD69 ______. Buprenorphine HCl. 1982. (NTIS order no. PB82-915901). [Information syntheses, Expert opinion, Epidemiological and other observational methods, Clinical trials, Bench testing]

FD70 ______. CaCl2, MgCl, Kcl, & NaCl. 1982. (NTIS order no. PB82-915902). [Information syntheses, Expert opinion, Epidemiological and other observational methods, Clinical trials, Bench testing]

FD71 ______. Carbamazepine. 1982. (NTIS order no. PB82-915901). [Information syntheses, Expert opinion, Epidemiological and other observational methods, Clinical trials, Bench testing]

FD72 ______. Cephradine. 1982. (NTIS order no. PB82-915901). [Information syntheses, Expert opinion, Epidemiological and other observational methods, Clinical trials, Bench testing]

FD73 ______. Ceruletide diethylamine. 1982. (NTIS order no. PB82-915901). [Information syntheses, Expert opinion, Epidemiological and other observational methods, Clinical trials, Bench testing]

FD74 ______. Cromolyn sodium. 1982. (NTIS order no. PB82-915903). [Information syntheses, Expert opinion, Epidemiological and other observational methods, Clinical trials, Bench testing]

FD75 ______. Desoximetasone. 1982. (NTIS order no. Pb82-915902). [Information syntheses, Expert opinion, Epidemiological and other observational methods, Clinical trials, Bench testing]

FD76 ______. Diflunisal. 1982. (NTIS order no. PB82-915904). [Information syntheses, Expert opinion, Epidemiological and other observational methods, Clinical trials, Bench testing]

FD77 ______. Digoxin. 1982. (NTIS order no. PB82-915904). [Information syntheses, Expert opinion, Epidemiological and other observational methods, Clinical trials, Bench testing]

FD78 ______. Disopyramide phosphate. 1982. (NTIS order no. PB82-915904). [Information syntheses, Expert opinion, Epidemiological and other observational methods, Clinical trials, Bench testing]

FD79 ______. Estramustine phosphate sodium. 1982. (NTIS order no. PB82-915901). [Information syntheses, Expert opinion, Epidemiological and other observational methods, Clinical trials, Bench testing]

FD80 ______. Ethynodiol diacetate with ethinyl estradiol. 1982. (NTIS order no. PB82-915901). [Information syntheses, Expert opinion, Epidemiological, and other observational methods, Clinical trials, Bench testing]

FD82 ______. Gemfibrozil. 1982. (NTIS order no. PB82-915901). [Information syntheses, Expert opinion, Epidemiological and other observational methods, Clinical trials, Bench testing]

FD82 ______. Gemfibrozil. 1982. (NTIS order no. PB82—915901). [Information syntheses, Expert opinion, Epidemiological and other observational methods, Clinical trials, Bench testing]

FD83 ______. Gonadorelin HCl. 1982. (NTIS order no. PB82-915904). [Information syntheses, Expert opinion, Epidemiological and other observational methods, Clinical trials, Bench testing]

FD84 ______. Hydrocortisone butyrate. 1982. (NTIS order no. PB82-915902). [Information syntheses, Expert opinion, Epidemiological and other observational methods, Clinical trials, Bench testing]

FD85 ______. Ibuprofen. 1982. (NTIS order no. PB82-915902). [Information syntheses, expert opinion, Epidemiological and other observational methods, Clinical trials, Bench testing]

FD86 ______. Indomethacin. 1982. (NTIS order no. PB82-915901). [Information syntheses, Expert opinion, Epidemiological and other observational methods, Clinical trials, Bench testing]

FD87 ______. Indomethacin. 1982. (NTIS order no. PB82-915902). [Information syntheses, Expert opinion, Epidemiological and other observational methods, Clinical trials, Bench testing]

FD88 ______. Intravenous fat emulsion. 1982. (NTIS order no. PB82-915901). [Information syntheses, Expert opinion, Epidemiological and other observational methods, Clinical trials, Bench testing]

FD89 ______. Isotretinoin. 1982. (NTIS order no. PB82-915903). [Information syntheses, Expert opinion, Epidemiological and other observational methods, Clinical trials, Bench testing]

FD90 ______. Malathion. 1982. (NTIS order no. PB82-915904). [Information syntheses, Expert opinion, Epidemiological and other observational methods, Clinical trials, Bench testing]

FD91 ______. Methoxsalen. 1982. (NTIS order no. PB82-915903). [Information syntheses, Expert opinion, Epidemiological and other observational methods, Clinical trials, Bench testing]

FD92 ______. Metoclopramide HC1. 1982. (NTIS order no. PB82-915903). [Information syntheses, Expert opinion, Epidemiological and other observational methods, Clinical trials, Bench testing]

FD93 ______. Metronidazole injection, 0.5%. 1982. (NTIS order no. PB82-915904). [Information syntheses, Expert opinion, Epidemiological and other observational methods, Clinical trials, Bench testing]

FD94 ______. Miconazole nitrate. 1982. (NTIS order no. PB82-915902). [Information syntheses, Expert opinion, Epidemiological and other observational methods, Clinical trials, Bench testing]

FD95 ______. Miconazole nitrate. 1982. (NTIS order no. PB82-915904). [Information syntheses, Expert opinion, Epidemiological and other observational methods, Clinical trials, Bench testing]

FD96 ______. Moxalactam disodium. 1982. (NTIS order no. PB82-915901). [Information syntheses, Expert opinion, Epidemiological and other observational methods, clinical trials, Bench testing]

FD97 ______. NaCl, KCl, MgSO4, NaPO4, & KPO4. 1982. (NTIS order no. PB82-915901). [Information syntheses, Expert opinion, Epidemiological and other observational methods, Clinical trials, Bench testing]

FD98 ______. Niclosamide. 1982. (NTIS order no. PB82-915903). [Information syntheses, Expert opinion, Epidemiological and other observational mehtods, Clinical trials, Bench testing]

FD99 ______. Nifedipine. 1982. (NTIS order no. PB82-915901). [Information syntheses, Expert opinion, Epidemiological and other observational methods, Clinical trials, Bench testing]

FD100 ______. Norethindrone & ethinyl estradiol. 1982. (NTIS order no. PB82-915902). [Information syntheses, Expert opinion, Epidemiological and other observational methods, Clinical trials, Bench testing]

FD101 ______. Pentazocine hydrochloride and acetaminophen. 1982. (NTIS order no. PB82-915904). [Information syntheses, Expert opinion, epidemiological and other observational methods, Clinical trials, Bench testing]

FD102 ______. Pentetate indium disodium In 111. 1982. (NTIS order no. PB82-915902). [Information syntheses, Expert opinion, Epidemiological and other observational methods, Clinical trials, Bench testing]

FD103 ______. Peritoneal dialysis solutions in plastic containers. 1982. (NTIS order no. PB82-915901). [Information syntheses, Expert opinion, Epidemiological and other observational methods, Clinical trials, Bench testing]

FD104 ______. Pindolol, 1982. (NTIS order no. PB82-915904). [Information syntheses, Expert opinion, Epidemiological and other observational methods, Clinical trials, Bench testing]

FD105 ______. Piroxicam. 1982. (NTIS order no. PB82-915903). [Information syntheses, Expert opinion, Epidemiological and other observational methods, Clinical trials, Bench testing]

FD106 ______. Salts solution plus dextrose and glutathione disulfides. 1982. (NTIS order no. PB82-915901). [Information syntheses, Expert opinion, Epidemiological and other observational methods, Clinical trials, Bench testing]

FD107 ______. Silver sulfadiazine. 1982. (NTIS order no. PB82-915902). [Information syntheses, Expert opinion, Epidemiological and other observational methods, Clinical trials, Bench testing]

FD108 ______. Sterile piperacillin sodium. 1982. (NTIS order no. PB82-915901). [Information syntheses, Expert opinion, Epidemiological and other observational methods, Clinical trials, Bench testing]

FD109 ______. Streptozocin. 1982. (NTIS order no. PB82-915903).

FD110 ______. Sucralfate. 1982. (NTIS order no. PB82-915901). [Information syntheses, Expert opinion, Epidemiological and other observational methods, Clinical trials, Bench testing]

FD111 ______. Sulfadoxine and pyrimethamine. 1982. (NTIS order no. PB82-915901). [Information syntheses, Expert opinion, Epidemiological and other observational methods, Clinical trials, Bench testing]

FD112 ______. Technetium Tc 99M succimer kit. 1982. (NTIS order no. PB82-915903). [Information syntheses, Expert opinion, epidemiological and other observational methods, Clinical trials, Bench testing]

FD113 ______. Technetium Tc 99m disofenin kit. 1982. (NTIS order no. PB82-915902). [Information syntheses, Expert opinion, Epidemiological and other observational methods, Clinical trials, Bench testing]

FD114 ______. Theophylline in 5% dextrose injection in plastic container. 1982. (NTIS order no. PB82-915904). [Information syntheses, Expert opinion, Epidemiological and other observational methods, Clinical trials, Bench testing]

FD115 ______. Timolol maleate & hydrochlorothiazide. 1982. (NTIS order no. PB82-915901). [Information syntheses, Expert opinion, Epidemiological and other observational methods, Clinical trials, Bench testing]

FD116 ______. Tobramycin. 1982. (NTIS order no. 82-915901). [Information syntheses, Expert opinion, Epidemiological and other observational methods, Clinical trials, Bench testing]

FD117 ______. Trazodone HCI. 1982. (NTIS order no. PB82-915901). [Information syntheses, Expert opinion, Epidemiological and other observational methods, Clinical trials, Bench testing]

FD118 ______. Trimethoprim tablets. 1982. (NTIS order no. PB82-915904). [Information syntheses, Expert opinion, Epidemiological and other observational methods, Clinical trials, Bench testing]

FD119 ______. Verapamil HCL. 1982. (NTIS order no. PB82-915902). [Information syntheses, Expert opinion, Epidemiological and other observational methods, Clinical trials, Bench testing]

FD120 ______. 0.45% sodium chloride injection, USP. 1981. (NTIS order no. PB81-915909). [Information syntheses, Expert opinion, Epidemiological and other observational methods, Clinical trials, Bench testing]

FD121 ______. 0.9% sodium chloride injection, USP. 1981. (NTIS order no. PB81-915909). [Information syntheses, Expert opinion, Epidemiological and other observational methods, Clinical trials, Bench testing]

FD122 ______. 10% Dextrose injection, USP. 1981. (NTIS order no. PB81-915909). [Information syntheses, Expert opinion, Epidemiological and other observational methods, Clinical trials, Bench testing]

FD123 ______. 5% Dextrose & 0.3% NaCl Inj., USP. 1981. (NTIS order no. PB81-915909). [Information syntheses, Expert opinion, Epidemiological and other observational methods, Clinical trials, Bench testing]

FD124 ______. 5% Dextrose & 0.9% NaCl Inj., USP. 1981. (NTIS order no. PB81-915909). [Information syntheses, Expert opinion, Epidemiological and other observational methods, Clinical trials, Bench testing]

FD125 ______. 5% Dextrose in lactated Ringer's injection in polyolefin bottle. 1981. [Information syntheses, Expert opinion, Epidemiological and other observational methods, Clinical trials, Bench testing]

FD126 ______. Aminoglutethimide. 1981. (NTIS order no. PB81-915901). [Information syntheses, Expert opinion, Epidemiological and other observational methods, Clinical trials, Bench testing]

FD127 ______. Amoxicillin. 1981. (NTIS order no. PB81-915901). [Information syntheses, Expert opinion, Epidemiological and other observational methods, Clinical trials, Bench testing]

FD128 ______. Atenolol. 1981. (NTIS order no. PB81-915911). [Information syntheses, Expert opinion, Epidemiological and other observational methods, Clinical trials, Bench testing]

FD129 ______. Azathioprine. 1981. (NTIS order no. PB81-915907). [Information syntheses, Expert opinion, Epidemiological and other observational methods, Clinical trials, Bench testing]

FD130 ______. Beclomethasone dipropionate. 1981. (NTIS order no. PB81-915912). [Information syntheses, Expert opinion, Epidemiological and other observational methods, Clinical trials, Bench testing]

FD131 ______. Bethanidine sulfate. 1981. (NTIS order no. PB81-915908). [Information syntheses, Expert opinion, Epidemiological and other observational methods, Clinical trials, Bench testing]

FD132 ______. Bromocriptine mesylate. 1981. (NTIS order no. PB81-915912). [Information syntheses, Expert opinion, Epidemiological and other observational methods, Clinical trials, Bench testing]

FD133 ______. Captopril. 1981. (NTIS order no. PB81-915907). [Information syntheses, Expert opinion, Epidemiological and other observational methods, Clinical trials, Bench testing]

FD134 ______. Chlorhexidine gluconate. 1981. (NTIS order no. PB81-915911). [Information syntheses, Expert opinion, Epidemiological and other observational methods, Clinical trials, Bench testing]

FD135 ______. Chlorpheniramine maleate pseudoephedrine sulfate. 1981. (NTIS order no.PB81-915906). [Information syntheses, Expert opinion, Epidemiological and other observational methods, Clinical trials, Bench testing]

FD136 ______. Clorazepate dipotassium. 1981. (NTIS order no. PB81-915904). [Information syntheses, Expert opinion, Epidemiological and other observational methods, Clinical trials, Bench testing]

FD137 ______. Cyclothiazide. 1981. (NTIS order no. PB81-915905). [Information syntheses, Expert opinion, Epidemiological and other observational methods, Clinical trials, Bench testing]

FD138 ______. DTIC (Dome). 1981. (NTIS order no. PB81-15907). [Information syntheses, Expert opinion, epidemiological and other observational methods, Clinical trials, Bench testing]

FD139 ______. Diazepam. 1981. (NTIS order no. PB81-915906). [Information syntheses, Expert opinion, Epidemiological and other observational methods, Clinical trials, Bench testing]

FD140 ______. Dopamine hydrochloride injection. 1981. (NTIS order no. PB81-915908). [Information syntheses, Expert opinion, Epidemiological and other observational methods, Clinical trials, Bench testing]

FD141 ______. Ergoloid mesylates. 1981. (NTIS order no. PB81-915904). [Information syntheses, Expert opinion, Epidemiological and other observational methods, Clinical trials, Bench testing]

FD142 ______. Erythromycin base (enteric-coated pellets). 1981. (NTIS order no. PB81-915904). [Information syntheses, Expert opinion, Epidemiological and other observational methods, Clinical trials, Bench testing]

FD143 ______. Extended purified beef insulin zinc suspension. 1981. (NTIS Order no. PB81-915909). [Information syntheses, Expert opinion, Epidemiological and other observational methods, Clinical trials, Bench testing]

FD144 ______. Furosemide injection. 1981. (NTIS order no. PB81-915908). [Information syntheses, Expert opinion, Epidemiological and other observational methods, Clinical trials, Bench testing]

FD145 ______. Furosemide tablets. 1981. (NTIS order no. PB81-915911). [Information syntheses, expert opinion, Epidemiological and other observational methods, Clinical trials, Bench testing]

FD146 ______. Halazepam. 1981. (NTIS order no. PB81-915912). [Information syntheses, Expert opinion, Epidemiological and other observational methods, Clinical trials, Bench testing]

FD147 ______. Hexachlorophene. 1981. (NTIS order no. PB81-915904). [Information syntheses, Expert opinion, Epidemiological and other observational methods, Clinical trials, Bench testing]

FD148 ______. Hexachlorophene. 1981. (NTIS order no. PB81-915909). [Information syntheses, Expert opinion, Epidemiological and other observational methods, Clinical trials, Bench testing]

FD149 ______. Ibuprofen. 1981. (NTIS order no. PB81-915908). [Information syntheses, expert opinion, Epidemiological and other observational methods, Clinical trials, Bench testing]

FD150 ______. Intravenous fat emulsion. 1981. (NTIS order no. 81-915904). [Information syntheses, Expert opinion, Epidemiological and other observational methods, Clinical trials, Bench testing]

FD151 ______. Iodoxamate meglumine. 1981. (NTIS order no. PB81-915911). [Information syntheses, Expert opinion, Epidemiological and other observational methods, Clinical trials, Bench testing.

FD152 ______. Iron dextran Inj. USP. 1981. (NTIS order no. PB81-915906). [Information syntheses, Expert opinion, Epidemiological and other observational methods, Clinical trials, Bench testing]

FD153 ______. Isophane purified beef insulin suspension. 1981. (NTIS order no. PB81-915909). [Information syntheses, Expert opinion, Epidemiological and other observational methods, Clinical trials, Bench testing]

FD154 ______. Isophane purified pork insulin suspension. 1981. (NTIS order no. PB81-915910). [Information syntheses, Expert opinion, Epidemiological and other observational methods, Clinical trials, Bench testing]

FD155 ______. Isosulfan blue. 1981. (NTIS order no. PB81-915910). [Information syntheses, Expert opinion, Epidemiological and other observational methods, Clinical trials, Bench testing]

FD156 ______. Ketoconazole. 1981. (NTIS order no. PB81-915909). [Information syntheses, Expert opinion, Epidemiological and other observational methods, Clinical trials, Bench testing]

FD157 ______. Lidocaine HCl in 5% dextrose in plastic container (PL-146). 1981. (NTIS order no. PB81-915907). [Information syntheses, Expert opinion, Epidemiological and other observational methods, Clinical trials, Bench testing]

FD158 ______. Lidocaine hydrochloride, USP sterile powder. 1981. (NTIS order no. PB81-915905. [Information syntheses, Expert opinion, Epidemiological and other observational methods, Clinical trials, Bench testing]

FD159 ______. Methyldopa. 1981. (NTIS order no. PB81-915911. [Information syntheses, Expert opinion, Epidemiological and other observational methods, Clinical trials, Bench testing]

FD160 ______. Metolazone. 1981. (NTIS order no. PB81-915905). [Information syntheses, Expert opinion, Epidemiological and other observational methods, Clinical trials, Bench testing]

FD161 ______. Mezlocillin sodium. 1981. (NTIS order no. PB81-915912). [Information syntheses, Expert opinion, Epidemiological and other observational methods, Clinical trials, Bench testing]

FD162 ______. Multiple electrolyte injection. 1981. (NTIS order no. PB81-915901). [Information syntheses, Expert opinion, Epidemiological and other observational methods, Clinical trials, Bench testing]

FD163 ______. Nitroglycerin for injection. 1981. (NTIS order no. PB81-915912). [Information syntheses, Expert opinion, Epidemiological and other observational methods, Clinical trials, Bench testing]

FD164 ______. Phenylpropanolamine hydrochloride chlorpheniramine maleate. 1981. (NTISorder no. PB81-915910). [Information syntheses, expert opinion, Epidemiological and other observational methods, Clinical trials, Bench testing]

FD165 ______. Potassium chloride 1981. (NTIS order no. PB81-915901). [Information syntheses, Expert opinion, Epidemiological and other observational methods, Clinical trials, Bench testing]

FD166 ______. Prompt purified beef insulin zinc suspension. 1981. (NTIS order no. PB81-915909). [Information syntheses, Expert opinion, Epidemiological and other observational methods, Clinical trials, Bench testing]

FD167 ______. Purified beef insulin zinc suspension. 1981. (NTIS order no. PB81-915909). [Information syntheses, Expert opinion, Epidemiological and other observational methods, Clinical trials, Bench testing]

FD168 ______. Purified pork insulin injection. 1981. (NTIS order no. PB81-915909). [Information syntheses, Expert opinion, Epidemiological and other observational methods, Clinical trials, Bench testing]

FD169 ______. Ringer's irrigation, USP in flex containers. 1981. (NTIS order no. PB81-915906). [Information syntheses, Expert opinion, Epidemiological and other observational methods, Clinical trials, Bench testing]

FD170 ______. Saralasin acetate. 1981. (NTIS order no. PB81-915908). [Information syntheses, Expert opinion, Epidemiological and other observational methods, Clinical trials, Bench testing]

FD171 ______. Secretin. 1981. (NTIS order no. PB81-915908). [Information syntheses, Expert opinion, Epidemiological and other observational methods, Clinical trials, Bench testing]

FD172 ______. Sisomicin sulfate. 1981. (NTIS order no. PB81-915901). [Information syntheses, Expert opinion, Epidemiological and other observational methods, Clinical trials, Bench testing]

FD173 ______. Sodium nitroprusside. 1981. (NTIS order no. PB81-915912) [Information syntheses, Expert opinion, Epidemiological and other observational methods, Clinical trials, Bench testing]

FD174 ______. Sterile cefotaxime sodium. 1981. (NTIS order no. PB81-915906). [Information syntheses, Expert opinion, Epidemiological and other observational methods, Clinical trials, Bench testing]

FD175 ______. Sterile water for injection, USP. 1981. (NTIS order no. PB81-915909). [Information syntheses, Expert opinion, Epidemiological and other observational methods, Clinical trials, Bench testing]

FD176 ______. Sulfamethoxazole and trimethoprim. 1981. (NTIS order no. PB81-915909). [Information syntheses, Expert opinion, Epidemiological and other observational methods, Clinical trials, Bench testing]

FD177 ______. Technetium 99m oxidronate kit. 1981. (NTIS order no. PB81-915905). [Information syntheses, Expert opinion, Epidemiological and other observational methods, Clinical trials, Bench testing]

FD178 ______. Technetium Tc 99m medronate kit. 1981. (NTIS order no. PB81-915905). [Information syntheses, Expert opinion, Epidemiological and other observational methods, Clinical trials, Bench testing]

FD179 ______. Temazepam. 1981. (NTIS order no. PB81-915905). [Information syntheses, Expert opinion, Epidemiological and other observational methods, Clinical trials, Bench testing]

FD180 ______. Trimethoprim/sulfamethoxazole. 1981. (NTIS order no. 81-915908). [Information syntheses, Expert opinion, Epidemiological and other observational methods, Clinical trials, Bench testing]

FD181 ______. Verapamil. 1981. (NTIS order no. PB81-915911). [Information syntheses, expert opinion, Epidemiological and other observational methods, Clinical trials, Bench testing]

FD182 ______. Zomepirac sodium. 1981. (NTIS order no. PB81-915901). [Information syntheses, Expert opinion, Epidemiological and other observational methods, Clinical trials, Bench testing]

Food and Drug Administration
Center for Food Safety and Applied Nutrition

Color for Drugs and Devices
200 C Street SW, HFF-214
Washington, DC 20204
202-485-0099

Special Purpose Infant Formulas
200 C Street SW, HFF-204
Washington, DC 20204
202-245-3117

Contact: Alan Rulis, Chief, Regulatory Chemistry Branch, (Colors for Drugs and Devices program) or Nicholas Duy, Chemist (Special Infant Formula program).

Overview: The FDA Center for Food Safety and Applied Nutrition (CFSAN) is primarily responsible for regulating foods and cosmetics. CFSAN is also responsible for assessment activities including: 1) the regulation of color additives in drugs and medical devices (as well as foods), and 2) the regulation of infant formulas that are prescribed as special diets. Both activities are federally mandated. The Special Infant Formulas program was implemented in 1986, pursuant to the Infant Formula Act of 1980, concerning special infant diets for inborn errors of metabolism and other special medical needs arising from such conditions as extreme low birthweight.

Purpose: To ensure the safety and suitability of colors added to foods, drugs, and devices and to ensure the safety and effectiveness of special purpose infant formulas.

Primary intended users: Health product manufacturers; health industry associations; government regulators.

Technologies: *Drug, device,* for color additives; *medical or surgical procedure* (i.e., special diet for medical reasons) for special infant formulas.

Intervention: *Treatment,* diagnosis, rehabilitation for color additives; *treatment* for special infant formulas.

Stage: *Emerging, new,* established or widespread practice for color additives and for special infant formulas.

Properties: *Safety* for color additives; *safety,* efficacy, effectiveness for special infant formulas.

Selection process: Manufacturers of both color additives and special infant formulas must request FDA assessment of their products. Exempted from this requirement are additives known as GRAS (generally recognized as safe) and "prior sanctioned." The latter are substances the FDA determined to be safe before the 1958 Food Additives amendment.

For color additives, the FDA is developing a program to reassess the safety of each previously approved additive in light of new scientific evidence and to remove unsafe ones from the market.

Reassessments of infant formulas are conducted if the agency receives information that infants are being harmed by a product or by a similar product.

Methods: *Information syntheses,* expert opinion, group judgment, bench testing.

For color additives, manufacturers submit test data that show the substance is safe and functional. The FDA then announces in the *Federal Register* that an additive petition has been filed. After experts have reviewed the data, CFSAN announces approval of the additive through a regulation, also published in the *Federal Register.* Under a provision that has become known as the "Delaney Clause," the agency is prohibited by law from approving any additive found to cause cancer in test animals. The agency conducts laboratory toxicology studies only in cases when already marketed products experience problems. Laboratory testing is also conducted for certification of purity of color additives that have potential for toxic contaminants.

For special infant formulas, the manufacturers submit the formulas for assessment. The formulas are assessed within the agency. The agency does conduct some laboratory analysis of special infant formula samples.

The approximate turnaround time from selection of assessment topic to reporting of findings varies widely.

Assessors: Experts in chemistry, toxicology, and environmental assessment review color additives.

Infant formulas are assessed within the CFSAN by experts in nutrition, diet, chemistry, medicine, and food technology.

Assessment reports include: The assessment's intended audience; the purpose of the assessment; relationship of this assessment to prior or concurrent assessments of the technology or other technologies intended for similar purposes; who sponsored/commissioned/supported the assessment; description of the technology; stage of life-cycle of technology when assessed; properties assessed; results; findings or conclusions; limitations of findings; implications of findings for practice; regulatory agency approval status; product recall history, environmental impact.

Dissemination: Advisories; press conferences/news releases, TV/radio broadcasts, video products.

Assessments of color additives are announced in the *Federal Register.*
Assessments of special infant formulas will be disseminated primarily through advisories to manufacturers and to foreign health agencies. Copies may be obtained by contacting the FDA's Freedom of Information Office or the CFSAN contact person given above.

Budget: Not provided. The approximate cost of an assessment is $40,000 for color additives and $10,000 for special infant formulas. Funding source for color additives: 97 percent parent organization, 3 percent manufacturers; funding source for special purpose infant formulas: 100 percent parent organization.

Use: The FDA uses the CFSAN's assessments to permit or deny use of the product or to require modifications. The assessments are also used by the manufacturers.

Program evaluation: The Colors for Drugs and Devices program is reviewed periodically by Congress.

Related activities: The CFSAN also certifies the purity of colors for drugs and devices that have a potential for problems with toxic contaminants.

Completed reports: The first assessment reports for special infant formulas should be available in 1988 or 1989.

Georgetown University Medical Center

Institute for Health Policy Analysis
2121 Wisconsin Avenue NW, Suite 220
Washington, DC 20007
202-625-2115

Contact: Seymour Perry, M.D., Deputy Director.

Overview: The Institute for Health Policy Analysis, a not-for-profit research institute, conducts research on and analyzes important national health policy issues. The Institute established its Technology and Health Care Program in 1983.

Purpose: To improve the public's understanding of national health policy issues and to aid the process by which policy is set within the government.

Primary intended users: General public; people concerned about their health; patients; providers, generally; physicians; health/medical professional associations; health industry associations; consumer associations; unions and other employee organizations; third party payers; reporters, writers, news media; policy-makers.

Technologies: Device, medical or surgical procedure.

Intervention: Diagnosis, treatment.

Properties: *Safety; effectiveness;* efficacy; cost; cost-benefit; cost-effectiveness; ethical, legal, social implications.

Selection process: Assessments may be requested by staff or by an outside organization. However, as a matter of policy, the Institute will not conduct an assessment for an outside group unless funding is obtained from multiple sources, so as to avoid any perception of bias. Requests are made either in writing or at a meeting, and Institute staff determine which assessment topics have priority.

Methods: *Group judgment,* information syntheses, expert opinion.

Workshops and conferences are the program's chief assessment method. The first step after selecting a topic is to establish a small planning committee of people outside the organization to develop the questions to be addressed, identify speakers, and plan other aspects of the workshop or conference. A neutral panel also is chosen. The approximate turnaround time from selection of assessment topic to reporting of findings is 4 to 6 months for a workshop and 12 to 18 months for a conference.

Assessors: Committee and panel members are experts in medical and technical areas or in other areas such as health economics, ethics, or law.

Assessment reports include: Abstract; the assessment's intended audience; the purpose of the assessment; relationship of this assessment to prior or concurrent assessments of the technology or other technologies intended for similar purposes; who sponsored/commissioned/supported the assessment; who conducted the assessment; description of the technology; stage of life-cycle of technology when assessed; properties assessed; procedure used for the assessment; sources of data/information; methods for collecting data/information; methods for analyzing/ synthesizing data/information; findings or conclusions; limitations of findings; implications of findings for practice; recommendations for practice, future assessments, technology development, research; where technology is in use; regulatory agency approval status; coverage/reimbursement status of the technology.

Dissemination: Printed reports, journal articles.

The Institute publishes a newsletter and maintains a mailing list. Results may also be reported in the lay press. The reports may be obtained, upon request, from the Institute.

Budget: $250,000. The approximate cost for a workshop is $25,000 to $30,000 and for a conference, $75,000 to $100,000. Funding sources: 50 percent parent organization; 10 percent government grants, contracts; 10 percent foundations, other private grants; 30 percent sponsors/members dues, contributions.

Use: The Institute's reports have been used in a variety of ways. The proceedings of two of its conferences on the reuse of disposable medical devices, for example, were used by several groups, including the Association for the Advancement of Medical Instrumentation, the American Society for Testing and Materials, and Congressional committees.

Related activities: The Institute also sponsors the following programs: Financial Compensation for Disease and Disability, a Unit of Advanced Studies, and the Program on Science and the Media.

Completed Reports

GU1 Georgetown University Medical Center, Institute for Health Policy Analysis. Reuse of disposable medical devices: legal liability and public policy issues. (In press) [Information syntheses, Expert opinion, Group judgment, Cost analyses]

GU2 Chu F, Novak N, Radany MH, Perry S. [Georgetown University Medical Center, Institute for Health Policy Analysis] Reuse and reprocessing of disposable medical devices. J Health Care Technol 1986;3:5-12. [Information syntheses, Expert opinion, Group judgment, Cost analyses]

GU3 Chu F. [Georgetown University Medical Center, Institute for Health Policy Analysis] Changing attitudes toward reusing medical devices. Health Span-Report of Health Bus Law 1986;3:14-8. [Information syntheses, Expert opinion, Group judgment, Cost analyses]

GU4 Georgetown University Medical Center, Institute for Health Policy Analysis. New medical technologies in a cost containment environment: implantable antitachyarrhythmia devices. Washington, DC: Institute for Health Policy Analysis, 1986. [Information syntheses, Expert opinion, Group judgment, Cost analyses]

GU5 Georgetown University Medical Center, Institute for Health Policy Analysis. National Health Services and Practice Patterns Survey. Report on fully automated blood pressure monitoring: current and future applications. Washington, DC: Institute for Health Policy Analysis, 1986. [Information syntheses, Expert opinion, Group judgment, Cost analyses]

GU6 Perry S. [Georgetown University Medical Center, Institute for Health Policy Analysis] Reuse of medical devices intended for single use only. Health Care Instrum 1985;1:4-8. [Information syntheses, Expert opinion, Group judgment, Cost analyses]

GU7 Perry S. [Georgetown University Medical Center, Institute for Health Policy Analysis] Reusing disposable medical devices raises ethical, legal and cost questions. Bus Health 1985;2:53-4. [Information syntheses, Expert opinion, Group judgment, Cost analyses]

GU8 Georgetown University Medical Center, Institute for Health Policy Analysis. Conference proceedings: International Conference on the Reuse of Disposable Medical Devices in the 1980s. Washington, DC: Institute for Health Policy Analysis, 1984. [Information syntheses, Expert opinion, Group judgment, Cost analyses]

Ongoing Assessments

GU9 ______. Therapeutic drug substitution: legal liability. Ongoing.

Planned Assessments

GU10 ______. Extended wear contact lenses. Planned.

GU11 ______. Home health technologies. Planned.

GU12 ______. Orphan devices in health care. Planned.

GU13 ______. Regionalization of medical technologies. Planned.

Harvard School of Public Health

Institute for Health Research
677 Huntington Avenue
Boston, MA 02115
617-729-5657

Contact: Howard S. Frazier, M.D.

Overview: The Institute for Health Research is a medical technology assessment program sponsored by Harvard University and the Harvard Community Health Plan. The technology assessment activities were initiated in 1965 by the Center for the Analysis of Health Practices of Harvard University, the precursor to the current Institute.

Purpose: To enhance the understanding of innovation and its consequences in the health sector.

Primary intended users: Providers, generally; physicians; acute facility administrators; other care givers; health/medical professional associations; third party payers; government regulators; public policy-makers, legislators.

Technologies: *Device,* medical or surgical procedure, support system, organizational or administrative system.

Intervention: *Treatment,* diagnosis.

Stage: *New,* established or widespread practice, obsolete.

Properties: *Efficacy;* safety; cost; cost-effectiveness; service requirements; system impact; economic implications; ethical, legal, social implications.

Selection process: An Institute investigator or nonmember (e.g., government agency) can request that assessments be conducted. The Institute Executive Committee sets assessment topic priorities based on research interest, opportunities for methodologic advances, or the potential impact of the technology or assessment. The Committee also examines the comparative advantage of the Institute over other organizations when setting priorities.

Methods: *Information syntheses,* expert opinion, group judgment, cost analyses, epidemiological and other observational methods, clinical trials, meta-analysis.

The turnaround time from selection of assessment topic to reporting of findings is 1 to 2 years.

Assessors: The assessors have expertise in the areas of medicine, surgery, dermatology, pediatrics, economics, statistics, policy analysis, psychology, law, and social psychology.

Assessment reports include: The purpose of the assessment; who sponsored/commissioned/supported the assessment; who conducted the assessment; description of the technology; stages of life-cycle of technology when assessed; properties assessed; procedure used for the assessment; sources of data/information; methods for collecting data/

information; methods for analyzing/synthesizing data/information; results; findings or conclusions; limitations of findings; implications of findings for practice; recommendations for practice, future assessments, technology development, research; how the technology works, including theory, principles.

Dissemination: *Journal articles,* printed reports.

Budget: $300,000. The cost per assessment is highly variable ranging from $5,000 to $250,000. Funding sources: 30 percent parent organization; 40 percent government grants/contracts; 30 percent foundations, other private grants.

Related activities: The Institute offers short postgraduate courses for medical educators and others. The courses include materials on aspects of technology assessment and cost effectiveness analysis.

Completed Reports

HA1 Hussain S, Belidegrun A, Seltzer SE, Feldstein ML, et al. [Harvard School of Public Health, Institute for Health Research] CT differentiation of malignant from benign adrenal masses. Am J Roentgenol, in press. [Epidemiological methods]

HA2 Stern RS and members of the 16-center PUVA Follow-up Study. [Harvard School of Public Health, Institute for Health Research] Long-term utilization of PUVA therapy for psoriasis—evidence for efficacy and cost savings. J Am Acad Dermatol, in press. [Clinical trials]

HA3 Stern RS, Pass TM, Komaroff AL. [Harvard School of Public Health, Institute for Health Research] Topical versus systemic agent treatment for papulopustular acne: A cost-effectiveness analysis. Arch Dermatol, in press. [Information syntheses]

HA4 Thompson M, Cohen A, Palmer H. [Harvard School of Public Health, Institute for Health Research] Decision making on clinical use of electronic fetal monitors. Semin Fam Med, in press. [Epidemiological methods]

HA5 Weinstein MC. [Harvard School of Public Health, Institute for Health Research] Economic techniques for technology assessment. In: Rutten F, Reiser S, eds. Economics of medical technology. Springer-Vering, in press. [Cost analyses]

HA6 Sandberg SI, Barnes BA, Weinstein MC, Braun P. [Harvard School of Public Health, Institute for Health Research] Elective hysterectomy: benefits, risks and costs. Med Care 1985;23:1067-1085. [Information syntheses]

HA7 Stason WB, Barnes BA. [Harvard School of Public Health, Institute for Health Research] Effectiveness and costs of continuous ambulatory peritoneal dialysis (CAPD). Washington, D.C.: U.S. Congress, Office of Technology Assessment, July 1985. (Health Technology Case Study 35, OTA-HCS-35) [Information syntheses]

HA8 Stason WB, Localio AR. [Harvard School of Public Health, Institute for Health Research] Magnetic resonance imaging: clinical efficacy, costs and policy considerations. Blue Cross and Blue Shield Association, 1985. [Information syntheses]

HA9 Li Tem, Sherman H, Cook EF, et al. [Harvard School of Public Health, Institute for Health Research] The selective impact of a cardiology data bank on physician's therapeutic recommendations. Medical Decision Making 1984;4(2):165-177. [Epidemiological methods]

HA10 Shepard DS, Karon SL. [Harvard School of Public Health, Institute for Health Research] The market for wheelchairs: innovations and federal policy. Washington, D.C.: U.S. Congress, Office of Technology Assessment, 1984. Health Technology Case Study 30, OTA-HCS-30) [Information syntheses]

HA11 Fineberg HV, Wittenberg J., Ferrucci J, Meuller P, Simeone J, Goldman J. [Harvard School of Public Health, Institute for Health Research] The clinical value of body computed tomography over time and technologic change. Am J Roentgenol 1983;141:1067-1072. [Epidemiological methods]

HA12 Berwick DM, Komaroff AL. [Harvard School of Public Health, Institute for Health Research] Cost effectiveness of lead screening. N Eng J Med 1982;306:1392-1398. [Information syntheses]

HA13 Fineberg HV, Stason WB. [Harvard School of Public Health, Institute for Health Research] Cost-effectiveness of alternative diagnostic strategies for coronary artery disease. Circulation 1982;66(III):80-86. [Information syntheses]

HA14 Kaufman SL, Shepard DS. [Harvard School of Public Health, Institute for Health Research] Costs of neonatal intensive care by day of stay. Inquiry 1982;19:167-178. [Epidemiological methods]

HA15 Liang M, Komaroff A. [Harvard School of Public Health, Institute for Health Research] Roentgenograms in primary care patients with acute low back pain. Arch Intern Med 1982;142:1108-1112. [Epidemiological methods]

HA16 Stason WB, Fortess E. [Harvard School of Public Health, Institute for Health Research] Case study #13: Cardiac radionuclide imaging and cost effectiveness. In: Implications of cost-effectiveness analysis of medical technology. Office of Technology Assessment, U.S. Congress, 1982. [Information syntheses]

HA17 Weinstein MC, Stason WB. [Harvard School of Public Health, Institute for Health Research] Cost-effectiveness of coronary artery bypass surgery. Circulation 1982;66(Suppl III):III56-III66. [Information syntheses]

HA18 Fineberg HV, Pearlman LA. [Harvard School of Public Health, Institute for Health Research] Benefit-and-cost analysis of medical interventions: the case of cimetidine and peptic ulcer disease. In: The implications of cost-effectiveness analysis of medical technology/background paper #2: case studies of medical technologies. Office of Technology Assessment, U.S. Congress. Washington, D.C.: U.S. Government Printing Office, 1981. [Information syntheses]

HA19 Thompson MS, Cohen AB. [Harvard School of Public Health, Institute of Health Research] Decision analysis: electronic fetal monitoring. In: Wortman PM, ed. Methods for evaluating health services. Beverly Hills: Sage, 1981. [Epidemiological methods]

HA20 Weinstein MC, Pearlman LA. [Harvard School of Public Health, Institute for Health Research] Case study on cost-effectiveness of automated multichannel chemistry analyzers. The implications of cost-effectiveness analysis of medical technology background paper #2: case studies of medical technologies. Office of Technology Assessment, U.S. Congress. Washington, D.C.: U.S. Government Printing Office, 1981. [Epidemiological methods]

HA21 Fineberg HV, Wittenberg J. [Harvard School of Public Health, Institute for Health Research] Evaluation of computed tomography in pancreatic cancer. Bull Cancer (Paris) 1980;67:390-394. [Epidemiological methods]

HA22 Wittenberg J, Fineberg HV, Ferrucci JT Jr, Simeone JF, Mueller PR, van Sonnenberg E, Kirkpatrick RH. [Harvard School of Public Health, Institute for Health Research] The clinical efficacy of computed body tomography. II. Am J Roentgenol 1980;134:1111-1120. [Epidemiological methods]

HA23 Fineberg HV, Wittenberg J, Ferruci JT, Jr. [Harvard School of Public Health, Institute for Health Research] The clinical value of diagnostic tests: CT as a prototype. IN: Margulis A, Burhenne HJ, eds. Alimentary tract radiology: abdominal imaging, v. 3. St. Louis, Missouri: C.V. Mosby, 1979. [Epidemiological methods]

HA24 Fineberg HV. [Harvard School of Public Health, Institute for Health Research] Assessing the diagnostic contribution of imaging tests: computed tomography and ultrasound of the pancreas. In: Alperovitch A, de Dombal FT, Gremy F, eds. Evaluation of efficacy of medical action. New York: Elsevier-North Holland, 1979. [Epidemiological methods]

HA25 Fineberg HV. [Harvard School of Public Health, Institute for Health Research] Gastric freezing: a study of diffusion of a medical innovation. In: Medical techonology and the health care system: a study of the diffusion of equipment-embodied technology. Washington, D.C.: National Academy of Sciences, 1979. [Epidemiological methods]

HA26 Fineberg HV. [Harvard School of Public Health, Institute for Health Research] Medical technology policies and computed tomography. Ann Intern Med 1979;90:114-115. [Information syntheses]

HA27 Koplan JP, Schoenbaum SC, Weinstein MC, Fraser DW. [Harvard School of Public Health, Institute for Health Research] Pertussis vaccine—an analysis of benefits, risks and costs. N Eng J Med 1979;301:906-911. [Information syntheses]

HA28 Thompson M. [Harvard School of Public Health, Institute for Health Research] Prenatal diagnosis and public policy. In: Milunsky A, ed. Genetic disorders and the fetus: diagnosis, prevention and treatment. New York: Plenum Press, 1979. [Information syntheses]

HA29 Weinstein MC. [Harvard School of Public Health, Institute for Health Research] Economic evaluation of medical procedures and technologies: progress, problems, and prospects. In: Medical technology. Washington, D.C.: National Center for Health Services Research, 1979. (NCHSR Research Proceedings Series, DHEW pub. no. (PHS) 79-3254) [Cost analyses]

HA30 Neuhauser D. [Harvard School of Public Health, Institute for Health Research] Cost effective clinical decision making: are routine pediatric preoperative chest X-rays worth it? Ann Radiol (Paris) 1978;21:80-83. [Information syntheses]

HA31 Neutra RR, Fienberg SE, Greenland S, Friedman EA. [Harvard School of Public Health, Institute for Health Research] Effect of fetal monitoring on neonatal death rates. N Eng J Med 1978;299:324-326. [Epidemiological methods]

HA32 Wittenberg J, Fineberg HV, Black EB, Kirkpatrick RH, Schaffer DL, Ikeda MK, Ferrucci JT Jr. [Harvard Medical School, Institute for Health Research] The clinical efficacy of computerized body tomography. Am J Roentgenol 1978;131:5-14. [Epidemiological methods]

HA33 Barnes BA, Barnes AB. [Harvard School of Public Health, Institute for Health Research] Evaluation of surgical therapy by cost-benefit analysis. Surgery 1977;82:21-33. [Information syntheses]

HA34 Bunker J, Barnes B, Mosteller F, eds. Costs, risks, and benefits of surgery. New York: Oxford University Press, 1977. [Information syntheses]

HA35 Fineberg HV, Bauman K, Sossman M. [Harvard School of Public Health, Institute for Health Research] Computerized cranial tomography: effect on diagnostic and therapeutic plans. JAMA 1977;238:224-227. [Epidemiological methods]

HA36 Fineberg HV, Parker GS, Pearlman LA. [Harvard School of Public Health, Institute for Health Research] CT scanners: distribution and planning status in the United States. N Eng J Med 1977;297:216-218. [Epidemiological methods]

HA37 Neuhauser D, Jonsson E. [Harvard School of Public Health, Institute for Health Research] Managerial response to new health care technology: coronary artery bypass surgery. In: Abernathy WJ, Sheldon A, Prahalad CK, eds. The management of health care. Cambridge: Ballinger Press, 1975. [Information syntheses]

HA38 Neuhauser D, Lewicki A. [Harvard School of Public Health, Institute for Health Research] What do we gain from the sixth stool guaiac? N Eng J Med 1975;293:226-228. [Epidemiological methods]

Hastings Center

255 Elm Road
Briarcliff Manor, NY 10510
914-762-8500

Contact: Paul Homer, Assistant to the Director.

Overview: The Hastings Center is a nonprofit corporation formerly known as the Institute of Society, Ethics and Life Sciences. Since its founding in 1969, the Center has addressed ethical issues arising from advances in health and medicine, the natural sciences, and the social and behavioral sciences. The Center has about 11,000 individual members, including 2,200 libraries. Membership fees range from $38 for students to $48 for institutions and libraries.

Purpose: To carry out nonpartisan research on pressing ethical issues; to develop educational programs and literature; and to assist universities, legislators, and professional organizations in coping with moral problems.

Primary intended users: General public; providers, generally; health/medical professional associations; third party payers; government regulators; public policy-makers, legislators; policy research organizations.

Technologies: Drug, device, medical or surgical procedure, support system, organizational or administrative system.

Most Hastings Center work is conducted by research groups that address certain technological areas. Among those currently active are groups on health policy research, chronic illness, neonatology, genetic screening, and organ transplantation.

Intervention: Prevention, diagnosis, treatment.

Stage: Emerging, new, established or widespread practice.

By examining technologies already in use—such as dialysis and heart transplants—and those currently under development, the members of the health policy research group aim to arrive at some consensus that may prove useful to researchers and policy-makers who face difficult decisions about the appropriate direction for financing and distributing new medical technologies.

Properties: Ethical, legal, social implications.

The Center is especially interested in highlighting the role played by regulatory agencies and committees in monitoring new technologies. Research groups have addressed the ethical, social, and legal issues in genetic counselling and genetic engineering; occupational health; death and dying; and alternative forms of care for the terminally ill.

The death and dying research group, established in 1970, has examined the moral, social, and legal issues of the care of the dying engendered by advanced medical technology. Subjects included organ transplantation and the definition of death, the termination of treatment of dying patients, and the allocation of scarce resources to the dying. A successor group examined the goals of medicine and their relationship to death, suffering, and well-being. It examined changing social attitudes and practices toward childbirth; the difficulties of treating pain that appears to be psychological in origin; and the nature of suffering in a life-threatening illness, including the role of hospices. The current group examines decisions to forgo various life-sustaining technologies.

Selection process: Subjects for assessments may originate from many sources, including Center staff, fellows of the Center, medical societies and professional organizations, government agencies, foundations, and subscribing members of the Center. The selection of project topics is generally made by Center staff, as approved by the board of directors. In some cases, final selection is made by foundation approval of project grant proposals made by the Center.

Methods: Information syntheses, expert opinion, group judgment.

The Center works primarily through small, multidisciplinary study groups of about 10 to 12 outside specialists. Each group is set up to address a particular set of problems, and may meet 4 or 5 times over 12 months or more. Groups usually meet first for informal planning in response to staff suggestions. Work plans are finalized and approved by groups, then approved by the Center director or associate director. Groups often discuss relevant case studies or case histories, and may use a consensus development format. Reports and guidelines go through numerous drafts by Center staff and subgroups.

Turnaround time from selection of assessment topic to reporting of findings varies among types of projects. Most studies range from 6 to 12 months, although some have taken 2 to 3 years. The Center must also respond quickly to certain types of requests, such as requests to present testimony at Congressional hearings and requests from State and local government agencies.

Dissemination: Printed reports, journal articles.

The bimonthly *Hastings Center Report* is devoted to case studies, court decisions, other news, and articles regarding ethical problems of the biomedical, behavioral, and social sciences and issues in professional and applied ethics. Published since 1971, this is the Center's primary means of communication with its members and the general public. Other publications include monographs, reports, and books resulting from project work. Also, Center staff publish papers on ethical issues in medical technology, speak at medical conferences, and respond to inquiries from attorneys and journalists.

Budget: The annual budget of the Center is about $1.5 million, including about $250,000 devoted to studies in health and medicine. Funding sources: 56 percent foundations, other private grants; 44 percent sponsors/members dues, contributions, publications, workshops, other sources.

Technology assessment activities are supported directly by foundations such as the General Electric Foundation, the Charles A. Dana Foundation, and the Pettus-Crowe Foundation and by general funds from the Hastings Center's budget.

Use: Use of studies varies. For example, the program on ethical problems of research on human subjects monitors government regulations regarding human subjects research, develops educational and training programs and related activities, and serves as a resource for institutional review boards. A 1981 Hastings report, *The Hastings Center: Ethics in the 80s.* listed a variety of activities in which it had participated to indicate both the scope of its work and range of possible impact. The Center is described in: Institute of Medicine, Committee on Evaluating Medical Technologies in Clinical Use. *Assessing medical technologies.* Washington, DC: National Academy Press, 1985.

Related activities: The Hastings Center conducts an educational workshop program for teachers and other professionals throughout the country, and sponsors study programs for graduate and undergraduate students and visiting scholars. The Center holds workshops on problems in the ethical and legal assessment of new technologies and week-long seminars on medical ethics.

Completed Reports

HC1 Caplan A. [The Hastings Center] Should fetuses or infants be used as organ donors? Bioethics, forthcoming.

HC2 Bermel J. [The Hastings Center] Mothers vs. their babies in fetal therapy. Dialog Pediat Urol 1986 Jan.

HC3 Callahan D. [The Hastings Center] How technology is reframing the abortion debate. Hastings Cent Rep 1986 Feb.

HC4 Callahan D. [The Hastings Center] Public policy and the cessation of nutrition. In: Lynn J, ed. By no extraordinary means: the choice to forgo life-sustaining food and water. University of Indiana Press, 1986.

HC5 Caplan A. [The Hastings Center] A new dilemma: quality, ethics and expensive medical technologies. NY Med Q 1986;6(1).

HC6 Caplan A. [The Hastings Center] Ethics of in vitro fertilization. Primary Care 1986 Jun.

HC7 Caplan A. [The Hastings Center] The morality and immorality of reuse. Renal Life. 1986 Oct.

HC8 Cohen C. [The Hastings Center] Autonomy and equity in the ICU. Hastings Cent Rep 1986.

HC9 Cohen C. [The Hastings Center] Ethical and legal considerations in the care of the infant with end stage renal disease whose parents elect conservative therapy. Pediatr Nephrol 1986.

HC10 Cohen C. [The Hastings Center] Ethical problems in the clinical practice of anesthesia. In: Dekornfeld T, ed. Textbook of anesthesia. 1986.

HC11 Wolf S. [The Hastings Center] Ethics committees in the courts. Hastings Cent Rep 1986 Jun.

HC12 The Hastings Center. Ethical, legal and policy issues pertaining to solid organ procurement: a report of the Project on Organ Transplantation. 1985 Oct.

Health Care Financing Administration
Bureau of Eligibility, Reimbursement, and Coverage

East Building, Room 401
6325 Security Boulevard
Baltimore, MD 21207
301-594-9690

Contact: Robert E. Wren, Director, Office of Coverage Policy; or Barton McCann, M.D., 301-594-9370.

Overview: The Health Care Financing Administration (HCFA) is responsible for administering the Medicare program, provided for in title XVIII of the Social Security Act, and Federal participation in the Medicaid program. HCFA will spend approximately $84 billion for Medicare and $27 billion for Medicaid in 1988. Almost 400 million individual Medicare claims were processed in 1987.

The Medicare law provides coverage for broad categories of benefits, including inpatient and outpatient hospital care, skilled nursing facility care, home health care, and physicians' services. It places general and categorical limitations on the coverage of the services furnished by certain health care practitioners. Medicare payment is prohibited for any expenses incurred for items and services "which are not reasonable and necessary for the diagnosis or treatment of illness or injury or to improve the functioning of a malformed body member." HCFA regulations do not define "reasonable and necessary," and the regulations do not denote a process for how this term is to be applied.

The process used for making Medicare coverage determinations is largely a decentralized one. Most decisions are made by the 35 carriers, 54 fiscal intermediaries, and 54 professional review organizations (PROs) that contract with DHHS to review and adjudicate Medicare claims. (In general, carriers administer hospital services and related aspects of Part A of Medicare, intermediaries administer physician claims and other aspects of Part B, and PROs review appropriateness of services, utilization, and related aspects of delivery of services under Medicare.)

Although most "reasonable and necessary" coverage issues can be decided by contractors based on the Medicare statute, regulations, and policy precedents, some cannot be resolved without seeking additional expertise. Some 20 to 30 procedures per year are subject to a centralized technology assessment process coordinated by the HCFA Central Office. These issues are referred within HCFA to the Bureau of Eligibility, Reimbursement and Coverage (BERC), which assists in development of national policy on coverage, payment, and eligibility of services under Medicare and Medicaid.

HCFA's Medicaid responsibilities deal primarily with guidelines for appropriate institutional settings for services, eligibility for services, payment limitation rates, and other administrative matters. HCFA does not set technology policy for Medicaid programs, which are administered by the States, although the States often look to Medicare coverage rules for guidance. State Medicaid programs do follow HCFA policy regarding discontinuation of coverage for certain drugs—generally old ones—found by the FDA to be less than effective and that are no longer to be marketed for certain indications.

Purpose: To determine whether items and services are, or continue to be, reasonable and necessary for Medicare coverage purposes.

Primary intended users: Patients; providers, generally; physicians; acute facility administrators; long-term care facility administrators; other care givers; health product manufacturers; third party payers; government regulators; public policy-makers, legislators.

Technologies: *Device, medical or surgical procedure,* drug, support system, organizational or administrative system.

Medicare coverage of drugs is treated differently from procedures. Current Medicare manual instructions provide for coverage of drugs that have been approved for marketing by FDA, except when a particular use has been expressly disapproved or withdrawn from the market by the FDA, or designated as not covered in a national HCFA instruction.

Intervention: *Diagnosis, treatment,* rehabilitation.

Stage: *New,* established or widespread practice, obsolete.

Coverage questions may concern either new or unusual technologies, or those that are believed to be outmoded and no longer reasonable and necessary.

Properties: *Safety; effectiveness;* efficacy; cost; cost-effectiveness; service requirements; acceptance/adoption level; system impact; economic implications; ethical, legal, social implications.

Selection process: Coverage inquiries normally come through the HCFA regional offices from a number of sources, usually Medicare contractors. Inquiries are also raised by individual beneficiaries, physicians and other health care providers, health product manufacturers, public officials, professional associations, and government agencies. Other coverage issues are raised during HCFA's ongoing review of medical practice, and in the course of hearings on disputed claims.

Medicare contractors have the discretion—within HCFA national coverage determinations, rulings, or manual instructions—to decide coverage issues identified in the claims review process. When a claim for a new or otherwise questionable technology is received for which national HCFA policy does not exist, contractors are authorized to make "reasonable or necessary" decisions with respect to the technology, taking into account the frequency, duration, and the setting in which it was furnished. Such decisions are usually made in consultation with the contractor's own medical staff and local medical specialty groups. Thus, coverage of any particular technology may vary among contractors.

If contractors cannot resolve a question locally, or believe a national coverage determination may be necessary, the issue is referred to the HCFA Central Office through a HCFA regional office. Assessment priorities are set by the HCFA Central Office, based on Medicare significance, potential expenses, diffusion, and level of controversy regarding the technology.

Technologies may be reassessed when new or forthcoming published information indicates the need for reconsideration of an assessment. HCFA may choose to reassess an item or service that is already excluded or covered under the Medicare program. This might occur if, in a previous assessment, PHS suggests a reevaluation of a technology at a later date.

Methods: *Information syntheses, group judgment,* expert opinion, cost analyses.

The assessment process involves the HCFA Central Office staff and Physicians Panel, the PHS, and the national medical community. Upon receiving a coverage issue, the BERC staff prepares a background paper based on a medical literature search, the status of any FDA action, administrative aspects of the issue, current applicable Medicare coverage guidelines, and any available assessments from other organizations.

The background paper is presented to the HCFA Physicians Panel for review. The Panel meets once every 6 to 8 weeks in closed session. Based on the background paper, other evidence, and discussion, the Panel may recommend that the technology be: (1) covered or not covered, (2) referred to PHS on either an informal inquiry basis or with a request for a full assessment, (3) covered or not at the discretion of the particular Medicare contractor pending receipt of more information, or (4) subject to a special study or action (e.g., as in the case of the special study on heart transplantation commissioned by HCFA.)

When a referral is made to PHS, it is made to the NCHSR Office of Health Technology Assessment (OHTA). In the case of an informal request (known as an inquiry) OHTA conducts a review of the medical literature, discusses the issue with other government agencies and medical groups, and responds to the specific questions raised by HCFA. Handling of requests for full assessments varies according to the topic, though usually involves an announcement in the *Federal Register* soliciting comments from interested parties, seeking information from other agencies and medical groups, an extensive literature search, and synthesis of this information. (This process is described in the profile on OHTA in this Directory.) HCFA coverage decisions are based on recommendations from the PHS and other available sources of public comment and expert opinion. For those issues referred to OHTA, HCFA coverage decisions have nearly always been consistent with OHTA's recommendations.

The time to complete an assessment generally ranges from 6 months to 2 years, depending upon the quality of available information, potential impact on the Medicare population, and availability of alternative technologies.

Reassessments are conducted as are those for new technologies, except that decisions to withdraw coverage call for publication of a notice in the *Federal Register* announcing that intent.

Assessors: The HCFA Physicians Panel includes about eight HCFA staff physicians, as well as other HCFA staff members with health financing expertise. Ex officio members of the Panel include representatives from OHTA, NIH, and FDA. Depending upon the assessment topic, other experts may be consulted as well. HCFA is establishing referral lists of experts in particular technological areas from other Federal agencies to be called upon for consultation on coverage decisions.

Assessment reports include: Description of the technology; findings or conclusions; coverage/reimbursement status of the technology.

National Medicare coverage decisions made by HCFA usually appear as guidelines in the *Medicare Coverage Issues Manual* provided to Medicare contractors. (Some coverage decisions require no revision of the manual.) Rather than being assessment reports as such, the guidelines in the *Manual* usually consist of at most several sentences describing a technology, whether it is covered or not, and if so, under what conditions it is covered. A few guidelines, such as those on cardiac pacemaker evaluation services (section 50-1 in the *Manual*) and magnetic resonance imaging (50-13), are 3 to 4 pages long. The background papers prepared by HCFA staff for the Physicians Panel and the OHTA assessments on which many HCFA coverage decisions are based are more detailed reports. See the Completed Reports section at the end of this profile for an example of a *Manual* coverage guideline.

Although most coverage guidelines derive from the assessment process described in this profile, the *Manual* includes some coverage guidelines set by statutory changes and other rulings. Examples are the guidelines on laser procedures (section 35-52 in the *Manual*), artificial hearts and related devices (65-15), and enteral and parenteral nutritional therapy (65-10); these guidelines are not associated with assessment reports. A coverage decision that was not subject to normal OHTA or HCFA assessment procedures was the 1986 ruling on heart transplantation, based in part on the findings of the special DHHS-sponsored study completed in 1984 by the Battelle Human Affairs Research Centers.

Dissemination: *Printed reports;* press conferences/news releases, TV/radio broadcasts, video products.

After a final HCFA coverage decision is made, the guidelines are disseminated via the *Medicare Coverage Issues Manual* and through public notice of rules, regulations, and informally through correspondence and public presentations. Background papers prepared for the Physicians Panel are for internal use only.

The *Medicare Coverage Issues Manual (HCFA Publication 6)* is available from the U.S. Government Printing Office, Washington, DC 20402. The *Manual* is updated about 15 to 20 times a year by transmittal sheets sent to its users. Individual guidelines are available from HCFA.

Budget: The budget for the HCFA Office of Coverage Policy was approximately $2,000,000 in 1986. This figure does not include the cost of OHTA assessments, the value of consultation from outside experts, and related assessment costs; and does include the cost of a variety of Medicare and Medicaid coverage activities not directly pertinent to technology assessment. Funding source: 100 percent parent organization.

Use: HCFA coverage decisions are used as a basis for Medicare coverage policy. Coverage decisions made by other government entities and private third party payers are also influenced by the guidelines.

The Medicare coverage process is described by HCFA in: Medicare Program; Procedures for Medical Services Coverage Decisions; Request for Comments, *Federal Register*; 52(82), April 29, 1987, 15560-62.

The HCFA assessment activity has been evaluated in the following two reports sponsored by DHHS:

Lewin and Associates. *A forward plan for Medicare coverage and technology assessment.* Prepared for the Assistant Secretary for Planning and Evaluation, Department of Health and Human Services, 1986.

Macro Systems, Inc. *Technology assessment and coverage decision-making in the Department of Health and Human Services.* Prepared for the Assistant Secretary for Planning and Evaluation, Department of Health and Human Services, 1984.

Related activities: BERC staff members participate in meetings and conferences sponsored by other organizations conducting technology assessment. BERC also convenes regular meetings with medical directors of HCFA contractors to discuss coverage, payment, and medical review issues.

Completed Reports:

As discussed above under Assessment Reports, HCFA coverage decisions appear as guidelines in the *Medicare Coverage Issues Manual* and normally do not generate assessment reports other than those provided by OHTA. Therefore, no listing of HCFA assessment reports is shown here; the reader may consult the profile on OHTA in this *Directory* for a listing of assessments conducted for HCFA.

For purposes of illustration, the following HCFA national coverage guideline appearing in the *Medicare Coverage Issues Manual* is reproduced here. This HCFA coverage decision followed a 1985 OHTA assessment report, *Implantable Automatic Cardioverter-Defibrillators*.

35-85 IMPLANTATION OF AUTOMATIC DEFIBRILLATORS (Effective for services performed on and after 1-24-86.)

The implantable automatic defibrillator is an electronic device designed to detect and treat life-threatening tachyarrhythmias. The device consists of a pulse generator and electrodes for sensing and defibrillating. The implantation of an automatic defibrillator is a covered service only when used as a treatment of last resort for patients who have had a documented episode of life-threatening ventricular tachyarrhythmia or cardiac arrest not associated with myocardial infarction. Patients must also be found, by electrophysiologic testing, to have an inducible tachyarrhythmia that proves unresponsive to medication or surgical therapy (or be considered unsuitable candidates for surgical therapy).

It must be emphasized that unless all of the above described conditions and stipulations are met in a particular case, including the inducibility of tachyarrhythmia, etc., implan- implantation of an automatic defibrillator cannot be covered.

Health Care Financing Administration
Office of Research and Demonstrations

Oak Meadows Building, Room 2-B-12
6325 Security Boulevard
Baltimore, MD 21207
301-597-1435

Contact: Joel Broida, Research Analyst.

Overview: The Office of Research and Demonstrations (ORD), Health Care Financing Administration (HCFA) is a Federal agency that directs more than 300 research, evaluation, and demonstration projects. ORD's activities are carried out by three major components—the Office of Research, the Office of Demonstrations and Evaluations, and the Office of Operations Support. The Office of Research conducts and supports data collection efforts and research on health care providers, reimbursement, beneficiary behavior, and health care utilization. The Office of Demonstrations and Evaluations funds, manages, and evaluates pilot programs that test new ways of delivering and financing Medicare and Medicaid services. The Office of Operations Support provides ORD-wide administrative direction for its research, demonstration, and evaluation projects, which includes the budget and accounting operations; grants, cooperative agreements, and contracts-award process; and publications and information resources program.

Purpose: To carry out research, evaluation, and demonstration projects related to the administration and operation of the Medicare and Medicaid programs. A major focus is on expenditures as they relate to reimbursement, coverage, eligibility, and management alternatives. Study activity also examines program impact on beneficiary health status, access to services, utilization, and out-of-pocket expenditures. The behavior and economics of health care providers and the overall health care industry are also topics of investigation.

Primary intended users: Providers, generally; acute facility administrators; long-term care facility administrators; health industry associations; employers; unions and other employee organizations; third party payers; government regulators; biomedical researchers; public policy-makers, legislators; policy research organizations.

Technologies: *Organizational or administrative system,* drug, device, medical or surgical procedure, support system.

Intervention: Prevention, diagnosis, treatment, rehabilitation.

Stage: New, established or widespread practice.

Generally, devices and procedures are assessed after they have been introduced in the clinical setting.

Properties: *Effectiveness, cost, cost-effectiveness,* safety, efficacy, cost-benefit, service requirements, acceptance/adoption level, system impact, economic implications.

Selection process: Requests for assessments may originate either within the agency or from outside it, through Medicare insurance contractors, other third party payers, physicians, intermediaries, and other persons. Some requests come in the form of unsolicited grant applications. Questions about reassessments are usually decided in HCFA's Bureau of Eligibility, Reimbursement, and Coverage.

Methods: Information syntheses, expert opinion, group judgment, modeling, cost analyses, epidemiological and other observational methods.

Assessments are conducted in-house or extramurally through contracts, grants, and cooperative agreements.

Assessment reports include: Abstract; the assessment's intended audience; the purpose of the assessment; relationship of this assessment to prior or concurrent assessments of the technology or other technologies intended for similar purposes; who conducted the assessment; description of the technology; stage of life-cycle of technology when assessed; properties assessed; procedure used for the assessment; sources of data/information; methods for collecting data/information; methods for analyzing/synthesizing data/information; results; findings or conclusions; limitations of findings; implications of findings for practice; recommendations for practice, future assessments, technology development, research; how much the assessment cost; how the technology works, including theory, principles; development of the technology; procurement/deployment information; where technology is in use; regulatory agency approval status; coverage/reimbursement status of the technology; product recall history, liability actions.

Dissemination: *Printed reports;* journal articles; advisories to members/constituents; press conferences/news releases, TV/radio broadcasts, video products; clearinghouses, data/citation bases, online services, specifically, the NTIS database.

As extramural projects are completed, the final reports are placed with the National Technical Information Service (NTIS). For those projects with final reports at NTIS, the accession number is necessary when ordering. Further information may be obtained from: NTIS, Document Sales, 5285 Port Royal Rd., Springfield, VA 22151, 703-487-4650.

A select number of final reports is published by HCFA under its *Grants and Contracts Reports Series.* These reports are available for sale from the U.S. Government Printing Office (GPO). Reports must be ordered by title and stock number directly from GPO: Superintendent of Documents, U.S. Government Printing Office, Washington, DC 20402.

In addition, results from intramural and extramural research projects and demonstrations are often featured in the *Health Care Financing Review,* the agency's quarterly journal. The journal also offers synopses on newly awarded research and demonstration projects being funded by HCFA. The *Review* is available on a subscription basis from the GPO for $18.00 ($22.50 foreign).

Budget: Not provided. Funding source: 100 percent parent organization.

Use: HCFA uses the assessment reports to assess new methods and approaches for providing quality health care while containing costs and to help make policy decisions on coverage and reimbursement of services for Medicare beneficiaries. The reports are also used by the research community, other Government agencies, universities, and other interested parties in the private sector such as private health insurers.

Completed Reports

HF1 A demonstration and evaluation of a preventive services package to provide early detection of illness and monitoring high-risk Medicare beneficiaries. In: Office of Research and Demonstrations, Health Care Financing Administration. Health care financing status report: research and demonstrations in health care financing. Jan 1986. (HCFA Pub. No. 03219).

HF2 A demonstration of cost control and patient satisfaction resulting from the relaxation of the maximum public enrollment rule for HMO's. In: ______.

HF3 A longitudinal study of case-mix outcomes and resource use in nursing homes. In: ______.

HF4 A national study of resource-based relative value scales for Physician Services. In: ______.

HF5 AFDC/Medicaid eligibility—impact on prenatal care use. In: ______.

HF6 Acquisition and analysis of state Medicaid data. In: ______.

HF7 Alcoholism services under Medicare and Medicaid: Illinois demonstration. In: ______.

HF8 Alcoholism services under Medicare and Medicaid: Michigan demonstration. In: ______.

HF9 Alcoholism services under Medicare and Medicaid: New Jersey demonstration. In: ______.

HF10 Alcoholism services under Medicare and Medicaid: New York demonstration. In: ______.

HF11 Alcoholism services under Medicare: Connecticut demonstration. In: ______.

HF12 Alcoholism services under Medicare: Oklahoma demonstration. In: ______.

HF13 Alternate models for prepaid capitation of health care services for Medicare beneficiaries—Oregon. In: ______.

HF14 American Association of Retired Persons' Informed Buyer Program. In: ______.

HF15 An analysis of long-run rate setting strategies for risk-based contracting under Medicare. In: ______.

HF16 An evaluation of "Life-Continuum of Care" residential centers in the United States. In: ______.

HF17 An independent evaluation of the reliability of the standardized Medreview Instrument. In: ______.

HF18 Analysis of Medicare routine costs under alternative assumptions. In: ______.

HF19 Analysis of NMCUES data. In: ______.

HF20 Analysis of long-term care payment systems. In: ______.

HF21 Analysis of physician fee information from several sources. In: ______.

HF22 Analysis of physician pricing behavior, third-party administrative practices. In: ______.

HF23 Analysis of the 1982 Long-Term Care Survey. In: ______.

HF24 Analysis of the 1982 survey of informal caregivers. In: ______.

HF25 Annual reports to Congress on the impact of the Medicare Hospital prospective payment system. In: ______.

HF26 Appropriateness of hospitalization: a comparative analysis of reliability and validity of the Appropriateness Evaluation Protocol and the Standardized Medreview Instrument. In: ______.

HF27 Aspects of physician behavior in Medicare and Medicaid. In: ______.

HF28 Assess (State) tax incentives as a means of strengthening the informal support system for the elderly. In: ______.

HF29 Assessment of emerging technologies for the treatment of end-stage renal disease. In: ______.

HF30 Assignment rates revisited. In: ______.

HF31 California State Copayment Project In: ______.

HF32 Can geriatric nurse practitioners improve nursing home care? In: ______.

HF33 Capitation payment system for all end-stage renal disease services. In: ______.

HF34 Case mix and resource use in hospital emergency room settings. In: ______.

HF35 Case-managed medical care for nursing home patients. In: ______.

HF36 Case-mix measure for long-term care Medicare patients. In: ______.

HF37 Changes in the distribution of Medicare expenditures. In: ______.

HF38 Children's Hospital Case-Mix Classification System Project. In: ______.

HF39 Comparative analysis of the costs and outcomes of kidney transplants. In: ______.

HF40 Comparison by state of SNF/ICF types: beds, staffing, utilization, and ownership. In: ______.

HF41 Comparison of quality of life of end-stage renal disease patients. In: ______.

HF42 Comparison of the cost and quality of home health and nursing home care. In: ______.

HF43 Competitive managed health plans for AFDC Medicaid recipients. In: ______.

HF44 Consumer as a partner in medical cost containment. In: ______.

HF45 Cost of care information to consumers. In: ______.

HF46 Costs, outcomes, and competition in the End-Stage Renal Disease Program. In: ______.

HF47 Creating diagnosis-related-group-based physician reimbursement schemes: a conceptual and empirical analysis. In: ______.

HF48 Demonstration and evaluation of competitive bidding as a method of purchasing durable medical equipment. In: ______.

HF49 Demonstration and evaluation of competitive bidding as a method to purchase clinical laboratory services. In: ______.

HF50 Demonstration of community-wide, alternative long-term care model. In: ______.

HF51 Determination of health maintenance organization capitation rates for Medicare beneficiaries. In: ______.

HF52 Develop the technology of aide sharing into a transferable form for use by home health agencies to reduce home health costs. In: ______.

HF53 Developing incentive systems to increase the supply of cadaveric kidneys for transplants. In: ______.

HF54 Development of a case-mix based reimbursement method for hospital outpatient departments and free-standing clinics. In: ______.

HF55 Development of staging for six rehabilitation conditions and a cross-reference system with their respective diagnois-related groups. In: ______.

HF56 Development, pilot testing, and refinement of valid outcome measures for the home care setting. In: ______.

HF57 Diagnosis-related groups and nursing resources. In: ______.

HF58 Diagnosis-related groups refinement for nursing care. In: ______.

HF59 Diagnosis-related groups refinement using measures of disease severity. In: ______.

HF60 Diagnostic mix, illness severity, and costs in teaching and nonteaching hospitals. In: ______.

HF61 Disease-specific severity adjustments to diagnosis-related groups. In: ______.

HF62 Disproportionate share hospitals: costs and case mix. In: ______.

HF63 Economic and clinical outcomes of three drug cost-containment strategies in Medicaid. In: ______.

HF64 Economics of diagnosis-related-group-based physician reimbursement. In: ______.

HF65 Effects of alternative family support strategies. In: ______.

HF66 Encouraging appropriate care for the chronically ill elderly: a controlled experiment to evaluate the impacts of incentive payments on nursing home admissions, discharges, case mix, care, outcomes,and costs. In: ______.

HF67 End-Stage Renal Disease Nutritional Therapy Study. In: ______.

HF68 End-stage renal disease annual report to Congress. In: ______.

HF69 End-stage renal disease competitive bidding demonstration. In: ______.

HF70 Enrollment of Medicare beneficiaries under a unique intra-health maintenance organization competition model. In: ______.

HF71 Evaluability assessment of the Medicare prospective payment system on long-term care. In: ______.

HF72 Evaluation of Massachusetts case-managed medical care for nursing home patients. In: ______.

HF73 Evaluation of Medicaid competition demonstrations. In: ______.

HF74 Evaluation of Medicare health maintenance organization demonstration projects. In: ______.

HF75 Evaluation of Municipal Health Services Program. In: ______.

HF76 Evaluation of National Rural Swing-Bed Program. In: ______.

HF77 Evaluation of Obstetrical Access Pilot Project. In: ______.

HF78 Evaluation of coordinated community-oriented, long-term care demonstration. In: ______.

HF79 Evaluation of health maintenance organization (HMO) capitation demonstrations. In: ______.

HF80 Evaluation of prepaid managed health care demonstration. In: ______.

HF81 Evaluation of prepaid risk-bearing care organization. In: ______.

HF82 Evaluation of social health maintenance organization demonstrations. In: ______.

HF83 Evaluation of the Arizona health care cost-containment system. In: ______.

HF84 Evaluation of the Medicare competition demonstrations. In: ______.

HF85 Evaluation of the Medicare mental health demonstration. In: ______.

HF86 Evaluation of the alcoholism services demonstration. In: ______.

HF87 Evaluation of the impact of second opinions for elective surgery. In: ______.

HF88 Evaluation of the urban health clinics demonstration. In: ______.

HF89 Evaluation of three-state demonstration in nursing home quality assurance. In: ______.

HF90 Feasibility of incorporating CPT-4 codes for physician billing into the diagnosis-related groups system for in-hospital Medicare surgical patients. In: ______.

HF91 Foot care coverage study. In: ______.

HF92 Further analysis of the medical doctor diagnosis-related groups algorithms. In: ______.

HF93 Geriatric Continence Research Project. In: ______.

HF94 Health Care Plus: the Lutheran Medical Center program for prepaid managed health care. In: ______.

HF95 Health Status at Discharge Research Project. In: ______.

HF96 Health care alternatives within Title XIX: evaluation of alternative reimbursement methods to providers of primary care medical services. In: ______.

HF97 Health care services for children under Medicaid. In: ______.

HF98 Health services utilization study. In: ______.

HF99 Home health agency prospective payment demonstration. In: ______.

HF100 Home respiratory therapy services. In: ______.

HF101 Home services for functionally disabled adults. In: ______.

HF102 Hospice patient outcomes and quality of care. In: ______.

HF103 Impact of DRG-based prospective payment system on quality of care for hospitalized Medicare patients. In: ______.

HF104 Impact of Medicare fee freeze and participation agreements on physicians. In: ______.

HF105 Impact of Medicare's prospective payment system and private sector initiatives: the Blue Cross and Blue Shield Organization's experiences. In: ______.

HF106 Impact of physician supply and regulation on physician fees and utilization of services. In: ______.

HF107 Impact of psychological intervention on health care utilization and costs: a prospective study. In: ______.

HF108 Impact of the prospective payment system on the quality of inpatient care. In: ______.

HF109 Implications of the National Hospice Study for hospice prospective reimbursement. In: ______.

HF110 Improving New York State's Nursing Home Quality Assurance Program. In: ______.

HF111 Incentive prospective payment system for hospitals through fiscal intermediaries (Massachusetts). In: ______.

HF112 Incentive reimbursement plan for Medicaid home health services. In: ______.

HF113 Incorporating the cost of ambulatory care into case-mix based hospital reimbursement. In: ______.

HF114 Independent broker: coordinating open enrollment for Medicare health maintenance organizations and competitive medical plans. In: ______.

HF115 Information for prudent insurance choices. In: ______.

HF116 Learning from and improving diagnosis-related groups for end-stage renal disease patients. In: ______.

HF117 Long-term care of aged individuals with hip fractures: public versus private costs. In: ______.

HF118 Long-term care residential services for developmentally disabled people. In: ______.

HF119 Longitudinal studies of local area hospital use. In: ______.

HF120 Longitudinal study of the impact of prospective reimbursement under Medicaid on nursing home care in Maine. In: ______.

HF121 Malpractice component of the Medicare economic index. In: ______.

HF122 Massachusetts Health Care Panel Study of Elderly—Wave IV. In: ______.

HF123 Measuring the cost of case mix using patient management categories. In: ______.

HF124 Medicaid child health care evaluation. In: ______.

HF125 Medicaid program evaluation. In: ______.

HF126 Medicaid program evaluation: cluster I. In: ______.

HF127 Medicaid program evaluation: cluster II. In: ______.

HF128 Medicaid program evaluation: cluster III. In: ______.

HF129 Medicaid tape-to-tape ambulatory services project. In: ______.

HF130 Medicaid tape-to-tape: data and analysis. In: ______.

HF131 Medicaid voucher demonstration. In: ______.

HF132 Medical doctor diagnosis-related groups algorithms. In: ______.

HF133 Medicare Prospective Capitation Demonstration Project. In: ______.

HF134 Medicare and Medicaid data book. In: ______.

HF135 Medicare automated data retrieval system. In: ______.

HF136 Medicare clinical social worker demonstration. In: ______.

HF137 Medicare competition demonstrations. In: ______.

HF138 Medicare health maintenance organization additional benefits. In: ______.

HF139 Medicare reimbursement regression to the mean. In: ______.

HF140 Medicare-Medicaid payment policies and capital formation. In: ______.

HF141 Medigap study of comparative effectiveness of state regulations. In: ______.

HF142 Methods of improving case mix and severity of illness classification for use in the Medicare prospective payment system. In: ______.

HF143 Metropolitan Comprehensive Care Program: a health systems organization demonstration. In: ______.

HF144 Missouri Medicaid Prepaid Health Demonstration Project. In: ______.

HF145 National Hospice Study. In: ______.

HF146 National Hospital Rate-Setting Study. In: ______.

HF147 National Kidney Dialysis and Kidney Transplantation Study. In: ______.

HF148 National and cross-national study of long-term care populations. In: ______.

HF149 New Jersey mobile intensive care system. In: ______.

HF150 New York Ambulatory Care Reimbursement Project. In: ______.

HF151 New York State case-mix, prospective reimbursement system for long-term care. In: ______.

HF152 Noncertified hospice cost analysis. In: ______.

HF153 Nonintrusive outcome measures: identification and validation. In: ______.

HF154 Organ Donor Education Project. In: ______.

HF155 Payment options for nonphysician anesthetists under the prospective payment system. In: ______.

HF156 Physician reimbursement and continuing care under Medicaid in Suffolk County, New York. In: ______.

HF157 Planning study: phase I of a major study of national long-term care policies. In: ______.

HF158 Population-based study of hospice. In: ______.

HF159 Post-surgical mortality among the aged for common operations. In: ______.

HF160 Prenatal care and its relationship to Medicaid costs. In: ______.

HF161 Prevention of falls in the elderly. In: ______.

HF162 Prevention of future utilization of health and long-term care services. In: ______.

HF163 Program for prepaid managed health care. In: ______.

HF164 Prospective payment beneficiary impact study. In: ______.

HF165 Prospective payment in rehabilitation hospitals and programs. In: ______.

HF166 Prospective payment of physicians. In: ______.

HF167 Prospective payment system and post-hospital care: use, cost, and market changes. In: ______.

HF168 Prospective payment system for acute and chronic care hospitals in Maryland. In: ______.

HF169 Prospective reimbursement system based on patient case mix for New Jersey hospitals. In: ______.

HF170 Quality and effectivness of preventive medical care. In: ______.

HF171 Quality assurance sampling: a statistical quality-control approach to inspection of care. In: ______.

HF172 Quality of life among life-care facility and community residents: A comparison. In: ______.

HF173 Reducing inappropriate use of inpatient medical, surgical, and pediatric services—extension of the Appropriateness Evaluation Protocol. In: ______.

HF174 Registered dietitians in home care. In: ______.

HF175 Rehospitalization after surgery among Medicare enrollees. In: ______.

HF176 Relative effectiveness and cost of transplantation and dialysis in end-stage renal disease. In: ______.

HF177 Research on competitive forces driving Medicare utilization. In: ______.

HF178 Resource utilization groups: validation and refinement of a case-mix system for long-term care reimbursement. In: ______.

HF179 Respite care co-op for impaired elderly. In: ______.

HF180 Response of Massachusetts acute-care hospitals to the Massachusetts Cost-Containment Act. In: ——

HF181 Responsibility of children for financing institutional care: potential response and possible adjustments. In: ______.

HF182 Section 1619 study on the working disabled. In: ______.

HF183 Selected analyses of the prospective payment system's impact on hospital's behavior In: ______.

HF184 Self-care home computer program to reduce health care costs. In: ______.

HF185 Senior Group Health Plan Waiver-Only Medicare Competition Demonstration Program. In: ______.

HF186 Severity of illness and diagnosis-related groups in selected cancers. In: ______.

HF187 Severity of illness in end-stage renal disease population in northern Florida. In: ______.

HF188 Social Health Maintenance Organization Project for long-term care. In: ______.

HF189 South Carolina Community Long-Term Care Project. In: ______.

HF190 State Medicaid nursing home policies, utilization, and expenditures. In: ______.

HF191 Statewide Medicaid competition demonstration. In: ______.

HF192 Studies evaluating Medicaid home- and community-based services: a report to Congress. In: ______.

HF193 Studies of Medicare use before death. In: ______.

HF194 Study of Medicare-funded heart transplants. In: ______.

HF195 Study of high-cost infants under Medicaid. In: ______.

HF196 Study of long-term care quality and reimbursement in teaching and nonteaching nursing homes. In: ______.

HF197 Study of the quality and effectiveness of experimental fixed-price Medicare Part A intermediary contracting. In: ______.

HF198 Systematic examination of factors that promote home care by the family. In: ______.

HF199 Test of the out-of-pocket cost savings as an incentive for changing beneficiary choice behavior. In: ______.

HF200 Texas Long-Term Care Case-Mix Reimbursement Project. In: ______.

HF201 The economy and efficacy of Medicare reimbursement for preventive services. In: ______.

HF202 The impact of Medicaid home and community-based waiver services for the mentally retarded in Maine. In: ______.

HF203 The nature, process, and modes of hospice care delivery. In: ______.

HF204 The relation of surgical volume and other factors to mortality after surgery. In: ______.

HF205 Title XVIII Hospice Benefit Program evaluation (Medicare). In: ______.

HF206 Urban health clinics demonstration. In: ______.

HF207 Use of Medicare services by disabled enrollees under 65 years of age. In: ______.

HF208 Use of services by the dually entitled (crossovers). In: ______.

HF209 Waiver-Only Competition Project for Southern California, Illinois, Indiana, and Texas. In: ______.

Health Council of The Netherlands

PO Box 90.517
2509 LM The Hague
The Netherlands
(31-70) 47-14-41

Contact: Dr. Henk Rigter, Executive Director.

Overview: The Health Council of The Netherlands is a not-for-profit, independent advisory council funded by the Government of The Netherlands. The Council was established in 1903 and its position was recomfirmed in the Health Act of 1956.

Purpose: To advise the government about the "state of science" with respect to health care and environmental protection.

Primary intended users: General public; people concerned about their health; patients; providers, generally; physicians; acute facility administrators; long-term care facility administrators; other care givers; health product manufacturers; health/medical professional associations; health industry associations; consumer associations; employers; unions and other employee organizations; third party payers; government regulators; voluntary associations, organizations; biomedical researchers; financial analysts, consultants; reporters, writers, news media; information/computer industry; labs, blood banks; public policy-makers, legislators; policy research organizations; lawyers.

Technologies: Drug, device, medical or surgical procedure, support system, organizational or administrative system, environmental protection technologies.

Intervention: *Prevention, treatment,* diagnosis, rehabilitation.

Stage: *New,* emerging, established or widespread practice, obsolete.

Properties: Safety; efficacy; effectiveness; cost; cost-benefit; cost effectiveness; service requirements; acceptance/adoption level; system impact; economic implications, ethical, legal, social implications; psychological issues.

Selection process: Although financed by the government, the Council operates as an independent agency. The Council selects assessment topics, sets priorities, and decides how an assessment should be conducted. The government may also formally request advice on specific topics. The Council is free to issue reports at its own initiative. Reports are updated regularly. Staff members, Council members, or committee members may suggest reassessments to the President of the Council.

Methods: *Group judgment,* information syntheses, expert opinion, modeling, cost analyses, epidemiological and other observational methods.

The Council's assessment activities emphasize state-of-the-art syntheses. For each subject, the President or Vice-President of the Council appoints a multidisciplinary committee of experts. At any given time, about 65 committees are at work, involving a total of approximately 600 persons (members and non-members of the Council). The approximate turnaround time from selection of assessment topic to reporting of findings is 18 months.

Assessors: Committee members have expertise in medical specialties, economics, psychology, sociology, law, ethics, management, physics, chemistry, and biology.

Assessment reports include: Abstract; the assessment's intended audience; the purpose of the assessment; relationship of this assessment to prior or concurrent assessments of the technology or other technologies intended for similar purposes; who sponsored/commissioned/supported the assessment; who conducted the assessment; description of the technology; stage of life-cycle of technology when assessed; properties assessed; procedure used for the assessment; sources of data/information; methods for collecting data/information; methods for analyzing/synthesizing data/information; results; findings or conclusions; limitations of findings; implications of findings for practice; recommendations for practice, future assessments, technology development, research; how the technology works, including theory, principles; development of the technology; procurement/deployment information; where technology is in use; coverage/reimbursement status of the technology.

Dissemination: *Printed reports;* journal articles; advisories to profession, hospitals; press conferences/news releases, TV/radio broadcasts, video products.

In general, the reports of the Council are public. They are printed and distributed by the Council and sent to the press and interested organizations and individuals. Most reports have an English summary; this is only the first step in making the publications accessible to an international audience. The Council plans to produce an English newsletter, to be published 3 times a year. The first issue is scheduled to appear in 1987.

Budget: $1.7 million. The approximate cost per assessment is $70,000. Funding sources: 90 percent government grants/contracts; 5 percent foundations, other private grants; 5 percent sales of assessments, consultant services.

Use: Although formally addressed to the government, some reports of the Council are directly relevant to health care professionals. For example, most hospitals in The Netherlands use reports issued by the Council as a reference source for radiation protection and prevention of hospital infections.

Program evaluations: In 1983, the government established a national commission to evaluate the Council. The evaluation consisted of interviews and the results were very positive.

Related activities: The Council publishes a newsletter, sponsors symposia, and serves a clearinghouse function for medical technology assessment in The Netherlands.

Completed Reports

HN1 Health Council of The Netherlands. CO2. 1987

HN2 ______. Transplantation issues. 1987.

HN3 ______. Ultrasound. 1987.

HN4 ______. Artificial procreation. 1986. (English summary only).

HN5 ______. Dialysis and kidney transplantation. 1986. [English summary only].

HN6 ______. Inhalation sedation in dentistry. 1986. [English summary only].

HN7 ______. Inhalation sedation in dentistry. 1986. [English summary only].

HN8 ______. Magnetic resonance spectroscopy. 1986. [English summary only].

HN9 ______. Mental health care. 1986. [English summary only].

HN10 ______. Monoclonal antibodies. 1986.

HN11 ______. Monoclonal antibodies. 1986. [English summary only].

HN12 ______. Otitis media. 1986. [English summary only].

HN13 ______. Pain treatment. 1986. [English summary only].

HN14 ______. Positron emission tomography. 1986. [English summary only].

HN15 ______. Sexually transmitted diseases. 1986. [English summary only].

HN16 ______. Suicide. 1986. [English summary only].

HN17 ______. Therapeutic hemapheresis. 1986. [English summary only].

HN18 ______. Very low energy diets. 1986. [English summary only].

HN19 ______. Allogenic bone marrow transplantation. 1985. (English summary only).

HN20 ______. Classification of and standards for radionuclide laboratories. 1985. (English summary only).

HN21 ______. Guidelines for radiation protection in hospitals and out-patient departments. 1985. (English summary only).

HN22 ______. Minimal brain dysfunction. 1985. (English summary only).

HN23 ______. Second report on AIDS: clinical, psychosocial and ethical aspects. 1985. (English summary only).

HN24 ______. Cardiac surgery. 1984.

HN25 ______. Brain death criteria. 1983.

HN26 ______. Hepatitis B. 1983.

HN27 ______. Neonatal intensive care. 1982.

HN28 ______. Hypertension. 1978.

HN29 ______. Recent developments in anesthesiology. 1978.

HN30 ______. Transsexualism. 1977.

HN31 ______. Use of antibiotics. 1977.

HN32 ______. Coronary heart surgery. 1976.

HN33 ______. Preventing hospital infections. 1976.

Ongoing Assessments

HN34 ______. AIDS (acquired immune deficiency syndrome). Ongoing.

HN35 ______. Admission of new sera and vaccines. Ongoing.

HN36 ______. Alternative medicine. Ongoing.

HN37 ______. Anorexia nervosa and boulimia. Ongoing.

HN38 ______. Biotechnology: new avenues of research. Ongoing.

HN39 ______. Bone marrow transplantation. Ongoing.

HN40 ______. Breast feeding (contamination of milk). Ongoing.

HN41 ______. Chymopapain. Ongoing.

HN42 ______. Diagnosis and treatment of the fetus. Ongoing.

HN43 ______. Dialysis. Ongoing.

HN44 ______. Endoscopy. Ongoing.

HN45 ______. Fetal surgery. Ongoing.

HN46 ______. Food irradiation. Ongoing.

HN47 ______. Hair analysis. Ongoing.

HN48 ______. In vitro fertilization. Ongoing.

HN49 ______. Innovations in medical technology. Ongoing.

HN50 ______. Lasers. Ongoing.

HN51 ______. Lithotryptor. Ongoing.

HN52 ______. Liver transplantation. Ongoing.

HN53 ______. Medical equipment: priorities in research and development. Ongoing.

HN54 ______. Minimal brain dysfunction. Ongoing.

HN55 ______. Monoclonal antibodies, advice on regulatory issues. Ongoing.

HN57 ______. NMR/MRI. Ongoing.

HN58 ______. National vaccination program. Ongoing.

HN59 ______. Osteoporosis. Ongoing.

HN60 ______. Otitis media. Ongoing.

HN61 ______. PET-scan. Ongoing.

HN62 ______. Pain treatment and clinics. Ongoing..

HN63 ______. Pediatric surgery. Ongoing.

HN64 ______. Prevention of hospital infections. Ongoing.

HN65 ______. Psychogeriatrics. Ongoing.

HN66 ______. Psychosurgery. Ongoing.

HN67 ______. Screening for breast cancer. Ongoing.

HN68 ______. Screening for neural tube defects. Ongoing.

HN69 ______. Stress and health. Ongoing.

HN70 ______. Suicide. Ongoing.

HN71 ______. Transplantation: ethical and legal; kidney; heart; liver; pancreas; bone marrow. Ongoing.

HN72 ______. Treatment of kidney stone disease. Ongoing.

HN73 ______. Ultrasound. Ongoing.

HN74 ______. Vaccination against haemophilus influenzae B. Ongoing.

HN75 ______. Vaccination against influenza. Ongoing.

Planned Assessments

HN76 ______. Home care. Planned.

HN77 ______. Lasers. Planned.

HN78 ______. Medical, ethical, and legal implications of advances in genetics. Planned.

HN79 ______. Post marketing surveillance of drugs. Planned.

HN80 ______. Radiation risks. Planned.

HN81 ______. Synthetic growth hormone. Planned.

Health and Welfare Canada

Health Services and Promotion Branch
Institutional and Professional Services Division
Guidelines for Institutional Programs
Ottawa, Ontario K1A 1B4
Canada
613-954-8623

Contact: David L. Martin, Consultant in Health Technology or Donald F. Moffatt, Director, Institutional and Professional Services Division.

Overview: The Institutional and Professional Services Division is a government agency that provides leadership in the development of Canada's health services system. The Guidelines for Institutional Programs is a technology assessment program that issues guidelines on specific health services.

Purpose: To provide guidelines for the planning, organization, staffing, and operation of institutional health programs.

Primary intended users: Providers, generally; physicians; acute facility administrators; long-term care facility administrators; health/medical professional associations; government regulators; labs, blood banks; public policy-makers; legislators; lawyers; provincial and regional health planners.

Technologies: Device, medical or surgical procedure, support system, organizational or administrative system.

Technologies with a major impact on institutional resources, provincial fiscal resources, or patient well-being are assessed.

Intervention: *Treatment,* diagnosis, rehabilitation.

Stage: *New,* established or widespread practice.

Assessments are generally conducted after the initial introduction of a technology; many assessments address how technologies should be implemented in established systems.

Properties: *Service requirements,* effectiveness.

A technology's requirements for medical and allied health staff preparation and maintenance of skills, support services, and other resources are assessed.

Selection process: Provincial ministries of health usually request that an assessment be conducted. Occasionally health professional associations, other institutions, or individuals initiate a request. Requests are submitted to the appropriate federal/provincial review committee for approval. The committee also sets assessment topic priorities. Anyone can suggest the periodic review of a guideline.

Methods: Group judgment, information syntheses.

Departmental staff prepares information syntheses on a specific technology. An expert panel meets on several occasions and then drafts a report. It requires 8 months to prepare the report and obtain the review committee's approval. An additional 6 months is needed to edit, translate, and publish the final report.

Assessors: The assessors' areas of expertise cover a broad range of disciplines.

Assessment reports include: Abstract; the assessment's intended audience; the purpose of the assessment; who sponsored/commissioned/supported the assessment; who conducted the assessment; description of the technology; stage of life-cycle of technology when assessed; properties assessed; results; findings or conclusions; limitations of findings; implications of findings for practice; recommendations for practice, future assessments, technology development, research; how the technology works, including theory, principles; development of the technology; minimum requirements in terms of workload support services.

Dissemination: Printed reports, journal articles.

Assessment results are disseminated using a mailing list and are publicized in professional journals. Copies of the reports may be requested from the provincial or federal health ministry.

Budget: $400,000. The approximate cost per assessment is $30,000 plus department staff time (1 man-year each). Funding source: 100 percent parent organization.

Use: The government uses the guidelines to promote uniform health care standards for all Canadians. Provincial ministries, hospital administrators, and others use the guidelines for planning purposes.

Program evaluation: The Division requested an evaluation of the program to determine relevance and to identify potential improvements. Funded by the government, a private consulting firm (RMS Consultants) conducted the evaluation from November

1985 to March 1986. Based on interviews with provincial and hospital administrators, it was learned that the program is well received but marketing of products needed improvement. Within current budget constraints, efforts are being made to increase awareness of the program. The evaluation's findings were distributed to the provincial ministries.

Related activities: The Division is involved in several related activities including consensus development conferences; surveys of hospital practices; and consultant services, particularly to interpret report recommendations.

Completed Reports

HW1 Subcommittee on Institutional Program Guidelines. [Health and Welfare Canada, Health Services and Promotion Branch, Institutional and Professional Services Division] Rehabilitation medicine program guidelines. 1986. [Information syntheses, Expert opinion, Group judgment]

HW2 ______. Spinal cord injury program guidelines. 1986. [Information syntheses, Expert opinion, Group judgment]

HW3 ______. Stroke program guidelines. 1986. [Information syntheses, Expert opinion, Group judgment]

HW4 ______. Burn unit guidelines. Revised 1985. [Information syntheses, Expert opinion, Group judgment]

HW5 ______. Child and youth long term services guidelines. 1985. [Information syntheses, Expert opinion, Group judgment]

HW6 ______. Nuclear medicine units in hospitals. 1985. [Information syntheses, Expert opinion, Group judgment]

HW7 ______. Prehospital emergency care services. 1985. [Information syntheses, Expert opinon, Group judgment]

HW8 Subcommittee on Special Services in Hospitals. [Health and Welfare Canada, Health Services and Promotion Branch, Institutional and Professional Services Division] The reuse of disposables: an information report. 1985. [Information syntheses, Expert opinion, Group judgment]

HW9 ______. Diagnostic ultrasound facilities in hospital guidelines. 1985. [Information syntheses, Expert opinion, Group judgment]

HW10 ______. Hospital day medicine unit guidelines. 1984. [Information syntheses, Expert opinion, Group judgment]

HW11 ______. Addiction services in hospitals guidelines. 1984. [Information syntheses, Expert opinion, Group judgment]

HW12 ______. Adult long-term institutional care. 1984. [Information syntheses, Expert opinion, Group judgment]

HW13 ______. Child and adolescent services in general hospitals. 1982. [Information syntheses, Expert opinion, Group judgment]

HW14 ______. Day surgery unit guidelines. 1982. [Information syntheses, Expert opinion, Group judgment]

HW15 ______. Pulmonary function laboratories guidelines. 1982. [Information syntheses, Expert opinion, Group judgment]

HW16 ______. Child adolescent psychiatric services provided by general hospitals. 1981. [Information syntheses, Expert opinion, Group judgment]

HW17 Subcommittee on Institutional Program Guidelines. [Health and Welfare Canada, Health Services and Promotion Branch, Institutional and Professional Services Division] Computed tomography guidelines. 1980. [Information syntheses, Expert opinion, Group judgment]

HW18 Subcommittee on Special Services in Hospitals. [Health and Welfare Canada, Health Services and Promotion Branch, Institutional and Professional Services Division] Regional Renal Failure Program. 1980. [Information syntheses, Expert opinion, Group judgment]

HW19 ______. Adult psychiatric services provided by general hospitals guidelines. 1979. [Information syntheses, Expert opinion, Group judgment]

HW20 ______. Geriatric units in hospitals, geriatric day hospital guidelines. 1979. [Information syntheses, Expert opinion, Group judgment]

HW21 ______. Intensive care unit guidelines. 1979. [Information syntheses, Expert opinion, Group judgment]

HW22 ______. Perinatal intensive care unit guidelines. 1979. [Information syntheses, Expert opinion, Group judgment]

HW23 ______. Diabetic day care unit guidelines. 1978. [Information syntheses, Expert opinion, Group judgment]

HW24 ______. Patient hostel unit guidelines. 1978. [Information syntheses, Expert opinion, group judgment]

HW25 ______. Respiratory technology service unit guidelines. 1978. [Information syntheses, Expert opinion, Group judgment]

Johns Hopkins Program for Medical Technology and Practice Assessment

Center for Hospital Finance and Management
624 North Broadway, Room 305
Baltimore, MD 21205
301-955-2300

Contact: Earl P. Steinberg, M.D., Director, Johns Hopkins Hospital, 624 North Broadway, Baltimore, MD, 21205.

Overview: The Johns Hopkins Program for Medical Technology and Practice Assessment was established in July 1986 to merge the functions of the Johns Hopkins Center for Hospital Finance and Management and the Johns Hopkins Office of Medical Practice Evaluation. As a collaborative effort of the Johns Hopkins School of Medicine, the Johns Hopkins School of Hygiene and Public Health, the Johns Hopkins Hospital, and the Johns Hopkins Health System, it draws together a multidisciplinary faculty to address both broad medical technology matters and issues of institutional concern.

Purpose: (1) To assess the clinical efficacy and financial implications of new and established medical technologies in order to assist hospitals and other providers in making informed decisions concerning the acquisition and use of certain technologies; (2) to evaluate the short- and long-term cost and quality implications of alternative technologies and practice patterns; (3) to assess the relative costs and benefits of alternative medical practices; (4) to examine the clinical and economic impacts of health care payment innovations; (5) to provide information to ensure that appropriate reimbursement is available for medical technologies, procedures and services; and (6) to influence State and Federal policy-makers concerning the financing and regulation of health care delivery with particular attention to technology use and medical practice patterns.

Primary intended users: Providers, generally; physicians; acute facility administrators; health product manufacturers; health/medical professional associations; health industry associations; employers; third party payers; government regulators; reporters, writers, news media; public policy-makers, legislators; policy research organizations.

Technologies: *Device,* drug, medical or surgical procedure, support system, organizational or administrative system.

Intervention: *Diagnosis,* prevention, treatment, rehabilitation.

Stage: *New,* emerging, established or widespread practice, obsolete.

Properties: *Cost-effectiveness;* safety; efficacy; effectiveness; cost; cost-benefit; service requirements; acceptance/adoption level; system impact; economic implications; ethical, legal, social implications.

Technologies are assessed for their clinical impacts, including their efficacy and effectiveness, effect on patient outcome and on physicians' use of other technologies and resources. Assessments also include evaluations of technologies' actual and potential economic effects from the perspective of providers, payers, patients, and society as a whole.

Selection process: Assessments are initiated by Program faculty after consultation with members of the medical staff and administration of the Johns Hopkins Medical Institutions. Outside parties, including hospitals, hospital systems or other providers, government agencies, insurers, employers, private industry, or foundations may suggest assessments that would be of particular interest to them. Requests for assessments are made by telephone call, memorandum, letter, or request for proposal. The Program faculty set assessment topic priorities based on several criteria: resources required, feasibility in terms of available data and funding timeliness, and relevancy. Decisions to initiate an assessment are also based on the recommendations of the Program's Advisory Board. Priority is given to issues that have important clinical, economic, and policy implications; capitalize on the multidisciplinary strengths of Program faculty; and have particular interest and concern to the Johns Hopkins Hospital and Health System. Final decisions regarding the performance of assessments are made by the Program's Director and Co-Director.

Methods: *Cost-analyses,* Information syntheses, expert opinion, group judgment, modeling, epidemiological and other observational methods, clinical trials.

The Program conducts original research and synthesizes existing knowledge from the health services and medical literature. Generally, assessments are conducted by teams of researchers under the direction of a project manager. Teams first develop a set of medically important and policy-relevant issues to be addressed in the assessment and then develop methods of addressing those issues. Frequently government or medical experts are consulted in developing the project's issues, approach, scope, and purpose.

Some assessments will be completed in 3 or 4 months, others in 12 to 15 months. The average turnaround time is expected to be 8 months.

Assessors: The assessors have expertise in medicine, health economics, health care financing, business, health policy, and public health, computer science, artificial intelligence, decision analysis, cost effectiveness analysis, clinical epidemiology and education. Each of the physicians involved in technology assessment also has clinical responsibilities at the Johns Hopkins Hospital and continues to be involved in the practice of medicine. Several of the analysts have previous experience in government policymaking. The Program's Advisory Board consists of a representative from each of the schools, from the Johns Hopkins Hospital, and from the Johns Hopkins Health System, so there is a direct link between the Program, the hospital, and the health system.

Assessment reports include: Abstract; the assessment's intended audience; the purpose of the assessment; relationship of this assessment to prior or concurrent assessments of the technology or other technologies intended for similar purposes; who sponsored/commissioned/supported the assessment; who conducted the assessment; description of the technology; stage of life-cycle of technology when assessed; properties assessed; procedure used for the assessment; sources of data/information; methods for collecting data/information; methods for analyzing/synthesizing data/information; results; findings or conclusions; limitations of findings; implications of findings for practice; recommendations for practice, future assessments, technology development, research; development of the technology; where technology is in use; regulatory agency approval status; coverage/reimbursement status of the technology.

Dissemination: *Journal articles;* printed reports; press conferences/news releases, TV/ radio broadcasts, video products.

Assessment results are disseminated through publication of articles and reports; seminars sponsored by the Johns Hopkins School of Hygiene and Public Health; presentations at professional society conferences; meetings with public and private officials; and press releases and press conferences. In some instances, project sponsors, such as manufacturers, are likely to publish or disseminate their own reports based on Program findings.

Budget: $165,000. The cost per assessment will depend on the type of assessment undertaken. Costs are expected to vary considerably, ranging from small ($15,000) contracts to $800,000 clinical trials. Most assessments are expected to cost $20,000 to $100,000. Funding source: 90 percent parent organization, 10 percent government grants/contracts. The School of Medicine, School of Hygiene and Public Health, and the Johns Hopkins Hospital each contributed $50,000 per year for the first 2 years of the Program. This funding is being used to initiate Program activities. it is expected that in the future the Program will be supported both by grants and contracts to perform specific assessments and contributions to support the Program more generally.

Use: The Program provides a means to assist the Johns Hopkins Hospital and the Johns Hopkins Health System administrators and medical staff in decisions regarding the acquisition of new technologies and optimal use of existing resources. Assessment results will be shared with administrators and medical staff.

Ongoing Assessments

JH1 Johns Hopkins Program for Medical Technology and Practice Assessment. A synthesis of the published literature regarding the comparative toxicity of high osmolar and low osmolar radiographic contrast dyes. Ongoing.

JH2 ______. An analysis of economic and policy issues related to the introduction of low osmolar radiographic contrast dyes. Ongoing.

JH3 ______. An assessment of the potential effects of changes in supply purchasing behavior and arrangements in hospitals on quality of care. Ongoing.

JH4 ______. Analysis of the comparative cost-effectiveness of alternative strategies for managing acute heart attacks, including use of thrombolytic drugs, such as tissue plasminogen activator and steptokinase, and emergency coronary angioplasty. Ongoing.

Planned Assessments

JH5 ______. A clinical trial at determining the comparative nephrotoxicity and comparative cost-effectiveness of low osmolar versus high osmolar radiographic contrast dyes. Planned.

JH6 ______. An analysis of automatic implantable cardiac defibrillators (AICDs). Planned.

JH7 ______. An analysis of the comparative costs of inpatient versus outpatient surgery for several types of surgery. Planned.

JH8 ______. An analysis of the potential cost implications of Medicare of unbundling of services (particularly diagnostic services provided by hospitals). Planned.

JH9 ______. An assessment of automatic blood pressure monitoring. Planned.

JH10 ______. An evaluation of patterns of utilization of CT scanners, with particular attention to variations in practice patterns. Planned.

Kings Fund Centre for Service Development

Kings Fund Forum Consensus and Controversies in Medicine
126 Albert Street
London NWI, England
(44-1) 267-6111

Contact: Dr. J. Spiby.

Overview: The Kings Fund Centre for Service Development is a not-for-profit foundation that promotes good practice in health care organizations. The first Kings Fund Forum Consensus and Controversies in Medicine conference was held in 1984.

Purpose: To produce consensus statements.

Primary intended users: General public; patients; providers, generally; physicians; acute facility administrators; long-term care facility administrators; other care givers; health/medical professional associations; consumer associations; government regulators; voluntary associations, organizations; biomedical researchers; financial analysts, consultants; reporters, writers, news media; public policy-makers, legislators; policy research organizations; lawyers.

Technologies: *Medical or surgical procedure,* support system, organizational or administrative system.

Intervention: Prevention, diagnosis, treatment, rehabilitation.

Stage: *Established or widespread practice,* new.

Properties: Efficacy; effectiveness; cost; cost-benefit; cost-effectiveness; service requirements; system impact; economic implications; ethical, legal, social implications.

Selection process: Suggestions for assessment topics are accepted from anyone, although the Steering Group provides major input to the selection process. The Steering Group sets assessment topic priorities.

Methods: *Group judgment.*

The assessment process is conducted as a consensus conference. The average turnaround time from selection of assessment topic to reporting of findings is 1 year.

Assessors: Consensus panels consist of medical professionals and laymen who represent mixed areas of expertise.

Assessment reports include: Consensus statement; the purpose of the assessment; relationship of this assessment to prior or concurrent assessments of the technology or other technologies intended for similar purposes; who sponsored/commissioned/supported the assessment; who conducted the assessment; properties assessed; procedure used for the assessment; sources of data/information; methods for collecting data/information; methods for analyzing/synthesizing data/information; results; findings or conclusions; recommendations for practice, future assessments, technology development, research.

Dissemination: Printed reports; journal articles; press conferences/news releases, TV/radio broadcasts, video products.

Budget: $30,000. The approximate cost per assessment is $15,000. Funding sources: 50 percent foundations, other private grants; 50 percent sponsors/members due, contributions.

Program evaluation: To review the usefulness of the Kings Fund Forum, the Project Coordinator is conducting a survey which was initiated in May 1986.

Completed Reports

KF1 King's Fund. [King's Fund Centre for Service Development. King's Fund Forum Consensus and Controversies in Medicine] Treatment of primary breast cancer: the Second King's Fund Forum. 1986.

KF2 King's Fund. [King's Fund Centre for Service Development. King's Fund Forum Consensus and Controversies in Medicine] Coronary artery bypass surgery: the First UK Consensus Development Conference. 1984.

Lewin and Associates, Inc.

Medical Technology Group
1090 Vermont Avenue NW, Suite 700
Washington, DC 20005
202-842-2800

Contact: Wayne Roe, Vice President.

Overview: Lewin and Associates is a for-profit consulting firm specializing in the health care field. It offers a range of services including hospital strategic planning; HMO, PPO, and insurance industry consulting; strategic market analysis for medical technology product firms; and health policy consulting for federal, state, and local governments and private sector organizations. The Medical Technology Group program was initiated in 1985; since then numerous retrospective and prospective studies have been conducted.

Purpose: To assist technology developers, providers, purchasers, and payers to develop objective, sophisticated, empirical analyses on the impacts of new and existing technologies.

Primary intended users: Providers, generally; physicians; health product manufacturers; health/medical associations; third party payers; government regulators; public policy-makers, legislators.

Technologies: Drug, device, medical or surgical procedure, support system, organizational or administrative system.

Intervention: *Treatment,* prevention, diagnosis, rehabilitation.

Stage: *New,* established or widespread practice.

Properties: *Cost,* safety, effectiveness, cost-effectiveness, service requirements, economic implications.

Properties assessed depend on the client's information need and audience.

Selection process: Anyone can request that an assessment be conducted. Requests are made through client inquiries and occasionally the program receives formal RFPs. Staff and clients set assessment topic priorities.

Methods: *Information syntheses, cost analyses, expert opinion, group judgment, modeling.*

As part of the assessment process, staff conduct statistical studies, prepare quantitative simulation models, collect primary data from prospective trials, and analyze Lewin databases and private insurance claims.

The approximate turnaround time from selection of assessment topic to reporting of findings depends on the study and ranges from 4 months to 2 years.

Assessors: The assessors have expertise in clinical medicine, economics, statistics, health policy, and modeling. Frequently, outside academic/research consultants are used.

Assessment report include: The assessment's intended audience; the purpose of the assessment; relationship of this assessment to prior or concurrent assessments of the technology or other technologies intended for similar purposes; who sponsored/commissioned/supported the assessment; who conducted the assessment; description of the technology; stage of life-cycle of technology when assessed; properties assessed; procedure used for the assessment; sources of data/information; methods for collecting data/information; methods for analyzing/synthesizing data/information; results; findings or conclusions; limitations of findings; implications of findings for practice; recommendations for practice, future assessments, technology development, research; where technology is in use; regulatory agency approval status; coverage/reimbursement status of the technology.

Dissemination: Printed reports; journal articles; advisories to members/constituents; public presentations; private meetings with policy-makers.

If an assessment report is not proprietary, copies may be obtained through the Lewin and Associates library.

Budget: Not available.

Use: Public and private third party payers use the assessment reports in formulating reimbursement policy. For example, Lewin and Associates recently conducted a reimbursement analysis of a new cardiovascular device. The results of the study have been used by public and private insurers to develop reimbursement policy. Other studies have been submitted to the Health Care Financing Administration and the Prospective Payment Assessment Commission.

Completed Reports

LE1 [Lewin and Associates, Inc.] The safety, efficacy, and cost effectiveness of home intravenous antibiotics. 1986 Feb. [Information syntheses, Modeling, Cost analyses]

LE2 Roe W, Anderson M, Strauss M, Arnold J, Gong J, Eresian K. [Lewin and Associates, Inc.] Technology assessment and coverage decision making. 1986 Oct. [Information syntheses, Modeling, Cost analyses]

Linköping University

Center for Medical Technology Assessment
S-581 83 Linköping, Sweden
(46-13) 28-10-00, Ext. 2310

Contact: Bengt Jonsson, Ph.D., Director; or Ann Bonair, Research Assistant.

Overview: The Center for Medical Technology Assessment (CMT) is an independent research unit at Linköping University. The Center was established in fall 1984 after an agreement between Linköping University and the Ostergotland County Council, the local government's health unit. Inauguration took place in April 1985.

Purpose: To develop a long-term knowledge base and methodology pertinent to medical technology assessment; to initiate, support and undertake medical technology assessment in a joint medical, economic, and social perspective; to identify areas of medical technology in need of evaluation in terms of cost, benefits, diffusion potential, and relevant social and ethical consequences; and to organize and support courses, seminars, conferences, and information exchange and dissemination in the field.

Primary intended audience: Providers, generally; physicians; health product manufacturers; health/medical professional associations; health industry associations; third party payers; government regulators; reporters, writers, news media; public policymakers, legislators.

Technologies: *Medical or surgical procedure,* drug, device, support system, organizational or administrative system.

Intervention: *Treatment,* prevention.

Stage: Emerging, new, established or widespread practice.

Properties: Safety; efficacy; effectiveness; cost; cost-benefit; cost-effectiveness; service requirements; acceptance/adoption level; system impact; economic implications; ethical, legal, social implications.

Selection process: Executive Committee members, health care providers, government agencies, and health product manufacturers can request, through formal and informal contacts with the CMT Director, that an assessment be conducted. Assessment topic priorities are guided by CMT's internal framework and objectives. The Director decides if the CMT will undertake a requested assessment after screening the proposed study. The screening process includes determination of resource and time requirements.

Methods: Information syntheses, expert opinion, modeling, cost analyses, epidemiological and other observational methods, clinical trials.

Drafts of assessments are presented at staff seminars before the final report is written. The turnaround time from selection of assessment topic to reporting of findings varies from 6 months to 2 years.

Assessors: CMT has a multidisciplinary staff representing economics, business administration, medicine, biomedical engineering, philosophy, and nursing. Depending on the assessment topic, experts from different areas may be added to the staff team on a temporary basis.

Assessment reports include: The purpose of the assessment; relationship of this assessment to prior or concurrent assessments of the technology or other technologies intended for similar purposes; who sponsored/commissioned/supported the assessment; who conducted the assessment; description of the technology; stage of life-cycle of technology when assessed; properties assessed; procedure used for the assessment; sources of data/information; methods for collecting data/information; methods for analyzing/synthesizing data/information; results; findings or conclusions; limitations of findings; implication of findings for practice; recommendations for practice, future assessments, technology development, research; how the technology works, including theory, principles; development of the technology; procurement/deployment information; where technology is in use; coverage/reimbursement status of the technology.

Dissemination: *Printed reports;* journal articles; advisories to members/constituents; press conferences/news releases, TV/radio broadcasts, video products.

Abstracts and lists of assessment reports are published in the *CMT Newsletter*. The *Newsletter* is distributed free of charge to approximately 1000 subscribers primarily in the health care sector. Five issues of the *CMT Newsletter* have been published; the first issue in English was published in January 1987. Assessment results are also disseminated at conferences and seminars. The CMT accepts telephone and written requests for copies of assessment reports.

Budget: $270,000. The approximate cost per assessment is $7,500. Funding sources: 60 percent parent organization; 10 percent government grants, contracts; 30 percent foundations, other private grants.

Use: Linköping University uses the CMT's assessment reports in courses and as background papers for conferences. Based on personal communications, CMT staff are aware that other researchers in the field, physicians, and health care administrators use the assessment reports for various purposes.

Related activities: An international conference on quality of life was held in September 1986; the proceedings will be published in English. Educational activities include undergraduate courses and a postgraduate course in medical technology assessment.

The CMT Director is the Associate Editor for the *Journal of Health Economics* and is also a member of the following committees: Nordic Planning Group for Health Services Research, the Government Committee for Research about the Public Sector, the Executive Committee of the European Association of Programmes in Health Service Studies, and the Scientific Advisory Board, National Board of Health and Welfare, Sweden.

In collaboration with the World Health Organization's European Program for Health Technology Assessment, the University Library, and the Health University in Linköping, the CMT is establishing a clearinghouse on the evaluation of medical technology literature. It is anticipated that the clearinghouse will be operational in late 1987.

Completed Reports

LU1 Bjork S, Bonair A. [Linköping University, Center for Medical Technology Assessment] Quality of life measurements. 1986. (Discussion series paper #7) (Swedish language only) [Information syntheses]

LU2 Carlsson P, Jonsson. [Linköping University, Center for Medical Technology Assessment] Medical technology assessment in a macroeconomic perspective—a study of the introduction of cimetidine for treatment of ulcers. 1986. (Discussion series paper #1) [Swedish language only] [Cost analyses, Epidemiological methods]

LU3 Carlsson P, Tiselius HG. [Linköping University, Center for Medical Technology Assessment] Evaluation of extracorporeal shock-wave lithotripsy treatment for upper urinary tract calculi—the first year experiences. 1986. (Discussion series paper #10) [Swedish language only] [Cost analyses, Clinical trials, Epidemiological methods]

LU4 Jonsson B. [Linköping University, Center for Medical Technology Assessment] Cost benefit analysis of hepatitis-B vaccination. 1986. (Discussion series paper #12) [Information syntheses]

LU5 Jonsson B. [Linköping University, Center for Medical Technology Assessment] Economic aspects of prevention as a health technology. 1986. (Discussion series paper #3) [Swedish language only] [Information syntheses]

LU6 Jonsson, B. [Linköping University, Center for Medical Technology Assessment] Economic aspects of health care provision—is there a current crisis? 1986. (Discussion series paper #4)

LU7 Jonsson, B. [Linköping University, Center for Medical Technology Assessment] The economics of drug regulation. 1986. (Discussion series paper #5) [Information syntheses]

LU8 Karlsson CT. [Linköping University, Center for Medical Technology Assessment] Economics of osseointegrated implants—a prestudy. 1986. (Discussion series paper #8) [Swedish language only] [Cost analyses, Epidemiological methods]

LU9 Levin, LA. [Linköping University, Center for Medical Technology Assessment] Economic consequences of postinfarction prophylaxis with beta-blockers: a cost effect study of metoprolol treatment. 1982. (Discussion series paper #2) [Swedish language only] [Cost analyses, Epidemiological methods]

Ongoing Assessments

LU10 Linköping University, Center for Medical Technology Assessment. Alternative treatments in stroke—assessment of cost and social implications. Ongoing.

LU11 ______. Assessment of quality of life and medical resource requirements in patients with rheumatoid arthritis—evaluation of cooperation between primary health care and specialized care. Ongoing.

LU12 ______. Economics of ossointegrated implants. Ongoing.

LU13 ______. Ethical issues in medical technology assessment. Ongoing.

LU14 ______. Health care information systems and cost-effectiveness: a review of methodological issues and assessment methods. Ongoing.

LU15 ______. Medical technology in primary health care—an explorative study. Ongoing.

LU16 ______. Quality of life and pharmacotherapy in angina pectoris. Ongoing.

LU17 ______. The cost of prostate cancer in a defined population. Ongoing.

Planned Assessments

LU18 ______. Development of simulation models for use in cost-effectiveness studies. Planned.

LU19 ______. Diffusion of innovations—methodological issues. Planned.

LU20 ______. Economic aspects of prevention as a health care technology. Planned.

LU21 ______. Methodological issues in quality of life measurements, health indicators, and utility index. Planned.

McGill University

Department of Epidemiology and Biostatistics
1020 Pine Avenue West
Montreal, Canada H3A 1A2
514-392-4740

Contact: Dr. Walter O. Spitzer, Chairman, Department of Epidemiology and Biostatistics 514-392-4741.

Overview: McGill University, a public institution, established its Department of Epidemiology and Biostatistics in 1964. Technology assessment is an integral part of the Department's research function.

Purpose: To provide teaching, research, and consultation in epidemiology, statistics, and community medicine.

Primary intended users: General public, people concerned about their health, patients, government regulators.

Technologies: Drug, medical or surgical procedure, organizational or administrative system.

Intervention: Prevention, diagnosis, treatment.

Stage: Emerging, new, established or widespread practice.

Properties: Safety, efficacy, effectiveness, cost, cost-effectiveness.

Selection process: Assessments are an integral part of the Department's research function. They are initiated as a result of interaction between the investigators and the person or organizations interested in the results. Assessment topic priorities also emerge from this interaction.

Methods: Information syntheses, expert opinion, group judgment, cost analyses, epidemiological and other observational methods, clinical trials.

The approximate turnaround time from selection of assessment topic to reporting of findings is 2 years.

Assessors: Assessors are experts in epidemiology, biostatistics, community medicine, and various substantive areas such as cancer, nephrology, and adverse drug reactions.

Assessment reports include: Abstract; the assessment's intended audience; the purpose of the assessment; relationship of this assessment to prior or concurrent assessments of the technology or other technologies intended for similar purposes; who sponsored/commissioned/supported the assessment; who conducted the assessment; description of the technology; stage of life-cycle of technology when assessed; properties assessed; procedure used for the assessment; sources of data/information; methods for collecting data/information; methods for analyzing/synthesizing data/information; results; findings or conclusions; limitations of findings; implications of findings for practice; recommendations for practice, future assessments, technology development, research; how the technology works, including theory, principles, where technology is in use.

Dissemination: Printed reports; journal articles; advisories to members/constituents; press conferences/news releases, TV/radio broadcasts, video products.

Copies of assessments can be acquired through the publishers, the authors, or the Chairman of the Department.

Budget: Variable. The cost of individual assessments varies. Funding sources: 75 percent government grants/contracts; 25 percent foundations, other private grants.

Completed Reports

MG1 Clark DC, Hanley JA, Geoghegan S, Vinet D. [McGill University, Department of Epidemiology and Biostatistics] The effectiveness of a desensitizing toothpaste in treating dentinal hypersensitivity. J Periodontol Res 1985;20:212-219.

MG2 Clark DC, Hanley JA, Stamm JW, Weinstein PL. [McGill University, Department of Epidemiology and Biostatistics] An empirically based system to estimate the effectiveness of caries-preventive agents: a comparison of the effectiveness estimates of APF gels and solutions and fluoride varnishes. Caries Res 1985;19:83-95.

MG3 Hutchinson TA, Harvey CE. [McGill University, Department of Epidemiology and Biostatistics] Survival with different forms of dialysis treatment—a prognostically controlled comparison. J Am Soc Artif Inter Organs 1985;8:13-17.

MG4 Hutchinson TA, Michaud L, Thomas DC. [McGill University, Department of Epidemiology and Biostatistics] Comparison of survival with dialysis and renal transplanation -the effect of the method of statistical analysis on results. J Am Soc Artif Intern Organs 1985;8:18-21.

MG5 Ostrowsky JT, Lippman A, Scriver CR. [McGill University, Department of Epidemiology and Biostatistics] Cost-benefit analysis of thalassemia disease prevention program. Am J Public Health 1985;75:732-736.

MG6 Parfrey PS, Hutchinson TA, Harvey C, Guttman RD. [McGill University, Department of Epidemiology and Biostatistics] Transplantation versus dialysis in diabetic patients with renal failure. Am J Kidney Dis 1985;5:112-116.

MG7 Parfrey PS, et al. [McGill University, Department of Epidemiology and Biostatistics] The impact of renal transplantation on the course of hepatitis B liver disease. Transplantation 1985;39:610-615.

MG8 Robitaille Y, Kramaer MS. [McGill University, Department of Epidemiology and Biostatistics] Does participation in prenatal courses lead to heavier babies? Am J Public Health 1985;75:1186-1189.

MG9 Strom BL, Melmon KL, Miettinen OS. [McGill University, Department of Epidemiology and Biostatistics] Post marketing studies of drug efficacy: why? Am J Med 1985;78:475-480.

MG10 Strom BL, Melmon KL, Miettinen OS. [McGill University, Department of Epidemiology and Biostatistics] Post-marketing studies of drug efficacy: a perspective. Arch Intern Med 1985;145:1791-1793.

MG11 Tousignant P, Hollomby D, Guttman RD. [McGill University, Department of Epidemiology and Biostatistics] Transplantation and home hemodialysis: their cost-effectiveness in the treatment of end stage renal disease. J Chronic Dis 1985;38.

MG12 [McGill University, Department of Epidemiology and Biostatistics] The nurse practitioner revisted: slow death of a good idea. (Editorial retrospective) N Engl J Med 1984;130:1049-1051.

MG13 Boivin JF, Hutchinson GB, Lyden M, Godbold J, Chorosh J, Schottenfeld D. [McGill University, Department of Epidemiology and Biostatistics] Second primary cancers following treatment of Hodgkin's disease. J Natl Cancer Inst 1984;72:233-241.

MG14 Fox ZR, Dupont C, Kramer MS, Stewart JH. [McGill University, Department of Epidemiology and Biostatistics] A double-blind crossover comparison between Phyllocontin and Theo-Dur in asthmatic children. In: Turner-Warwick M, Levy J, eds. New perspectives in theophylline therapy. London: Royal Society of Medicine, 1984:29-37.

MG15 Hutchinson TA, Thomas DC, Lemieux JC, Harvey CF. [McGill University, Department of Epidemiology and Biostatistics] A prognostically controlled comparison of dialysis and renal transplantation. Kidney Int 1984;26:44-51.

MG16 Kramaer MS, Naimark LE, Leduc DG. [McGill University, Department of Epidemiology and Biostatistics] Is antipyresis harmful? Proceedings of the Ambulatory Pediatric Association 1984 annual meeting, San Francisco. 1984:88.

MG17 Parfrey PS, Hutchinson TA, Lowry RP, Knaack J, Guttman RD. [McGill University, Department of Epidemiology and Biostatistics] Causes of late allograft failure and the role of azathioprine reduction. Transplant Proc 1984;16:1100-1102.

MG18 Parfrey PS, et al. [McGill University, Department of Epidemiology and Biostatistics] The diagnostic and prognostic value of renal allograft biopsy. Transplantation 1984;38(6):586-590.

MG19 Shamian J, Clarfield AM, Maclean J. [McGill University, Department of Epidemiology and Biostatistics] A randomized trial of intra-hospital relocation of geriatric patients in a tertiary-care teaching hospital. J Am Geriatr Soc 1984;32:794-800.

MG20 Spitzer WO. [McGill University, Department of Epidemiology and Biostatistics] The periodic health examination: 1. Introduction. Can Med Assoc J 1984;130:1376-1278

MG21 The Task Force on the Periodic Health Examination. W.O. Spitzer, Chairman. [McGill University, Department of Epidemiology and Biostatistics] The periodic health examination: 2. 1984 update. Can Med Assoc J 1984;130:1278-1285.

MG22 Williams JI, Hanley JA. [McGill University, Department of Epidemiology and Biostatistics] Assessing and diffusing today's medical technologies. Dimens Health Serv 1984;61(7):10-14.

MG23 Wood-Dauphinee SS, et al. [McGill University, Department of Epidemiology and Biostatistics] A randomized trial of team care following stroke. Stroke 1984;15:864-872.

MG24 Battista RN, Spitzer WO. [McGill University, Department of Epidemiology and Biostatistics] Adult cancer prevention in primary care: contrasts among primary care settings in Quebec. Am J Public Health 1983;73(9):1040-1041.

MG25 Battista RN. [McGill University, Department of Epidemiology and Biostatistics] Adult cancer prevention in primary care: patterns of practice in Quebec. Am J Public Health 1983;73(9):1036-1039.

MG26 Grover S, Gagnon G, Flegel K, Hoey JR. [McGill University, Department of Epidemiology and Biostatistics] Improving appointment-keeping by patients new to a hospital medical clinic with telelphone or mailed reminders. Can Med Assoc J 1983;129:1101-1103.

MG27 Loeser J, Zvagulis I, Hercz L, Pless IB. [McGill University, Department of Epidemiology and Biostatistics] The organization and evaluation of a computer-assisted centralized immunization registry. Am J Public Health 1983;73(11):1298-1301.

MG28 McNeil BJ, Hanley JA. [McGill University, Department of Epidemiology and Biostatistics] Critical questions regarding a new diagnostic technology: a case study using computed tomography (CT) of the head. In: Culyer AJ, Horisberger, eds. Economic and medical evaluation of health care technologies, proceedings of Wolfsberg Conference. 1983.

MG29 Thomson ME, Kramer MS. [McGill University, Department of Epidemiology and Biostatistics] Methodological standards for controlled clinical trials of perinatal contact: studies of early contact and maternal-infant behavior. Pediatrics 1983;73:294-300.

MG30 Hutchinson TA, Cole CH, Kaye M. [McGill University, Department of Epidemiology and Biostatistics] Chronic ambulatory peritoneal dialysis versus other dialysis therapy—a matched cohort study. Clin Res 1982;30:431A.

McMaster University

Department of Clinical Epidemiology and Biostatistics
1200 Main Street
Hamilton, Ontario L8N 325
Canada
416-525-9140, Ext. 2425

Contact: Dr. Peter Tugwell, Chairman, Department of Clinical Epidemiology and Biostatistics. Telex 061-8347.

Overview: The Department of Clinical Epidemiology and Biostatistics was founded as part of the medical school at McMaster University in 1967. The University provides health care services, research, and education.

Purpose: To provide rigorous evidence on the effectiveness and efficiency of health care interventions and to improve medical practice.

Primary intended users: Providers, generally; physicians; acute facility administrators; long-term care facility administrators; other care givers; health product manufacturers; health/medical professional associations; third party payers; government regulators; voluntary associations, organizations; biomedical researchers; financial analysts, consultants; reporters, writers, news media; information/computer industry; public policy-makers, legislators; policy research organizations.

Technologies: *Medical or surgical procedure,* drug, device, support system, organizational or administrative system.

Intervention: *Treatment,* prevention, diagnosis, rehabilitation.

Stage: *New,* emerging, established or widespread practice.

Although technologies have been assessed at a variety of points in their life-cycles, the focus is usually upon emerging technologies or major established ones for which there is not rigorous evidence.

Properties: *Effectiveness,* safety, efficacy, cost, cost-benefit, cost-effectiveness, service requirements, acceptance/adoption level, system impact, economic implications.

The evaluative focus is on efficiency, effectiveness, community effectiveness and efficiency in both pecuniary and quality of life terms.

Selection process: An assessment may be requested by clinical colleagues, funding agencies, public policy authorities. Assessments are made by clinical colleagues approaching members of the Department for methodological assistance; or external agencies may invite grant and contractual arrangements. Assessment topic priorities are based on external interest and support, internal expertise, and availability of appropriate investigators.

Methods: *Clinical trials,* information syntheses, expert opinion, group judgment, modeling, cost analyses, epidemiological and other observational methods.

Randomized controlled clinical trials and the utilization of other prospective designs are the primary methods used. Most assessments are done in the context of "management" trials with randomization. The approximate turnaround time from selection of assessment topic to reporting of findings is 3 years.

Assessors: The assessors have expertise in the areas of study and trial design; data collection, management, analysis, interpretation; economic evaluation; and quality of life assessment.

Assessment reports include: Abstract; the assessment's intended audience; the purpose of the assessment; relationship of this assessment to prior or concurrent assessments of the technology or other technologies intended for similar purposes; who sponsored/commissioned/supported the assessment; who conducted the assessment; description of the technology; stage of life-cycle of technology when assessed; properties assessed; procedure used for the assessment; sources of data/information; methods for collecting data/information; methods for analyzing/synthesizing data/information; results; findings or conclusions; limitations of findings; implications of findings for practice; recommendations for practice, future assessments, technology development, research.

Dissemination: *Journal articles;* printed reports; press conferences/news releases, TV/ radio broadcasts, video products; clearinghouses, data/citation bases, on-line services.

Assessment results are disseminated primarily through published journal articles, supplemented by reports, testimony, media interviews, and continuing medical education. Copies of assessments are available in the open scientific literature.

Budget: $4,000,000. The approximate cost of each assessment is $90,000. Funding sources: 25 percent parent organization; 25 percent government grants/contracts; 25 percent foundations, other private grants; 25 percent sponsors/members, contributions.

Use: Reports and publications are made available to clinicians, hospital administrators, and other interested parties. These assessment reports have had an impact in several areas. For example, the results of hypertension screening studies have influenced public health policy in Canada; related studies on compliance and treatment have contributed to the increasing effectiveness of hypertension control; and rigorous studies on the detection and treatment of deep vein thrombosis have also influenced clinical practice but have had a less pervasive impact.

Related activities: The Department of Clinical Epidemiology and Biostatistics offers, within the Faculty of Health Sciences, a Master's of Health Science in Design, Measurement, and Evaluation. Through the Rockefeller Foundation it participates as a training center for the International Clinical Epidemiology Network for medical school faculty members in less developed countries.

Completed Reports

MM1 Birkett NJ, Evans CE, Haynes RB, et al. [McMaster University, Department of Clinical Epidemiology and Biostatistics] Hypertension control in two Canadian communities: evidence for better treatment and overlabelling. J Hypertension 1986;4:369-374.

MM2 Haynes RB. [McMaster University, Department of Clinical Epidemiology and Biostatistics] Physician interventions to improve compliance. Geriatr Consultant 1986 Jul/Aug:20.

MM3 Haynes RB. [McMaster, Department of Clinical Epidemiology and Biostatistics] Is weight loss an effective treatment for hypertension? The evidence against. Can J Physiol Pharmacol 1986;64:825-830.

MM4 EC/IC Bypass Study Group. [McMaster University, Department of Clinical Epidemiology and Biostatistics] Failure of extracranial-intracranial arterial bypass to reduce the risk of ischemic stroke. New Eng J Med 1985;313:1191-1200.

MM5 Gent M, Blakely JA, Hachinski V, et al. [McMaster University. Department of Clinical Epidemiology and Biostatistics] A secondary prevention, randomized trial of suloctidil in patients with a recent history of thromboembolic stroke. Stroke 1985;16(3).

MM6 Haynes RB. [McMaster University, Department of Clinical Epidemiology and Biostatistics] Office management of patient compliance in the treatment of hypertension. Pract Cardiol 1985;11:63.

MM7 Haynes RB. [McMaster University, Department of Clinical Epidemiology and Biostatistics] Initial therapy for patients with uncomplicated hypertension. Can Fam Physician 1985;31:321.

MM8 Hull RD, Hirsch J, Carter CJ, et al. [McMaster University, Department of Clinical Epidemiology and Biostatistics] Diagnostic value of ventilation-perfusion lung scanning in patients with suspected pulmonary embolism. Chest 1985;88:819.

MM9 Evans CE, Haynes RB, Gilbert JR, Taylor DW, Sackett DL, Johnston M. [McMaster University, Department of Clinical Epidemiology and Biostatistics] Educational package on hypertension for primary care physicians. Can Med Assoc J 1984;130:719.

MM10 Johnston ME, Gibson ES, Terry CW, et al. [McMaster University, Department of Clinical Epidemiology and Biostatistics] Effects of labelling on income, work and social function among hypertensive employees. J Chron Dis 1984;37(6):417-423.

MM11 McDonald LA, Sackett DL, Haynes RB, Taylor DW. [McMaster University, Department of Clinical Epidemiology and Biostatistics] Labelling in hypertension: a review of the behavioral and psychological consequences. J Chron Dis 1984;37(12):933-942.

MM12 Gafni A, Gibson ES, Johnston M, et al. [McMaster University, Department of Clinical Epidemiology and Biostatistics] Is there a trade-off between income and health? the case of hypertensive steelworkers in Canada. Inquiry 1983;20:343-349.

MM13 Hull R, Delmore T, Carter C, et al. [McMaster University, Department of Clinical Epidemiology and Biostatistics] Adjusted subcutaneous heparin versus warfarin sodium in the long-term treatment of venous thrombosis. New Eng J Med 1982;306:189-194.

MM14 Hull R, Hirsch J, Sackett DL, et al. [McMaster University, Department of Clinical Epidemiology] Replacement of venography in suspected venous thrombosis by impedance plethysmography and I-fibrinogen leg scanning. Ann Intern Med 1981;94:12-15.

MM15 Hull R, Hirsh J, Sackett DL, et al. [McMaster University, Department of Clinical Epidemiology and Biostatistics] Clinical validity of a negative venogram in patients with clinically suspected venous thrombosis. Circulation 1981;64:622.

MM16 Logan AG, Milne BJ, Achber C, Campbell WP, Haynes, RB. [McMaster University, Department of Clinical Epidemiology and Biostatistics] Cost-effectiveness of a worksite hypertension treatment program. Hypertension 1981;3(2):211-218.

MM17 Gent M, Barnett HJM, Sackett DL, Taylor DW. [McMaster University, Department of Clinical Epidemiology and Biostatistics] A randomized trial of aspirin and sulfinpyrazone in patients with threatened stroke: results and methodologic issues. Circulation 1980;62(Suppl V):V-97.

MM18 Haynes RB, Sackett DL, Gibson ES, et al. [McMaster University, Department of Clinical Epidemiology and Biostatistics] Improvement of medication compliance in uncontrolled hypertension. Lancet 1976;(June 12):1265.

Medical Research Council

National Health and Welfare Canada
Jeanne Mance Building, Tunney's Pasture
Ottawa, Ontario K1A OW9
Canada
613-954-1959

Contact: Lewis Slotin, Ph.D., Director, Programs Branch.

Overview: The Medical Research Council of Canada (MRC) is one of three Federal granting agencies responsible for supporting research conducted primarily in universities and their affiliated institutions. The other agencies, the Natural Sciences and Engineering Research Council (NSERC) and the Social Sciences and Humanities Research Council (SSHRC), are responsible for the areas indicated by their names. Both the MRC and the NSERC operated originally within the framework of the National Research Council of Canada; the first became fully autonomous in 1969, the second in 1978. The SSHRC, also established in 1978, encompasses programs administered originally by the National Research Council of Canada. The MRC does not conduct research programs of its own; it is dedicated entirely to the provision of grants and awards for the support of extramural research.

Purpose: According to the Medical Research Act (R.S., c.M-9), the Council's function is to: "(a) promote, assist, and undertake basic, applied, and clinical research in Canada in the health sciences; and (b) advise the Minister of National Health and Welfare Canada in respect of such matters relating to such research as the Minister may refer to Council for its consideration."

Primary intended users: Biomedical researchers.

Technologies: Drug; device; medical or surgical procedure.

Generally, MRC supports basic primary research rather than evaluations of technologies or interventions. (The National Health Research and Development Program is the major source of funds within the Department of National Health and Welfare for the support of extramural research and related scientific activities in public health, health care organization, and health care delivery.)

Intervention: Diagnosis, treatment.

Stage: *Emerging,* new, established or widespread practice.

Properties: Efficacy; effectiveness; ethical, legal, social implications.

Ethical considerations are addressed in an agreement between MRC and the applicant regarding investigations involving human subjects, care and use of experimental animals, and research involving biohazards.

Selection process: The Council accepts applications designed to achieve the objectives set out in the Federal Main Estimates, which are: "to help attain the quality and scale of research in the health sciences essential to the maintenance and improvement of health services." Application forms are available from the Council or from the dean's office at any Canadian school of medicine, dentistry, pharmacy, or veterinary medicine. Further information on specific types of grants, application requirements, and deadlines is found in the MRC's *Grants and Awards Guide,* issued annually. The guide is available by contacting the MRC.

Methods: *Group judgment,* expert opinion, clinical trials.

The Council is comprised of 22 members representing the scientific and lay community, and its programs are administered by a staff of 53. In carrying out its grant-making functions, it is assisted by 37 peer review committees drawn chiefly from universities in Canada. The Council also makes wide use of external referees from Canada and other countries. For some applications, the Council may arrange for a site visit and ask reviewers to prepare a report following such a visit.

Dissemination: Grants awarded by the MRC are listed in *Reference List of Health Science Research in Canada 1984-1985.* Single copies are available upon request from the Council. The Council does not disseminate research results or final reports. Findings or results of MRC-sponsored research should be obtained directly from the individual or organization conducting the research.

Budget: $164,236,000. Funding source: 100 percent parent organization.

Completed reports: Cited below are a selection of the grants that the Council awarded in 1984-1985. Grants were selected from the *Reference List* based on their relevance to technology assessment as used in this Directory.

Completed Reports

MR1 Albisser AM. [Hospital for Sick Children, Toronto] [Medical Research Council—Canada] Clinical applications of an artificial pancreas. (Grant period 1975-1985).

MR2 Allen PS. [Department Medicine, University Alberta] [Medical Research Council—Canada] In-vivo medical applications of nuclear magnetic resonance. (Grant period 1984-1985).

MR3 Barbeau A. [Clinical Research Institute of Montreal] [Medical Research Council—Canada] Etiology and treatment of Parkinson's disease (with a study of efficacy and side effects of levodopa therapy). (Grant period 1973-1985).

MR4 Bergeron C. [Department Pathology, University Toronto] [Medical Research Council—Canada] Canadian brain tissue bank. (Grant period 1983-1985).

MR5 Bitter-Suermann H. [Department Surgery, Dalhousie University] [Medical Research Council—Canada] Liver preservation. (Grant Period 1984-1985).

MR6 Bronskill MJ. [Princess Margaret Hospital, Toronto] [Medical Research Council—Canada] Physical studies of NMR imaging (Grant period 1983-1985).

MR7 Chang EJH. [Department Computer Science, University Victoria] [Medical Research Council—Canada] Computer assisted medical reasoning. (Grant period 1984-1985).

MR8 Chernick V. [Department Pediatrics, University Manitoba] [Medical Research Council—Canada] Clinical trial of naloxone in birth asphyxia. (Grant period 1983-1985).

MR9 Chouinard G. [Department Psychiatry, McGill University] [Medical Research Council-Canada] A clinical trial of L-dopa in the prevention of tardive dyskinesia and in the long-term treatment of Parkinsonian side effects induced by neuroleptics. (Grant period 1982-1985).

MR10 Chouinard G. [Department Psychiatry, McGill University] [Medical Research Council—Canada] Controlled clinical trials of lithium and tryptophan in the treatment of patients with bipolar affective disorders. (Grant period 1982-1985).

MR11 Chouinard G. [Louis-H. La Fontaine Hospital, Montreal] [Medical Research Council—Canada] A controlled clinical trial of rubidium in chronic schizophrenia. (Grant period 1983-1985).

MR12 Clark DC. [Department Dentistry, McGill University] [Medical Research Council—Canada] The preventive effect of fluoride varnishes on dental caries: three year community trial. (Grant period 1981-1985).

MR13 Daniel RK. [Department Plastic Surgery, McGill University] [Medical Research Council—Canada] Surgical reconstruction utilizing microsurgical tissue transplants. (Grant period 1984-1985).

MR14 Fenster A. [Princess Margaret Hospital, Toronto] [Medical Research Council—Canada] Investigations of new imaging system and dose reduction. (Grant period 1979-1985).

MR15 Garfinkel PE. [Department Psychiatry, University Toronto] [Medical Research Council-Canada] Bulimia: Neuroendocrine evaluation, relationship to effective disorder and treatment with carbamazepine. (Grant period 1983-1985).

MR16 Guttman FM. [Montreal Children's Hospital] [Medical Research Council—Canada] Long term organ preservation. (Grant period 1979-1985).

MR17 Inch WR. [Department Radiation Oncology, University Western Ontario] [Medical Research Council—Canada] Nuclear magnetic resonance to monitor lung injury. (Grant period 1983-1985).

MR18 Jugdutt, BI. [Department Medicine, University Alberta] [Medical Research Council—Canada] Preservation of ischemic myocardium. (Grant period 1983-1985).

MR19 Man GCW. [Department Medicine, University Alberta] [Medical Research Council—Canada] The effect of high frequency oscillatory ventillation. (Grant period 1983-1985).

MR20 Mclachlan KR. [Department Dentistry, University Manitoba] [Medical Research Council-Canada] The effectiveness of loops and auxiliary appliances in continuous arch orthodontic therapy.

MR21 Miller JE. [Montreal General Hospital Research Institute] [Medical Research Council—Canada] Optimization of fixation of artificial joint components to bone—the prevention of loosening in total joint arthroplasty.

MR22 Milner M. [Department Biomedical Engineering, University Toronto] [Medical Research Council—Canada] Therapeutic and orthotic aspects of electrostimulation in paediatric cerebral palsy. (Grant period 1981-1985).

MR23 Morales A. [Department Urology, Queens University] [Medical Research Council—Canada] The validation of nocturnal and sexual erections in the etiological diagnosis of impotence. (Grant period 1984-1985).

MR24 Morales A. [Department Urology, Queens University] [Medical Research Council—Canada] A controlled clinical trial of yohimbine in the treatment of impotence. (Grant period 1981-1985).

MR25 Nattel S. [Department Pharmacology and Therapeutics, McGill University] [Medical Research Council—Canada] Effects of antiarrhythmic drugs on arrhythmias related myocardial infarction. (Grant period 1981-1985).

MR26 Pape KE. [Hospital for Sick Children, Toronto] [Medical Research Council—Canada] A prospective study of the evolution and outcome of cystic brain damage in the preterm infant utilizing diagnostic ultrasound brain scans.

MR27 Paty DW. [Department Medicine, University British Columbia] [Medical Research Council—Canada] A therapeutic trial of interferon in multiple sclerosis (MS). (Grant period 1983-1985).

MR28 Paty DW. [Department Medicine, University British Columbia] [Medical Research Council—Canada] Interferon therapeutic trial in MS—supplemental application. (Grant Period 1984-1985).

MR29 Paty DW. [Department Medicine, University British Columbia] [Medical Research Council—Canada] NMR imaging in MS, I: The nature of the lesion. (Grant period 1984-1985).

MR30 Paty DW. [Department Medicine, University British Columbia] [Medical Research Council—Canada] NMR imaging in MS, II, diagnosis of the disease and quantitation. (Grant period 1984-1985).

MR31 Podgorsak EB. [Department Radiation Oncology, McGill University] [Medical Research Council—Canada] Noninvasive thermometry and hyperthermia in cancer treatment. (Grant period 1982-1985).

MR32 Podgorsak FB. [Department Radiation Oncology, McGill University] [Medical Research Council—Canada] Radiographic imaging by solid state electrostatic techniques. (Grant period 1981-1985).

MR33 Pomier-Layrargues G. [Department Medicine, University Montreal] [Medical Research Council—Canada] Treatment of portal hypertension—a randomized clinical trial. (Grant period 1984-1985).

MR34 Poznansky MJ. [Department Physiology, University Alberta] [Medical Research Council—Canada] Soluble enzyme-albumin polymers: new approaches to enzyme therapy. (Grant period 1976-1985).

MR35 Price M. [Department Ophthalmology, University British Columbia] [Medical Research Council—Canada] The development of electrodiagnostic tests to detect early chronic open angle glaucoma. (Grant period 1983-1985).

MR36 Pritchard KI. [Department Medicine, University of Toronto] [Medical Research Council—Canada] A trial of adjuvant therapy in post menopausal women with axillary node positive breast cancer. (Grant period 1984-1985).

MR37 Racz WJ. [Department Pharmacology, Queens University] [Medical Research Council—Canada] Acetaminophen induced hepatotoxicity. (Grant period 1983-1985).

MR38 Roder JC. [Department Microbiology and Immunology, Queens University] [Medical Research Council—Canada] The application of human hybridoma technology to cancer and autoimmune disease. (Grant period 1983-1985).

MR39 Schachar NS. [Department Surgery, University Calgary] Investigation of optimal methods of cryopreservation of osteoarticular allografts for transplantation. (Grant period 1984-1985).

MR40 Sherwin BB [Sir Mortimer B. Davis-Jewish General Hospital, Montreal] [Medical Research Council-Canada] Long-term effects of androgen and/or estrogen on psychosexual functioning, hormone levels, and lipid metabolism in surgically menopausal women. (Grant period 1984-1985)

MR41 Szarek W. [Department Chemistry, Queens University] Radiopharmaceutical development for positron imaging. (Grant period 1981-1985).

MR42 Trachtenberg J. [Department Surgery, University Toronto] [Medical Research Council—Canada] Hormonal control of human prostatic cancer. (Grant period 1980-1985).

MR43 Trevithick JR,. [Department Biochemistry, University Western Ontario] [Medical Research Council—Canada] Microwave and heat-induced cataracts: prevention by vitamin E and chronic studies of low level pulsed irradiation. (Grant period 1983-1985).

MR44 Tugwell P. [Department Medicine, McMaster University] [Medical Research Council—Canada] Clinical trials computer network. (Grant period 1984-1985).

MR45 Viviani GR. [Department Surgery, McMaster University] [Medical Research Council—Canada] Biomechanical studies of surgical systems to correct spinal deformities. (Grant period 1982-1985).

MR46 Ward RH. [Medical Genetics, University British Columbia] [Medical Research Council—Canada] Identifying pregnancies at high risk for neural tube defects. (Grant period 1984-1985).

Medical Technology and Practice Patterns Institute

National Health Services and Practice Patterns Survey
2233 Wisconsin Avenue NW, Suite 302
Washington, DC 20007
202-333-8841

Contact: Dennis J. Cotter, Director.

Overview: The Medical Technology and Practice Patterns Institute (MTPPI) was initiated at the Institute for Health Policy Analysis, Georgetown University Medical Center. In July 1986, MTPPI was established as an independent entity, separate from Georgetown, to allow broad participation by the health care industry. MTPPI is in the process of affiliating with organizations representing the health care industry. The National Health Services and Practice Patterns Survey (NHSPPS) was the first MTPPI program.

Purpose: To provide current information regarding adoption and use of new medical technologies to health care providers, hospital administrators, and policy makers to assist them in making appropriate payments for new and emerging technologies. The objective is to avoid financial barriers to these technologies for all categories of patients. NHSPPS seeks to accomplish this through collection and analysis of primary data, education, and the exchange of information on resource requirements and changes in practice patterns resulting from use of new medical technologies.

Primary intended users: Providers, generally; acute facility administrators; health product manufacturers; health/medical professional associations; health industry associations; third party payers; government regulators.

Technologies: Drug, device, medical or surgical procedure.

Intervention: Diagnosis, treatment.

Stage: Emerging, new, established or widespread practice.

Properties: Cost, cost-effectiveness, service requirements, economic implications.

In order to encourage the optimal use of a technology, the NHSPPS is primarily concerned with assessing a technology's costs, charges, practice pattern variation, and utilization.

Selection process: Requests for assessments come from hospitals, third party payers, clinicians, medical specialty societies, and industry. NHSPPS reports include mail-in forms that recipients may use to suggest assessment topics. Assessment topics are approved by the MTPPI Governing Boards.

Methods: Information syntheses, cost analyses.

Approximately 50 medical centers/hospitals participate in the NHSPPS Program. The process includes four activities: 1) collection and analysis of hospital cost and utilization information; 2) solicitation of judgment by participating hospitals reporting appropriate applications and costs of new technologies; 3) development and distribution to participating hospitals of reports on study findings; and 4) submission of NHSPPS results to appropriate government agencies for their consideration of diagnosis-related group (DRG) assignment and reimbursement. Anonymity of individual hospital data is maintained in all NHSPPS studies.

Each NHSPPS project monitors a specific new or emerging technology over a 3 to 4 year period during the early phase of diffusion. Individual projects end when there is general agreement among providers regarding third party payment or other policy concerns for a specific technology. Reports for each technology involved in the survey are updated and generated annually. NHSPPS reports are comprised of hospital data collected during the previous year.

MTPPI reports are conducted by a core staff and associates from other institutions with expertise relevant to particular assessments.

Assessors: Staff and associates have expertise in bioengineering, medicine, law, public health, and economics. Once the new MTPPI governing board is appointed, it will have approximately 18 members representing medical professionals, insurers, hospitals, manufacturers, others from the health care industry, and community representatives.

Assessment reports include: Abstract; who sponsored/ commissioned/supported the assessment; who conducted the assessment; description of the technology; properties assessed; procedure used for the assessment; sources of data/information; results; findings or conclusions; recommendations for practice, future assessments, technology development, research; regulatory agency approval status; coverage/reimbursement status of the technology.

Dissemination: Printed reports; journal articles; advisories to member/constituents; press conference/news releases.

MTPPI publishes two types of reports. *NHSPPS Public Policy Reports* are available to the public. Approximately 20 to 50 pages in length, they include aggregate and average cost, payment, and utilization data on technologies used by the national sample of participating hospitals and related narrative discussion. *NHSPPS National Average Amounts Reports* are available only to participating hospitals; they provide the hospitals with information comparing their respective experiences with national averages. Public policy report prices range from $19 to $40; rates are discounted for member hospitals that participate in the surveys. NHSPPS reports can be ordered from MTPPI. MTPPI mails notices about report availability and related information to over 4,000 health care related organizations and professionals. Reports are also distributed to congressional and executive branches of government and insurance companies.

Budget: The annual budget for all MTPPI activities is $425,000, including $250,000 for NHSPPS. Funding sources: 10 percent foundations, other private grants; 75 percent sponsors/members dues, contributions; 15 percent sales of assessments, consultant services.

Use: The first NHSPPS public policy report on extracorporeal shockwave lithotripsy was used in reassigning DRG levels by the Prospective Payment Assessment Commission. Findings have appeared in such publications as: *Technology Reimbursement Reports—Beige Sheet, COTH Report, Hospitals, Washington Actions on Health, Trends in Health Business,* and reports of the Prospective Payment Assessment Commission.

Related Activities: The Medical Technology Forum is a new program that sponsors conferences on selected medical technology topics. It serves as a catalyst to focus the expertise of public and private organizations on issues such as costs and quality of care, third party payer coverage and reimbursement policy, equitable access to care, and regulating the distribution and use of major medical technologies. The first forum was held on fully automated ambulatory blood pressure monitoring. Forum reports are made public.

The Hospital Stay Charge Profile (HSCP) is a new service that provides MTPPI client hospitals with computer analysis of: (1) current demand for acute-care services, (2) resources consumed during the hospital stay, and (3) practice pattern information related to the care given Medicare beneficiaries. This includes analyses of public and private health care costs and utilization databases (e.g., Medicare's MEDPAR and PATBILL data) and data collected from client hospital discharge records. HSCP reports that address public policy issues may be made public subject to agreement by the client and MTPPI.

Completed Reports

MT1 Medical Technology and Practice Patterns Institute. Ambulatory blood pressure monitoring. 1987.

MT2 ______. Bone marrow transplantation. 1987.

MT3 ______. Cochlear implantation. 1987.

MT4 ______. Cochlear implants outpatient training. 1987.

MT5 ______. Dialysis treatment for end stage renal disease (inpatient). 1987.

MT6 ______. Dialysis treatment for end stage renal disease (outpatient). 1987.

MT7 ______. End tidal carbon dioxide monitoring. 1987.

MT8 ______. Endocardial electrical stimulation. 1987.

MT9 ______. Extracorporeal shockwave lithotripsy (inpatient). 1987.

MT10 ______. Extracorporeal shockwave lithotripsy (outpatient). 1987.

MT11 ______. Fetal heart monitoring. 1987.

MT12 ______. Gastric bubble for treatment of morbid obesity. 1987.

MT13 ______. Heart transplantation. 1987.

MT14 ______. Left ventricular assist device. 1987.

MT15 ______. Liver transplantation. 1987.

MT16 ______. Magnetic resonance imaging (inpatient). 1987.

MT17 ______. Magnetic resonance imaging (outpatient). 1987.

MT18 ______. Percutaneous lithotripsy. 1987.

MT19 ______. Percutaneous transluminal coronary angioplasty. 1987.

MT20 ______. Pulse oximetry. 1987.

MT21 ______. Total parenteral nutrition (inpatient). 1987.

MT22 ______. Total parenteral nutrition (outpatient). 1987.

National Center for Health Services Research and Health Care Technology Assessment

Parklawn Building, Room 18-05
5600 Fishers Lane
Rockville, MD 20857
301-443-5650

Individual profiles on two assessment-related programs of the National Center for Health Services Research and Health Care Technology Assessment, the Division of Extramural Research and the Office of Health Technology Assessment, follow this overview of the agency. In addition, the agency's National Advisory Council on Health Care Technology Assessment is described in the organizational resources section of this Directory.

The National Center for Health Services Research and Health Care Technology Assessment (NCHSR/HCTA) is part of the Office of the Assistant Secretary for Health, Public Health Service (PHS), U.S. Department of Health and Human Services (DHHS). NCHSR/HCTA is the primary source of federal support for research on problems related to the quality and delivery of health services. NCHSR/HCTA programs evaluate health services, assess technologies, and improve access to new scientific and technical information for research users. NCHSR/HCTA's research is targeted to the needs of health care policy-makers, those who operate hospitals and other health care institutions, and those who are responsible for health care expenditures.

NCHSR/HCTA's extramural research program is directed toward health promotion and disease prevention, technology assessment, the role of market forces in the delivery of health care, primary care, and state and local health problems. It provides support for investigator-initiated projects in these areas conducted at universities, nonprofit organizations and institutions, and by industry.

The NCHSR/HCTA intramural research program conducts studies that have immediate as well as long-term policy relevance. It addresses four major health care issues in the following programs: the Hospital Studies Program, the Health Services for the Aged Studies Program, the National Health Care Expenditures Study, and the Health Status and Health Promotion Studies Program.

The Office of Health Technology Assessment (OHTA) conducts evaluation of the safety and clinical effectiveness of medical technologies in order to provide federally funded agencies such as the Health Care Financing Administration (HCFA) with medical and scientific information to assist in policy formulation involving issues related to Medicare or other coverage.

The NCHSR/HCTA has a National Advisory Council on Health Care Technology Assessment to advise the Secretary of DHHS and the Director of NCHSR/HCTA with respect to the performance of NCHSR/HCTA technology assessment activities. The National Advisory Council is described in another section of this Directory.

Inquiries about NCHSR/HCTA and its programs may be directed to the NCHSR/HCTA Publications and Information Branch, 301-443-4100. NCHSR/HCTA research reports are available for sale through the U.S. Department of Commerce, National Technical Information Service (NTIS), 703-487-4650. Reports are announced in the NTIS *Government Reports Announcements and Index* and *NTIS Abstract Series 44*. Abstracts may be accessed directly through two online databases: the NTIS database, and the National Library of Medicine's MEDLARS Health Planning and Administration file.

Research reports of particular interest are published by NCHSR/HCTA in its own publication series. Information materials are available on various topics, including *NCHSR/HCTA Research Activities*, which announces the availability of NCHSR/HCTA research results in journals, books, reports, and papers. A publications list will be sent on request.

National Center for Health Services Research and Health Care Technology Assessment
Division of Extramural Research

5600 Fishers Lane, Room 18A-19
Rockville, MD 20857
301-443-2080

Contact: James R. Ullom; or Maria Friedman, Publications and Information Branch 301-443-4100.

Overview: The National Center for Health Services Research and Health Care Technology Assessment (NCHSR/HCTA) is the primary source of federal support for research on problems related to the quality and delivery of health services. NCHSR/

HCTA programs evaluate health services, assess technologies, and improve access to new scientific and technical information for research users.

This profile addresses the NCHSR/HCTA Division of Extramural Research. An overview of the NCHSR/HCTA is provided immediately preceding this profile. Another profile in this section describes the NCHSR/HCTA Office of Health Technology Assessment. The NCHSR/HCTA National Advisory Council of Health Technology Assessment is described in the organizational resources section of this Directory.

NCHSR/HCTA's extramural research program is directed toward health promotion and disease prevention, technology assessment, the role of market forces in the delivery of health care, primary care, and state and local health problems. It provides support for investigator-initiated projects in these areas conducted at universities, nonprofit organizations and institutions, and by industry.

Purpose: To provide support for health services research, including investigations on specific health care technologies, methods to improve technology assessment, and ways to monitor and affect the introduction and use of health care technologies.

Primary intended users: General public; patients; providers, generally; physicians; acute facility administrators; long-term care facility administrators; health/medical professional associations; health industry associations; consumer associations; employers; unions and other employee organizations; third party payers; government regulators; voluntary associations, organizations; biomedical researchers; reporters, writers, news media; information/computer industry; public policy-makers, legislators; policy research organizations.

Technologies: *Device,* drug, medical or surgical procedure, support system, organizational or administrative system.

Intervention: *Treatment,* prevention, diagnosis.

Stage: *Established or widespread practice,* new, obsolete.

Properties: *Effectiveness; cost-effectiveness; system impact;* safety; efficacy; cost; cost-benefit; service requirements; acceptance/adoption level; economic implications; ethical, legal, social implications.

Selection process: Most projects are initiated by outside investigators through the formal grant application process established by NCHSR/HCTA. Applications are reviewed by nonfederal peer panels and by the National Advisory Council on Health Care Technology, and are selected for funding based on their scientific merit and their potential for improving the cost-effectiveness and quality of health services. Dissertation research grants are available. Assessment topic priorities are developed by the Director of NCHSR/HCTA with the input and advice of the Director of Extramural Research, senior NCHSR/HCTA staff, advisory councils, study sections, and health services researchers.

Methods: *Epidemiological and other observational methods,* information syntheses, expert opinion, group judgment, modeling, cost analyses, clinical trials, bench testing.

Grant project periods can be as long as 5 years, but most projects are completed within 3 years.

Assessors: Assessors are experts in the areas of medicine, health, nursing, economics, epidemiology, biostatistics, computer sciences, informatics, and sociology.

Assessment reports include: Abstract; the purpose of the assessment; relationship of this assessment to prior or concurrent assessments of the technology or other technologies intended for similar purposes; who sponsored/commissioned/supported the assessment; description of the technology; stage of life-cycle of technology when assessed; properties assessed; procedure used for the assessment; sources of data/information; methods for collecting data/ information; methods for analyzing/synthesizing data/ information; results; findings or conclusions; limitations of findings; implications of findings for practice; recommendations for practice, future assessments, technology development, research; where technology is in use.

Dissemination: *Journal articles;* printed reports; clearinghouses, data/citation bases, online services, specifically, the National Library of Medicine MEDLARS and National Technical Information Service (NTIS) databases.

Results are also disseminated through NCHSR/HCTA publications and presentations at professional meetings. Reports are disseminated to State and local users. Copies of reports may be obtained by contacting the NCHSR/HCTA Publications and Information Branch.

Budget: $4,000,000. Grant awards vary greatly, with the average being approximately $500,000 for a 3-year study. Funding source: 100 percent parent organization.

Use: NCHSR/HCTA uses assessment reports as the basis for policy recommendations and testimony before Congress. Based on references in the literature, the reports are also used outside the agency.

The general programs of the Division of Extramural Research are described in the *Catalog of Federal Domestic Assistance* and in the *NCHSR/HCTA Program Note,* September 1986.

Completed Reports

NA1 McDonald CJ, Tierney WM. [National Center for Health Services Research and Health Care Technology Assessment, Division of Extramural Research] The medical gopher: a microcomputer system to help find, organize, and decide about patient data. West J Med, in press.

NA2 Anderson JG. [______] Use of an HIS by physicians and nurses. 1985 Aug. (NTIS order no. PB86-121126/AS)

NA3 Antczak AA, Tang J, Chalmers TC. [______] Quality assessment of randomized control trials in dental research. I. Methods. J Periodont Dis 1986;21:305-314.

NA4 Antczak AA, Tang J, Chalmers TC. [______] Quality assessment of randomized control trials in dental research. II Results. J Periodent Res 1986;21:315-321.

NA5 Eisenberg JM, et al. [______] Derived thresholds in medical decision making. 1986 Mar.(NTIS order no.PB86-219359/AS)

NA6 Frankel N, et al. [______] Utilization of lung scans by clinicians. J Nucl Med 1986 Mar;27(3):366-369.

NA7 Henderson MG. [______] Resource utilization in alternative ambulatory care sites. 1986. (NTIS order no. PB86-102662)

NA8 Lee KL, et al. [______] Predicting outcome in coronary disease: statistical models versus expert clinicians. Am J Med 1986 Mar;27(3):366-369.

NA9 Perrin JM, Valvona J, Sloan FA. [______] Changing patterns of hospitalization for children requiring surgery. Pediatrics 1986 Apr;77(4):587-592.

NA10 Ray WA, et al. [______] Reducing long-term diazepam prescribing in office practice: a controlled trial of educational visits. JAMA 1986 Nov;256(18):2536-2539.

NA11 Rovner DR, et al. [______] Validity of structured cases to study clinical judgment. 1986 Jan. (NTIS order no. PB86-226222/AS)

NA12 Schaffner W, Ray WA, Federspiel CF. [______] Improving prescribing in outpatient practice. 1985 Oct. (NTIS order no. PB86-218997/AS)

NA13 Shwartz M et al. [______] A deep model of the incidence of dental caries on proximal surfaces. Med Decision Making 1986 Jan-Mar;b(1):42-48.

NA14 Sloan FA, Perrin JM, Valvona J. [______] In-hospital mortality of surgical patients: is there an empiric basis for standard setting? Surgery 1986 Apr;99(4):446-453.

NA15 Smith CC. [______] Microchip medicine. Ambassador 1986 Apr;19(4):20-22.

NA16 Tierney WM, Hui SC, McDonald CJ. [______] Delayed feedback of physician performance versus immediate reminders to perform preventive care. Med Care 1986 Aug;24(8):659-666.

NA17 Zimmerman JE, et al. [______] The use and implications of do not resuscitate orders in intensive care units. JAMA 1986 Jan 17;255(3):351-356.

NA18 Bleich HC. [______] Clinical computing in a teaching hospital. N Engl J Med 1985 Mar 31(12):756-764.

NA19 Bunker JP. [______] Outcomes of total hip replacement using northern California claims data: a pilot study. 1985 Aug. (NTIS order no. PB86-129574/as, inventory only)

NA20 Burton BK, Dillard RG, Clark EN. [______] MSAFP screening: the effect of participation on anxiety and attitudes toward pregnancy in women with normal results. Am J Obset Gynecol 1985;152:540-543.

NA21 Burton BK, Dillard RG, Clark EN. [______] The psychological impact of "false positive" MSAFP elevations. Am J Obstet Gynecol 1985;151:77-82.

NA22 Califf RM, et al. [______] Prognostic value of a coronary artery jeopardy score. J Am Coll Cardiol May 1985;5(5):1055-1063.

NA23 Christian CL. [______] Total knee replacement study. 1985 Apr. (NTIS order no. PB85-236909/AS)

NA24 Darnell JC, et al. [______] After hours telephone access to physicians with access to computerized medical records. Med Care 1985 Jan;23(1):20-26.

NA25 Doubilet P, et al. [______] Probabilistic sensitivity analysis using Monte Carlo simulation. Med Decision Making 1985 Feb;5(2):157-177.

NA26 Eisenberg MS, Hallstrom A, Bergner LG. [______] Defibrillation by emergency medical technicians. 1983 May. (NTIS order no. PB85-163632/AS).

NA27 Feinstein AR, Sosin DM, Wells CK. [______] The Will Rogers phenomenon: stage migration and new diagnostic techniques as a source of misleading statistics for survival in cancer. N Engl J Med 1985 Jun 20;312(25):1604-1608.

NA28 Fineberg HV, Marks H. [______] Development and diffusion of automated chemistry analyzers. 1985 Feb. (NTIS order no. PB85-105696)

NA29 Fineberg HV. [______] Technology assessment: achievements, capabilities and future directions. Med Care 1985 May;23(5):663-671.

NA30 Harrell FE, Lee KL. [______] In: Sen PK, ed. Biostatistics: statistics in biomedical, public health and environmental sciences. North Holland: Elsevier Science Publishers,1985:333-433.

NA31 Harris PJ, et al. [______] Nonfatal myocardial infarction in medically treated patients with coronary artery disease. Am J Cardiol 1980 Dec;46:937-942.

NA32 Hlatky MA, et al. [______] Am J Cardiol 1985 Feb;55:325-329.

NA33 Kaplan EB, et al. [______] The usefulness of preoperative laboratory screening. JAMA 1985 Jun;253(24):3576-3589.

NA34 Komaroff Al, et al. [______] Cost-effective strategies in ambulatory care. 1985. (NTIS order no. PS85-135366)

NA35 Lasch KE. [______] Political culture of medical technology assessment. 1985 Feb. (NTIS order no. PB86-119054/AS)

NA36 Pryor DB, et al. [______] Clinical databases—accomplishments and unrealized potential. Med Care 1985 May 23(5):648-662.

NA37 Pryor DB. [______] In: Califf RM, Wagner GS, eds. Acute coronary care: principles and practice. 1985:473-478.

NA38 Ray WA, Schaffner W, Federspiel CF. [______] Persistence of improvement in antibiotic prescribing practice. JAMA 1985 Mar;253(12):1774-1776.

NA39 Ray WA, Schaffner W, Federspiel CF. [______] Persistence of improvement in antibiotic prescribing practice. JAMA 1985 Mar;253(12):1774-1776.

NA40 Ray WA, et al. [______] Improving antibiotic prescribing in outpatient practice: nonassociation of outcome with prescriber characteristics and measures of receptivity. Med Care 1985 Nov;23(11):1307-1313.

NA41 Reddecord KM, Taylor RB. [______] Education, training, professional certification, and work patterns of directors in interstate laboratories. Am J Clin Pathol 1985 Apr;83(4):480-485.

NA42 Russell LB. [______] Evaluating preventive medical care as a health strategy. 1985. (NTIS order no. PB85-208163/AS)

NA43 Scitovsky AA. [______] Medical cost changes of selected illnesses, 1971-1981. 1985 Jul. (NTIS order no. PB86-155553/AS)

NA44 Showstack JA, Stone MH, Schroeder SA. [______] Changes in the use of medical technologies, 1972-1982: a study of ten inpatient diagnoses. 1985. (NTIS order no. PB85-183929/AS)

NA45 Sloan FA. [______] Diffusion of surgical technology. 1985 Jul. (NTIS order no. PB86-124559/AS)

NA46 Tierney WM, McDonald CJ, McCabe C. [______] Serum potassium testing in diuretic-treated outpatients: a multivariate approach. Med Decision Making 1985;5(1):89-104.

NA47 Wagner GS. [______] The effectiveness of mobile intensive care. 1985. (NTIS order no. PB85-191211/AS)

NA48 Weinstein MC, Stason WB.[______] Cost-effectiveness of interventions to prevent or treat coronary heart disease. Annu Rev Public Health 1985 Jun;6:41-63.

NA49 Whiting-O'Keefe QE, et al. [______] A computerized summary medical record system can provide more information than the standard medical record. JAMA 1985 Sep 6;254(9):1185-1192.

NA50 Winickoff RN, et al. [______] Limitations of provider interventions in hypertension quality assurance. Am J Public Health 1985 Jan;75(1):43-46.

NA51 Wortman PM, Yeaton WH. [______] Cumulating quality of life results in controlled clinical trials of coronary artery bypass graft surgey. Controlled Clin Trials 1985 Dec;6(4):289-305.

NA52 Yeaton WH and Wortman PM. [______] Medical technology assessment: the evaluation of coronary artery bypass graft surgery using data synthesis techniques. Int J Technol Assessment Health Care 1985 Jan; 1(1):125-1416.

NA53 Avorn J. [______] De-marketing and administrative strategies in prescription drug use. 1984. (NTIS order no. PB84-182781)

NA54 Avorn JL. [______] Benefit and cost analysis in geriatric care: turning age discrimination into health policy. N Engl J Med 1984 May;310(20):1294-1301.

NA55 Avorn, JL. [______] Drug revolution places prescribing practices in question. Bus Health 1984 Mar;1(4):353-39.

NA56 Barnett GO. [______] The application of computer-based medical record systems in ambulatory practice. N Engl J Med 1984 Jun;310(25):1643-1650.

NA57 Brand DA. [______] An x-ray screening protocol for extremity injuries. 1984. (NTIS order no. PB84-111384)

NA58 Braun P. [______] Elective hysterectomy: benefits, risks, and costs. 1984. (NTIS order no. PB84-240126)

NA59 Cohen, S. [______] Development, implementation and preliminary evaluation of monitoring and intervention of therapeutic actions system (MINERVA). 1984 Jun. (NTIS order no. PB85-138493/AS)

NA60 Conrad D, Milgrom P, Kiyak A. [______] Insurance plan effects on dental provider treatment for elderly patients. Med Care 1984 May;22(5):;430-445.

NA61 Cox JR. [______] A medical information systems design methodology. 1984 Aug. (NTIS order no. PB86-212388/AS)

NA62 Eisenberg MS, et al. [______] Treatment of ventricular fibrillation: emergency medical technician defibrillation and paramedic services. JAMA 1984 Apr;251(13):1723-26.

NA63 Fries JF. [______] Assessment of technology in chronic disease. 1984. (NTIS order no. PB84-200237)

NA64 Fries JF. [______] The chronic disease data bank: first principles to future directions. J Med and Philos 1984 May;9(2):161-180.

NA65 Gehlbach SH, et al. [______] Improving drug prescribing in a primary care practice. Med Care 1984 Mar;22(3):193-201.

NA66 Grossman M, et al. [______] An economic analysis of community health centers. 1984. (NTIS order no. PB84-159185)

NA67 Mackenzie EJ. [______] Injury severity scales: overview and directions for future research. Am J Emerg Med 1984 Nov;2(6):537-549.

NA68 Payne BC. [______] Burn care facility study. 1984. (NTIS order no. PB84-240688)

NA69 Poddercord M, Taylor RN. [______] Evaluation of laboratory quality assurance activities. 1984. (NTIS order no. PB84-205913)

NA70 Pryor DB, et al. [______] Am J Cardiol 1984 Jan;53:18-22

NA71 Pryor DB, et al. [______] Prognostic indicators from radionuclide angiography in medically treated patients with coronary artery disease. Am J Cardiol 1984 Jan;53:18-22.

NA72 Rikli AE, Leonard MS. [______] End stage renal disease: resource forecasting by predictive model. 1981. (NTIS order no. PB81-141665)

NA73 Seigel. [______] The effects of a computerized drug order review system. 1984. (NTIS order no. PB84-156199)

NA74 Sherman H. [______] The dollar rank order of diagnostic tests used with specific problems in primary medical encounters. 1984. (NTIS order no. PB85-113843)

NA75 Sherman H. [______] Surveillance effects on community physician test ordering. Med Care 1984 Jan;22(1):80-83.

NA76 Simborg DW. [______] Evaluation of a summary medical record system. 1984 (NTIS order no. PB84-100247)

NA77 Soumerai SB, Avorn JL. [______] Efficacy and cost-containment in hospital pharmacotherapy: state-of-the-art and future directions. Milbank Mem Fund Q 1984;63(3).

NA78 Stead EA. [______] A medical database approach to evaluate technology. 1984. (NTIS order no. PB84-200559)

NA79 Thomas KAJ. [______] The influence of incubator air temperature on the respiratory responses of preterm infants. 1986 Mar. (NTIS order no. Pb86-218096/AS)

NA80 Wagner DP, Draper EA. [______] Acute Physiology and Chronic Health Evaluation (APACHE II) and Medicare reimbursement. Health Care Finance Rev 1984 Nov;annual suppl:91-105.

NA81 Wayne DP, et al. [______] International use of APACHE. Med Decision Making 1984 Fall;4(3):297-313.

NA82 Widerhold G. [______] Automated ambulatory medical record systems in the U.S. 1984. (NTIS order no. PB84-118884)

NA83 [______] MEDIPHOR: drug interaction facts. St. Louis, MO: JB Lippinott Co, 1983.

NA84 Avorn JL, Soumerai SB. [______] Improving drug-therapy decisions through educational outreach: a randomized controlled trial of academically based "detailing." N Engl J Med 1983 Jun; 308(24):1457-1463.

NA85 Barnett GO, et al. [______] A computer-based monitoring system for follow-up of elevated blood pressure. Med Care 1983 Apr;21(4):400-409.

NA86 Beardsley RS, Freeman JM, Appel FA. [______] Anticonvulsant serum levels are useful only if the physician appropriately uses them: an assessment of the impact of providing serum level to physician data. Epilepsia 1983 Jun;24(6):330-335.

NA87 Blazer DG, et al. [______] The risk of anticholinergic toxicity in the elderly: a study of prescribing practices in two populations. J Cardiol 1983 Jan;38(1):31-35.

NA88 Brand DA, et al. [______] A protocol for selecting patients with injured extremities who need x-rays. N Engl J Med 1983 Feb;306(6):333-339.

NA89 Brian EW. [______] Evaluation of automated hospital data management systems in 100-300 bed hospitals. 1983. (NTIS order no. PB83-153437).

NA90 Fine EG [______] An evaluation of the 911 system. 1983 (NTIS order no. PB83-137968).

NA91 Gibbons RJ, et al. [______] The use of radionuclide angiography in the diagnosis of coronary artery disease; a logistic regression analysis. Circulation 1983 Oct;68(4):740-746.

NA92 Hanky JA, McNeil BJ. [______] A method of comparing the areas under receiver operating characteristic curves derived from the same cases. Radiology 1983 Sep;148(3):839-843.

NA93 Knaus WA. [______] Changing the cause of death. JAMA 1983 Feb;249(8):1059-1060.

NA94 Koespell TD, et al. [______] The Seattle evaluation of computerized drug profiles: effect on provider activities. Med Care 1983 May 21(5):498-507.

NA95 McDonald CJ, Mazzuca SA, McCabe GP. [______] How much of the "placebo effect" is really statistical regression? Stat Med 1983 Feb;2:417-427.

NA96 Newman M. [______] J Emerg Med Serv 1983 Jan;8(1):74-78.

NA97 Polister P. [______] The evaluation and use of repeated medical tests: logical and statistical considerations. 1983. (NTIS order no. PB83-173716)

NA98 Pryor DB, et al. [______] Early discharge after myocardial infarction. Ann Intern Med 1983 Oct;99(4):528-538.

NA99 Ruthow IM. [______] Surgical decision making and operative rates. 1983. (NTIS order no. PB83-141929)

NA100 Schaffner W, et al. [______] Improving antibiotic prescribing in office practice. JAMA 1983 Oct;250(13):1728-1732.

NA101 Wagner DP, Wineland TD, Knaws WA. [______] Health Care Financ Rev 1983 Fall;5(1):81-86

NA102 Wagner DP, et al. [______] Identification of low-risk monitoring patients within a medical-surgical intensive unit. Med Care 1983 May;21(4):4425-434.

NA103 Wheller JRC, et al. [______] The effects of burn severity and institutional differences on the costs of care. Med Care 183 Dec;21(12):1192-1203.

NA104 [______] The effect of immediate access to a computerized medical record on physician test ordering: a controlled clinical trial in the emergency room. Am J Public Health 1982 Jul;72(7):698-702.

NA105 Avorn JL, Chen M, Hartley R. [______] Scientific versus commercial sources of influence on the prescribing behavior of physicians. Am J Med 1982 Jul;72:4-8.

NA106 Blum RL. [______] Discovery, confirmation, and incorporation of causal relationships from a large time-oriented clinical data base: the RX Project. Comput Biomed Res 1982;15(2):164-187.

NA107 Brand DA. [______] A computer audit to improve ER drug prescribing. 1982. (NTIS order no. PB82-253188).

NA108 Champion HR. [______] Measurement of patient illness severity. Crit Care Med 1982 Aug;10(8):552-553.

NA109 Cohen, SN, et al. [______] Development, implementation and evaluation of drug interactions by a pharmacy oriented reporting system. 1982 (NTIS order no. PB82-140757)

NA110 Dibner AS, Lowry L, Morris JN. [______] Usage and acceptance of an emergency alarm system by the elderly. Gerontologist 1982;22(6):538-539.

NA111 Knaus WA, et al. [______] A comparison of intensive care in the USA and France. Lancet 1982 Sep:642-646.

NA112 Knaus WA, et al. [______] Evaluating outcome from intensive care: a preliminary multihospital comparison. Crit Care Med 1982;10(8):491-496.

NA113 Lubeck D. [______] Cost-benefit analysis of heart disease research. 1982. (NTIS order no. PB82-194556)

NA114 McDonald CJ. [______] A controlled trial of a quality assurance mechanism. 1982. (NTIS order no. PB82-265539)

NA115 Mosteller F. [______] Improving the precision of clinical trials. Am J Public Health 1982 May;72(5):430.

NA116 Scheffler RM, et al. [______] Severity of illness and the relationship between intensive care and survival. Am J Public Health 1982 May;72(5):449-454

NA117 Simborg DW, et al. [______] A hospital local area communication network: the first year's experience. IEEE 1982:479-481.

NA118 Tompkins RK, Koepsell TO. [______] Experimental evaluation of computerized drug profiles. 1982. (NTIS no. PB82-265257)

NA119 Wagner D, Knaws W, Draper E. [______] In: Blum B, ed. Proceedings: Sixth Annual Symposium on Computer Applications in Medical Care, October 30-November 2, 1982, IEEE Computer Society, 727-731.

NA120 Berwich DM, Cretin S, Keeler E. [______] Cholesterol, children, and heart disease: analysis of alternatives. Pediatrics 1981 Nov;68(5):721-730, 1981.

NA121 Bly J, et al. [______] Short procedure units: impact and performance factors. 1981. (NTIS order no. PB81-195851)

NA122 Draper EA, Wagner DP, Knaws WA. [______] The use of intensive care: a comparison of a university and community hospital. Health Care Financ Rev 1981 Dec;3(2):49-64.

NA123 Eisenberg M, Hallstrom A, Bergner L. [______] The ACLS score: predicting survival from out of hospital cardiac arrest. JAMA 1981 Jul;246(1):50-52.

NA124 Evans RW. [______] Quality of self-care (home) and facility hemodialysis. 1981. (NTIS order no. PB81-140477)

NA125 Hallstrom A, Eisenberg MS, Bergner L. [______] Modeling the effectiveness and cost-effectiveness of an emergency service system. Soc Sci Med 1981 Mar;15c(1):13-17.

NA126 Keller MD, et al. [______] The impact of mobile coronary care units. 1981. (NTIS order no. PB81-13381)

NA127 Pittman JT. [______] Health information system transferability evaluation. 1981. (NTIS order no. PB81-206500)

NA128 Ruchlin HS, Morris JN. [______] Cost-benefit analysis of an emergency alarm and response system: a case study of a long term care program. Health Serv Res 1981 Spring;16(1):65-80.

NA129 Sherwood S. [______] Effects of an emergency alarm and response for the aged. 1981. (NTIS order no. PB81-137259)

NA130 Strauss J, et al. [______] Evaluation of emergency room referral system. 1981. (NTIS order no. PB81-231755)

NA131 Wiederhold GC, Blum RL. [______] Integrating medical knowledge and clinical data banks. 1981. (NTIS order no. PB81-227233)

NA132 Eisenberg MS, Bergner L, Hallstrom A. [______] Out-of-hospital cardiac arrest: improved survival with paramedic services. Lancet 1980 Apr 12:812-814.

NA133 Harris PJ, et al. [______] The prognostic significance of 50% coronary stenosis in medically treated patients with coronary artery disease. Circulation 1980 Aug:62(2):240-248.

NA134 Harris PJ, et al. [______] Outcome in medically treated coronary artery disease. Ischemic events: nonfatal infarction and death. Circulation 1980 Oct;62(4):718-726.

NA135 Stiles GL, Rosati RA, Wallace AG. [______] Clinical relevance of exercise-induced ST segment elevation. Am J Cardiol 1980 Dec;46:936.

National Center for Health Services Research and Health Care Technology Assessment
Office of Health Technology Assessment

5600 Fishers Lane, Room 18A-27
Rockville, MD 20857
301-443-4990

Contact: Enrique D. Carter, M.D., Director; or Morgan N. Jackson, M.D., Deputy Director. Telex 301-443-6463, 301-443-1719, or 301-443-1726. Telefax 301-443-2706.

Overview: The National Center for Health Services Research and Health Care Technology Assessment (NCHSR/HCTA) is the primary source of federal support for research on problems related to the quality and delivery of health services. NCHSR/HCTA programs evaluate health services, assess technologies, and improve access to new scientific and technical information for research users.

This profile addresses the NCHSR/HCTA Office of Health Technology Assessment. An overview of the NCHSR/HCTA is provided immediately preceding the profile on the NCHSR/HCTA Division of Extramural Research. The NCHSR/HCTA National Advisory Council on Health Technology Assessment is described in the organizational resources section of this Directory.

The NCHSR/HCTA Office of Health Technology Assessment (OHTA) has direct responsibility for assessing technologies and making Public Health Service (PHS) recommendations in response to requests from federally funded programs such as the Health Care Financing Administration (HCFA) and the Office of the Civilian Health and Medical Program of the Uniformed Services (OCHAMPUS). OHTA (originally as the Office of Health Research, Statistics, and Technology) assumed these responsibilities following the dissolution of the National Center for Health Care Technology in 1981. OHTA also collects and maintains data on organ transplants in the U.S.

Purpose: To provide the clinical and scientific basis on which federally reimbursed health programs may develop coverage policies.

Primary intended users: Providers, generally; physicians; acute facility administrators; long-term care facility administrators; other care givers; health/medical professional associations; consumer associations; employers; unions and other employee organizations; third party payers; government regulators; biomedical researchers; public policy-makers, legislators; policy research organizations; Federal health programs.

Technologies: *Device, medical or surgical procedure,* drug.

Intervention: *Diagnosis, treatment,* prevention, rehabilitation.

Stage: *Established or widespread practice,* emerging, new, obsolete.

Properties: *Safety, effectiveness,* efficacy, cost, cost-effectiveness, acceptance/adoption level.

Selection process: Assessments are requested by federally reimbursed programs, such as HCFA and OCHAMPUS. In the case of HCFA, the first step in the selection process is a joint discussion of the issues by the Physicians Panel, a formal HCFA review board. The second step is a written interagency memorandum to the OHTA, by the requester. HCFA and the OHTA Program Director determine priorities for assessment topics.

Reassessments are also requested through HCFA and reviewed by the Physicians Panel, which decides whether there is enough new information to warrant reassessment. In other cases, OHTA itself makes plans to reopen an issue after a specified time period, with HCFA concurrence.

Methods: *Information syntheses,* expert opinion, cost analyses.

When the HCFA Physicians Panel decides that a technology warrants an assessment, a formal written request is submitted to the OHTA. The OHTA announces impending assessments in the *Federal Register,* inviting comments from appropriate federal agencies. It seeks advice from medical associations, manufacturers' groups, and experts in the medical and life sciences. A literature search is also performed. The OHTA staff then synthesizes the available information and develops the PHS recommendation. Once HCFA has made its coverage decision, the OHTA disseminates its findings in an assessment report. The average turnaround time from selection of topic to reporting of findings is 10 months.

Assessors: Assessments are conducted by OHTA staff in cooperation with outside experts and other federal agencies. OHTA is staffed by approximately 7 physicians and 2 non-physician professionals, as well as support staff.

Assessment reports include: Abstract; the purpose of the assessment; relationship of this assessment to prior or concurrent assessments of the technology or other technologies intended for similar purposes; who sponsored/commissioned/supported the assessment; who conducted the assessment; description of the technology; properties assessed; sources of data/information; methods for collecting data/information; results; findings or conclusions; how the technology works, including theory, principles; regulatory agency approval status.

Dissemination: Printed reports, advisories to members/constituents, memoranda of recommendation.

Reports are disseminated through direct mailings. They may be requested by contacting NCHSR/HCTA Publications and Information Branch, 5600 Fishers Lane, Room 18-12, Rockville, MD 20857, 301-443-4100. Reports are also available through the

National Technical Information Service, 5285 Port Royal Rd., Springfield, VA 22161, 703-487-4650. Reports are published occasionally in the professional literature.

Budget: $789,000. The approximate cost per assessment is $15,000 to $20,000. Funding source: 100 percent parent organization.

Use: Assessment reports are used by the OHTA to make policy recommendations to HCFA and OCHAMPUS. Third party reimbursers, providers, hospital administrators, health policy-makers and analysts, and government officials have reported using the assessments as well. The impact of the OHTA's assessments is exemplified by *Liver Transplants,* which constitutes the formal basis for federal policy on this procedure. The program has been described in:

Marshall JE, Carter ED. The role of the OHTA in medicine coverage decisions. *J Health Care Technol* 1986;3(2):75-78.

Institute of Medicine, Committee on Evaluating Medical Technologies in Clinical Use. *Assessing medical technologies.* Washington, DC: National Academy Press, 1985.

Program evaluation: The OHTA program has been evaluated by several groups and individuals including a 1984 study conducted by Macro Systems, Inc., and a 1986 study conducted by Lewin and Associates, both for the Office of the Assistant Secretary for Planning and Evaluation, Department of Health and Human Services. The program is also described in SN Finkelstein et al., *J Health Care Technol* 1984;1(2):89-102.

Completed Reports

NC1 National Center for Health Services Research and Health Care Technology Assessment, Office of Health Technology Assessment. Angelchik anti-reflux prosthesis. 1986.

NC2 ———. Apheresis in the treatment of systemic lupus erythematosus (SLE). 1986.

NC3 ———. Cochlear implants. 1986.

NC4 ———. Continuous positive airway pressure (CPAP) for the treatment of obstructive sleep apnea. 1986.

NC5 ———. Dual photon absorptiometry for measuring bone mineral density. 1986.

NC6 ———. Endoscopic electrocoagulation of upper gastrointestinal bleeding. 1986.

NC7 ———. Fully automated blood pressure monitoring of hypertension. 1986.

NC8 ———. Hemodialyzer reuse. 1986.

NC9 ———. Hemofiltration as a substitute for hemodialysis. 1986.

NC10 ———. Hemoperfusion in conjunction with deferoxamine for the treatment of aluminum toxicity or iron overload in ESRD patients. 1986.

NC11 ———. Laboratory tests for the management of ESRD dialysis patients. 1986.

NC12 ———. Single photon absorptiometry for measuring bone mineral density. 1986.

NC13 ———. 24-hour ambulatory esophageal pH monitoring. 1985.

NC14 ———. Allogenic bone marrow transplantation for indications other than aplastic anemia and leukemia. 1985.

NC15 ———. Apheresis in the treatment of Guillain-Barré syndrome. 1985.

NC16 ———. Autologous bone marrow transplantation (ABMT). 1985.

NC17 ———. Bilateral carotid body resection. 1985.

NC18 ———. Debridement and other treatment of mycotic toenails. 1985.

NC19 ———. Extracorporeal shock wave lithotripsy (ESWL) procedures for the treatment of kidney stones. 1985.

NC20 ———. Implantable automatic cardioverter-defibrillators. 1985.

NC21 ———. Magnetic resonance imaging (MRI). 1985.

NC22 ______. Patient selection criteria for percutaneous coronary angioplasty of a stenotic lesion in a single coronary artery. 1985.

NC23 ______. Percutaneous ultrasound procedures for the treatment of kidney stones. 1985.

NC24 ______. Portable hand-held x-ray instrument (lixiscope). 1985.

NC25 ______. Reassessment of cardiokymography. 1985.

NC26 ______. Stereotactic cingulatomy as a means of psychosurgery. 1985.

NC27 ______. Transurethral ureteroscopic lithotripsy procedures for the treatment of kidney stones. 1985.

NC28 ______. 13CO2 breath test for diagnosing bile acid malabsorption. 1984.

NC29 ______. 13CO2 breath test for diagnosing fat malabsorption. 1984.

NC30 ______. Ambulatory electroencephalographic (EEG) monitoring. 1984.

NC31 ______. Apheresis in the treatment of chronic relapsing polyneuropathy. 1984.

NC32 ______. Apheresis used in preparation for kidney transplant. 1984.

NC33 ______. Carbon dioxide lasers in head and neck surgery. 1984.

NC34 ______. Diagnostic endocardial electrical stimulation. 1984.

NC35 ______. Electrotherapy for treatment of facial nerve paralysis. 1984.

NC36 ______. External counterpulsation. 1984.

NC37 ______. External open-loop pump for the subcutaneous infusion of insulin in diabetics. 1984.

NC38 ______. Hyperbaric oxygen for treatment of chronic peripheral vascular insufficiency. 1984.

NC39 ______. Hyperbaric oxygen in treatment of severed limbs. 1984.

NC40 ______. Hyperbaric oxygen therapy for acute cerebral edema. 1984.

NC41 ______. Implantable pump for chronic heparin therapy. 1984.

NC42 ______. Intraoperative ventricular mapping. 1984.

NC43 ______. Laser trabeculoplasty (LTP) for open angle glaucoma. 1984.

NC44 ______. Local hyperthermia for treatment of superficial and subcutaneous malignancies. 1984.

NC45 ______. Nd:YAG laser for posterior capsulotomies. 1984.

NC46 ______. Neuromuscular electrical stimulation in the treatment of disuse atrophy in the absence of nervous system involvement. 1984.

NC47 ______. Noninvasive method of monitoring cardiac output by doppler ultrasound. 1984.

NC48 ______. Percutaneous transluminal angioplasty for obstructive lesions of arteriovenous dialysis fistulas. 1984.

NC49 ______. Percutaneous transluminal angioplasty for obstructive lesions of the aortic arch vessels. 1984.

NC50 ______. Streptokinase infusion for acute myocardial infarction. 1984.

NC51 ______. Transcutaneous electrical nerve stimulation for acute pain treatment for ambulatory patients. 1984.

NC52 ______. Transillumination light scanning for the diagnosis of breast cancer. 1984.

NC53 ______. Transplantation of the pancreas. 1984.

NC54 ______. Anti-gastroesophageal reflux implantation. 1983.

NC55 ______. Apheresis for the treatment of Goodpasture's syndrome and membranous proliferative glomerulonephritides. 1983.

NC56 ______. Cardiokymography. 1983.

NC57 ______. Closed-loop blood glucose control device. 1983.

NC58 ______. Computer enhanced perimetry. 1983.

NC59 ______. Diathermy as a physical therapy modality. 1983.

NC60 ______. EEG monitoring during open heart surgery. 1983.

NC61 ______. Electroversion therapy for the treatment of alcoholism. 1983.

NC62 ______. External infusion pump for heparin. 1983.

NC63 ______. Fully automated ambulatory blood pressure monitoring of hypertension. 1983.

NC64 ______. Hyperbaric oxygen for treatment of actinomycosis. 1983.

NC65 ______. Hyperbaric oxygen therapy for treatment of crush injury and acute traumatic peripheral ischemia. 1983.

NC66 ______. Implantable chemotherapy infusion pump for the treatment of liver cancer. 1983.

NC67 ______. Lactose breath hydrogen test for the diagnosis of lactose malabsorption.

NC68 ______. Lactulose breath hydrogen test for small bowel bacterial overgrowth and small bowel transit time. 1983.

NC69 ______. Liver transplantation. 1983.

NC70 ______. Negative pressure respirators. 1983.

NC71 ______. Photokymography. 1983.

NC72 ______. Plasma perfusion of charcoal filters for treatment of pruritis of cholestatic liver disease. 1983.

NC73 ______. Thermography for breast cancer detection. 1983.

NC74 ______. Topical oxygen therapy in the treatment of decubitus ulcers and persistent skin lesions. 1983.

NC75 ______. Ambulatory blood pressure monitoring in hypertensives using semiautomatic, patient-activated portable devices. 1982.

NC76 ______. Apheresis for multiple sclerosis. 1982.

NC77 ______. Bendien's test for cancer and tuberculosis. 1982.

NC78 ______. Bolen's test for cancer. 1982.

NC79 ______. Bone mineral studies. 1982.

NC80 ______. Carbon dioxide laser surgery for selected conditions. 1982.

NC81 ______. Electrotherapy for treatment of facial nerve paralysis (Bell's Palsy). 1982.

NC82 ______. Endothelial cell photography. 1982.

NC83 ______. Gastric freezing for peptic ulcer disease. 1982.

NC84 ______. Home blood glucose monitors. 1982.

NC85 ______. Hyperbaric oxygen therapy for treatment of arthritic diseases. 1982.

NC86 ______. Hyperbaric oxygen therapy for treatment of chronic refractory osteomyelitis. 1982.

NC87 ______. Hyperbaric oxygen therapy for treatment of multiple sclerosis. 1982.

NC88 ______. Hyperbaric oxygen therapy for treatment of organic brain syndrome (senility).

NC89 ______. Hyperbaric oxygen therapy for treatment of soft tissue radionecrosis and osteoradionecrosis. 1982.

NC90 ______. Melodic intonation therapy. 1982.

NC91 ______. Obesity and protein supplemented fasting. 1982.

NC92 ______. Percutaneous transluminal angioplasty for treatment of stenotic lesionsof a single coronary artery. 1982.

NC93 ______. Percutaneous transluminal angioplasty in treatment of stenotic lesions of the renal arteries. 1982.

NC94 ______. Photoplethysmography. 1982.

NC95 ______. Plasmapheresis and plasma exchange for thrombotic thrombocytopenic purpura. 1982.

NC96 ______. Rehfuss test for gastric acidity. 1982.

NC97 ______. Rheumatoid vasculitis therapeutic apheresis. 1982.

NC98 ______. Serum seromucoid assay. 1982.

NC99 ______. Alcohol aversion therapy. 1981.

NC100 ______. B-mode scan in peripheral arterial disease. 1981.

NC101 ______. Cytotoxic leukocyte test for the diagnois of food allergy. 1981.

NC102 ______. Desoxyribonucleic acid-bentonite flocculation for the diagnosis of rheumatoid arthritis. 1981.

NC103 ______. Ethylenediamine-tetra-acetic acid (EDTA) chelation therapy for atherosclerosis. 1981.

NC104 ______. Hydrotherapy (whirlpool) baths for treatment of decubitus ulcers. 1981.

NC105 ______. Intracranial pressure measurement. 1981.

NC106 ______. Intracutaneous (intradermal) and subcutaneous provocative and neutralization testing and neutralization therapy for food allergies. 1981.

NC107 ______. Percutaneous transluminal angioplasty in treatment of the lower extremities. 1981.

NC108 ______. Shortwave diathermy. 1981.

NC109 ______. Stereotaxic depth electrode implantation prior to surgical treament of focal epilepsy. 1981.

NC110 ______. Sublingual provocative testing and neutralization therapy for food allergies. 1981

NC111 ______. The Kunkel test for estimating total serum gamma globulin levels in patients with rheumatoid arthritis. 1981.

NC112 ______. The of use anti-inhibitor coagulant complex (activated prothrombin-complex concentrate) in the treatment of patients with hemophilia A and antibodies to factor VIII. 1981.

NC113 ______. The role of joint scans using technetium-99m pertechnetate in diagnosing and assessing therapeutic gain in arthritis. 1981.

NC114 ______. The use of human tumor stem cell drug sensitivity assays for predicting anticancer drug effects. 1981.

NC115 ______. The use of the bentonite flocculation test in the diagnosis of rheumatoid arthritis. 1981.

NC116 ______. The use of the mycoplasma complement fixation test in the diagnosis of rheumatoid arthritis. 1981.

NC117 ______. Therapeutic apheresis for rheumatoid arthritis. 1981.

NC118 ______. Tinnitus maskers. 1981.

NC119 ______. Transcutaneous electrical nerve stimulation for acute postoperative incision pain. 1981.

NC120 ______. Transsexual surgery. 1981.

NC121 ______. Ultraviolet absorbing or reflecting spectacle lenses for aphakic and pseudophakic patients. 1981.

NC122 ______. Ultraviolet light for treatment of decubitus ulcers. 1981.

NC123 ______. Urine autoinjection (autogenous urine immunization). 1981.

Ongoing Assessments

NC124 ______. Adult liver transplantation. Ongoing.

NC125 ______. Bone mineral density studies: computed tomography. Ongoing.

NC126 ______. Bone mineral density studies: radiographic absorptiometry. Ongoing.

NC127 ______. Cardiac catheterization in a freestanding setting. Ongoing.

NC128 ______. Cardiac rehabilitation program services. Ongoing.

NC129 ______. Cardiointegram as an alternative to stress test or thallium stress test. Ongoing.

NC130 ______. Cardiokymography. Ongoing.

NC131 ______. Carotid endarterectomy. Ongoing.

NC132 ______. Chemical aversion therapy for treatment of alcoholism. Ongoing.

NC133 ______. Coverage of gating devices and the use of surface radio frequency coils in conjunction with magnetic resonance imaging (MRI) procedures. Ongoing.

NC134 ______. Development of criteria for speech pathologist's services for dysphagia. Ongoing.

NC135 ______. Diagnostic tests for impotency: devices (Snap-gauge, Rigi-scan). Ongoing.

NC136 ______. Diagnostic tests for impotency: papaverine injections. Ongoing.

NC137 ______. Diagnostic tests for impotency: plethysmography. Ongoing.

NC138 ______. Drug delivery systems: external infusion pumps for IV antibody therapy. Ongoing.

NC139 ______. Drug delivery systems: external infusion pumps for rehydration therapy. Ongoing.

NC140 ______. Drug delivery systems: external pump for chemotherapy for other than liver cancer. Ongoing.

NC141 ______. Drug delivery systems: external pumps for morphine for pain of nonmalignant origin. Ongoing.

NC142 ______. Drug delivery systems: implantable pumps for chemotherapy for other than liver cancer. Ongoing.

NC143 ______. Drug delivery systems: implantable pumps for infusion of drugs for congestive heart failure. Ongoing.

NC144 ______. Drug delivery systems: implantable pumps for morphine (analgesia) intractable cancer pain. Ongoing.

NC145 ______. Drug delivery systems: implanted pumps for morphine for pain of nonmalignant origin. Ongoing.

NC146 ______. Endoscopic photocoagulation for upper gastrointestinal hemorrhage. Ongoing.

NC147 ______. Extra-intracranial artery bypass surgery in the treatment of strokes. Ongoing.

NC148 ______. Intermittent positive pressure breathing (IPPB therapy). Ongoing.

NC149 ______. Percutaneous transluminal coronary angioplasty when multi-vessel disease is involved (reassessment). Ongoing.

NC150 ______. Real time cardiac monitors. Ongoing.

NC151 ______. Reassessment of autologous bone marrow transplantation (ABMT). Ongoing.

NC152 ______. Thermography for indications for other than breast lesions. Ongoing.

NC153 ______. Transillumination light scanning for use in detection of diseases of the breast. Ongoing.

NC154 ______. Treatment of kidney stones—transurethral ureteroscopic lithotripsy. Ongoing.

NC155 ______. Treatments for impotency: surgical treatments. Ongoing.

NC156 ______. Treatments for impotency: Erect-aid system. Ongoing.

NC157 ______. Treatments for impotency: drug injections. Ongoing.

NC158 ______. Treatments for impotency: other significant therapeutic modalities. Ongoing.

NC159 ______. Treatments for impotency: papaverine. Ongoing.

NC160 ______. Treatments for impotency: penile artery bypass. Ongoing.

National Health Research and Development Program

Jeanne Mance Building, Room 513
Tunney's Pasture
Ottawa, Ontario K1A 1B4
Canada
613-954-8543

Contact: Sheena M. Lee, Director, Research Administration Division; or Information Officer 613-954-8549.

Overview: The National Health Research and Development Program (NHRDP) is a government agency that supports scientific activities to provide the Department of National Health and Welfare with the information needed to fulfill its statutory functions and responsibilities. The NHRDP funds extramural research focusing on public health and health services delivery issues. The technology assessment activities are an integral part of the extramural research program.

Purpose: To fund public health and health services management research through the competitive grant process.

Primary intended users: General public; health/medical professional associations, government regulators; voluntary associations, organizations; biomedical researchers; public policy-makers, legislators; policy research organizations.

Technologies: *Organizational or administrative system,* drug, device, medical or surgical procedure, support system.

Intervention: *Treatment,* prevention, diagnosis, rehabilitation.

Stage: *Established or widespread practice,* new.

Drugs and specific treatments are assessed usually after clinical efficacy has been established and biomedical studies have been completed. Rehabilitation devices are assessed after the basic engineering phases have been completed.

Properties: *Effectiveness,* safety, cost, cost-benefit, cost-effectiveness, service requirements, system impact, economic implications.

Selection process: Any Canadian researcher can submit a research protocol to the NHRDP. The protocol must be submitted as part of a formal research application. Peer review competition is used to evaluate the protocol's methodological acceptability. Department officials assess the relevance to Department programs.

Methods: *Epidemiological and other observational methods,* modeling, cost analyses.

A variety of assessment methods may be selected at the discretion of the investigators. The approximate turnaround time from selection of assessment topic to reporting of findings is 3 to 4 years.

Assessors: The assessors are usually university or hospital faculty.

Dissemination: The NHRDP does not use a standard format for reporting assessment results. All research projects are required to submit five copies of a final report. The final reports are available through interlibrary loan. Further dissemination is primarily the researchers responsibility. Most results are published in academic journals.

Budget: $19,000,000. The approximate cost for a 3-year project is $60,000 to $80,000. Funding source: 100 percent parent organization.

Use: The NHRDP uses the reports to assist in the planning and delivery of health care services in Canada. Based on interlibrary loan requests, the library has some potential data on outside use of the reports. After 10 years of supporting research in this area, the number of published reports and references to NHRDP-funded research are too numerous to mention.

Related activities: The NHRDP directly supports the research community through other activities including training and career grant awards and funding for conferences and workshops. The conferences and workshops must be sponsored by Canadian organizations, held in Canada, and address health care research issues.

Completed Reports

ND1 Aierre YN, Waters BGH. [National Health Research and Development Program—Canada] Erythrocyte membrane enzyme and lithium in manic-depressive disorder. 1986. (Grant No. 6606-2149-52).

ND2 Broder I. [______] A study of the health status of residents in homes insulated with urea formaldehyde foam, before and after remedial measures are undertaken. 1986. (Grant No. 6606-2286-03).

ND3 Brown RE, Schipper, H. [______] Electronic diaphanography (E/DPG) as an adjunct to the early diagnosis of breast cancer. 1986. (Grant No. 6607-1304-07).

ND4 Buchanan WW, Kragg G, Tugwell R. [______] A trial to assess the efficacy of peer group rehabilitative counselling in patients with rheumatoid arthritis. 1986. (Grant No. 6606-1941-43).

ND5 Burrunham RC, Binns B. [______] Etiology and therapy of acute salpingitis. 1986. (Grant No. 6607-1323-54).

ND6 Burton HJ. [______] Factors influencing outcome of home and satellite care dialysis. 1986. (Grant No. 6606-2304-05).

ND7 Byles JA. [______] An assessment of a survey instrument designed to diagnose children's behavioural disorders. 1986. (Grant No. 6606-2245-04).

ND8 Cadman D. [______] Mental health problems associated with chronic physical disability in children: prerequisites for a family-focused preventive mental health strategy. 1986. (Grant No. 6606-2899-43).

ND9 Cameron R, Horlick L, Shepel L. [______] Toward an economical, broadly accessible weight control program: the refinement and evaluation of a correspondence approach. 1986. (Grant No. 6606-2588-42).

ND10 Chamberg LW, Mohide AE, Tugwell P, Bayne R, Pill ML, Nightingale H. [______] Randomized trial of resident care quality assurance by criteria mapping in nursing homes. 1986. (Grant No. 6606-2450-44).

ND11 Chandra RK. [______] Influence of nutritional counselling and support on immunocompetence, nutritional status and illness in the elderly. 1986. (Grant No. 6601-1063-56).

ND12 Chapman JS, Pike R, Segalowitz S. [______] Incidence and degree of laterality preference and cerebral dominance for speech as related to prematurely born 5 1/2 year olds' degree of perinatal stress and cognitive functioning. Effects of hospital and home intervention programmes in preventing deficits of language comprehension skills in prematurely born 5 1/2 year olds. 1986. (Grant No. 6606-1956-43).

ND13 Chipman ML. [______] Population-based studies of corneal graft outcome. 1986. (Grant No. 6606-2671-46).

ND14 Chretien M, M'Bikay M. [______] Screening of bronchogenic adenocarcinoma: development of a model to use tumour markers. 1986. (Grant No. 6605-2299-52).

ND15 Cohen MM. [______] A population-based study of cervical screening in Manitoba. 1986. (Grant No. 6607-1401-53).

ND16 Cole EH, Cattran DC. [______] A controlled trial of plasmapheresis in idiopathic rapidly progressive glomerulonephritis. 1986. (Grant No. 6606-2372-52).

ND17 Colle E. [______] Study of siblings of patients with type I insulin dependent diabetes mellitus: tests which predict the development of disease. 1986. (Grant No. 6605-2390-54).

ND18 Collins J. [______] An evaluation of infertility therapy in Canadian infertility clinics. 1986. (Grant No. 6606-2628-44).

ND19 Conine TA. [______] A controlled randomized trial of two seat cushions in the prevention of decubitus ulcers in institutionalized elderly persons. 1986. (Grant No. 6610-1493-55).

ND20 Conrath DW. [______] The effect of health care practice and environmental factors on the health of, and the use of health care services by, Native Canadians. 1986. (Grant No. 6606-2309-05).

ND21 Cott A. [______] Intervention in disability and chest pain associated with (a) mitral valve prolapse and (b) no known cardiac disease: a cognitive-behavioral approach. (Grant No. 6606-2250-05).

ND22 Crawhall, J. [______] Effect of D-penicillamine on circulating immune complexes and rheumatoid factor. What is the mechanism of its therapeutic action? 1986. (Grant No. 6605-1758-52).

ND23 Cunningham AJ. [______] A randomized control trial of a brief behavioural training group programme for alleviating psychological distress in cancer patients. 1986. (Grant No. 6606-2884-44).

ND24 Curry L. [______] Improving physician manpower distribution and cost effectiveness of training: an application of individual difference theory. 1986. (Grant No. 6606-2982-55).

ND25 D'Arcy C. [______] Phobia, anxiety and alcoholism: evaluating a behavioural treatment program. 1986. (Grant No. 6608-1182-43).

ND26 Detsky A, Baker JP, Jeejeebhoy KN. [______] Predicting nutrition-associated complications in hospitalized patients. 1986. (Grant No.6606-2362-42).

ND27 Doehring DG [______] Reading in hearing-impaired children: word recognition skills of children educated by auditory-oral methods. 1986. (Grant No. 6605-2452-45).

ND28 Dubois S. [______] Validity of food records and dietary recalls in elderly subjects. 1986. (Grant No. 6605-2284-42).

ND29 Duncan PG. [______] The influence of anesthesia and surgery on the outcome of pregnancy—pilot analysis. 1986. (Grant No. 6607-1289-53).

ND30 Durance JP. [______] Modular sockets in the prosthetic fitting of below-knee amputees (evaluation). 1986 (Grant No. 6606-2315-01).

ND31 Edgar LJ. [______] Implementation and evaluation of a rehabilitative approach as a part of normal nursing care of cancer patients. 1986. (Grant No. 6605-2223-46).

ND32 Eyssen GE. [______] Methods of assessing neurological abnormality for use in remote areas. 1986. (Grant No. 6606-2216-55).

ND33 Fancott T. [______] A prototype ambulatory ECG tape analysis system. 1986. (Grant No. 6605-2052-51).

ND34 Ferguson HB. [______] Assessment of cognitive functioning in learning disabled children. 1986. (Grant No. 6606-2096-46).

ND35 Fernie GR. [______] An evaluation of computer-aided design of trans-tibial prosthetic sockets. 1986. (Grant No. 6606-3024-51).

ND36 Fernie GR. [______] Balance training device for stroke rehabilitation. 1986. (Grant No. 6606-3023-45).

ND37 Fernie GR. [______] High speed dimensional shape sensor for clinical application. 1986. (Grant No. 6606-2404-51).

ND38 Fernie GR. [______] Use of trunk shape measurements to quantify scoliotic deformity. 1986. (Grant No. 6606-2995-51).

ND39 Foort J. [______] A modular exoskeletal system for supporting heavy disabled people in the sitting position. 1986. (Grant No. 6610-1291-51).

ND40 Foort J. [______] Amputee fitting—standard shape processing. 1986. (Grant No. 6610-1289-51).

ND41 Foort J. [______] Tabular orthoses for stabilizing body joints. 1986. (Grant No. 6610-1290-51).

ND42 Frasure-Smith N. [______] The long-term outcomes of the ischemic heart disease life stress monitoring program. 1986. (Grant No. 6605-2388-44).

ND43 Frasure-Smith N. [______] The psychosocial outcomes of coronary bypass surgery: a study of patient and spouse adjustment during the first post-surgical year. 1986. (Grant No. 6605-2021-44).

ND44 Fried PA. [______] Long-term effects of maternal soft drug use on the development of pre-school children. 1986. (Grant No. 6606-1887-46).

ND45 Friel JK. [______] Trace element supplementation of pre-term infants. 1986. (Grant No. 6602-1087-56).

ND46 Frost BL, Mason JL. [______] The development and evaluation of a portable vibrotactile auditory prosthetic device for the profoundly deaf. 1986. (Grant No. 6606-1959-51).

ND47 Garner DM. [______] Cognitive therapy for anorexia nervosa and bulimia. 1986. (Grant No. 6606-2666-46).

ND48 Gartrell JW. [______] Evaluation study of community-based health demonstration programs at Alexsis. Hobbema, and Saddle Lake Reserves. 1986. (Grant No. 6609-1361-55).

ND49 Gillam S. [______] Development of subunit vaccine against rubella virus by recombinant DNA technology. 1986. (Grant No. 6610-1314-08).

ND50 Gilman JP. [______] Methods survey—genetic toxicology tests using cultured mammalian cells. 1986. (Grant No. 6606-3145-55).

ND51 Glueckauf RL. [______] Assertion training for disabled persons in wheelchairs. 1986. (Grant No. 6606-2255-01).

ND52 Gravel RA. [______] Genetic complementation analysis in clinical diagnosis. 1986. (Grant No. 6606-1932-52).

ND53 Halliday ML. [______] Investigation to determine the usability of existing statistical data gathering systems to describe and monitor hepato bilary disease in Ontario and other provinces. 1986. (Grant No. 6606-239743).

ND54 Harding GRM. [______] Epidemiology and strategies for management of hospital-acquired catheter-associated urinary tract infections in women after catheter removal. 1986. (Grant No. 6607-1351-54).

ND55 Hirst M. [______] Toward a non-invasive screen for susceptibility to alcoholism. 1986. (Grant No. 6606-2676-52).

ND56 Humphries TW. [______] The effects of sensory integrative therapy on selected aspects of functioning in learning disabled children. 1986. (Grant No. 6606-2441-43).

ND57 Hunter A. [______] The use of chorionic villi biopsy for the first trimester diagnosis of genetic diseases. 1986. (Grant No. 6606-2681-52).

ND58 Irvine EJ. [______] A prospective study to compare diagnostic agreement and cost-effectiveness of air contrast barium enema plus flexible sigmoidoscopy with colonoscopy in rectal bleeding. 1986. (Grant No. 6606-2974-42).

ND59 Jamieson DG. [______] Assessment and rehabilitation of hearing impairment: a phoneme oriented approach.1986. (Grant No. 6609-1298-51).

ND60 Jamieson DG. [______] Optimizing procedures for prescribing and fitting hearing aids. 1986. (Grant No. 6609-1343-45).

ND61 Jewett M. [______] Evaluation of oxybutynin chloride and metoclopramide in the treatment of detrusor instability in the elderly. 1986. (Grant No. 6606-2677-53).

ND62 Johnston CC. [______] Comparison of preparation for surgery in children undergoing major and minor surgery. 1986. (Grant No. 6605-1955-04).

ND63 Jones BD, Chouinarad G. [______] Clinical application of the neuroleptic radio receptor assay in the management of schizophrenia. 1986. (Grant No. 6605-1867-44).

ND64 Jongbloed L. [______] Leisure skills training program with stroke survivors: a double blind study. 1986. (Grant No. 6610-1455-45).

ND65 Kaplan BJ. [______] Nutrition and behavior in hyperactive children. 1986. (Grant No. 6609-1211-44).

ND66 Kragg GR, Stokes B. [______] The effects of comprehensive home physiotherapy and supervision on patients with ankylosing spondylitis—A randomized controlled trial. 1986. (Grant No. 6606-2385-43).

ND67 Kramer MS. [______] Infant determinants of childhood adiposity: the effectiveness of prophylactic nutrition. 1986. (Grant No. 6605-1693-43).

ND68 Larson C. [______] Perinatal intervention project: the effectiveness of prenatal and postpartum home visiting. 1986. (Grant No. 6605-1878-44).

ND69 Laxdal OE. [______] A study of the effectiveness of continuing medical education in improving physician performance. 1986. (Grant No. 6608-1144-07).

ND70 LeTouze D. [______] "Hospital of the future" forum development. 1986. (Grant No. 6613-1280-X).

ND71 Lederman S. [______] Adapting a descriptive analysis of hand movements during identification of object properties for use with patients with sensory impairment of the hand. 1986. (Grant No. 6606-2850-55).

ND72 Levison H. [______] The effects of home care chest physiotherapy on the pulmonary function of patients with cystic fibrosis—a three year study to evaluate the effects of postural drainage with mechanical percussion. 1986. (Grant No. 6606-2355-44).

ND73 Love E, Cruickshank B. [______] A study in Canadian women of the clinical efficacy and acceptability of the cervical cap as a method of reversible contraception. 1986. (Grant No. 6613-1232-X).

ND74 Lupien PJ, Dagenais GR, Moorjani S. [______] An approach to reversibility of atherosclerosis. 1986. (Grant No. 6605-2079-52).

ND75 Lytton H. [______] Effects of short-term interaction coaching with mothers of preterm infants. 1986. (Grant No. 6609-1275-44).

ND76 Maclean HM. [______] Mothering in the context of multiple roles: preventive health implications. 1986. (Grant No. 6606-2696-42).

ND77 Martin BA, Kedwood HB, Kramer PM. [______] Electroconvulsive therapy for psychogeriatric patients: evaluation of new stimulus waveform technology. 1986. (Grant No. 6606-2460-44).

ND78 Martin RH. [______] The effect of cryopreservation on the frequency of chromosome abnormalities in human sperm. 1986. (Grant No. 6609-1319-52).

ND79 Mathias RG. [______] To evaluate the effectiveness of a syndromic approach to treatment of sexually transmitted infections in Northern communities. 1986. (Grant No. 6610-1463-54).

ND80 Matthews VL. [______] Assessment of the feasibility of estimating incidence of ischemic heart disease (from available data-sets). 1986. (Grant No. 6608-1162-55).

ND81 McGrath P. [______] Development of a self-administered treatment for adolescent migraine. 1986. (Grant No. 6606-2674-44).

ND82 McGrath PA. [______] Paediatric pain and behavioural medicine: pain assessment and the role of an endogenous opiate system in pain relief by psychological intervention. 1986. (Grant No. 6606-2244-04).

ND83 McLachlan DR, Dalton AJ. [______] Aluminum chelation in Alzheimer's disease: a therapeutic proposal. 1986. (Grant No. 6606-2330-08).

ND84 Miller AB. [______] National study of screening for breast cancer. 1986. (Grant No. 6613-1149-X).

ND85 Miller RS. [______] Psychological preparation for stressful medical procedures: heart catheterization. 1986. (Grant No. 6606-2640-44).

ND86 Milner M, Levison H. [______] Evaluation of relaxed breathing and its augmentation with biofeedback upon bronchospasm induced by methacholine in paediatric patients with chronic asthma. 1986. (Grant No. 6606-2113-53).

ND87 Milner M, Lotto W, McNaughton SH, Parnes PH. [______] Creative programming by non-speaking physically disabled persons through computer and interface adaptations. 1986. (Grant No. 6606-2116-51).

ND88 Milner M. [______] The effects of proximal tibial osteotomy and tibial tubercle elevation on knee and ankle joint loading. 1986. (Grant No. 6606-2740-51).

ND89 Mitchell A. [______] Pilot study: a randomized controlled trial of supportive care for patients with ulcerative colitis. 1986. (Grant No. 6606-2769-43).

ND90 Morrison JB. [______] Online clinical assessment of muscular activity in lower limb disability. 1986. (Grant No. 6610-1309-51).

ND91 Nicholson RL. [______] Nuclear magnetic resonance imaging: clinical evaluation and future impact on health care. 1986. (Grant No. 6606-2240-03).

ND92 Oldridge NB. [______] Comprehensive early rehabilitation after myocardial infarction (MI). 1986. (Grant No. 6606-2724-44).

ND93 Overburg O, Jackson WB, West ML. [______] Determinates of successful use of low vision aids: an interdisciplinary study to correlate ophthalmological and psychological variables. 1986. (Grant No. 6605-1799-43).

ND94 Pabst HF. [______] BCG vaccine take in babies with and without maternal PPD sensitization. 1986. (Grant No. 6609-1205-54).

ND95 Parnes PH. [______] Towards development of a modular universal wheelchair tray system for communication control and ADL. 1986. (Grant No. 6605-3006-51).

ND96 Patla AE. [______] Development and implementation of an adapted movement notation system for clinical use. 1986. (Grant No. 6606-2399-51).

ND97 Patrick J. [______] Nutritional resuscitation of children with cerebral palsy: does the amount and type of dietary lipid in enteral feeds influence membrane function? 1986. (Grant No. 6606-2684-52).

ND98 Patrick J. [______] The nutritional requirements for energy, potassium and zinc for rapid "catch-up" growth in children with cystic fibrosis. 1986. (Grant No. 6606-2303-07).

ND99 Perlman K. [______] Dietary studies with new insulin delivery systems for the treatment of diabetes mellitus. 1986. (Grant No. 6606-2451-52).

ND100 Piper WE. [______] A controlled study of patient suitability and outcome in short term, individual psychotherapy. 1986. (Grant No. 6609-1367-46).

ND101 Pless IB. [______] Social support & counselling in the prevention of psychosocial maladjustment in children with chronic illness. 1986. (Grant No. 6605-2060-43).

ND102 Postl BD. [______] Epidemiology and therapy of group A streptococcal disease in northern Native communities. 1986. (Grant No. 6607-1320-54).

ND103 Prato FS. [______] Effects on human and rat learning and behavior of radio frequency waves and magnetic fields associated with NMR imaging. 1986. (Grant No. 6606-2300-03).

ND104 Putman RW, Curry L. [______] An assessment of the impact on health outcomes of patient care appraisal in the ambulatory setting. 1986. (Grant No. 6603-1138-46).

ND105 Ramsey RA. [______] Multi-dimensional response of chronic low-back pain patients to a multimodal treatment program: a controlled study. 1986. (Grant No. 6605-2311-46).

ND106 Rang MC, Milner M. [______] Preoperative and postoperative gait assessments as a guide in planning tendon transfers about the ankle joint in children with cerebral palsy. 1986. (Grant No. 6606-2110-51).

ND107 Richardson MF. [______] Construction and testing of a motorized variable-height wheelchair. 1986. (Grant No. 6606-2123-55).

ND108 Robertson JMD. [______] Does supplementary vitamin E prevent cataracts? 1986. (Grant No. 6606-2445-43).

ND109 Robinson, GC. [______] The impact of paediatric hospital-based ambulatory care upon paediatric hospital utilization in B.C. during the past decade. 1986. (Grant No. 6610-1411-46).

ND110 Rock GA. [______] A clinical research project to study the role of plasma exchange and plasma infusion in the treatment of thrombotic thrombocytopenic purpura. 1986. (Grant No. 6613-1158-46).

ND111 Rock GA. [______] An evaluation of the effects of various plasticizers and/or leachables contained in plastic medical devices on blood components, blood donors, and patients. 1986. (Grant No. 6613-1239-52).

ND112 Rock GA. [______] Development of an improved procedure for the production of factor VIII for use in the treatment of hemophilia A. 1986. (Grant No. 6613-1209-52).

ND113 Rock GA. [______] Development of immunoradiometric assay for the measurement of factor VIII procoagulant antigen using monoclonal antibodies to procoagulant factor VIII. 1986. (Grant No. 6613-1178-52).

ND114 Rock GA. [______] Storage of platelets for 5 days—optimization of conditions by factorial analysis. 1986. (Grant No. 6613-1208-52).

ND115 Rock GA. [______] The role of plasma exchange in the management of immune thrombocytopenia. 1986. (Grant No. 6613-1164-52).

ND116 Rock GA. [______] Toxicological evaluation of plasticizers and their metabolites leaching from plastic medical devices into human plasma. 1986. (Grant No. 6613-1177-52).

ND117 Roos LL, Ross NP. [______] A collaborative analysis of common surgical procedures. 1986. (Grant No. 6607-1197-44).

ND118 Roos NP, Howens B, Mossey JM. [______] Health services use, morbidity & mortality among the elderly: longitudinal study of the relationship between needs, psycholog. & social factors & health service use, morbidity & mortality among the elderly in Manitoba. 1986. (Grant No. 6607-1157-46).

ND119 Rooser W. [______] Evaluation of a patient, nurse and physician reminder system for screening procedures in family practice. 1986. (Grant No. 6606-2374-43).

ND120 Roy EA. [______] Disruptions to limb, oral and verbal praxis: assessment and remediation. 1986. (Grant No. 6606-2459-51).

ND121 Sacks S. [______] Prevention of neonatal herpes simplex virus infection: a cost-effectiveness comparison of low risk versus high risk screening. 1986. (Grant No. 6610-1421-54).

ND122 Saunders CG, Morrison JB, Foort J. [______] Amputee fitting standard shape processing (sealing) Part II. 1986. (Grant No. 6610-1369-51).

ND123 Scherer K, Farrell P. [______] A project for measuring the quality of nursing care in Manitoba. 1986. (Grant No. 6607-1238-46).

ND124 Schipper H, Levitt M. [______] Development and validation of a cancer specific quality of life index. 1986. (Grant No. 6607-1284-06).

ND125 Schneider BH. [______] Individualized intervention for social competence. 1986. (Grant No. 6606-2264-07).

ND126 Schnell BR. [______] The development of a Canadian hospital pharmacy workload measurement system. 1986. (Grant No. 5608-1113-46).

ND127 Schwartzman AE, Serbin LA, Ledingham JE. [______] Identification of children at risk for adult schizophrenia for preventive and early treatment programs: a longitudinal study. 1986. (Grant No. 6605-1865-44).

ND128 Schwarz RD. [______] An assessment of the need for radiological evaluation of all girls with recurrent urinary infection. 1986. (Grant No. 6603-1201-42).

ND129 Scott KE. [______] Evaluation of enhanced community reproductive care—a randomized clinical trial of a community reproductive care program. 1986. (Grant No. 6603-1127-44).

ND130 Scott RN, Dunfield VA. [______] Design and evaluation of myoelectric controls. 1986. (Grant No. 6604-1029-51).

ND131 Scott RN. [______] Functional tests for upper extremity amputees. 1986. (Grant No. 6604-1048-51).

ND132 Scott RN. [______] Infants and myoelectric prostheses. 1986. (Grant No. 6604-1056-51).

ND133 Seshia SS, Shwedyk E. [______] Computerized EEG data base from prolonged ambulatory 4 channel (cassette) recordings in children. 1986. (Grant No. 6607-1257-42).

ND134 Seshua SS. [______] Prediction of outcome in nontraumatic coma in children. 1986. (Grant No.6607-1358-44).

ND135 Sharp AR. [______] Resolution enhanced pulsed NMR investigation of normal, preneoplastic and neoplastic systems. 1986. (Grant No. 6604-1042-03).

ND136 Shephard RJ, Ward GR. [______] Training responses of blind and of deaf children. 1986. (Grant No. 6606-2279-55).

ND137 Short RH. [______] The role of problem-solving in the readjustment of closed head injured adults. 1986. (Grant No. 6609-1238-46).

ND138 Shwedyk E, Quanbury AO, Marinic J. [______] Sequential myoelectric processor evaluation. 1986. (Grant No. 6607-1332-51).

ND139 Shwedyk E, Sesha S. [______] Pattern recognition system for ambulatory electroencephalograms: design and evaluation. 1986. (Grant No. 6607-1352-51).

ND140 Simeon JG. [______] Biological and behavioural factors associated with methylphenidate therapy of attention deficit and conduct disorders in children. 1986. (Grant No. 6606-2407-52).

ND141 Skinner HA. [______] Computerized lifestyle assessment of medical patients: early intervention for alcohol problems. 1986. (Grant No. 6606-3002-43).

ND142 Smith A, MacMurray SB, Goodman JT. [______] A comparison of crib-o-gram and brainstem electric response audiometry in the screening of hearing loss in high risk neonates. 1986. (Grant No. 6606-1924-43).

ND143 Soldin S. [______] Development of a definitive procedure for the measurement of digoxin. 1986. (Grant No. 6606-2709-52).

ND144 Spence L, Bishai FR, Sekla LH. [______] Application of ELISA to monitoring for activity of western equine encephalitis. 1986. (Grant No. 6606-2368-54).

ND145 Spevack MG,, Monks RC. [______] Assessment of cognitive abilities in severe closed head injury patients. 1986. (Grant No. 6605-1851-46).

ND146 Spitzer WO. [______] Evaluation of factors affecting reintegration of cancer patients to normal working patterns. 1986. (Grant No. 6605-1926-05).

ND147 Stancer HC, Persad E. [______] A study to determine genetic vulnerability to depressive illnesses. Strategies for prevention. 1986. (Grant No. 6606-2280-04).

ND148 Stewart M. [______] Illness after measles-mumps-rubella (MMR) vaccination—a study using the health diary method. 1986. (Grant No. 6606-3028-43).

ND149 Stich HF. [______] Application of the micronucleus test to exfoliated human urinary cells for quantitating exposures to lifestyle factors and industrial carcinogens. 1986. (Grant No. 6610-1329-52).

ND150 Stuchly SS. [______] Radiowave and microwave dosimetry in human models. 1986. (Grant No. 6606-2455-52).

ND151 Sullivan SJ. [______] Electromyographic biofeedback and the learning process in the treatment of hemiplegia. 1986. (Grant No. 6605-2415-45).

ND152 Tefft BM. [______] Public beliefs, attitudes, and behavioural intentions regarding the mentally ill and community mental health services. 1986. (Grant No. 6607-1395-42).

ND153 Telner J, Knott V. [______] Early neurochemical and neurophysiological predictors of antidepressant response outcome. 1986. (Grant No. 6606-2710-52).

ND154 Tevaarwerk GJM. [______] An evaluation of treatment modalities and adjuncts in diabetes mellitus. 1986. (Grant No. 6606-2646-44).

ND155 Thibert RJ, Draisey TF. [______] Development of new reagents for the determination of serum bilirubin in neonates. 1986. (Grant No. 6606-2131-52).

ND156 Tomkins DJ. [______] Validation of in vivo somatic cell mutation tests in human populations. 1986. (Grant No. 6606-2688-52).

ND157 Tredwell SJ, Saunders CG. [______] A clinical study of shadow moire contourography as a useful assessment of the effects of orthotic treatment of curvature of the spine. 1986. (Grant No. 6610-1366-51).

ND158 Tredwell SJ. [______] Pelvic stabilizer for postural control. 1986. (Grant No. 6610-1422-51).

ND159 Urbach GI. [______] Immunodiagnosis of human ovarian cancer. 1986. (Grant No. 6606-2908-54).

ND160 Voelker CA, Martin JC. [______] Management Information Systems Project. 1986. (Grant No. 6613-1195-X).

ND161 Wainberg MA. [______] Development of an antigen detection assay and a neutralization assay for HTLV-III. Studies on transmission and infectivity. 1986. (Grant No. 6605-2450-X).

ND162 Walker MC. [______] The development of human monoclonal antibodies against HLA antigens. 1986. (Grant No. 6605-2035-52).

ND163 Wall JC. [______] An evaluation of out-patient physiotherapy and a home exercise program in the restoration and improvement of locomotor function in residual hemiplegia. 1986. (Grant No. 6603-1161-01).

ND164 Warrington RJ. [______] Assessment of the migration inhibition test in the diagnosis of hypersensitivity to food additives and salicylates in chronic urticaria. 1986. (Grant No. 6607-12878-08).

ND165 White DR. [______] Evaluation of a behavioral-development treatment for childhood obesity. 1986. (Grant No. 6605-1876-42).

ND166 Wiens E, Kumpula VW, Hill GB. [______] Early detection of colorectal cancer in Northern Alberta. 1986. (Grant No. 6609-1243-53).

ND167 Wong J. [______] Effects of an experimental program on post-hospital adjustment of early discharged patients. 1986. (Grant No. 6603-1198-46).

ND168 Woogh CM. [______] Kingston psychiatric record linkage system. 1986. (Grant No. 6606-2880-43).

ND169 Wright LA, Breckenridge WC. [______] Development of a definitive method for serum cholesterol. 1986. (Grant No. 6606-2331-52).

ND170 Zemore R, Shepel LF. [______] Coping with breast cancer and mastectomy. 1986. (Grant No. 6608-1170-42).

ND171 Zerr SJ. [______] The evaluation of child care in the home. 1986. (Grant No. 6606-2238-55).

ND172 Browne RB, Salanta PA, Bryne CM, Streiner DL, Roberts RS, Truscott. [______] Long term follow-up of burn victims psychosocial adjustment: a historical perspective cohort analytic study to estimate avoidable need. 1985. (Grant No. 6606-2349-43).

ND173 Cooper BA. [______] Evaluation and development of assays for B12 and folate. 1985. (Grant No. 6605-1784-52).

ND174 Feldman W, Corber ST, Quinn A. [______] Assessment of ambulatory health needs of adolescents. 1985. (Grant No. 6606-2289-07).

ND175 Fontaine R, Chouinard G. [______] Long term study of different treatment modalities in chronically anxious patients. 1985. (Grant No. 6605-1870-44).

ND176 Gauthier L, Gauthier S. [______] Group rehabilitation as an adjunct to medical therapy in idiopathic Parkinson's disease. 1985. (Grant No. 6605-1946-05).

ND177 Gray JD, Renton KW. [______] Drug elimination during respiratory tract infections. 1985. (Grant No. 6603-1150-52).

ND178 Gripton J. [______] A social research and development project on adolescent contraceptive practice. 1985. (Grant No. 6609-1264-X).

ND179 Hillman E. [______] Evaluation of an outreach program to promote utilization of health and developmental screening for three-year-old children. 1985. (Grant No. 6601-1042-44).

ND180 Hislop TG. [______] Coordinated studies of the courses, methods of diagnosis, prognosis and impact on lifestyle of breast cancer in British Columbia. 1985. (Grant No. 6610-1215-44)

ND181 Jewett M, Fernie G. [______] Evaluation of neuropharmacologic agents in the management of urinary dysfunction of the elderly. 1985. (Grant No. 6606-2141-53).

ND182 Larochelle P. [______] Long-term clinical trial on the treatment of hypertension in patients above the age of 55 years and with signs of arterio-atherosclerosis. 1985. (Grant No. 6605-1933-X).

ND183 Lotto WN, Milner M. [______] Evaluations and development of powered mobility aids for two-to-five year olds with neuromusculoskeletaal disorders. 1985. (Grant No. 6606-2114-51).

ND184 McGrath P, Durieux Smith A, Goodman JT. [______] Compliance to hearing aid use in the classroom. 1985. (Grant No. 6606-2297-51).

ND185 Mowat DL. [______] An outreach program to promote utilization of health and developmental screening for three-year-old children (Demonstration). 1985. (Grant No. 6601-1041-44).

ND186 Newell E. [______] Development of a clinical evaluation scheme to test the efficacy of shoe insole materials used in the treatment of metatarsalgia associated with rheumatoid arthritis. 1985. (Grant No. 6606-2144-51).

ND187 Penner DW. [______] Quality control (quality evaluation) for diagnostic surgical pathology and cytopathology. 1985. (Grant No. 6607-1279-55).

ND188 Penner JL. [______] Development of a serotyping scheme for campylobacter fetus subspecies jejuni for epidemiological investigations. 1985. (Grant No. 6606-1832-54).

ND189 Piper MC. [______] Effect of early physical therapy on the neuromotor status of the high risk infant. 1985. (Grant No. 6605-1754-51).

ND190 Rickert WS, Robinson JC. [______] Development of a practical and inexpensive technique for large scale monitoring of exposure to cigarette tar. 1985. (Grant No. 6606-2360-52).

ND191 Rock GA. [______] A clinical research project to study the role of plasma exchange in the treatment of Rh disease. 1985. (Grant No. 6613-1156-52).

ND192 Sauter WF, Galway RH, Gillespie R. [______] Development of onionized (layered) upper extremity prosthetic sockets for juvenile amputees. 1985. (Grant No. 6606-2115-55).

ND193 Scott RN. [______] Evaluation of moire topography in sclerosis monitoring. 1985. (Grant No. 6604-1055-51).

ND194 Scott RN. [______] Moire topography in scoliosis monitoring. 1985. (Contract No. 6604-1049-51).

ND195 Tomkins DJ. [______] In vivo tests for somatic cell mutation in man. 1985. (Grant No. 6606-2074-52).

ND196 Williams CN. [______] Prevalence and pathogenesis of cholesterol gallstones in Halifax: prevention of recurrence by diet changes after medical dissolution therapy. 1985. (Grant No. 6603-1125-44).

ND197 Winter DA. [______] Ambulation profiles: correlation with biomechanical variables as a quantifier of gait dysfunction. 1985. (Grant No. 6606-2313-01).

ND198 Zemore R, Shepel LF. [______] Psychosocial adjustment to breast cancer. 1985. (Grant No. 6608-1128-42).

National Heart, Lung, and Blood Institute

National Heart, Blood Vessel, Lung, and Blood Program
Office of Program Planning and Evaluation
National Institutes of Health
Building 31, Room 5A-11
9000 Rockville Pike
Bethesda, MD 20892
301-496-3620

Contact: Carl A. Roth, Ph.D, J.D., Chief, Program Analysis and Evaluation Branch.

Overview: The National Institutes of Health (NIH) is the principal biomedical research agency of the Federal government. NIH is composed of 12 bureaus and institutes and six research and support divisions. The National Heart, Lung, and Blood Institute (NHLBI) is the second largest in terms of funding. It was established in 1948 as the National Heart Institute. With a growing awareness of national health problems, it was redesignated the National Heart and Lung Institute in 1969 and in 1976 was redesignated the National Heart, Lung, and Blood Institute.

Purpose: To serve the overriding strategy of the Institute's national program. This strategy is represented by the biomedical research and clinical applications spectrum in which the products of research flow from basic research and clinical research to applied research and development and practical health care.

Primary intended users: General public; people concerned about their health; patients; providers, generally; physicians; health product manufacturers; health/medical professional associations; health industry associations; consumer associations; employers; unions and other employee organizations; voluntary associations, organizations; biomedical researchers; reporters, writers, news media; labs, blood banks.

Technologies: *Medical or surgical procedure,* drug, device, support system.

NHLBI also devotes considerable attention to the roles of smoking, diet, and other aspects of lifestyle and the environment in heart and vascular diseases, lung diseases, and blood diseases.

Intervention: *Treatment,* prevention, diagnosis.

Stage: *New,* emerging, established or widespread practice, obsolete.

According to the Institute, emerging technologies are those under development that appear likely to be used in the practice of medicine within 4 years. New technologies are those that may have passed the stage of clinical trials but are not yet widely disseminated, or those that are moving into general use without benefit of clinical trials. The last group are those established technologies that are currently undergoing or likely to undergo major changes in use or costs as a result of new research findings, or for which serious concerns have been raised concerning safety and effectiveness.

Properties: *Effectiveness;* safety; efficacy; ethical, legal, social implications.

The principal concerns of NHLBI assessment activities are safety and efficacy. The planning and conduct of research reported by NHLBI, particularly clinical trials, are subject to detailed review of ethical considerations. The Institute does conduct some cost studies, such as in-house studies to demonstrate the cost-effectiveness of its clinical trials. It must also evaluate the cost-effectiveness of the Federal investment in the National Heart, Blood Vessel, Lung, and Blood Program, and make recommendations regarding future resource allocations.

Selection process: Large-scale clinical trials are usually initiated by Institute staff, advisory groups, and other biomedical scientists and health care researchers. The smaller, grant-supported clinical trials are usually initiated by investigators who apply for grants. Consensus development conferences are initiated by the Institute, Office of Medical Applications of Research (OMAR), other government agencies, or the public.

If the concept of a large-scale clinical trial is approved by the Institute, a request for proposal (RFP) or request for application (RFA) is prepared and advertised. The RFP or RFA defines the program requirements and describes the criteria by which the proposals will be evaluated. Consensus development conferences may be requested by the Institute, OMAR, other government agencies, and the public.

Institute Advisory Groups, Institute staff, and the National Heart, Lung, and Blood Advisory Council all set assessment topic priorities throughout the processes of concept development and initiation of assessments.

The NHLBI reassesses technologies in light of new scientific evidence of efficacy or of long-term adverse effects not apparent in short-term studies, and gives suggested new uses for established technologies.

Methods: *Clinical trials,* information syntheses, expert opinion, group judgment, epidemiological and other observational methods, bench testing.

If NHLBI makes a commitment to conduct a trial, subject recruitment and clinical intervention begin. Generally subjects are not recruited simultaneously, and thus the recruitment and intervention activities proceed together.

Once the trial is under way, it is managed by a complex of committees composed of the investigators, advisors, and Institute staff. Often, the central organizational element of the trial is a steering committee that provides overall scientific direction for the study at the operational level. Various subcommittees appointed by the steering committee are responsible for reviewing such matters as patient adherence, quality control, nonfatal events, natural history, mortality classification, bibliography, and editorial review. An assembly of investigators representing all of the clinical and logistical coordinating centers reports to the steering committee. A policy data-monitoring board which does not include any of the trial investigators acts in a senior advisory capacity to the NHLBI on policy matters throughout the trial's duration. It periodically reviews study results and evaluates the study treatments for beneficial and adverse effects, and consults on such major policy decisions as trial safety and termination, changes in protocol, measurement procedures, and publication.

Analysis continues during the trial. By the time the trial is ended, much of the analysis concerning the major question may already have been completed. However, only in rare cases such as those in which a trial is not double-blind and the trends are extraordinary, might the findings of a trial be published during its course.

The duration of clinical trials supported by NHLBI has ranged from 2 to 18 years (including patient follow-up), averaging about 6.6 years, although interim assessments and other reports are made during the longer trials. Consensus conferences, state-of-the-art conferences, and workshops generally take about 1 year to plan.

Assessors: NHLBI technology assessment activities entail the participation of the full complement of biomedical research and health care delivery personnel. Various advisory groups also include representatives of other professions. As noted above, members of the National Heart, Lung, and Blood Advisory Council include scientists and others who are lay community members with a demonstrated interest in health areas relevant to the program area of the Institute. The study sections that review proposals are composed of nonfederal scientists selected for their competence in the particular scientific areas for which a study section has review responsibilities.

Assessment reports include: Abstract; the purpose of the assessment; relationship of this assessment to prior or concurrent assessments of the technology or other technologies intended for similar purposes; who sponsored/commissioned/supported the assessment; who conducted the assessment; description of the technology; stage of lifecycle of technology when assessed; properties assessed; procedure used for the assessment; sources of data/information; methods for collecting data/information; methods for analyzing/synthesizing data/information; results; findings or conclusions; limitations of findings; implications of findings for practice; recommendations for practice, future assessments, technology development, research.

Dissemination: *Journal articles;* printed reports; press conferences/news releases, TV/radio broadcasts, video products.

NHLBI promotes and disseminates assessment findings through workshops; information centers; and prevention, education, and control programs. The Institute also disseminates information through professional societies, educational programs such as the National High Blood Pressure Education Program, clearinghouses such as the High Blood Pressure Information Center, interactions with industry representatives, and activities of the Institute's Office of Prevention, Education, and Control.

Copies of assessments are available in the open scientific literature. Many special reports can be obtained from the Communications and Public Information Branch, NHLBI, NIH, Building 31 Room 4A-31, 9000 Rockville Pike, Bethesda, MD 20892.

Budget: $29,000,000. The cost of large scale clinical trials ranges between $1.6 million and $142.3 million. Funding source: 100 percent parent organization.

Use: The NHLBI uses the assessment reports for planning and evaluation. The NIH and NHLBI conducted an evaluation of the impact of clinical trials on medical practice. The study evaluated the relationship between the dissemination of the clinical trial results and subsequent physician knowledge and medical practice. The two trials, both supported by NHLBI, were the Coronary Drug Project (CDP) reported in 1976 and the Aspirin Myocardial Infarction Study (AMIS) which was completed in 1979 with results disseminated in 1980. Following AMIS, there was a small increase in the number of physicians who said aspirin was of unproven benefit for post-myocardial infarction use, but most physicians still heavily prescribed aspirin.

NHLBI assessment activities are described in Institute of Medicine, Committee on Evaluating Medical Technologies. *Assessing medical technologies.* Washington, DC: National Academy Press, 1985.

Program evaluations: NHLBI has sponsored several evaluations of its assessment program and clinical trials. Listed below are the evaluation project names followed by citations to published documents about the evaluation or its findings.

1. Evaluation of Clinical Trial Coordinating Center Model Project. The University of Maryland conducted this study from June 1976 to June 1979.

The following reports were submitted to the NHLBI.

- I. *Study design and methods*
- II. *RFPs for coordination centers: a content evaluation*
- III. *The contract process for selecting coordination centers*
- V. *Terminology*
- VI. *Phases of a multicenter clinical trial*
- X. *Management of coordinating centers*
- XIV. *Enhancement of methodological research in the field of clinical trials*
- XVI. *CCMP manuscripts presented at the Annual Symposia on Coordinating Clinical Trials*

2. Evaluation of the Impact of Clinical Trials on Medical Practice. Market Facts, Inc. conducted this study from September 1978 to January 1982.

Markets Facts, Inc. *The impact of clinical trials on physician knowledge and practice.* 1982 Mar.

3. Evaluation of the Impact of Adenine on Blood Banking. JRB Associates conducted this study from June 1979 to June 1983.

Cummings PD, Cerveny RP, Wallace EL, et al. *Impact of adenine on blood banking.* 1983 Jul.

4. Evaluation of Regimen Compliance in Long-term Clinical Trials. The University of Maryland conducted this study from June 1979 to September 1984.

Howard J, Whittemore AS, Hoover JJ, Panos M, and the Aspirin Myocardial Infarction Study Research Group. How blind was the patient blind in AMIS? *Clin Pharmacol Ther* 1982;32:543-553.

Mattson ME, Friedman LM. Issues in medication adherence assessment in clinical trials of the National Heart, Lung, and Blood Institute. *Controlled Clin Trials* 1984;5:488-496.

Mattson ME, Curb JD, McArdle R, and the AMIS and BHAT Research Groups. Participation in a clinical trial: the patients' point of view. *Controlled Clin Trials* 1985;6:156-167.

Byington AP, Curb JD, Mattson ME for the Beta-Blocker Heart Attack Trial Research Group. Assessment of Double-Blindness at the conclusion of the Beta-Blocker Heart Attack Trial. *JAMA* 1985;253:1733-1736.

5. Assessment of the Impact of the Hypertension Detection and Follow-up Program (HDFP). NHLBI Staff conducted this study from January 1981 to October 1982.

National Heart, Lung, and Blood Institute. *Conference on the implications of the Hypertension Detection and Follow-up Program, November 30, 1982.*

6. Evaluation of the Impact of the Coronary Primary Prevention Trial: Baseline Measurement of Practice Before Release of Clinical Trial Results. National Capitol Systems conducted this study from July 1983 to June 1984.

National Capitol Systems, Inc. *Determination of medical practice regarding coronary heart disease risk factors: baseline measurements of practice before release of results of the Coronary Primary Prevention Trial. final report.* 1984 Apr.

7. Evaluation of the Impact of the Coronary Primary Prevention Trial (CPPT) on Clinical Practice: Measurement of Practice after Release of Clinical Trial Results. National Capitol Systems conducted this study from October 1985 to October 1986. The findings have not yet been published.

8. Evaluation of the Impact of the Coronary Primary Prevention Trial (CPPT) on Public Attitudes, Knowledge, and Behavior Regarding Serum Cholesterol and Other Risk Factors for Coronary Heart Disease. This study was conducted by the Food and Drug Administration and NHLBI staff from January 1984 to September 1985. The findings have not yet been published.

Completed Reports

NH1 Curb JD, Borhani NO, Blaszkowski TP, et al. [National Heart, Lung, and Blood Institute] Patient perceived side effects to antihypertensive drugs. J Community Health, accepted for publication.

NH2 Beta-Blocker Heart Attack Study Group. [______] The Beta-Blocker Heart Attack Trial: cooperative trial-preliminary report. JAMA 1986;246:2073-2074.

NH3 Friedman LM, Byington RP, Capone RJ, et al. for the Beta-Blocker Heart Attack Trial Research Group. [______] Effect of propranolol in patients with myocardial infarction and ventricular arrhythmia. J Am Coll Cardiol 1986;7:1-8.

NH4 Hulley SB, Feigal DW, Ireland CC, et al. [______] The Systolic Hypertension in the Elderly Program (SHEP): the first three months. 1986. J Am Ger Soc 1986;34:101-105.

NH5 Muller JE, Turi ZG, Store PH, et al. and the MILIS Study Group.[______] Digoxin therapy and mortality after myocardial infarction. Experience in the MILIS Study. N Eng J Med 1986;314:265-271.

NH6 Wheelan K, Mukharji J, Rude RE, et al. and the MILIS Study Group.[______] Sudden death and its relation to QT-internal prolongation after acute myocardial infarction: two year follow-up. Am J Cardiol 1986;57:745-750.

NH7 Buchwald H, Fitch L, Varco RL. [______] Ileal bypass for hyperlipidemia. World J Surg 1985:9;850-859.

NH8 Buchwald H, Fitch L, Varco RL. [______] Partial ileal bypass; hypercholesterolemia; atherosclerosis. In: Nyhus LM, Nelson RL, (eds): Blackwell Scientific Publ Inc, Boston, MA, 1985, in press.

NH9 Buchwald H, Fitch L, Varco RL. [______] Surgical intervention in atherosclerosis: partial ileal bypass and the Program of Surgical Control of the Hyperlipidemias (POSCH). Int Encyclo Pharm Therapy, 1985 (in press).

NH10 Buchwald H. [______] Partial ileal bypass: a surgical approach to cholesterol lowering. In: Perspectives in lipid disorders. New York: McGraw-Hill Publishing Co., 1985:Vol 3.

NH11 Byington R, Goldstein S, for the BHAT Research Group. [______] Association of digitalis therapy with mortality in survivors of acute myocardial infarction: observation in the Beta-Blocker Heart Attack Trial. J Am Coll Cardiol 1985;6:976-982.

NH12 Byington RP, Curb DJ, Mattson ME for the Beta-Blocker Heart Attack Trial Research Group. [______] Assessment of double-blindness at the conclusion of the Beta-Blocker Heart Attack Trial. JAMA 1985;253(12):1733-1766.

NH13 Collaborative Group on Antenatal Steroid Therapy. [______] Prevention of respiratory distress syndrome: effect of antenatal dexamethasone administration. Hospital and follow-up studies. 1985 [NIH Publication No. 85-2695]

NH14 Curb DJ, Borhani NO, et al. [______] Long-term surveillance for adverse effects of antihypertensive drugs. JAMA 1985;253:3263-3268.

NH15 Cutler JA, Neaton JD, Hulley SB et al. [______] Coronary heart disease and all-cause mortality in the Multiple Risk Factor Intervention Trial: subgroup findings and comparisons with other trials. Prev Med 1985;14:293-311.

NH16 Gersh BJ, Kronmal RA, Schaff HV, et al. [______] Comparison of coronary artery bypass surgery and medical therapy in patients 65 years of age or older. a nonrandomized study from the Coronary Artery Surgery Study (CASS) registry. N Engl J Med 1985;313:217-224.

NH17 Grimm RH, Neaton JD, McDonald M, et al for the Multiple Risk Factor Intervention Trial Research Group. [______] Beneficial effects from systematic dosage reduction of the diuretic chlorthalidone: a randomized study within a clinical trial. Am Heart J 1985;109:858-864.

NH18 Grimm RH, Neaton JD, McDonald M, et al. [______] Beneficial effects from systematic dosage reduction of the diuretic, chlorthalidone: a randomized study within a clinical trial. Am Heart J 1985;109:858-864.

NH19 Hennekens C, Eberlein K. [______] A randomized trial of aspirin and beta-carotene among U.S. physicians. Prev Med 1985:Appendix VI.

NH20 Hillis LD, Borer J, Braunwald E, et al. [______] High dose intravenous streptokinase for acute myocardial infarction: preliminary results of a multicenter trial. J Am Coll Cardiol 1985;6:957-962.

NH21 Hulley SB, Furberg CD, Gurland BJ, et al for the SHEP Research Group. [______] The Systolic Hypertension in the Elderly Program (SHEP): antihypertensive efficacy of chlorthalidone. Am J Cardiol 1985;56:913-920.

NH22 Hypertension Detection and Follow-up Program Cooperative Group. [______] Five-year findings of the Hypertension Detection and Follow-up Program. Prevention and reversal of left ventricular hypertrophy with antihypertensive drug therapy. Hypertension 1985;7:105-112.

NH23 Hypertension Detection and Follow-up Program Cooperative Research Group. [______] Mortality findings for stepped-care and referred-care participants in the Hypertension Detection and Follow-up Program, stratified by other risk factors. Prev Med 1985;14:312-335.

NH24 Karnegis JN, Matts JP, Tuna N and the POSCH Group. [______] Development and evolution of electrocardiographic Minnesota Q-Qs codes in patients with acute myocardial infarction. Am Heart J 1985;110:452-459.

NH25 Karnegis JN, Matts JP, Tuna N, et al and the POSCH Group. [______] Quantitative assessment of left ventricular function after myocardial infarction using the Minnesota Q-Qs codes for resting electrocardiograms. Cathet Cardiovasc Diagn 1985;11:393-400.

NH26 Kuller L, Farrier N, Borhani N, et al. [______] Relationship of diuretic therapy and serum magnesium levels among participants in the Multiple Risk Factor Intervention Trial. Am J Epidemiol 1985;122:1045-1059.

NH27 Langford HG, Blaufox MD, Oberman A, et al. [______] Dietary therapy slows the return of hypertension after stopping prolonged medication. JAMA 1985;5:657-664.

NH28 Long JM. [______] Discovery and confirmation of causal relationships in a large medical record database: a POSCH experiment. Society for Clinical Trials, Annual Conference, 1985.

NH29 Long, JM. [______] The POSCH secondary intervention trial. Proc Int Cong Prev Cardiology, Moscow, 1985.

NH30 Mattson M, Curb JD, McArdle R and the AMIS and BHAT Research Group. [______] Participation in a clinical trial: the patient's point of view. Controlled Clin Trial 1985;6:156-167.

NH31 Morganroth J, Lichstein E, Byington R. [______] Beta-Blocker Heart Attack Trial: impact of propranolol therapy on ventricular arrhythmias. Prev Med 1985;14:346-357.

NH32 Multiple Risk Factor Intervention Trial Research Group. [______] Baseline rest electrocardiographic abnormalities, antihypertensive treatment, and mortality in the Multiple Risk Factor Intervention Trial. Am J Cardiol 1985;55:1-15.

NH33 Multiple Risk Factor Intervention Trial Research Group. [______] Exercise electrocardiogram and coronary heart disease mortality in the Multiple Risk Factor Intervention Trial. Am J Cardiol 1985;55:16-24.

NH34 Passamani E, David B, Gillespie MJ, et al. [______] A randomized trial of coronary artery bypass surgery: survival of patients with a low ejection fraction. N Engl J Med 1985;312:1655-1671.

NH35 Rifkind BM. [______] The Lipid Research Clinics Coronary Primary Prevention Trial. Heartbeat 1985;1:7-8.

NH36 Shekelle RB, Gale M, Norusis M for the Aspirin Myocardial Infarction Study Research Group. [______] Type A score (Jenkins activity survey) and risk of recurrent coronary heart disease in the Aspirin Myocardial Infarction Study. Am J Cardiol 1985;56:221-225.

NH37 TIMI Study Group. [______] Special report. The Thrombolysis in Myocardial Infarction (TIMI) Trial. Phase I findings. N Engl J Med 1985;312:932-936.

NH38 Brensike JF, Levy RI, Kelsey SF, et al. [______] Effects of therapy with cholestyramine on progression of coronary arteriosclerosis: results of the NHLBI Type II Coronary Intervention Study. Circulation 1984:69;313-324.

NH39 Byington RP for the Beta-Blocker Heart Attack Trial Research Group. [______] Beta-Blocker Heart Attack Trial—design, methods and baseline results. Controlled Clin Trials 1984;4:382-437.

NH40 CASS Principal Investigators and Their Associates. [______] Coronary Artery Surgery Study (CASS): a randomized trial of coronary artery bypass surgery: myocardial infarction and mortality in the randomized trial. N Engl J Med 1984;310:750-758.

NH41 Collaborative Group on Antenatal Steroid Therapy. [______] Effects of antenatal dexamethasone administration in the infant: long-term follow-up. J Pediatr 1984;104:259-267.

NH42 Connett JE, Stamler J. [______] Responses of Black and white males to the special intervention program of the Multiple Risk Factor Intervention Trial. Am Heart J 1984;108(3):839-849.

NH43 Croft CH, Rude RE, Lewis SE, et al. [______] Comparison of left ventricular function and infarct size in patients with and without positive technetium-99m pyrophosphate myocardial scintigrams after myocardial infarction: analysis of 357 patients. Am J Cardiol 1984;53:421-428.

NH44 DeMets DL, Hardy R, Friedman LM, et al. [______] Statistical aspects of early termination in the Beta-Blocker Heart Attack Trial. Controlled Clin Trials 1984;5:362-372.

NH45 Furberg CD, Hawkins CM, Lichstein E for the Beta-Blocker Heart Attack Study Group. [______] Effect of propranolol in postinfarction patients with mechanical or electrical complications. Circulation 1984;69:761-765.

NH46 Goldstein S, Friedman L, Hutchinson, R et al and the Aspirin Myocardial Infarction Study Research Group. [______] Timing, mechanism and clinical setting of witnessed deaths in postmyocardial infarction patients. J Am Coll Cardiol 1984;3:1111-1117.

NH47 Hypertension Detection and Follow-up Program Cooperative Group. [______] Five-year findings of the Hypertension Detection and Follow-up Program: mortality by race-sex and blood pressure level: a further analysis. J Community Health 1984;9:314-327.

NH48 Hypertension Detection and Follow-up Program Cooperative Research Group. [______] The effect of antihypertensive drug treatment on mortality in the presence of testing electrocardiographic abnormalities at baseline: the HDFP experience. Circulation 1984;70:996-1003.

NH49 Hypertension Detection and Follow-up Program. [______] Effect of stepped-care treatment on the incidence of myocardial infarction of the Hypertension Detection and Follow-up Program. Hypertension 1984;6(Suppl 1).

NH50 Langford HG, Blaufox MD, Oberman A, et al. [______] Effect of weight loss on the return of hypertension after withdrawal of prolonged antihypertensive therapy. In: Nutritional Prevention of Cardiovascular Disease. 1984:311-315.

NH51 Langford HG, Oberman A, Borhani NO, et al. [______] Black-white comparison of indices of coronary heart disease and myocardial infarction in the stepped-care cohort of the Hypertension Detection and Follow-Up Program. Am Heart J 1984;108(3):797-801.

NH52 Langford HG, Schlundt D, Levine K. [______] Sodium restriction in hypertension. Compr Ther 1984;10:6-11.

NH53 Lasser N, Grandits G, Caggiula A, et al. [______] Effects of antihypertensive therapy on plasma lipids and lipoproteins in the Multiple Risk Factor Intervention Trial. Am J Med 1984;76:52-66.

NH54 Levy RI, Brensike JF, Epstein SF, et al. [______] The influence of changes in lipid values induced by cholestyramine and diet on progression of coronary artery disease: results of the NHLBI Type II Coronary Intervention Study. Circulation 1984;69:325-337.

NH55 Lipid Research Clinics Program. [______] The Lipid Research Clinics Coronary Primary Prevention Trial results. I. Reduction in incidence of coronary heart disease. JAMA 1984;251:351-364.

NH56 Lipid Research Clinics Program. [______] The Lipid Research Clinics Coronary Primary Prevention Trial results. II. The relationship of reduction in incidence of coronary heart disease to cholesterol-lowering. JAMA 1984;251:365-374.

NH57 Muller JE (ed), Braunwald E, Mock MB, et al. (assoc. eds). [______] ______ Multicenter Investigation of the Limitation of Infarct Size (MILIS). Design and methods of the clinical trial. An investigation of beta-blockade and myaluronidase for treatment of acute myocardial infarction. Am Heart Assoc Monograph 1984;100:1-134.

NH58 Rifkind BM. [______] The Lipid Research Clinics Coronary Primary Prevention Trial: results and implication. Am J Cardiol 1984;54:30C-34C.

NH59 Roberts R, Croft C, Gold HK, et al. and the MILIS Study Group.[______] Effect of propranolol on myocardial-infarct size in a randomized blinded multicenter trial. N Eng J Med 1984;311:218-225.

NH60 Shekelle R. [______] Diuretic treatment of hypertension and changes in plasma lipids over six years in the Multiple Risk Factor Intervention Trial. In: Paolette R et al. (eds). Endpoints for cardiovascular drug studies. New York: Raven, 1984:216.

NH61 Wing R, Caggiula A, Nowalk M, et al. [______] Dietary approaches to the reduction of blood pressure: the independence of weight and sodium/potassium interventions. Prev Med 1984;13:233-234.

NH62 Beta-Blocker Heart Attack Trial Research Group. [______] A randomized trial of propranolol in patients with acute myocardial infarction. II. Morbidity results. JAMA 1983;250:2814-2819.

NH63 Buchwald H, Moore RB, Rucker Rd, et al. [______] Clinical angiographic regression of atheroscerosis after partial ileal bypass. Artherosclerosis 1983;46:117.

NH64 CASS Principal Investigators and Their Associates. [______] Coronary Artery Surgery Study (CASS): a randomized trial of coronary artery bypass surgery: quality of life in patients randomly assigned to treatment groups. Circulation 1983;68:951-960.

NH65 CASS Principal Investigators and Their Associates. [______] Coronary Artery Surgery Study (CASS): randomized trial of coronary artery bypass surgery: survival data. Circulation 1983;68:939-950.

NH66 CASS Principal Investigators and Their Associates. [______] Coronary Artery Surgery Study (CASS): a randomized trial of coronary artery bypass surgery: comparability of entry characteristics and survival in randomized patients and nonrandomized patients meeting randomization criteria. J Am Coll Card 1983;3:114-128.

NH67 Davis KB, Chatman BR, Killip T, et al. [______] Effect of coronary bypass surgery on operative mortality and survival patterns in subsets of patients with left main coronary artery disease. In: Hammermeister KE, ed. Coronary bypass surgery. New York: Praeger Scientific, 1983:99-127.

NH68 Davis KB, Kennedy JW, Berger RL, et al. [______] Operative mortality in the CASS registry. In: Hammermeister KE ed. Coronary bypass surgery. New York: Praeger Scientific, 1983:99-127.

NH69 Frommer PL, Fisher LD, Moek MB, et al. [______] The Coronary Artery Surgery Study: a randomized trial in the context of the registry. In: Hammermeister KE, ed. Coronary bypass surgery. New York: Praeger Scientific, 1983:57-82.

NH70 Furberg CD, Byington RP for the BHAT Research Group. [______] What do subgroup analyses reveal about differential response to beta-blocker therapy? The Beta-Blocker Heart Attack Trial experience. Proceedings of the Workshop on Implications of Recent Beta-Blocker Trials for Post-Myocardial Infarction Patients. Circulation 1983;67(Supplement I):I-98.

NH71 Gersh BJ, Kronmal RA, Frye RL, et al. [______] Coronary arteriography and coronary artery bypass surgery: morbidity and mortality in patients ages 65 years or older: a report from the Coronary Artery Surgery Study. Circulation 1983;67:483-490.

NH72 Goldstein, S. [______] Propranolol therapy in patients with acute myocardial infarction: the Beta-Blocker Heart Attack Trial. Circulation 1983;67(Suppl 1):53-57.

NH73 Hardy RJ, Hawkins CM. [______] The impact of selected indices of anti-hypertensive treatment on all-cause mortality. Am J Epidemiol 1983;117:566-574.

NH74 Heaton RK, Grant I, McSweeny J, et al. [______] Psychologic effects of continuous and nocturnal oxygen therapy in hypoxemic chronic obstructive pulmonary disease. Arch Intern Med 1983;143:1941-1947.

NH75 Holmes DR, Vliestra RE, Fisher LD, et al. [______] Follow-up of patients from the Coronary Artery Surgery Study (CASS) potentially suitable for percutaneous transluminal coronary angioplasty. Am Heart J 1983;106:981-988.

NH76 Hughes GH, Schnaper HW. [______] The Systolic Hypertension in the Elderly Program. Int J Mental Health 1983;11:76-97.

NH77 Intermittent Positive Pressure Breathing Trial Group. [______] Intermittent positive pressure breathing therapy of chronic obstructive pulmonary disease—a clinical trial. Ann Intern Med 1983;99:612-620.

NH78 Keogh BA, Bernardo J, Hunninghake GW, et al. [______] Effect of intermittent high dose parenteral corticosteroids on the alveolitis of idiopathic pulmonary fibrosis. Am Rev Respir Dis 1983;127:18-27.

NH79 Lichstein E, Morganroth J, Harrest R, et al. [______] Effect of propranolol on ventricular arrhythmia: the Beta-Blocker Heart Attack Trial Experience. Circulation 1983;67(Suppl I):5-10.

NH80 Ryan TJ, Bailey KR, McCabe CH, et al. [______] The effects of digitalis on survival in high-risk patients with coronary artery disease: the Coronary Artery Surgery Study (CASS). Circulation 1983;67:735-742.

NH81 Smith WM. [______] Isolated systolic hypertension in the elderly. In: Mild hypertension. New York: Raven Press, 1983.

NH82 Wassertheil-Smoller S, Langford HG, Blaaufox MD, et al. [______] Diuretics and salt-restriction in blood pressure control. In: Winick M ed. Nutrition and drugs. New York: John Wiley and Sons Inc, 1983:175-189.

NH83 Brensike JF, Kelsey SF, Passamani ER, et al. [______] National Heart, Lung, and Blood Institute Type II Coronary Intervention Study: design, methods, and baseline characteristics. Controlled Clin Trials 1982:3;91-111.

NH84 Buchwald H, Fitch L, Moore RL. [______] Overview of clinical trials of lipid intervention for atherosclerotic cardiovascular disease. Controlled Clin Trials 1982;3:271-283.

NH85 Buchwald H, Moore RB, Matts JP, et al. [______] The Program on the Surgical Control of the Hyperlipidemias: a status report. Surgery 1982;92:654.

NH86 Buchwald H, Moore RB, Varco RL. [______] Surgery in the therapy of atherosclerosis: partial ileal bypass. In: Arteriosclerosis: clinical evaluation and therapy. MTP Press Limited, International Medical Publication, 1982.

NH87 Buchwald H, Rucker RD Jr, Moore RB, et al. [______] Regression of atherosclerosis by surgical cholesterol reduction. In: Noseda CI, et al. eds. Lipoproteins and coronary atherosclerosis. Elsevier Biomedical Press, 1982:417.

NH88 Curb JD, Hardy RJ, Labarthe DR, et al. [______] Reserpine and breast cancer in the Hypertension Detection and Follow-up Program. Hypertension 1982;4(2):307-311.

NH89 Fisher LD, Lundberg ED, McBride R, et al. [______] The design of a database management system, C2, for research use in the Coronary Artery Surgery Study (CASS). In: Proceedings of the Fifteenth Hawaii International Conference on Systems Sciences, 1982, Volume II, Software, Hardware, Decision Support Systems, Special Topics. North Hollywood, CA: Western Periodicals Co., 1982.

NH90 Hymowitz N. [______] The Multiple Risk Factor Intervention Trial: a four year evaluation. Int J Ment Health 1982;11:44-67.

NH91 Hypertension Detection and Follow-up Program Cooperative Group. [______] Five-year findings of the Hypertension Detection and Follow-Up Program.III. Reductions in stroke incidence among persons with high blood pressure. JAMA 1982;247:633-638.

NH92 Hypertension Detection and Follow-up Program Cooperative Group. [______] The effect of treatment on mortality in "mild" hypertension: results of the Hypertension Detection and Follow-up Program. N Engl J Med 1982;307:976-980.

NH93 Lipid Research Clinics Program. [______] Recruitment for clinical trials: the Lipid Research Clinics Coronary Primary Prevention Trial experience. Its implications for future trials. (AHA Monograph No. 93) Circulation 1982;66:IV1-IV78.

NH94 Long JM, Brasshear JR, Matts JP, et al. [______] The evolution of a large clinical database. Proceedings of Medcomp 1982;82:224-229.

NH95 Lundberg ED, McBride R, Rawson TE, et al. [______] A data base management system developed for the Coronary Artery Surgery Study (CASS) and other clinical studies. In: Riddle K, Thurber P, Keen P, et al. eds. Proc of the 15th Hawaii Internat Conf on Systems Sciences, 1982, Vol II, Software, Hardware, Decision Support Systems, Special Topics, North Hollywood, CA: Western Periodicals Co, 1982:484-500.

NH96 Mock MB, Ringvist I, Fisher LD, et al. [______] Survival of medically treated patients in the Coronary Artery Surgery Study (CASS) registry. Circulation 1982;66:562-568.

NH97 Multiple Risk Factor Intervention Trial Research Group. [______] Multiple Risk Factor Intervention Trial: risk factor changes and mortality results. JAMA 1982;248:1465-1477.

NH98 Ockene J, Hymowitz N, Sexton M, Broste S. [______] Comparison of patterns of smoking behavior change among smokers in the Multiple Risk Factor Intervention Trial (MRFIT). Prev Med 1982;11:621-638.

NH99 Shulman N, Cutter G, Daugherty R, et al. [______] Correlates of attendance and compliance in the Hypertension Detection and Follow-Up Program. Controlled Clin Trials 1982;3:13-27.

NH100 Smith EO, Curp JD, Hardy RJ, et al. [______] Clinic attendance in the Hypertension Detection and Follow-Up Program.' Hypertension 1982;4:710-715.

NH101 Vlietstra RE, Kronmal RA, Frye RL, et al. [______] Factors affecting the extent and severity of coronary artery disease in patients enrolled in the Coronary Artery Surgery Study. Arteriosclerosis 1982;2:208-215.

NH102 Wassertheil-Smoller S, Langford HG, Blaufox MD et al. [______] Rate of hypertension return after withdrawal of prolonged antihypertensive therapy. Clin Sci 1982;63(Suppl 8):4235-4255.

NH103 Benfari R, Sherwin R. [______] The Multiple Risk Factor Intervention Trial after 4 years: a summing-up. Prev Med 1981;10:544-546.

NH104 Berger RL, Davis KB, Kaiser GC, et al. [______] Preservation of the myocardium during coronary artery bypass grafting. Circulation 1981;64 (Supplement II):II61-II66.

NH105 Beta-Blocker Heart Attack Trial Research Group. [______] A randomized trial of propranolol in patients with acute myocardial infarction. l. Mortality results. JAMA 1982;247:1707-1713.

NH106 Beta-Blocker Heart Attack Trial Research Group. [______] Beta-Blocker heart attack trial—design features. Controlled Clin Trials 1981;2:275-285.

NH107 Caggiula A, Christakis G, Farrand M, et al. [______] The Multiple Risk Factor Intervention Trial (MRFIT). IV. Intervention on blood lipids. Prev Med 1981;10:443-475.

NH108 Chaitman BR, Bourassa MG, Davis K, et al. [______] Angiographic prevalance of high-risk coronary artery disease patient subjects (CASS). Circulation 1981;64:360-367.

NH109 Chaitman BR, Fisher LD, Bourassa MG, et al. [______] Effect of coronary bypass surgery on survival patterns in subsets of patients with left main coronary artery disease. Report of the collaborative study in Coronary Artery Surgery (CASS). Am J Cardiol 1981;48:765-777.

NH110 Cohen J, Grimm R Jr, Swith W. [______] Multiple Risk Factor Intervention Trial (MRFIT). VI. Intervention on blood pressure. Prev Med 1981;10:501-518.

NH111 Collaborative Group on Antenatal Steroid Therapy. [______] Effect of antenatal dexamethasone administration on the prevention of respiratory distress syndrome. Am J Obstet Gynecol 1981;141:276-287.

NH112 Coronary Drug Project Research Group. [______] Implications of findings in the Coronary Drug Project for secondary prevention trials in coronary heart disease. Circulation 1981;63:1342-1350.

NH113 Fisher LD, Kennedy JW, Chaitman BR, et al. [______] Diagnostic quantification of CASS (Coronary Artery Surgery Study) clinical and exercise test results in determining presence and extent of coronary artery disease: a multivariate approach. Circulation 1981;63:987-1000.

NH114 Hodgkin JE and Zorn EG. [______] Intermittent positive pressure breathing (IPPB) in the outpatient management of chronic obstructive pulmonary disease (COPD): description of the NIH clinical trial. Respir Care 1981;26:1095-1104.

NH115 Howard JM, DeMets D, and the BHAT Research Group. [______] How informed is informed consent? The BHAT experience. Controlled Clin Trials 1981;2:287-303.

NH116 Hughes G, Hymowitz N, Ockene J, et al. [______] The Multiple Risk Factor Intervention Trial (MRFIT). V. Intervention on smoking. Prev Med 1981;10:476-500.

NH117 Kennedy JW, Kaiser GC, Fisher LD, et al. [______] Clinical and angiographic predictors of operative mortality from the collaborative study in Coronary Artery Surgery (CASS). Circulation 1981;63;793-802.

NH118 Neaton J, Broste S, Cohen L, et al. [______] The Multiple Risk Factor Intervention Trial (MRFIT). VII. A comparison of risk factor changes between the two study groups. Prev Med 1981;10:519-543.

NH119 Principal Investigators of CASS and Their Associates. [______] National Heart, Lung, and Blood Institute Coronary Artery Surgery Study. Circulation 1981;63 (AHA Monograph No. 79):I1-I81.

NH120 Strauss RG, Connett JE, Gale RP, et al. [______] A controlled trial of prophylactic granulocyte transfusions during initial induction chemotherapy for acute myelogenous leukemia. N Eng J Med 1981;305:597-603.

NH121 Winston DJ, Ho WG, Gale RP. [______] Prophylactic granulocyte transfusions during chemotherapy of acute nonlymphocytic leukemia. Ann Intern Med 1981;94:616-622.

NH122 Zukel PO, Schnaper H. [______] The Multiple Risk Factor Intervention Trial (MRFIT). I. Historical perspectives. Prev Med 1981;10:387-401.

NH123 Aspirin Myocardial Infarction Research Group. [______] Aspirin Myocardial Infarction Study: design, methods and baseline results. DHEW Pub. No. (NIH) 80-2106, 1980.

NH124 Aspirin Myocardial Infarction Research Group. [______] A randomized controlled trial of aspirin in persons recovered from myocardial infarction. JAMA 1980;243:661-669.

NH125 Aspirin Myocardial Infarction Study Research Group. [______] The Aspirin Myocardial Infarction Study: final results. Circulation 1980;60(Suppl V)V79-V84.

NH126 Beta-Blocker Heart Attack Trial Study Group. [______] Beta-Blocker Heart Attack Trial Study protocol. DHHS Pub No. (NIH)81-2209, 1980.

NH127 Borhani NO. [______] Clinical ramifications of the Hypertension Detection and Follow-Up Program: SC yields lower mortality and morbidity. Symposia Reporter 1980;4(2):16.

NH128 Coronary Drug Research Group. [______] Aspirin in coronary heart disease. Circulation 1980;62(Suppl V):V59-V62.

NH129 Coronary Drug Research Project Group. [______] Influence of adherence to treatment and response of cholesterol on mortality in the Coronary Drug Project. N Eng J Med 1980;303:1038-1041.

NH130 Cowan L, Detels R, Farbar M, et al. [______] Residential mobility and long-term hypertension. J Community Health 1980;5:159-166.

NH131 Cutter G, Heyden S, Kasteler J, et al. [______] Mortality surveillance in collaborative trials. Am J Public Health 1980;70:394-400.

NH132 Farrand ME, Majonnier L, (for the MRFIT Group). [______] Nutrition in the Multiple Risk Factor Intervention Trial (MRFIT). J Am Dietetic Assn 1980;76:347-351.

NH133 Gosselin AJ, Fisher L, Judkins MP, et al. [______] An estimate of the number of possible candidates from the CASS registry. Proceedings of the workshop on percutaneous transluminal coronary angioplasty June 15-16, 1979, March 1980:89-100. (U.S. Department of Health, Education and Welfare, NIH Publication No. 80-2030).

NH134 Kennedy JW, Kaiser GC, Fisher LD, et al. [______] Multivariate discriminant analysis of the clinical and angiographic predictors of operative mortality from the Collaborative Study in Coronary Artery Surgery (CASS). J Thorac Cardiovasc Surg 1980;80:876.

NH135 Knopp RH. [______] Test of the lipid hypothesis: the Coronary Primary Prevention Trial (CPPT) of the Lipid Research Clinics Program. In: Gotto AM, Jr., ed. Proceedings of the Fifth International Symposium on Atherosclerosis. Springer-Verlag 1980:509-512.

NH136 Kuller L, Neaton J, Caggiula A, et al (for the MRFIT Group). [______] Primary prevention of heart attacks: the Multiple Risk Factor Intervention Trial. Am J Epidemiol 1980;112:185-199.

NH137 Langford HG. [______] Clinical ramifications of the Hypertension Detection and Follow-Up Program: HDFP methodology and results: overview. Symposia Reporter 1980;4(2):3-6.

NH138 Long JM, Brashear JR, Matts JP, et al. [______] The POSCH Information Management System: experience with alternative approaches. J Med Systems 1980;4:355-366.

NH139 Lusher JM, Shapiro SS, Palascak JE, et al. [______] Efficiency of prothrombin-complex concentrates in hemophiliacs with antibodies to Factor VIII. N Eng J Med 1980;303:421.

NH140 Moore RB, Buchwald H, Varco RL, and the Participants in the Program on the Surgical Control of the Hyperlipidemias. [______] The effect of partial ileal bypass on plasma lipoproteins. Circulation 1980;62:469-476.

NH141 Nocturnal Oxygen Therapy Trial Group. [______] Continuous or nocturnal oxygen therapy in hypoxemic chronic obstructive lung disease: a clinical trial. Ann Intern Med 1980;93:391-398.

NH142 Nocturnal Oxygen Therapy Trial Study Group. [______] Is 12-hour oxygen as effective as 24-hour oxygen in advanced chronic obstructive pulmonary disease with hypoxemia? (The Nocturnal Oxygen Therapy Trial—NOTT). Chest 1980;78:419-420.

NH143 Remmell PS, Benfari RC (for the MRFIT Group). [______] Assessing dietary adherence in the Multiple Risk Factor Intervention Trial (MRFIT). II. Food record rating as an indicator of compliance. J Am Dietetic Assn, 1980;76:357-360.

NH144 Remmell PS, Gorder DD, Hall Y, et al (for the MRFIT Group). [______] Assessing dietary adherence in the Multiple Risk Factor Intervention Trial (MRFIT). I. Use of a dietary monitoring tool. J Am Dietetic Assn 1980;76:351-356.

NH145 Rifkind B, Goor R. [______] Lipid Research Clinics Coronary Primary Prevention Trial. In: Fumagalli R, Kritchevsky D, Paoletti R, eds. Drugs affecting lipid metabolism. Elsevier, North Holland Biomedical Press, 1980:151-157.

NH146 Russell RO, Wayne JB, Kronenfeld J, et al. [______] Surgical versus medical therapy for treatment of unstable angina: changes in work status and family income. Am J Cardiology 1980;45:134-140.

NH147 Stamler J, Borhani NO. [______] Interview: HDFP mortality and morbidity. Hypertension Report 1980;1(1):12-14.

NH148 Stamler J. [______] Clinical ramifications of the Hypertension Detection and Follow-Up Program: benefits of treatment outweigh risks. Symposia Reporter 1980;4(2):12-14.

NH149 Szmuness W, Stevens CE, Harley EJ, et al. [______] Hepatitis B vaccine: demonstration of efficacy in a controlled clinical trial in high-risk population in the United States. N Eng J Med 1980;303:833-841.

NH150 Unstable Angina Pectoris Study Group. [______] Unstable Angina Pectoris Study National Cooperative Study Group to compare medical and surgical therapy. III. Results in patients with S-T segment elevation during pain. Am J Cardiology 1980;45:819-824.

NH151 Hypertension Detection and Follow-Up Program Cooperative Group. [______] Five year findings of the Hypertension Detection and Follow-Up Program. I. Reduction in mortality of persons with high blood pressure including mild hypertension. JAMA 1979;242:2562-2571.

NH152 Hypertension Detection and Follow-Up Program Cooperative Group. [______] Five-year findings of the Hypertension Detection and Follow-Up Program: II. Mortality by race-sex and age. JAMA 1979;242:2572-2577.

NH153 Unstable Angina Pectoris Study Group. [______] Unstable Angina Pectoris National Cooperative Study Group to compare medical and surgical therapy. II. In-hospital experience and initial follow-up results in patients with one, two and three vessel disease. Am J Cardiol 1978;42:839-848.

NH154 Williams DO, Passamani ER, et al. [______] Intravenous recombinant tissue-type plasminogen activator in patients with acute myocardial infarction: a report from the NHLBI Thrombolysis in Myocardial Infarction Trial. Circulation 1986;73:338-346.

National Institute of Child Health and Human Development

Office of Planning and Evaluation
Building 31, Room 2A10
9000 Rockville Pike
Bethsda, MD 20892
301-496-1877

Contact: James G. Hill, Chief Office of Planning and Evaluation. Telex 494-8446.

Overview: The National Institute of Child Health and Human Development (NICHD) supports and conducts research to help families have healthy children at the time they are wanted, to prevent disease and disability among children, to foster normal development, and to insure that each child will have a healthy and productive life. The NICHD Technology Assessment/Transfer program was initiated in 1978.

Purpose: To maintain an awareness of technologies used in fields related to NICHD's mission and to conduct assessments of technologies with high public interest and importance.

Primary intended users: General public; people concerned about their health; patients; providers, generally; physicians; other care givers; health product manufacturers; health/medical professional associations; health industry associations; consumer associations; third party payers; government regulators; voluntary associations, organizations; biomedical researchers; reporters, writers, news media; public policy-makers, legislators; policy research organizations; lawyers; liability, malpractice insurers.

Technologies: *Medical or surgical procedure,* drug, device, support system.

Intervention: *Prevention,* diagnosis, treatment, rehabilitation.

Stage: *New,* emerging, established or widespread practice.

Properties: *Effectiveness;* safety; efficacy; cost; cost-benefit; ethical, legal, social implications.

Selection Process: Requests for assessment can come from any source, but most suggestions come from Institute staff, advisory groups, and professional associations within the scope of the Institute's mission. In addition, an annual request for assessment topics is sent to the NICHD research programs and the primary professional organizations within the Institute's mission.

Topics submitted are reviewed and analyzed by the Office of Planning and Evaluation (OPE) according to the criteria for selection of consensus topics developed by the Office of Medical Applications of Research (OMAR), NIH. In addition, relevance to the NICHD mission and research priorities are considered. The OPE Analysis of the suggested topics is reviewed by the Director, NICHD and a list of topics (usually two or three) are selected for formal assessment during the year. The selected topics are reviewed with OMAR to determine which will be consensus development conferences. Remaining topics are subjected to full scale assessment (e.g. prenatal and perinatal factors in brain injury, contents of prenatal care) or a workshop (e.g. malpractice issues in childbirth).

Technologies are reassessed when, in the judgment of Institute staff, sufficient new information is available. For example, when the clinical trial on chorion villi sampling is complete, antenatal diagnosis will be reassessed.

Methods: *Group judgment,* information synthesis, expert opinion, cost analyses, epidemiological and other observational methods, clinical trials.

Task Force, expert panels and workshops are used for conducting assessments. Once a topic is selected, a planning meeting is held. Three tasks are completed: 1) selection of a chairperson; 2) specification of the types of individuals to serve on the panel; and 3) identification of the questions to be answered by the panel. With the assistance of the National Library of Medicine, a major literature search is undertaken. The panel meets for the first time. Armed with their questions, the results of the literature search, and other information (e.g. hearings or new data sets), the panel drafts a report containing the draft consensus statement. The draft report is circulated among interested organizations and individuals who are encouraged to submit written comments and/or give oral testimony at the consensus meeting. The next step is a consensus conference that is open to the public. It consists of a summary presentation of the draft report by the members of the panel, invited comments, presentation of additional data not considered by the panel, testimony from individuals and organizations, and a closed executive session in which the panel resolves and includes additional information and prepares the final statement. The panel chairperson concludes the conference by delivering the final consensus statement in an open session.

The approximate turnaround time from selection of assessment topic to reporting of findings ranges from 1 to 2 years.

Assessors: The expertise of the panel members varies with the technology. At a minimum the group is composed of basic scientists, academic physicians, epidemiologists, practicing physicians, and consumer representatives.

Assessment reports include: The assessment's intended audience; the purpose of the assessment; relationship of this assessment to prior or concurrent assessments of the technology or other technologies intended for similar purposes; who sponsored/commissioned/supported the assessment; who conducted the assessment; description of the technology; stage of life-cycle of technology when assessed; properties assessed; procedure used for the assessment; sources of data/information; methods for collecting data/information; methods for analyzing/synthesizing data/information; results; findings or conclusions; limitations of findings; implications of findings for practice; recommendations for practice, future assessments, technology development, research; how the technology works, including theory, principles; development of the technology.

Dissemination: Printed reports, journal articles; advisories to members/constituents; press conferences/news releases, TV/radio broadcasts, video products.

Results are disseminated using mailing lists, working with professional organizations such as the American Academy of Pediatrics and the American College of Obstetricians and Gynecologists, and at professional and lay meetings. Copies of assessment reports can be obtained from the Office of Research Reporting, NICHD, Bldg. 31, Room 2A32, 9000 Rockville Pike, Bethsda, MD 20892, (301)496-5133.

Budget: $200,000. The approximate cost per assessment is $200,000. Funding source: 100 percent parent organization.

Use: Based on an analysis of requests, practicing physicians, health consumers, researchers, and physician residency training programs use the assessment reports.

The following articles reference the NICHD program:

Hill, JG. Technology assessment at the National Institute of Child Health and Human Development: an alternative model. In: Wisniewski HM, Snider DA, eds. *Mental retardation: research, education, and technology transfer.* New York: Annals of the New York Academy of Sciences 1986;477: 351-355.

Shino, et al. Recent trends in C/B and trial of labor rates in the U.S. *JAMA* 1987;257(4).

Completed Reports

NK1 National Institute of Child Health and Human Development. Infantile apnea and home monitoring. Bethesda, MD: National Institute of Child Health and Human Development, 1987 (in press). [Group judgment, Expert opinion]

NK2 International Childbirth Education Association, National Institute of Child Health and Human Development, Division of Maternal and Child Health. Malpractice issues in childbirth. Minneapolis, MN: International Childbirth Education Association, 1985. [Group judgment, Expert opinion]

NK3 National Institute of Child Health and Human Development, National Institute of Neurological and Communicative Disorders and Stroke. Prenatal and perinatal factors associated with brain disorders. Bethesda, MD: National Institutes of Health, 1985. (NIH publication no. 85-1149) [Group judgment, Expert opinion]

NK4 National Institute of Child Health and Human Development. Diagnostic ultrasound imaging in pregnancy. Bethesda, MD: National Institute of Child Health and Human Development, 1984. (NIH publication no. 84-667) [Group judgment, Expert opinion]

NK5 ______. Cesarean childbirth. Bethesda, MD: National Institute of Child Health and Human Development, 1981. (NIH publication no. 82-2067) [Group judgment, Expert opinion]

NK6 ______. Antenatal diagnosis. Bethesda MD: National Institute of Child Health and Human Development, 1979. (NIH publication no. 80-1973) [Group judgment, Expert opinion]

Ongoing Assessments

NK7 ______, Division of Maternal and Child Health. Content of prenatal care. Ongoing. [Group judgment, Expert opinion]

Planned Assessments

NK8 ______. Antenatal diagnosis of hereditary disease (an update of the 1979 Conference on Antenatal Diagnosis). Planned. [Group judgment, Expert opinion]

NK9 ______. Modification of inappropriate behavior in the mentally retarded. Planned. [Group judgment, Expert opinion]

NK10 ______. Safety and efficacy of oral contraceptives. Planned. [Group judgment, Expert opinion]

National Institutes of Health

Consensus Development Program
Building 1, Room 210
9000 Rockville Pike
Bethesda, MD 20892
301-496-1143

Contact: Michael J. Bernstein, Director of Communications, Office of Medical Applications of Research.

Overview: The National Institutes of Health (NIH) is the principal biomedical research agency of the Federal Government. The NIH Office of Medical Applications of Research (OMAR) operates the NIH Consensus Development Program which conducts consensus conferences. The conferences are jointly sponsored by OMAR and one or more of the NIH Institutes; other Public Health Service (PHS) agencies occasionally join in the sponsorship.

Purpose: To evaluate in a public forum the use of biomedical technologies, to publish a consensus statement relevant to the public at large that provides guidelines for practitioners on the use of the technology, and to disseminate this information to the intended audience.

Primary intended users: General public; providers, generally; physicians; biomedical researchers.

Technologies: Drug, device, medical or surgical procedure, support system.

Intervention: Prevention, diagnosis, treatment, rehabilitation.

Stage: *New,* established or widespread practice.

Most often the program focuses on new information. This information can pertain to existing technologies, making them obsolete, or to emerging technologies.

Properties: Safety, efficacy, effectiveness, service requirements.

Selection process: Most often topics are selected by the NIH leadership as part of the NIH-wide planning process. At times topics are requested for consideration by other PHS agencies or organizations outside the government. Requests are submitted to OMAR. Assessment topic priorities are set by the OMAR Director in consultation with the NIH Coordinating Committee on Assessment and Transfer of Technology. Meetings can be held to reassess topics; for example adjuvant chemotherapy for breast cancer was recently reexamined.

Methods: *Group judgment,* information syntheses, modeling.

OMAR uses consensus conferences as its assessment method. A consensus panel, after listening to expert presentations, develops a consensus statement. This statement is a response to a set of questions presented to the panel.

The average turnaround time from selection of assessment topic to reporting of findings is 1 year.

Assessors: The assessors' areas of expertise include biomedical research, clinical practice, biostatistics, epidemiology, and public policy.

Assessment reports include: The assessment's intended audience; the purpose of the assessment; relationship of this assessment to prior or concurrent assessments of the technology or other technologies intended for similar purposes; who sponsored/commissioned/supported the assessment; who conducted the assessment; description of the technology; stage of life-cycle of technology when assessed; properties assessed; procedure used for the assessment; sources of data/information; methods for collecting data/information; methods for analyzing/synthesizing data/information; results; findings or conclusions; limitations of findings; implications of findings for practice; recommendations for practice, future assessments, technology development, research.

Dissemination: *Printed reports;* journal articles; advisories to members/constituents; press conferences/news releases, TV/radio broadcasts, video products.

The consensus statements are widely disseminated through targeted mailing lists, dedicated TV networks such as the Hospital Satellite Network, and professional journals such as the *Journal of the American Medical Association* Copies of consensus statements are available from OMAR.

Budget: $900,000. The approximate, all-inclusive cost per conference is $95,000. Funding source: 100 percent parent organization.

Use: Summary statements are widely used by practitioners as well as the public in considering care and patient management. Impact has been shown recently by the significant sales increases of certain drugs following the consensus conferences on osteoporosis and blood cholesterol. The use of these drugs was recommended in the summary statements.

The following articles describe the Consensus Development Program:

Institute of Medicine, Committee on Evaluating Medical Technologies in Clinical Use. *Assessing medical technologies.* Washington, DC: National Academy Press, 1985.

Jacoby I, Mullan F. The town meeting for technology: the maturation of consensus conferences. *JAMA* 1985 Aug;254(8).

Jacoby, I. The Consensus Development Program of the National Institutes of Health: current practices and historical perspectives. *Internl J Technol Assessment Health Care* 1985 Jun;1(2).

A Rand note: "Treatment of eight NIH Consensus Development Conferences in the biomedical literature." 1986 Sep.

Program evaluation: During 1982 to 1986, the Rand Corporation conducted an evaluation of the Consensus Development Program's impact. Funded by OMAR, the study included lengthy questionnaires responded to by physicians, a detailed hospital chart-audit, and analyses based upon literature searches. The findings suggested that while the program has a positive impact, some elements of the process can be improved. Evaluation results are continuously introduced to improve topic selection, synthesis of data, the conduct of the group process, and dissemination methods.

The Rand Corporation report will be available shortly upon request from the Rand Corporation, Santa Monica, California. See also: Wortman P, Vinokura A, and Sechrest L. *Evaluation of NIH consensus development process: phase I: final report.* Center for Research on Utilization of Scientific Knowledge, Institute for Social Research, University of Michigan, Ann Arbor. 1982;Sep.

Completed Reports

NL1 National Institutes of Health, Consensus Development Program. Assessment methods for decisions about long-term care. (Consensus Development Conference Statement, Oct 19-21, 1987). [Group judgment]

NL2 ______. Differential diagnosis of dementing diseases. (Consensus Development Conference Statement, Jul 6-8, 1987). [Group judgment]

NL3 ______. Magnetic resonance imaging. (Consensus Development Conference Statement, Oct 26-28, 1987). [Group judgment]

NL4 ______. Management of clinically localized prostate cancer. (Consensus Development Conference Statement, Jun 15-17 1987). [Group judgment]

NL5 ______. Newborn screening for sickle cell disease and other hemoglobinopathies. (Consensus Development Conference Statement, Apr 6-8 1987). [Group judgment]

NL6 ______. Diet and exercise in noninsulin-dependent diabetes mellitus. (Consensus Development Conference Statement, Dec 8-10 1986). [Group judgment]

NL7 ______. Impact of routine HTLV-III antibody testing of blood and plasma donors on the health of the public. (Consensus Development Conference Statement, Jul 7-9 1986). [Group judgment]

NL8 ______. Infantile apnea and home monitoring. (Consensus Development Conference Statement, Sep 29-Oct 1 1986). [Group judgment]

NL9 ______. Integrated approach to the management of pain. (Consensus Development Conference Statement, May 19-21 1986). [Group judgment]

NL10 ______. Platelet transfusion therapy. (Consensus Development Conference Statement, Oct 6-8 1986). [Group judgment]

NL11 ______. Prevention of venous thrombosis and pulmonary embolism. (Consensus Development Conference Statement, Mar 24-26 1986). [Group judgment]

NL12 ______. The utility of therapeutic plasmapheresis for neurological disorders. (Consensus Development Conference Statement, Jun 2-4 1986). [Group judgment]

NL13 ______. Adjuvant chemotherapy for breast cancer. (Consensus Development Conference Statement, Sep 9-11 1985). [Group judgment]

NL14 ______. Anesthesia and sedation in the dental office. (Consensus Development Conference Statement, Apr 22-24 1985). [Group judgment]

NL15 ______. Electroconvulsive therapy. (Consensus Development Conference Statement, Jun 10-12 1985). [Group judgment]

NL16 ______. Health implications of obesity. (Consensus Development Conference Statement, Feb 11-13 1985). [Group judgment]

NL17 ______. Travelers' diarrhea. (Consensus Development Conference Statement, Jan 28-30 1985). [Group judgment]

NL18 ______. Analgesic-associated kidney disease. (Consensus Development Conference Statement, Feb 27-29 1984). [Group judgment]

NL19 ______. Diagnostic ultrasound imaging in pregnancy. (Consensus Development Conference Statement, Feb 6-8 1984). [Group judgment]

NL20 ______. Fresh frozen plasma: indications and risks. (Consensus Development Conference Statement, Sep 24-26 1984). [Group judgment]

NL21 ______. Limb-sparing treatment of adult soft-tissue sarcomas and osteosarcomas. (Consensus Development Conference Statement, Dec 3-5 1984). [Group judgment]

NL22 ______. Lowering blood cholesterol to prevent heart disease. (Consensus Development Conference Statement, Dec 10-12 1984). [Group judgment]

NL23 ______. Mood disorders: pharmacologic prevention of recurrences. (Consensus Development Conference Statement, Apr 24-26 1984). [Group judgment]

NL24 ______. Osteoporosis. (Consensus Development Conference Statement, Apr 2-4 1984). [Group judgment]

NL25 ______. Critical care medicine. (Consensus Development Conference Statement, Mar 7-9 1983). [Group judgment]

NL26 ______. Dental sealants in the prevention of tooth decay. (Consensus Development Conference Statement, Dec 5-7 1983). [Group judgment]

NL27 ______. Drugs and insomnia: the use of medications to promote sleep. (Consensus Development Conference Statement, Nov 15-17 1983). [Group judgment]

NL28 ______. Liver transplantation. (Consensus Development Conference Statement, Jun 20-23 1983). [Group judgment]

NL29 ______. Precusors to malignant melanoma. (Consensus Development Conference Statement, Oct 24-26 1983). [Group judgment]

NL30 ______. Treatment of hypertriglyceridemia. (Consensus Development Conference Statement, Sep 27-29 1983). [Group judgment]

NL31 ______. Clinical applications of biomaterials. (Consensus Development Conference Statement, Nov 1-3 1982). [Group judgment]

NL32 ______. Defined diets and childhood hyperactivity. (Consensus Development Conference Statement, Jan 13-15 1982). [Group judgment]

NL33 ______. Total hip joint replacement. (Consensus Development Conference Statement, Mar 1-3 1982). [Group judgment]

NL34 ______. Computed tomographic scanning of the brain. (Consensus Development Conference Statement, Nov 4-6 1981). [Group judgment]

NL35 ______. Diagnosis and treatment of Reye's syndrome. (Consensus Development Conference Statement, Mar 2-4 1981). [Group judgment]

NL36 ______. Adjuvant chemotherapy of breast cancer. (Consensus Development Conference Statement, Jul 14-16 1980). [Group judgment]

NL37 ______. CEA as a cancer marker. (Consensus Development Conference Statement, Sep 29-Oct 1 1980). [Group judgment]

NL38 ______. Cervical cancer screening: the pap smear. (Consensus Development Conference Statement, Jul 23-25 1980). [Group judgment]

NL39 ______. Cesarean childbirth. (Consensus Development Conference Statement, Sep 22-24 1980). [Group judgment]

NL40 ______. Coronary artery bypass surgery: scientific and clinical aspects. (Consensus Development Conference Statement, Dec 3-5 1980). [Group judgment]

NL41 ______. Endoscopy in upper GI bleeding. (Consensus Development Conference Statement, Aug 20-22 1980). [Group judgment]

NL42 ______. Febrile seizures. (Consensus Development Conference Statement, May 19-21 1980). [Group judgment]

NL43 ______. Thrombolytic therapy in thrombosis. (Consensus Development Conference Statement, Apr 10-12 1980). [Group judgment]

NL44 ______. Amantadine: does it have a role in the prevention and treatment of influenza? (Consensus Development Conference Statement, Oct 15-16 1979). [Group judgment]

NL45 ______. Antenatal diagnosis. (Consensus Development Conference Statement, Mar 5-7 1979). [Group judgment]

NL46 ______. Estrogen use and postmenopausal women. (Consensus Development Conference Statement, Sep 13-14 1979). [Group judgment]

NL47 ______. Improving clinical and consumer use of blood pressure measuring devices. (Consensus Development Conference Statement, Apr 26-27 1979). [Group judgment]

NL48 ______. Intraocular lens implantation. (Consensus Development Conference Statement, Sep 10-11 1979). [Group judgment]

NL49 ______. Pain, discomfort, and humanitarian care. (Consensus Development Conference Statement, Feb 16 1979). [Group judgment]

NL50 ______. Removal of third molars. (Consensus Development Conference Statement, Nov 28-30 1979). [Group judgment]

NL51 ______. Steroid receptors in breast cancer. (Consensus Development Conference Statement, Jun 27-29 1979). [Group judgment]

NL52 ______. The treatment of primary breast cancer: management of local disease. (Consensus Development Conference Statement, Jun 5 1979). [Group judgment]

NL53 ______. The use of microprocessor-based "intelligent" machines in patient care. (Consensus Development Conference Statement, Oct 17-19 1979). [Group judgment]

NL54 ______. Transfusion therapy in pregnant sickle cell disease patients. (Consensus Development Conference Statement, Apr 23-24 1979). [Group judgment]

NL55 ______. Availability of insect sting kits to non physicians. (Consensus Development Conference Statement, Sep 14 1978). [Group judgment]

NL56 ______. Dental implants: benefit and risk. (Consensus Development Conference Statement, Jun 13-14 1978). [Group judgment]

NL57 ______. Indications for tonsillectomy and adenoidectomy: phase I. (Consensus Development Conference Statement, Jul 20 1978). [Group judgment]

NL58 ______. Mass screening for colo-rectal cancer. (Consensus Development Conference Statement, June 26-28 1978). [Group judgment]

NL59 ______. Mass screening for lung cancer. (Consensus Development Conference Statement, Sep 18-20 1978). [Group judgment]

NL60 ______. Supportive therapy in burn care. (Consensus Development Conference Statement, Nov 10-11 1978). [Group judgment]

NL61 ______. Surgical treatment of morbid obesity. (Consensus Development Conference Statement, Dec 4-5 1978). [Group judgment]

NL62 ______. Treatable brain diseases in the elderly. (Consensus Development Conference Statement, Jul 10-11 1978). [Group judgment]

NL63 ______. Breast cancer screening. (Consensus Development Conference Statement, Sep 14-16 1977). [Group judgment]

National Library of Medicine

Building 38, Room 2S-18
8600 Rockville Pike
Bethesda, MD 20894
301-496-8834

Contact: Elliot R. Siegel, Ph.D., Special Assistant for Operations Research; or Robert Mehnert, Chief, Office of Public Inquiries and Publications Management 301-496-6308.

Overview: The National Library of Medicine (NLM) was established in 1836 as the Library of the Army Surgeon General's Office. Transferred in 1956 to the National Institutes of Health in the U.S. Public Health Service, the Library today collects materials exhaustively in all major areas of the health sciences. To aid in the dissemination and exchange of information, the Library produces specialized medical bibliographies such as *Index Medicus,* and the computer-based Medical Literature Analysis and Retrieval System (MEDLARS).

One component of the Library, the Lister Hill National Center for Biomedical Communications, conducts and supports research in techniques for recording, storing, retrieving, and communicating health information. Another, the Division of Extramural Programs, supports research on the generation, organization, and utilization of health information. Both are concerned with technology assessment.

Purpose: To evaluate new and existing biomedical information technologies that help disseminate information and facilitate its use by health professionals and others.

Primary intended users: Patients; providers, generally; physicians; acute facility administrators; long-term care facility administrators; other care givers; health product manufacturers; health/medical professional associations; health industry associations; third party payers; government regulators; voluntary associations, organizations; biomedical researchers; reporters, writers, news media; information/computer industry; labs, blood banks; public policy-makers, legislators; policy research organizations.

Technologies: Support system.

Assessments include, but are not limited to, systems for information storage, retrieval, and dissemination; teaching/learning systems; artificial intelligence or expert systems; and the management of health information.

Stage: *New,* emerging, established or widespread practice, obsolete.

Properties: *Effectiveness,* cost, cost-benefit, cost-effectiveness, service requirements, acceptance/adoption level, system impact, economic implications.

Selection process: Assessments may be requested by intramural research and development staff; NLM management; and officials of the National Institutes of Health, the Department of Health and Human Services, and Congress. Selection is influenced by the source of the request, the information needs of the biomedical community, potential impact on the performance of the Library's statutory mission, and availability of funds. Technologies involved in NLM's own internal operations, such as MEDLARS, are evaluated and improved periodically.

Methods: *Epidemiological and other observational methods,* information syntheses, expert opinion, group judgment, cost analyses, bench testing.

Assessments are performed in-house by research and development and operations staff and extramurally through grants. Whenever feasible, evaluations are designed to allow for the participation of those who will be affected by the product or service, including health professionals and researchers. Assessments are generally carried out within a period of 6 to 8 months. Evaluations lasting up to 3 years may be appropriate in certain instances, when the study design incorporates both formative and summative features.

Assessment reports include: Abstract; the assessment's intended audience; the purpose of the assessment; relationship of this assessment to prior or concurrent assessments of the technology or other technologies intended for similar purposes; who sponsored/commissioned/supported the assessment; who conducted the assessment; description of the technology; stage of life-cycle of technology when assessed; properties assessed; procedure used for the assessment; sources of data/information; methods for collecting data/information; methods for analyzing/synthesizing data/information; results; findings or conclusions; limitations of findings; recommendations for practice, future assessments, technology development, research; how much the assessment cost; how the technology works, including theory, principles; development of the technology; procurement/deployment information; where technology is in use.

Dissemination: Printed reports; journal articles; advisories to members/constituents; press conferences/news releases, TV/radio broadcasts, video products; clearinghouses, data/citation bases, on-line services.

Reports are routinely sent to the original requestor. Study reports may be filed with the National Technical Information Service (NTIS), the Educational Resources Information Center (ERIC), and similar document distribution centers. NLM staff report study findings at meetings and in the professional literature, as well.

Budget: $500,000. The approximate cost of an assessment ranges from $25,000 to $125,000, depending on the nature and amount of external support services required. Funding source: 100 percent parent organization.

Use: Evaluation studies have affected NLM's research and development activities as well as its products and services. For instance, 1) a field test and evaluation of the Hepatitis Knowledge Base System resulted in the adoption of computer conferencing technology as an important feature of the NLM information systems; 2) a survey of the users of the Library's Videocassette Loan Program led to an expansion of the program; and 3) a comparative study of the coverage of the medical behavioral services by MEDLARS and other databases resulted in the NLM's reconsidering its indexing and coverage policies.

Colleagues in the information and computer science communities keep abreast of the latest research and development activities at NLM. In addition, the Nation's biomedical library network uses NLM as a leader and role model for technological advancements affecting information transfer.

Research scientists at the OCLC adapted the NLM's methodology and evaluation strategy in the design of an evaluation of alternative searching strategies for online catalogs. For a discussion see: Markey K. The Dewey decimal classification as a library user's tool in an online catalog. In: Flood B, Witiak J, Hogan TH, comps. *Proceedings of the American Society for Information Science 47th annual meeting, 1984.* White Plains, NY: Knowledge Industry Publications, 1984:121-5.

Frequent reference is made in the literature to NLM's development and assessment of the Hepatitis Knowledge Base System and to other assessment activities at the Library.

NLM assessment activities are described in Institute of Medicine, Committee on Evaluating Medical Technologies in Clinical Use. *Assessing medical technologies.* Washington, DC: National Academy Press, 1985.

Completed Reports

NM1 [National Library of Medicine] Health professionals use of MEDLINE. Bethesda, MD: National Library of Medicine, 1987. [Epidemiological and other observational methods]

NM2 La Croix EM. [National Library of Medicine] A comparison of interlibrary loan requests received by the National Library of Medicine: 1959 and 1984. Bull Med Libr Assoc 1987 Jan (in press). [Epidemiological and other observational methods]

NM3 [National Library of Medicine] Medical education in the information age. Proceedings of the Symposium on Medical Informatics. Washington, DC: Association of American Medical Colleges, 1986. [Epidemiological and other observational methods]

NM4 [National Library of Medicine] Evaluation of medical information science in medical education. Adopted by the Executive Council of the Association of American Medical Colleges, Washington, DC, January 23, 1986. J Med Educ 1986;61:487-543. [Epidemiological and other observational methods]

NM5 Griffith BC, White HD, Drott MC, Saye JD. [National Library of Medicine] Tests of methods for evaluating bibliographic databases—an analysis of the National Library of Medicine's handling of literatures in the medical behavioral sciences. J Am Soc Info Sci 1986;37:261-70. [Epidemiological and other observational methods]

NM6 Bratton B, Brooks CM, Holland GJ, Weinholtz D, Jackson J. [National Library of Medicine] Study of the audiovisual selection and acquisition process in health professions education. Ames, IA: Iowa State University, 1985. (NTIS order no. PB86-10813/XAB) [Epidemiological and other observational methods]

NM7 Kopp JJ. [National Library of Medicine] Research and writing in the history of health sciences, 1970-1982: a quantitative analysis of NLM's HISTLINE database. Bull Med Libr Assoc 1985;73:146-152. [Epidemiological and other observational methods]

NM8 Siegel ER, Spann M, Collins KA, Hazard G, Woodsmall RM. [National Library of Medicine] Report on the CHEMLINE evaluation study. Bethesda, MD: National Library of Medicine, 1985. [Epidemiological and other observational methods]

NM9 Woelfel JC, Tesorero J. [National Library of Medicine] An evaluation of CHEMLINE: the results of a survey of users by the National Library of Medicine. Vienna, VA: Market Dynamics, Inc, 1985. [Epidemiological and other observational methods]

NM10 [National Library of Medicine] An analysis of the National Library of Medicine's (NLM) handling of the medical behavioral sciences' (MBS) literatures. Final report. (Five volumes plus executive summary). Bethesda, MD: National Library of Medicine, 1984. [Epidemiological and other observational methods]

NM11 Siegel ER, Kameen K, Sinn SK, Weise FO. [National Library of Medicine] A comparative evaluation of the technical performance and user acceptance of two prototype online catalog systems. Info Technol Libr 1984;3:35-46. [Epidemiological and other observational methods]

NM12 Ullmer E, Kuenz M, Seibert W. [National Library of Medicine] Audiovisual evaluation survey final report. Bethesda, MD: Lister Hill Center, National Library of Medicine, 1983. [Epidemiological and other observational methods]

NM13 Watson L. [National Library of Medicine] NLM videocassette interlibrary loan program report. Bethesda, MD: Audiovisual Resources Section, National Library of Medicine, 1983. [Epidemiological and other observational methods]

NM14 Roderer NK, King DW, McDonald DD, Bush CG. [National Library of Medicine] Evaluation of the Hepatitis Knowledge Base System. Rockville, MD: King Research, Inc., 1981. [Epidemiological and other observational methods]

NM15 [National Library of Medicine] Performance evaluation of a satellite-linked experimental network. IEEE Trans Aerosp Electron Syst 1980;16:771-82. [Epidemiological and other observational methods]

NM16 [National Library of Medicine] Biomedical communications experiments using the communications technology satellite: technical evaluation. Bethesda, MD: Lister Hill Center, National Library of Medicine, 1979. (NTIS order no. PB-80-111-016/GBB). [Epidemiological and other observational methods]

Ongoing Assessments

NM17 [National Library of Medicine] Development of evaluation methodologies to assess NLM's coverage of new biomedical literatures. Bethesda, MD: National Library of Medicine. Ongoing. [Epidemiological and other observational methods]

NM18 [National Library of Medicine] Evaluation of PC-oriented training packages for the NLM chemical and toxicological online files. Bethesda, MD: National Library of Medicine. Ongoing. [Epidemiological and other observational methods]

NM19 [National Library of Medicine] Evaluation of the Technological Innovations in Medical Education (TIME) Project. Bethesda, MD: Lister Hill Center, National Library of Medicine. Ongoing. [Epidemiological and other observational methods]

NM20 [National Library of Medicine] Evaluation of the scope and coverage of NLM's TOXLINE. Bethesda, MD: National Library of Medicine. Ongoing. [Epidemiological and other observational methods]

NM21 [National Library of Medicine] Field test and evaluation of MEDLINE on optical disk. Bethesda, MD: National Library of Medicine. Ongoing. [Epidemiological and other observational methods]

NM22 [National Library of Medicine] Testing of a general methodology for the evaluation of expert systems in medicine. Bethesda, MD: Lister Hill Center, National Library of Medicine. Ongoing. [Epidemiological and other observational methods]

Netherlands Organization for Applied Scientific Research

Medical Technology Unit (TNO)
PO Box 188
2300 AD Leiden
The Netherlands
(31-71) 21-4441

Contact: G.J. van Keulen.

Overview: The Netherlands Organization for Applied Scientific Research is an independent, not-for-profit organization created by law. It conducts research in the health, nutrition, industrial, and defense areas. The Medical Technology Unit (TNO) is a medical technology assessment program that evaluates medical devices.

Purpose: To establish the safety, efficiency, and effectiveness of medical devices; to examine the technical and ergonomic properties of medical devices; and to give information and advice to health care institutions.

Primary intended users: Acute facility administrators; long-term care facility administrators; health product manufacturers; government regulators; liability, malpractice insurers; clinical engineers.

Technologies: *Device.*

Intervention: *Diagnosis, treatment.*

Stage: *New, established or widespread practice.*

Properties: *Safety, efficacy, effectiveness.*

Selection process: There are no strict procedures established for requesting an assessment. Any party who can pay for an assessment can request that one be conducted. The Medical Technology Unit (TNO) sets assessment topic priorities in consultation with the National Hospital Institute or the party funding the assessment.

Methods: *Expert opinion, group judgement, bench testing.*

The approximate turnaround time from selection of assessment topic to reporting of findings is 1 year.

Assessment reports include: The purpose of the assessment; relationship of this assessment to prior or concurrent assessments of the technology or other technologies intended for similar purposes; who sponsored/commissioned/supported the assessment; who conducted the assessment; description of the technology; properties assessed; procedure used for the assessment; sources of data/information; methods for collecting data/information; methods for analyzing/synthesizing data/information; results; findings or conclusions; how the technology works, including theory, principles; procurement/deployment information; regulatory agency approval status; product recall history, liability actions.

Dissemination: *Printed reports.*

An online network to Dutch hospitals is planned. Copies of assessment reports may be ordered from the Advisory Center of the Medical Technology Unit (TNO).

Budget: $1.5 million. The approximate cost per assessment varies between $50,000 to $100,000. The cost depends on the complexity of the device and the number of different types of devices to be evaluated. Funding sources: 70 percent parent organization; 30 percent sales of assessments, consultant services.

The annual budget amount includes the following activities: evaluating a single device for the manufacturer; testing devices for manufacturers to prove compliance with regulations; developing functional specifications for devices with respect to safety, efficacy, and effectiveness; advising hospital technicians and administrators in the safe and effective use of devices; and offering courses for hospital technicians in quality control.

Completed Reports

NS1 Netherlands Organization for Applied Scientific Research, Medical Technology Unit (TNO). Syringe pumps for non-ambulatory use. 1986.

NS2 ———. Drip-rate controlled and volumetric infusion pumps. 1984.

NS3 ———. Defibrillators. 1983.

NS4 ———. Portable defibrillators. 1983.

NS5 ———. Bloodwarmers for use during transfusion. 1981.

NS6 ———. Electro-encephalographs. 1981.

NS7 ———. Heart monitors. 1981.

NS8 ———. Intensive care convection incubators. 1981.

NS9 ———. External pacemakers. 1978.

NS10 ———. Sphygmomanometers. 1978.

NS11 ———. Three channel (phono) electrocardiographs. 1977.

NS12 ———. One channel electrocardiographs. 1975.

Ongoing Assessments

NS13 ______. Ambulatory insulin pumps. Ongoing. [Expert opinion, Group judgment, Bench testing]

NS14 ______. Ultra-sound physiotherapy equipment. Ongoing. [Expert opinion, Group judgment, Bench testing]

Policy Analysis, Inc.

Medical Technology Cost-Effectiveness Program
1577 Beacon Street
Brookline, MA 02146
617-232-4400

Contact: Gerry Oster, Vice President.

Overview: Policy Analysis, Inc. is a business, founded in 1973, that conducts cost-benefit and cost-effectiveness analyses for organizations in both the public and private sectors. Its Medical Technology Cost-Effectiveness Program was started in 1982.

Purpose: To provide state-of-the-art analyses of the cost-effectiveness of new and existing medical technologies, including drugs, devices, and diagnostic products.

Primary intended users: Patients; providers, generally; physicians; acute facility administrators; health product manufacturers; health/medical professional associations; health industry associations; third party payers; government regulators; reporters, writers, news media; public policy-makers, legislators; policy research organizations.

Technologies: *Drug,* device, medical or surgical procedure, organizational or administrative system.

Intervention: Prevention, diagnosis, treatment.

Stage: New, established or widespread practice.

Properties: *Cost-effectiveness,* safety, efficacy, effectiveness, cost, cost-benefit, economic implications.

Selection process: Any funding organization, private or public, may request an evaluation, beginning usually with informal discussions that lead to a formal written request. Assessment topic priorities are generally set by the funding organization.

Methods: Information syntheses, modeling, cost analyses, epidemiological and other observational methods, clinical trials.

The approximate turnaround time from selection of assessment topic to reporting of findings is 6 months to 2 years.

Assessors: Assessors typically are experts in medicine, economics, and epidemiology.

Assessment reports include: Abstract; the purpose of the assessment; relationship of this assessment to prior or concurrent assessments of the technology or other technologies intended for similar purposes; who sponsored/commissioned/supported the assessment; who conducted the assessment; description of the technology; properties assessed; procedure used for the assessment; sources of data/information; methods for collecting data/information; methods for analyzing/synthesizing data/information; results; findings or conclusions; limitations of findings; implications of findings for practice; recommendations for practice, future assessments, technology development, research; coverage/reimbursement status of the technology.

Dissemination: Journal articles.

Reprints are available upon request.

Budget: $750,000. Costs of assessments start at $50,000. Funding sources: 10 percent government grants/contracts; 90 percent sales of assessments, consultant services.

Use: Funding organizations use the reports to address issues of concern regarding the cost-effectiveness of particular drugs, devices, or diagnostic products among patients, providers, and third-party payers.

Completed Reports

PA1 Oster G, Epstein AM. [Policy Analysis, Inc.] The cost-effectiveness of cholestyramine in the prevention of coronary heart disease: whom should we treat? JAMA, submitted for publication.

PA2 Oster G, Huse DM, Delea TE, Savage DD, Colditz GA. [Policy Analysis, Inc.] Cost effectiveness of labetalol and propranolol in the treatment of hypertension among blacks. 1987 Mar.

PA3 Oster G, Tuden RL, Colditz GA. [Policy Analysis, Inc.] A cost-effectiveness analysis of prophylaxis against deep-vein thrombosis in major or orthopedic surgery. JAMA 1987;257:203-208.

PA4 Oster G, Tuden RL, Colditz GA. [Policy Analysis, Inc.] Prevention of venous thromboembolism after general surgery: a cost effectiveness analysis of alternative approaches to prophylaxis. Am J Med 1987 (in press)

PA5 Oster G, Epstein AM. [Policy Analysis, Inc.] Primary prevention and coronary heart disease: the economic benefits of lowering serum cholesterol. Am J Public Health 1986;76:647-656.

PA6 Oster G, Huse DM, Delea TE, Colditz GA. [Policy Analysis, Inc.] Cost-effectiveness of nicotine gum as an adjunct to physician's advice against cigarette smoking. JAMA 1986;256:1315-1318.

Project HOPE

Center for Health Affairs
2 Wisconsin Circle, Suite 500
Chevy Chase, MD 20815
301-656-7401

Contact: Gail Wilensky, Ph.D., Vice President; or Louis P. Garrison, Jr., Ph.D., Deputy Director.

Overview: Project HOPE (Health Opportunity for People Everywhere) is the principal activity of the People-to-People Health Foundation, Inc., an independent, nonprofit corporation headquartered in Millwood, Virginia. Founded in 1958, Project HOPE is currently conducting health sciences education and training programs in 18 countries.

This profile addresses a division of Project HOPE, the Center for Health Affairs (CHA), which conducts research and policy analysis primarily related to issues of the U.S. health care system, as well as those of other countries.

Purpose: To conduct health policy research and analysis for private and public sector needs. With regard to assessment, CHA examines the interaction of technologies and their financing, and presents options regarding technologies to policy makers. In particular, CHA provides technical assistance to the Prospective Payment Assessment Commission (ProPAC) for updating and improving the Medicare Prospective Payment System (PPS), such as modifying diagnosis-related groups (DRGs) and studying the impact of the PPS on utilization of technologies.

Primary intended users: Providers, generally; physicians; acute facility administrators; long-term care facility administrators; third party payers; government regulators; public policy-makers, legislators; policy research organizations.

Technologies: *Organizational or administrative system,* medical or surgical procedure, device.

Intervention: *Treatment,* prevention, diagnosis.

Stage: *New,* established, widespread.

Properties: *Cost, cost-effectiveness,* service requirements, system impact, economic implications.

Selection process: Under its task order agreement with ProPAC, CHA responds to assessment requests that originate with ProPAC commissioners or staff.

Methods: *Cost analyses,* information syntheses, expert opinion, group judgment, modeling.

CHA reports are written primarily by staff members who draw upon a variety of experts and information sources in industry and the medical community. In addition, CHA is studying the use of physician panels, in face-to-face settings and using Delphi-style mail surveys, as a means for making adjustments in the PPS. These panels have been used in such exercises as developing lists of complications and comorbidities for DRGs in order to improve the ability of the system to capture variations in cost among patients, modifying surgical classes and hierarchies in selected diagnostic categories, and determining the scientific and technological component of the discretionary adjustment factor used in the PPS to account for changes in the cost of hospital services. Turnaround time for assessments ranges from 2 to 8 months, averaging about 6 months.

Assessors: CHA staff members have backgrounds in such fields as economics, health policy administration and management, political science, public policy, sociology, and computer science. Physicians and other experts are used for panels and as consultants as needed.

Assessment reports include: Abstract; assessment's intended audience; purpose of the assessment; who sponsored/commissioned/supported the assessment; who conducted the assessment; description of the technology; stage of life-cycle of technology when assessed; properties assessed; procedure used for the assessment; sources of data/information; methods for collecting data/information; methods for analyzing/synthesizing data/information; results; findings or conclusions; limitations of findings; implications of findings for practice; recommendations for practice, future assessments, technology development, research; how the technology works, including theory, principles; regulatory agency approval status; coverage/reimbursement status of the technology.

Dissemination: Reports are presented in monographs to ProPAC and other organizations, in journal articles, and in oral presentations. Reports are available from CHA.

Budget: The CHA budget is approximately $1.5 million, about one-third of which is devoted to assessment activities described here. Funding sources: 67 percent government grants/contracts; 33 percent foundations, other private grants.

Use: A number of CHA report recommendations have been adopted by ProPAC and used by the Department of Health and Human Services (DHHS) in making adjustments in the PPS. For example, as a result of the CHA analysis of PPS payments for expensive prosthetic and implantable devices, ProPAC recommended to DHHS that adjustments be made to the labor portion of the standardized amount for some DRGs involving these devices. The CHA analysis of heterogeneity of DRGs involving lymphomas and leukemias prompted ProPAC to recommend to DHHS that a separate DRG be created for acute leukemia patients and that other modifications to the assignment of the remaining patients be made. DHHS adopted one part of the recommendation that acute leukemias be assigned to a newly created DRG. Based on CHA recommendations regarding cardiac pacemakers, ProPAC recommended reclassification of cases based on pacemaker type and reassignment of some cases involving pacemaker replacement.

Related activities: Among its related activities, CHA is evaluating the impact of worksite health promotion programs at several major corporations. CHA is also studying the impact of corporate intervention in health benefits redesign and utilization review on the use of health services by employees. CHA has assisted DHHS in outlining recommendations for coverage of catastrophic illness. Staff members are examining the potential impact of HMOs and other competitive medical plans on quality of care and access to technology.

Completed Reports

PH1 Project HOPE, Center for Health Affairs. A pilot study in the use of physican panels to develop-specific lists of complications and comorbidities for Medicare diagnosis-related groups (for Prospective Payment Assessment Commission). 1987 Jan. [Group judgment]

PH2 ______. A technology-specific approach to estimating the scientific and technological component of the discretionary adjustment factor for excluded hospitals: options and issues. (for Prospective Payment Assessment Commission). 1987 Feb. [Cost analyses]

PH3 ______. A technology-specific approach to estimating the scientific and technological component of the discretionary adjustment factor: options and issues. (for the Prospective Payment Assessment Commission). 1987 Feb. [Cost analyses]

PH4 Garrison LP, Wilensky GR. [Project Hope Center for Health Affairs] Cost containment and technology. Health Affairs 1986;Summer:46-58. [Information syntheses]

PH5 Project Hope, Center for Health Affairs. A pilot study in the use of physician panels; to modify surgical classes and hierarchies in selected major diagnostic categories. (for Prospective Payment Assessment Commission). 1986 Dec. [Group judgment]

PH6 ______. Developing alternative DRG classifications for Medicare cases involving cardiac pacemakers. (for Prospective Payment Assessment Commission). 1986 Aug. [Information syntheses, Cost analyses]

PH7 ______. Evaluating the heterogeneity of DRGs involving lymphomas, leukemias, and chemotherapy and developing alternative classifications of discharges. (for Prospective Payment Assessment Commission). 1986 Aug. [Information syntheses, Cost analyses]

PH8 ______. PPS payments for expensive devices: issues and evidence. (for Prospective Payment Assessment Commission). 1986 Aug. [Cost analyses]

PH9 ______. Paying for heart transplantation under Medicare. (for Prospective Payment Assessment Commission). 1986 Feb. [Information syntheses, Cost analyses]

PH10 ______. Review of evidence in literature relevant to the measurement of hospital case mix index. (for Prospective Payment Assessment Commission). 1986 Jul. [Information syntheses]

PH11 ______. Background paper on cataract surgery and physician payment under the Medicare program. (for U.S. Congress, Office of Technology Assessment). 1985 Oct. [Information syntheses, Cost analyses]

Ongoing Assessments

PH12 ______. A review of the cost-effectiveness of home health care services. Ongoing, expected 1987. [Information syntheses, Cost analyses]

PH13 ______. Access to technology and quality of care in capitated plans. Ongoing. expected completion 1987. [Information syntheses]

PH14 ______. Evaluating the clinical and resource heterogeneity in DRG 468. (for Prospective Payment Assessment Commission). Ongoing; expected 1987. [Information syntheses]

PH15 ______. The effect of PPS on the diffusion and use of medical technologies. (for Prospective Payment Assessment Commission). Ongoing, expected 1987. [Information syntheses]

PH16 ______. Work site health promotion program evaluation. Ongoing, expected 1987. [Information syntheses]

Prospective Payment Assessment Commission

300 Seventh Street SW, Suite 301B
Washington, DC 20024
202-453-3986

Contact: Donald A. Young, Executive Director; or Judith D. Moore 202-453-3871.

Overview: The Prospective Payment Assessment Commission (ProPAC) is an independent agency that was established by Congress under the Social Security Act Amendments of 1983 (PL 98-21). The Commission is an advisory body and does not exercise regulatory or appeals functions.

Purpose: To recommend to the Congress and the Secretary of Health and Human Services (HHS) an appropriate percentage change in the payments made under the Medicare prospective payment system (PPS) for in-patient hospital services, and to recommend adjustments to the diagnosis-related groups (DRG) classification and weighting factors. These recommendations may concern specific technologies or practice patterns.

Primary intended users: Third party payers; public policy-makers, legislators.

Technologies: *Organizational or administrative system,* drug, device, medical or surgical procedure, support system.

ProPAC is primarily interested in those technologies having the greatest impact on the Medicare population.

Intervention: *Treatment,* diagnosis, rehabilitation.

Stage: *New,* emerging, established or widespread, obsolete.

The Commission withholds making recommendations until the technology is FDA-approved and is covered or about to be covered by Medicare.

Properties: *System impact;* safety; efficacy; effectiveness; cost; cost-benefit; cost-effectiveness; service requirements; acceptance/adoption level; economic implications; ethical, legal, social implications.

Other attributes that are assessed include number and distribution of Medicare patients affected, number and distribution of hospitals affected; financial impact on hospitals; financial impact on Medicare beneficiaries; estimate of impact on quality of care, access to care, or innovation and technology changes; complexity of the analysis that would be required; availability of data; and the likelihood improvements could be made in DRG classification and weights.

Selection process: Requests for assessments are made through telephone contact, correspondence, meetings, and public comment at Commission meetings. Commissioners on the Diagnostic and Therapeutic Practices Subcommittee prioritize topics brought to their attention by ProPAC staff and then send them to the full Commission for final approval. ProPAC monitors ongoing activities and performs reassessments as necessary. Permanent DRG assignment should be reconsidered within a period not to exceed 3 years.

Methods: *Cost analyses,* information syntheses, expert opinion, group judgment, modeling.

The assessment process consists of 3 stages: 1) identification of topics for consideration, 2) initial staff review, and 3) indepth analysis. There are two types of indepth analyses: 1) a comprehensive analysis of a specific technology or a practice pattern, and 2) a comprehensive analysis of generic issues related to case-mix measurement or payment. The approximate turnaround time from selection of assessment topic to reporting of findings varies from a few weeks to over a year.

Assessors: The assessors have expertise in medical/clinical specialties, economics, computer programming, medical record coding, and statistics.

Assessment reports include: The purpose of the assessment; relationship of this assessment to prior or concurrent assessments of the technology or other technologies intended for similar purposes; who sponsored/commissioned/supported the assessment; who conducted the assessment; description of the technology; stage of life-cycle of technology when assessed; properties assessed; procedure used for the assessment; sources of data/information; methods for collecting data/information; methods for analyzing/synthesizing data/information; results; findings or conclusions; limitations of findings; implications of findings for practice; recommendations for practice, future assessments, technology development, research; how the technology works, including theory, principles; development of the technology; where technology is in use; regulatory agency approval status; coverage/reimbursement status of the technology; technology's impact on the Medicare population.

Dissemination: *Printed reports;* advisories to members/constituents; press conferences/ news releases; open public meetings.

ProPAC accepts telephone and written requests for copies of assessment reports. A mailing list is maintained for those interested in receiving meeting announcements, agendas, and reports.

Budget: $1.5 million. The approximate cost per assessment is $50,000 to $100,000. Funding source: 100 percent Congressional appropriations.

Use: ProPAC is mandated to report annually to the Congress and the Secretary of HHS its recommendations on the prospective payment system. The technology assessments are incorporated into the recommendations. The recommendations made in ProPAC's annual reports are reviewed by the Secretary of HHS as potential areas for PPS modification. These modifications, based upon selected ProPAC recommendations, can be found in the final Medicare PPS regulations for fiscal year 1986 and fiscal year 1987 published in the September 3, 1985 and September 3, 1986 *Federal Register,* respectively. Congressional committees also use ProPAC's assessments.

ProPAC is described in Institute of Medicine, Committee on Evaluating Medical Technologies in Clinical Use. *Assessing medical technologies.* Washington, DC: National Academy Press, 1985.

Program evaluation: The U.S. Congress Office of Technology Assessment (OTA) is required to report annually on all phases of ProPAC's operations, including technology assessment. The first OTA report covered ProPAC's first year in operation and was issued in March 1985. The second OTA report was issued in March 1986. The OTA Health Program Advisory Committee provided advice and comment to the OTA on its oversight activities related to ProPAC; however, the content is the responsibility of the OTA and does not constitute consensus or endorsement by the advisors. General conclusions from both the first and second OTA reports find ProPAC's overall performance to be exceptionally high. OTA concluded that "the process by which ProPAC conducts its analyses and delivers them to the Congress is an effective one." ProPAC has continued its assessment program without major modifications. The following documents present OTA's findings: Office of Technology Assessment, *First report on the Prospective Payment Assessment Commission (ProPAC).* Washington, DC: Office of Technology Assessment, 1985. Office of Technology Assessment. *Second report on the Prospective Payment Assessment Commission (ProPAC).* Washington, DC: Office of Technology Assessment, 1986.

Related Activities: The Commission is required to collect and assess information on regional variations in medical practice; the length of hospitalization; and the safety, efficacy, and cost-effectiveness of new and existing medical and surgical procedures, practices, services, and technologies. In meeting this requirement, ProPAC has, among other things, convened panels of experts and organized conferences.

Completed Reports

PP1 Burn DRGs. In: Prospective Payment Assessment Commission. Technical appendixes to the report and recommendations to the Secretary, U.S. Department of Health and Human Services, April 1, 1986. Washington, DC: Government Printing Office, 1986:124-126. [Information syntheses, Cost analyses]

PP2 Cardiac pacemakers. In: Prospective Payment Assessment Commission. Technical appendixes to the report and recommendations to the Secretary, U.S. Department of Health and Human Services, April 1, 1986. Washington, DC: Government Printing Office, 1986:99-101. [Information syntheses, Cost analyses]

PP3 Extracorporeal shockwave lithotripsy. In: Prospective Payment Assessment Commission. Technical appendixes to the report and recommendations to the Secretary, U.S. Department of Health and Human Services, April 1, 1986 Washington, DC: Government Printing Office, 1986:112-114. [Information syntheses, Cost analyses]

PP4 Implantable defibrillator. In: Prospective Payment Assessment Commission. Technical appendixes to the report and recommendations to the Secretary, U.S. Department of Health and Human Services, April 1, 1986. Washington, DC: Government Printing Office, 1986:103. [Information syntheses, Cost analyses]

PP5 Lymphomas, leukemia, and chemotherapy. In: Prospective Payment Assessment Commission. Technical appendixes to the report and recommendations to the Secretary, U.S. Department of Health and Human Services, April 1, 1986. Washington, DC: Government Printing Office, 1986:121-123. [Information syntheses, Cost analyses]

PP6 Magnetic resonance imaging. In: Prospective Payment Assessment Commission. Technical appendixes to the report and recommendations to the Secretary, U.S. Department of Health and Human Services, April 1, 1986. Washington, DC: Government Printing Office, 1986:107-111.

PP7 PPS payments for expensive prosthetic and implantable devices and other medical supplies. In: Prospective Payment Assessment Commission. Technical appendixes to the report and recommendations to the Secretary, U.S. Department of Health and Human Services, April 1, 1986. Washington, DC: Government Printing Office, 1986:87-96 [Information syntheses, Cost analyses]

PP8 Penile prostheses. In: Prospective Payment Assessment Commission. Technical appendixes to the report and recommendations to the Secretary, U.S. Department of Health and Human Services, April 1, 1986. Washington, DC: Government Printing Office, 1986:104-106. [Information syntheses, Cost analyses]

PP9 Upper extremity procedures. In: Prospective Payment Assessment Commission. Technical appendixes to the report and recommendations to the Secretary, U.S. Department of Health and Human Services, April 1, 1986. Washington, DC: Government Printing Office, 1986:115-117. [Information syntheses, Cost analyses]

PP10 Prospective Payment Assessment Commission. Medicare prospective payment and the American health care system: report to the Congress, February 1986. Washington, DC: Government Printing Office, 1986. [Information systheses, Cost analyses]

PP11 ______. Report and recommendataions to the Secretary, U.S. Department of Health and Human Services, April 1, 1986. Washington, DC: Government Printing Office, 1986. [Information syntheses, Cost analyses]

PP12 ______. Technical appendixes to the report and recommendations to the Secretary, U.S. Department of Health and Human Services, April 1, 1986. Washington, DC: Government Printing Office, 1986. [Information syntheses, Cost analyses]

PP13 Intraocular lens implants. In: Prospective Payment Assessment Commission. Technical appendixes to the report and recommendations to the Secretary, U.S. Department of Health and Human Services, April 1, 1985. Washington, DC: Government Printing Office, 1985:101-105. [Information syntheses, Cost analyses]

PP14 Percutaneous transluminal coronary angioplasty. In: Prospective Payment Assessment Commission. Technical appendixes to the report and recommendations to the Secretary, U.S. Department of Health and Human Services, April 1, 1985. Washington, DC: Government Printing Office, 1985:105-111. [Information syntheses, Cost analyses]

PP15 Prospective Payment Assessment Commission. Report and recommendations to the Secretary, U.S. Department of Health and Human Services, April 1, 1985. Washington, DC: Government Printing Office, 1985. [Information syntheses, Cost analyses]

PP16 ______. Technical appendixes to the report and recommendations to the Secretary, U.S. Department of Health and Human Services, April 1, 1985. Washington, DC: Government Printing Office, 1985. [Information syntheses, Cost analyses]

Steering Committee on Future Health Scenarios

Commission on Future Health Care Technology
Room BCB 203
PO Box 5406
2280 HK Rijwijk
The Netherlands
(31-70) 40-72-05

Contact: R.F. Schreuder, LL.M, Secretary Ministry of Welfare, Health and Cultural Affairs; or David Banta, (31-70) 47-14-41.

Overview: The Steering Committee on Future Health Scenarios (STG) was set up in 1983 by the State Secretary of Welfare, Health and Cultural Affairs. The Committee's chief task is to create "scenarios" of possible and desirable futures in the field of public health and health care. A scenario may be defined as a description of the current situation in a society (or part of it), or potential and desirable future situations and a description of a series of events which could lead from the former to the latter. The health scenarios are used to increase the anticipatory and priority-setting ability of policy-making in the field of health and health care. The findings are incorporated in strategic policy documents and also serve as a basis for future planning.

The Steering Committee decides on topics to be studied, setting priorities on the basis of social relevance and the opportunities for research into future developments. For each topic an independent scenario committee is established; the STG appoints the chairman and its members. Attached to each committee is a research team comprised of experts in the relevant field as well as experts in scenario research.

The activities of each scenario committee are divided into five stages: preliminary research, formulation of draft report, organization of symposia to discuss results, draft of final report, and the development of a monitoring system to update the information collected.

The STG has established scenario committees on the following topics: aging (1983), cardiovascular diseases (1983), life styles (1983), oncology (1983), accidents and traumas (1985), care of the elderly, and Amsterdam in the year 2010 (1985). Currently, the STG is considering the feasibility of scenario committees on the following topics: health and environment, health and labor, mental health, chronic diseases, primary health care, and dental care.

The scenario project on medical technology is known as the Commission on Future Health Care Technology and was established in 1983. Renewal of Commission activities following the end of the scenario project in September 1987 is under consideration. This profile describes the Commissions's activities.

Purpose: To identify future health care technologies and to conduct prospective assessments of health care technologies of the future.

Primary intended users: General public; providers, generally; consumer associations; third party payers; government regulators; reporters, writers, news media; public policy-makers, legislators; policy research organizations.

Technologies: Drug, device, medical or surgical procedure.

Intervention: Prevention, diagnosis, treatment.

Stage: Emerging, future.

Properties: Cost; service requirements; system impact; economic implications; ethical, legal, social implications.

Methods: Information syntheses, expert opinion, group judgment, modeling, cost analyses.

The staff prepare a draft paper on the assessment topic using the scientific literature, consultation with experts, and modeling, if appropriate. Outside reviewers discuss the paper and it is revised as necessary. The revised paper undergoes a second external review by a broad-based group of experts. Any revisions are incorporated and the final paper is then submitted to the Commission for approval.

The approximate turnaround time from selection of assessment topic to reporting of findings is 1 year.

Assessors: The assessors' areas of expertise include technology assessment, medicine, law, and pharmacology.

Assessment reports include: The purpose of the assessment; who sponsored/commissioned/supported the assessment; who conducted the assessment; description of the technology; stage of life-cycle of technology when assessed; properties assessed; procedure used for the assessment; sources of data/information; methods for collecting data/information; methods for analyzing/synthesizing data/information; results; findings or conclusions; limitations of findings; implications of findings for practice; how the technology works, including theory, principles; where technology is in use; regulatory agency approval status; coverage/reimbursement status of the technology.

Dissemination: *Printed reports;* journal articles; advisories to members/constituents; press conferences/news releases, TV/radio broadcasts, video products.

Copies of assessment reports are available, on request, from the Steering Committee on Future Health Scenarios. Copies may also be purchased directly from the publisher: Kluwers Publishers, Bohn Scheltema, PO Box 13079, 3507 LB Utrecht, The Netherlands.

Budget: $300,000. The approximate cost per assessment is $25,000. Funding source: 90 percent parent organization, 10 percent World Health Organization.

Use: The Steering Committee relies on the assessment reports when formulating policy recommendations. The World Health Organization, the Health Council of the Netherlands, students, and faculty have also used the reports.

Completed Reports

SC1 Steering Committee on Future Health Scenarios, Commission on Future Health Care Technology (Netherlands). Prospective assessment of future health care technology: applications of the neurosciences. 1987.

SC2 ______. Prospective assessment of future health care technology: biotechnology and new vaccines. 1987.

SC3 ______. Prospective assessment of future health care technology: digital imagery. 1987.

SC4 ______. Prospective assessment of future health care technology: genetic screening. 1987.

SC5 ______. Prospective assessment of future health care technology: home care technology. 1987.

SC6 ______. Prospective assessment of future health care technology: lasers in cardiovascular surgery. 1987.

SC7 ______. Prospective assessment of future health care technology: monoclonal antibodies and diagnostic kits. 1987.

Swedish Planning and Rationalization Institute of the Health Services

Technology Assessment and Health Economics
Box 27310
102 54 Stockholm, Sweden
(46-8) 663-05-60

Contact: Stefan Hakansson Ph.D. Director; Pia Maria Jonsson, M.D.; or Eric Paulson, M.D. Telfax 46-8-60 35 10.

Overview: The Technology Assessment and Health Economics program is sponsored by the Swedish Planning and Rationalization Institute of the Health Services (SPRI). SPRI is a government agency that provides health authorities in the Swedish county councils with recommendations for health care.

Purpose: To provide the county councils with recommendations on new and established medical technologies.

Primary intended users: General public, physicians, acute facility administrators, health product manufacturers, health/medical professional associations, government regulators, public policy-makers, legislators.

Technologies: *Medical or surgical procedure.*

Preventive, diagnostic, and therapeutic technologies are assessed.

Intervention: *Diagnosis.*

Stage: *New.*

Properties: *Cost-effectiveness.*

Selection process: Program staff, board members, and clinicians can request that an assessment be conducted. The requests are usually generated by the staff. In collaboration with clinicians, the staff set the assessment topic priorities. This process is based on actual or perceived problems in the health services.

Methods: *Cost analyses;* surveys; interviews, before and after investigations; randomized controlled trials.

Working with clinicians, program staff conduct assessments. There is a 2-year turnaround time from selection of assessment topic to reporting of findings.

Assessors: The assessors have expertise in economics, medicine, and statistics.

Assessment reports include: Abstract; the assessment's intended audience; the purpose of the assessment; relationship of this assessment to prior or concurrent assessments of the technology or other technologies intended for similar purposes; who sponsored/supported the assessment; who conducted the assessment; description of the technology; properties assessed; procedure used for the assessment; sources of data/information; methods for collecting data/information; methods for analyzing/synthesizing data/information; results; findings or conclusions; implications of findings for practice; recommendations for practice, future assessments, technology development, research; how technology works, including theory principles; development of the technology; where technology is in use; coverage/reimbursement status of the technology.

Dissemination: *Printed reports.*

Using internal files reports are mailed to predetermined target groups in the health services. Copies of assessment reports may be obtained by writing to SPRI.

Budget: $500,000. The approximate cost per assessment is $100,000. Funding source: 100 percent parent organization.

Use: The assessment reports are frequently used in health planning within Sweden. For an example see: Lindgren E, Jonsson E, Neuhauser D. Controlling medical technology in Sweden. In: *Implications of cost-effectiveness analysis of medical technology.* Washington DC: Office of Technology Assessment, U.S. Congress, 1980.

Related activities: SPRI and its equivalent institutes in other Scandinavian countries, i.e. Finish Hospital League, Norwegian Institute of Hospital Research, and the Danish Hospital Institute, have jointly set up a body for collaboration on technology assessment activities. This body is called NEMT: Nordic Evaluation of Medical Technology. NEMT is presently finishing a study on nuclear magnetic resonance in the Nordic countries. SPRI, in collaboration with the Swedish Medical Research Council, is also responsible for the Consensus Development Conferences Program in Sweden. Conference topics have included: the artificial hip, treatment of myocardial infarction, treatment of depressive disorders, sight improving surgery, diagnostic imaging of liver cancer, diagnosis and treatment of stroke, and urinary incontinence among adults.

The technology assessment program at SPRI is related to a small program of technology assessment at the Karolinska Institute (The Stockholm School of Medicine). The Karolinska Institute program includes one ongoing project on treatment methods for obesity—costs, risks, and benefits. A randomized controlled trial for the treatment of leukemia is also planned. This project will examine bone marrow transplantation versus chemotherapy.

Completed Reports

SP1 Swedish Planning and Rationalization Institute of the Health Services. Spri technology report 8: treatment with insulin infusion pump: cost and effects. 1987. [Cost analyses, Epidemiological and other observational methods]

SP2 Swedish Planning and Rationalization Institute of the Health Services and the Swedish Medical Research Council. Diagnosing and treatment of stroke. 1986. [Cost analyses, Epidemiological and other observational methods]

SP3 ______. Urinary incontinence in adults. 1986. [Cost analyses, Epidemiological and other observational methods]

SP4 Swedish Planning and Rationalization Institute of the Health Services. Spri technology report 7: MRT—magnetic resonance tomography: experience in Sweden. 1986. [Cost analyses, Epidemiological and other observational methods]

SP5 Swedish Planning and Rationalization Institute of the Health Services and the Swedish Medical Research Council. Diagnostic imaging of liver cancer. 1985. [Cost analyses, Epidemiological and other observational methods]

SP6 Swedish Planning and Rationalization Institute of the Health Services. Spri technology report 6: digital subtraction angiography—economical, medical, technical and planning aspects. 1985. [Swedish language only] [Cost analyses, Epidemiological and other observational methods]

SP7 ______. Spri technology report 5: how can we assess medical technology? 1984. [Cost analyses, Epidemiological and other observational methods]

SP8 Swedish Planning and Rationalization Institute of the Health Services and the Swedish Medical Research Council. Sight improving surgery. 1984. [Cost analyses, Epidemiological and other observational methods]

SP9 ______. Treatment of depressive diseases. 1984. [Cost analyses, Epidemiological and other observational methods]

SP10 ______. Treatment of myocardial infarction. 1983. [Cost analyses, Epidemiological and other observational methods]

SP11 ______. The artificial hip. 1982. [Cost analyses, Epidemiological and other observational methods]

SP12 Swedish Planning and Rationalization Institute of the Health Services. Spri technology report 4: must we assess medical technology? 1982. [Cost analyses, Epidemiological and other observational methods]

SP13 ______. Spri technology report 2: CT scanning in Sweden—costs and effectiveness. 1981. (Spri report 73) [Cost analyses, Epidemiological and other observational methods]

SP14 ______. Spri technology report 3: cost effectiveness analysis in health care. 1981. [Cost analyses, Epidemiological and other observational methods]

Ongoing Assessments

SP15 ______. Artificial lens implantation: a cost-effectiveness analysis. Ongoing. [Cost analyses, Epidemiological and other observational methods]

SP16 ______. Mammography screening for breast cancer: a randomized controlled cost-effectiveness analysis. Ongoing. [Cost analyses, Epidemiological and other observational methods]

United Kingdom Department of Health and Social Security

Supplies Technology Division
Medical Devices Evaluation Programme
14 Russell Square
London WC1B SEP
England
(44-1) 636-6811, Ext. 3248

Contact: Derek E. Weston. Telex 88 3669. Telefax 01 637 8990.

Overview: The United Kingdom Department of Health and Social Security (DHSS) operates the Medical Services Evaluation Programme. The DHSS started the evaluation

Programme in the 1960s to satisfy the growing need within the National Health Service (NHS) for guidance in selecting suitable medical devices. The DHHS promotes the production and supply of safe and effective medical equipment; supports the research, development, and evaluation of equipment; and provides technical advice to equipment suppliers and users in the NHS.

Purpose: To assist prospective purchasers of medical devices in making an informed choice from the products available.

Primary intended users: Providers, generally; physicians; acute facility administrators; long-term care facility administrators; other care givers; health product manufacturers; health/medical professional associations; health industry associations; labs, blood banks.

Technologies: *Device.*

Devices related to a wide range of technologies are assessed. They are frequently, although not exclusively, electrically powered.

Intervention: *Treatment,* diagnosis, rehabilitation.

Stage: *New,* emerging, established or widespread practice.

Devices are usually evaluated when they become established in the marketplace, but sometimes when a production model is first available.

Properties: *Safety,* efficacy, effectiveness, costs.

The following attributes of a device are assessed: safety in use for both operators and patients, performance (against specifications), standard of construction, ease of repair, availability and cost of spare parts, standard of user information, and user reactions.

Selection process: The DHSS accepts written and verbal requests for assessments from all segments of the National Health Service. The Supplies Technology Division, DHSS in consultation with the NHS set assessment topic priorities using the following criteria: the equipment is 1) widely used, 2) relatively expensive, 3) complex (making technical judgment difficult), and 4) available in a variety of models (making selection difficult).

Methods: *Bench testing,* expert opinion, epidemiological and other observational methods.

Assessment methods vary according to the type of device being evaluated. Physical tests for safety and performance are conducted and are supplemented by user questionnaires. In the last 10 years, Centers of Continuous Evaluation have been established within the NHS to continually examine a single equipment category. A list of the current Centers and the equipment category evaluated is provided at the end of this profile. Each Center familiarizes itself with the category of equipment; develops test methods; and produces relevant, well-informed, and up-to-date information. Generally, reports from the Centers discuss several models of competing equipment, identify the advantages/disadvantages of each model, and give recommendations on models preferred in different circumstances. The equipment is not evaluated in clinical use, which limits the value of the information somewhat. The evaluation activity is based on these continuous assessments and is supplemented by individual examinations of single items of equipment. Approximately 50 evaluations are conducted annually.

In most cases, each item of equipment is subjected to each of the following assessment procedures: 1) a technical assessment against current safety and performance standards, using draft versions if final standards do not yet exist; a subjective assessment of the construction quality, the serviceability and the likely reliability; and 3) a period of user experience to establish its clinical acceptability, in operational and ergonomic terms. All findings and results relating to a particular model are discussed with the manufacturer or suppliers, who are given an opportunity to comment in writing.

Assessors: The assessors are scientists, engineers, technicians, nurses, and clinicians in the National Health Service units and specialized evaluation centers. The approximate turnaround time from selection of assessment topic to reporting of findings is 18 months for a full evaluation including user experience and 9 to 12 months for technical evaluation.

Assessment reports include: The assessment's intended audience; the purpose of the assessment; relationship of this assessment to prior or concurrent assessments of the technology or other technologies intended for similar purposes; who sponsored/commissioned/supported the assessment; who conducted the assessment; description of the technology; properties assessed; procedure used for the assessment; results; findings or conclusions; limitations of findings; implications of findings for practice; procurement/deployment information; where technology is in use.

Dissemination: *Printed reports,* journal articles.

Assessment results are published in *Health Equipment Information.* Each issue is intended to be a "buyer's guide," covering all models which have been evaluated and are still on the market in the United Kingdom. Full reports on any recent models are also included. Summaries are presented for all models, together with a photograph, current price, country of origin, and a reference to where the reader can find the full report.

Reports are available to anyone at their cover price. For details on individual report prices or for subscription information, contact: DHSS Leaflets Unit, PO Box 21, Stanmore, Middlesex, HA7 1AY, United Kingdom.

Budget: $3.2 million. Funding source: 100 percent parent organization.

Use: Based on feedback from the NHS, equipment manufacturers, and suppliers the assessment reports are widely used by the NHS when selecting equipment for purchase.

Program evaluation: To ensure that the Programme meets the NHS needs for information, the DHHS evaluates the Programme on a continuous basis.
Centers of Continuous Evaluation

Bath
Institute of Medical Engineering
Equipment category: infusion pumps and controllers, breathing system connectors.

Birmingham
Dudley Road Hospital
Equipment category: humidifiers, $CO2$ expired gas analysers

Cardiff
Medical Physics Department, South Glamorgan Health Authority
Equipment category: surgical diathermy units, baby incubators, infant warmers.

University of Wales
College of Medicine
Equipment category: lung ventilators, ventilator alarms, resuscitators.

London
St. Mary's Hospital, Paddington
Equipment category: fetal monitors.

Newcastle
Regional Engineer's Department, Northern Regional Health Authority
Equipment category: ECG monitors, automatic non-invasive blood pressure monitors.

Oxford
Regional Engineer's Department, Oxford Regional Health Authority
Equipment category: ECG recorders, ambulatory ECG (Holter) systems.

Sheffield
University and Health Authority, Department of Medical Physics and Clinical Engineering
Equipment category: dialysis and associated equipment (not dialysers).

Completed Reports

UA1 United Kingdom Department of Health and Social Security, Medical Devices Evaluation Programme. Assessment of Elscint Mam LS3 mammographic unit. 1986 Jan. (Report no. STB6E/86/3) [Epidemiological and other observational methods, Bench testing]

UA2 ______. Assessment of IGE L/U arm angiograph unit. 1986 Feb. (Report no. STB/86/7) [Epidemiological and other observational methods, Bench testing]

UA3 ______. Assessment of Siemens Optilux 57 intensifier associated with the Sircam 100mm camera and Polyphos 300E generator. 1986 Jan. (Report no. STB6E/86/4) [Epidemiological and other observational methods, Bench testing]

UA4 ______. Assessment of Wolverson X-ray (Acoma) MXR 102 mammography unit. 1986 Jan. (Report no. STB6E/86/1) [Epidemiological and other observational methods, Bench testing]

UA5 ______. Assessment of medical X-ray supplies (Soredex) Mammex DC mammographic unit. 1986 Jan. (Report no. STB6E/86/2) [Epidemiological and other observational methods, Bench testing]

UA6 ______. Comparison of imaging performance of CT scanners (Issue four). 1986 Mar. (Report no. STB/86/10) [Epidemiological and other observational methods, Bench testing]

UA7 ______. Evaluation of Don Whitley Mark II anaerobic cabinet/work station. 1986 Mar. (Report no. STB/86/11) [Epidemiological and other observational methods, Bench testing]

UA8 ______. Performance assessment of gamma cameras, part four. 1986 Mar. (Report no. STB/86/9) [Epidemiological and other observational methods, Bench testing]

UA9 ______. An evaluation of eight non-invasive electronic KV measuring instruments which are commercially available in the UK. 1985 Jun. (Report no. STB6E/85/19) [Epidemiological and other observational methods, Bench testing]

UA10 ______. An evaluation of the Beckman Astra 8 with enzymes. 1985 Jul. (Report no. STB3A/85/32) [Epidemiological and other observational methods, Bench testing]

UA11 ______. An evaluation of the Hamilton Microlab 2100. 1985 Apr. (Report no. STB3A/85/18) [Epidemiological and other observational methods, Bench testing]

UA12 ______. An evaluation of the Kone Process selective chemistry analyser. 1985 Jul. (Report no. STB3A/85/31) [Epidemiological and other observational methods, Bench testing]

UA13 ______. Assessment of Kodak M8 radiographic film processor. 1985 Jun. (Report no. STB6E/85/24) [Epidemiological and other observational methods, Bench testing]

UA14 ______. Assessment of Lixiscop hand held imager with radioactive source. 1985 Sep. (Report no. STB6E/85/33) [Epidemiological and other observational methods, Bench testing]

UA15 ______. Assessment of Philips Medical Systems Saturn 500 and Saturn 850 generators. 1985 Aug. (Report no. STB6E/85/28) [Epidemiological and other observational methods, Bench testing]

UA16 ______. Assessment of Picker Clinix C servo chest unit. 1985 Jun. (Report no. STB6E/85/14) [Epidemiological and other observational methods, Bench testing]

UA17 ______. Assessment of Picker Modulex T for radiography, tomography and occasional peripheral angiography. 1985 Dec. (Report no. STB6E/85/45) [Epidemiological and other observational methods, Bench testing]

UA18 ______. Assessment of Siemens basic radiological system (BRS) to WHO modified specification. 1985 Sep. (Report no. STB6E/85/34) [Epidemiological and other observational methods, Bench testing]

UA19 ______. Assessment of Sine Mobil 3N and 3H mobile imaging intensifiers. 1985 Sep. (Report no. STB6E/85/30) [Epidemiological and other observational methods, Bench testing]

UA20 ______. Assessment of Todd Research BRS to WHO modified specification. 1985 Sep. (Report no. STB6A/85/36) [Epidemiological and other observational methods, Bench testing]

UA21 ______. Assessment of Wolverson Mylo X radiographic unit, Royal Preston Hospital, North Manchester. 1985 Apr. (Report no. STB6E/85/8) [Epidemiological and other observational methods, Bench testing]

UA22 ______. Assessment of a Siemens Polydoros 80 X-ray generator. 1985 Aug. (Report no. STB6E/85/27) [Epidemiological and other observational methods, Bench testing]

UA23 ______. Comparative evaluation of free thyroxine assay kits. 1985 Nov. (Report no. STB3A/85/44) [Epidemiological and other observational methods, Bench testing]

UA24 ______. Comparative evaluation of prostatic acid phosphatase kits. 1985 May. (Report no. STB3A/85/21) [Epidemiological and other observational methods, Bench testing]

UA25 ______. Evaluation of Analogue LM3 analyser. 1985 May. (Report no. STB3/85/25) [Epidemiological and other observational methods, Bench testing]

UA26 ______. Evaluation of sickle cell haemoglobin (HBS) screening methods. 1985 Sep. (Report no. STB3A/85/41) [Epidemiological and other observational methods, Bench testing]

UA27 ______. Evaluation of the Autobac IDX. 1985 Dec. (Report no. STB3A/85/46) [Epidemiological and other observational methods, Bench testing]

UA28 ______. Evaluation of the IQ Bio Microlite Floteskan system. 1985 Oct. (Report No. STB3A/85/43) [Epidemiological and other observational methods, Bench testing]

UA29 ______. Evaluation of the Matascan. 1985 May. (Report no. STB3A/85/23) [Epidemiological and other observational methods, Bench testing]

UA30 ______. Evaluation of the Syra Advance (summary report). 1985 May. (Report no. STB3A/85/22) [Epidemiological and other observational methods, Bench testing]

UA31 ______. Evaluation of the Syva advance automated fluorescence immuno-assay system. Final report. 1985 Dec. (Report no. STB3A/85/47) [Epidemiological and other observational methods, Bench testing]

UA32 ______. Introduction to imaging cameras with assessment of Matric HPC 1010/4. 1985 Nov. (Report no. STB6E/85/42) [Epidemiological and other observational methods, Bench testing]

UA33 ______. PHLS & DHSS evaluation of five anti-HTLV3/LAV assay kits. 1985 Sep. (Report no. STB3A/85/40) [Epidemiological and other observational methods, Bench testing]

UA34 ______. Physical evaluation of the imaging performance of the Agfa Gevaert range of screen film systems. 1985 Aug. (Report no. STB6E/85/26) [Epidemiological and other observational methods, Bench testing]

UA35 ______. Survey of bench top centrifuges. 1985 May. (Report no. STB3A/85/20) [Epidemiological and other observational methods, Bench testing]

U.S. Administrators Inc.

Professional Policy Committee
5016 North Parkway Calabasas
Calabasas, CA 91302
800-872-7526, Ext. 173

Contact: Marvin J. Shapiro, M.D., Medical Director.

Overview: The U.S. Administrators Inc. is a for-profit corporation that manages self-funded medical care programs of corporations, unions, and government entities. It is sponsered by the Crownx Corporation of Canada and Samuel X. Kaplan and family. The Professional Policy Committee was organized in spring 1983 to obtain timely information on which daily reimbursement decisions could be based.

Purpose: To guide reimbursement policies.

Primary intended users: Physicians; acute facility administrators; long-term care facility administrators; other care givers; employers; unions and other employee organizations; third party payers; financial analysts, consultants; lawyers.

Technologies: *Medical or surgical procedure,* drug, device, support system, organizational or administrative system.

Any technology is assessed that requires a decision as to whether or not it should be reimbursed and/or under what circumstances it should be reimbursed.

Intervention: *Treatment,* prevention, diagnosis, rehabilitation.

Stage: *Established or widespread practice,* emerging, new, obsolete.

As soon as the Committee has knowledge of a new technology not yet released for general use it seeks to develop a policy. Technologies are also evaluated if evidence from claims indicates that there may be misuse of a technology, or a technology may become obsolete.

Properties: *Effectiveness;* safety; efficacy; cost; cost-benefit; cost-effectiveness; system impact; economic implications; ethical, legal, social implications.

Technologies are assessed from the perspective of their contribution to patient care. Does a technology contribute significantly to diagnosis or treatment? Does it do a better job than other technologies in that it is more convenient, causing less patient distress, and/or is less expensive?

Selection process: Account executives, clients, health benefit coordinators, claims personnel, committee members, the Medical Director, or physician consultants may request that an assessment be conducted. Requests may be either written or oral. Assessment topic priorities are set by the Medical Director. An assessment is performed if a problem with a procedure or a technology is identified. The staff presents the problem and a proposed resolution to the Policy Committee for discussion, evaluation, and final resolution.

Methods: *Group judgment,* information syntheses, expert opinion.

The Medical Director and his staff prepare a literature review and an agenda. This material is sent to the Committee members 4 to 6 weeks prior to the meeting. The Committee meets to consider and recommend actions. The Medical Director prepares the minutes, which are reviewed and approved by all Committee members. The results are presented in language suitable for clients and internal personnel and are then circulated in written form. The approximate turnaround time from selection of assessment topic to reporting of findings is 6 to 9 months.

Assessors: The assessors are physicians with various associations in the medical and academic communities.

Assessment reports include: Abstract; the assessment's intended audience; the purpose of the assessment; relationship of this assessment to prior or concurrent assessments of the technology or other technologies intended for similar purposes; description of the technology; stage of life-cycle of technology when assessed; properties assessed; procedure used for the assessment; sources of data/information; methods for collecting data/information; methods for analyzing/synthesizing data/information; results; findings or conclusions; limitations of findings; implications of findings for practice; recommendations for practice, future assessments, technology development, research; how the technology works, including theory, principles; development of the technology; where technology is in use; regulatory agency approval status; coverage/reimbursement status of the technology.

Dissemination: Advisories to members/constituents.

The assessment policies are called "Professional Policy Committee Recommendations." The recommendations are sent to all clients and concerned personnel within the organization. Copies of the assessments may be obtained by contacting Marvin J. Shapiro at U.S. Administrators.

Budget: $150,000. The approximate cost per assessment is $5,000. Funding source: 100 percent parent organization.

Use: The information is used by the parent organization to adjudicate the payment of claims for services. Claims personnel, professional review departments, and physician advisors all make use of the recommendations.

Program evaluation: There have been no formal evaluations, but the program is under constant review by the internal personnel who use the recommendations, and by clients. The ongoing review seems to be very positive, since the recommendations have, almost without exception, been accepted, and found helpful in adjudicating claims, dealing with providers, and educating claims personnel of clients as well as employees.

Completed Reports

UB1 U.S. Administrators, Professional Policy Committee. A.I.D.S. [7/86] [Group judgment]

UB2 ______. Adjuvant chemotherapy for breast cancer. [7/86] [Group judgment]

UB3 ______. Admission screening—hospital. [7/86] [Group judgment]

UB4 ______. Allergy—new tests for treatment. [7/86] [Group judgment]

UB5 ______. Alopecia areata. [7/86] [Group judgment]

UB6 ______. Arthritis—diagnostic procedures. [7/86] [Group judgment]

UB7 ______. Arthritis—medical therapy. [7/86] [Group judgment]

UB8 ______. Arthritis—surgical intervention. [7/86] [Group judgment]

UB9 ______. Arthritis, low-dose methotrexate therapy. [7/86] [Group judgment]

UB10 ______. Arthroscopy of joints other than the knee. [7/86] [Group judgment]

UB11 ______. Arthroscopy of knee. [7/86] [Group judgment]

UB12 ______. B.E.A.M. [7/86] [Group judgment]

UB13 ______. Biofeedback. [7/86] [Group judgment]

UB14 ______. Bone marrow transplantation. [7/86] [Group judgment]

UB15 ______. Breast imaging. [7/86] [Group judgment]

UB16 ______. CT scans—head. [7/86] [Group judgment]

UB17 ______. CT scans cervical and lumbar spine. [7/86] [Group judgment]

UB18 ______. Cardiac rehabilitation programs. [7/86] [Group judgment]

UB19 ______. Cardioverter defibrillator, implantable. [7/86] [Group judgment]

UB20 ______. Carotid artery disease. [7/86] [Group judgment]

UB21 ______. Cerebral artery anastomosis, superficial temporal-middle. [Group judgment]

UB22 ______. Cerebral artery anastomosis, superficial temporal-middle. [7/86] [Group judgment]

UB23 ______. Chemotherapy. [7/86] [Group judgment]

UB24 ______. Chest pain—chronic. [7/86] [Group judgment]

UB25 ______. Chiropractic services. [7/86] [Group judgment]

UB26 ______. Cholangiography, routine operative. [7/86] [Group judgment]

UB27 ______. Cholecystectomy. [7/86] [Group judgment]

UB28 ______. Cochlear implants. [7/86] [Group judgment]

UB29 ______. Coronary arteriography. [7/86] [Group judgment]

UB30 ______. Coronary artery angioplasty. [7/86] [Group judgment]

UB31 ______. Coronary care units, admission to. [7/86] [Group judgment]

UB32 ______. Decubitus surgery. [7/86] [Group judgment]

UB33 ______. Diabetes mellitus—diagnosis and management. [7/86] [Group judgment]

UB34 ______. Digital subtraction angiography—intravenous. [7/86] [Group judgment]

UB35 ______. Dilatation and curettage. [7/86] [Group judgment]

UB36 ______. E.S.W.L. [7/86] [Group judgment]

UB37 ______. Echocardiography in atherosclerotic coronary artery disease. [7/86] [Group judgment]

UB38 ______. Emergency rooms. [7/86] [Group judgment]

UB39 ______. Epikeratophakia grafts. [7/86] [Group judgment]

UB40 ______. Exercise training for chronic obstructive lung disease. [7/86] [Group judgment]

UB41 ______. Eye surgery. [7/86] [Group judgment]

UB42 ______. Fertilization, in vitro. [7/86] [Group judgment]

UB43 ______. Fetal monitoring—non-stress training. [7/86] [Group judgment]

UB44 ______. Gastric bubble, Garren-Edwards. [7/86] [Group judgment]

UB45 ______. Genetic counselling and screening. [7/86] [Group judgment]

UB46 ______. Growth hormone—human. [7/86] [Group judgment]

UB47 ______. Hodgkin's disease, routine lymphangiography. [7/86] [Group judgment]

UB48 ______. Hodgkin's disease, routine staging laparotomy. [7/86] [Group judgment]

UB49 ______. Holter monitoring. [7/86] [Group judgment]

UB50 ______. Hypertension, evaluation and management. [7/86] [Group judgment]

UB51 ______. Hyperthermia. [7/86] [Group judgment]

UB52 ______. Immunoaugmentative therapy. [7/86] [Group judgment]

UB53 ______. Incentive spirometry. [7/86] [Group judgment]

UB54 ______. Intermittent positive pressure breathing. [7/86] [Group judgment]

UB55 ______. Investigations (clinical). [7/86] [Group judgment]

UB56 ______. Kyphoscoliosis surgery. [7/86] [Group judgment]

UB57 ______. Laser therapy. [7/86] [Group judgment]

UB58 ______. Linear Pump, Wright. [7/86] [Group judgment]

UB59 ______. Maternity benefits. [7/86] [Group judgment]

UB60 ______. Metastatic neoplasms. [7/86] [Group judgment]

UB61 ______. Morbid obesity. [7/86] [Group judgment]

UB62 ______. Multiple views—diagnostic radiology. [7/86] [Group judgment]

UB63 ______. Nail bed transplants. [7/86] [Group judgment]

UB64 ______. Non-invasive testing—lower extremities. [7/86] [Group judgment]

UB65 ______. Non-invasive testing—peripheral artery disease. [7/86] [Group judgment]

UB66 ______. Nuclear magnetic resonance imaging. [7/86] [Group judgment]

UB67 ______. Organ transplantation. [7/86] [Group judgment]

UB68 ______. Orthoptic training. [7/86] [Group judgment]

UB69 ______. Pain rehabilitation programs. [7/86] [Group judgment]

UB70 ______. Periodic health screening. [7/86] [Group judgment]

UB71 ______. Peripheral pulmonary lesions. [7/86] [Group judgment]

UB72 ______. Physical therapy. [7/86] [Group judgment]

UB73 ______. Preadmission/presurgical screening. [7/86] [Group judgment]

UB74 ______. Psychiatric disorders—testing. [7/86] [Group judgment]

UB75 ______. Radionuclide scans (post-operative). [7/86] [Group judgment]

UB76 ______. Radionuclide scans (pre-operative). [7/86] [Group judgment]

UB77 ______. Research grants—investigational. [7/86] [Group judgment]

UB78 ______. Somatization disorder. [7/86] [Group judgment]

UB79 ______. Spinal stenosis. [7/86] [Group judgment]

UB80 ______. Streptokinase. [7/86] [Group judgment]

UB81 ______. Stress tests. [7/86] [Group judgment]

UB82 ______. Subcutaneous (subareolar) mastectomy (bilateral). [7/86] [Group judgment]

UB83 ______. Swan Ganz. [7/86] [Group judgment]

UB84 ______. Thallium and/or equilibrium-gated myocardial imaging. [7/86] [Group judgment]

UB85 ______. Therapeutic apheresis (plasmapheresis). [7/86] [Group judgment]

UB86 ______. Transfusion—preparation of blood. [7/86] [Group judgment]

UB87 ______. Unbundling. [7/86] [Group judgment]

UB88 ______. Upper G-I endoscopy. [7/86] [Group judgment]

UB89 ______. Urography (excretory). [7/86] [Group judgment]

Ongoing Assessments

UB90 ______. Autologous blood transfusions. Ongoing. [Group judgement]

UB91 ______. Bone healing/electromagnetic stimulation. Ongoing. [Group judgment]

UB92 ______. Bone marrow transplant—reconsideration. Ongoing. [Group judgment]

UB93 ______. CEA testing. Ongoing. [Group judgment]

UB94 ______. Carotid endarterectomy. Ongoing. [Group judgment]

UB95 ______. Chronic backache—diagnosis and therapy. Ongoing. [Group judgment]

UB96 ______. Echocardiography/re-evaluation. Ongoing. [Group judgment]

UB97 ______. Environmental illness and testing. Ongoing. [Group judgment]

UB98 ______. Evoked potential monitoring. Ongoing. [Group judgment]

UB99 ______. Guidelines for reimbursement policies for inpatient and outpatient therapy for alcoholism and psychiatric disorders. Ongoing. [Group judgment]

UB100 ______. Guidelines of appropriate indications for "oscopies". Ongoing. [Group judgment]

UB101 ______. Hospice care/Alzheimer's. Ongoing. [Group judgment]

UB102 ______. Hyperbaric oxygen therapy. Ongoing. [Group judgment]

UB103 ______. Intrapartum fetal monitoring. Ongoing. [Group judgment]

UB104 ______. Intrauterine fetal shunts. Ongoing. [Group judgment]

UB105 ______. Lithotripsy—reconsideration re expanded indications. Ongoing. [Group judgment]

UB106 ______. Liver/spleen scans. Ongoing. [Group judgment]

UB107 ______. Pain clinics. Ongoing. [Group judgment]

UB108 ______. Penile implants. Ongoing. [Group judgment]

UB109 ______. Programmed electronic stimulation—post-myocardial infarct. Ongoing. [Group judgment]

UB110 ______. Protocol for use of multiple EKG's and chest X-rays in CCUs and ICUs. Ongoing. [Group judgment]

UB111 ______. Radiation therapy for lung carcinoma. Ongoing. [Group judgment]

UB112 ______. Relaxation therapy for hypertension. Ongoing. [Group judgment]

UB113 ______. Sclerosing therapy for esophageal varices. Ongoing. [Group judgment]

UB114 ______. Screening tests for osteoporosis. Ongoing. [Group judgment]

UB115 ______. Sleep testing and therapy of sleep apnea. Ongoing. [Group judgment]

University of California, San Francisco

Institute for Health Policy Studies
1326 Third Avenue
San Francisco, CA 94143
415-476-4921

Contact: Jonathan Showstack, Associate Professor of Health Policy; or Phyllis Fetto, Program Administrator.

Overview: The Institute for Health Policy Studies (IHPS) is an academic and research unit of the University of California, San Francisco (UCSF). It was established in 1972 as the Health Policy Program. In 1982, the name officially changed to the IHPS when it was formally designated an Organized Research Unit within the School of Medicine, UCSF.

Purpose: The IHPS has a threefold purpose. First, IHPS provides education and training programs for students and practitioners in the health professions; for students and faculty in other disciplines; and for policy-makers, program managers, and others in the health field. Second, the IHPS faculty conduct health services research and policy analysis projects. Third, the IHPS gives advice on effective and efficient health care delivery systems to federal and state governments and other policy-making bodies.

Primary intended users: Physicians, third party payers, government regulators, public policy-makers, legislators, policy research organizations.

Technologies: *Medical or surgical procedure,* device, support system, organizational or administrative system.

In recent years, IHPS's priorities in research and policy analysis have been health maintenance organizations and other organized health care delivery systems, cost containment, impact of medical technology on health care, ethical issues in health care, reproductive health, the aged, child health, prescription drugs, health manpower, health planning, health promotion and disease prevention, and health care for disadvantaged persons.

Intervention: *Treatment,* diagnosis.

Stage: *Established or widespread practice,* new.

Properties: *Cost-effectiveness;* efficacy; effectiveness; cost; cost-benefit; service requirements; acceptance/adoption level; system impact; economic implications; ethical, legal, social implications.

Selection process: Faculty and staff members generally select assessment topics. Projects must be within a faculty/staff member's area of interest; consistent with the purposes of IHPS; and subject to university policies regarding grants, contracts, and other arrangements with outside parties.

Methods: *Cost analyses,* information syntheses, expert opinion, group judgment, modeling, epidemiological and other observational methods.

Through its formal relationships with other university institutions, IHPS has access to clinical data. The turnaround time from selection of assessment topic to reporting of findings varies according to the type of study conducted or other assistance provided. For instance, the case studies on various technologies conducted for the Congressional Office of Technology Assessment took approximately 6 months to complete. Responses to requests for technical assistance may take 1 day to several weeks and formal health services research projects are often 2 to 3 years long.

Assessors: The IHPS has approximately 30 faculty members and 28 affiliated faculty, over 20 full-time research staff, 40 predoctoral and postdoctoral fellows and visiting scholars, and approximately 20 full-time support staff. This multidisciplinary staff represents the fields of law, pharmacology, philosophy and ethics, medicine, economics, public policy and administration, planning, statistics, sociology, epidemiology, political science, medical anthropology, and medical information sciences.

Assessment reports include: Abstract; the purpose of the assessment; who sponsored/commissioned/supported the assessment; who conducted the assessment; description of the technology; stage of life-cycle of technology when assessed; properties assessed; procedure used for the assessment; source of data/information; methods for collecting data/information; methods for analyzing/synthesizing data/information; results; findings or conclusions; limitations of findings; implications of findings for practice; recommendations for practice, future assessments, technology development, research; how the technology works, including theory, principles; development of the technology; regulatory agency approval status; coverage/reimbursement status of the technology.

Dissemination: Printed reports; journal articles; press conferences/news releases, TV/radio broadcasts, video products.

A comprehensive dissemination program exists to communicate information on health policy issues and research findings to four major audiences: federal, state and local policy-makers; the health services research and health policy research communities; representatives of not-for-profit and for-profit organizations that provide health services; and the general public.

Faculty and research staff place a high priority on the development of publications including books, monographs, discussion papers, book chapters, and journal articles. There are three internal publication series: a discussion paper series; a monograph series; and a reprint series.

The Institute's semiannual newsletter *IHPS Report,* is designed to communicate Institute research findings. The Institute's Center for Population and Reproductive Health Policy produces the semiannual newsletter *Research Highlights.*

Institute faculty and research staff organize conferences on national, state, and local health policy issues. The conferences bring selected groups together to share research findings and to analyze the implications of these findings for key policy questions.

Budget: Research, $1,500,000, technology assessment, $750,000. Funding sources: 50 percent government grants/contracts, 50 percent foundations, other private grants.

Use: It is difficult to measure directly the impact of IHPS activities, because IHPS acts as an analytic and advisory body, not a policy-making body. Results of health services research and policy analyses projects have had wide circulation through publication in peer-reviewed journals and are often cited by other investigators. Technical assistance and policy analyses provided by IHPS have been used in augmenting and guiding legislative efforts and various policy changes.

From 1977 through 1983, IHPS faculty and research staff responded to approximately 800 requests for technical assistance. Over 50 percent of the requests were from federal policy-makers and staff.

The primary users have been Congress and Congressional offices, the Executive Office of the President, the Department of Health and Human Services, and the Federal Trade Commission. For these and other federal agencies, IHPS analyses have contributed to research agendas and policy options in such areas as prescription drugs, health manpower, health promotion and disease prevention, and health planning and regulation.

For the state of California, IHPS provided analyses of MediCal reform options, the impact of prepaid medical care plans, health and social service policy options in long-term care, the cost-effectiveness of prenatal care, and other areas. The health provider community—individual providers, institutions, and service programs—have benefited from IHPS technical assistance, information, and educational programs.

The expansion of IHPS research and analyses activities has augmented its role in education and training. IHPS faculty have developed some 20 courses in health policy and related areas for students on the UCSF and University of California, Berkeley campuses.

IHPS has been instrumental in several major developments in academic programs at UCSF, including the establishment of the Division of General Internal Medicine; the Division of Medical Ethics; the Aging Health Policy Center; and postgraduate programs in health policy research, health policy management, and clinical epidemiology.

The IHPS is described in Institute of Medicine, Committee on Evaluating Medical Technologies in Clinical Use. *Assessing medical technologies.* Washington, DC: National Academy Press, 1985.

Completed Reports

UF1 Showstack JA, Hughes Stone M, Schroeder SA. [University of California, San Francisco, Institute for Health Policy Studies] The role of changing clinical practices in the rising costs of hospital care. N Engl J Med 1985;313:1201-1207.

UF2 Korenbrot CC, Aalto LH, Laros RK. [University of California, San Francisco, Institute for Health Policy Studies] The cost effectiveness of stopping preterm labor with beta-adrenergic treatment. N Engl J Med 1984;310:691-696.

UF3 Nevitt MD, Epstein WV, Masem M, Murray WR. [University of California, San Francisco, Institute for Health Policy Studies] Work disability before and after total hip arthroplasty: assessment of effectiveness in reducing disability. Arthritis Rheum 1984;27:410-421.

UF4 Schroeder SA, Myers LP, McPhee SJ, et al. [University of California, San Francisco, Institute for Health Policy Studies] The failure of physician education as a cost containment strategy: report of a prospective controlled trial at a university hospital. JAMA 1984;252:225-230.

UF5 Budetti P, McManus P. [University of California, San Francisco, Institute for Health Policy Studies] Assessing the effectiveness of neonatal intensive care. Med Care 1982;20:1027-1039.

UF6 McPhee SJ, Myers LP, Schroeder SA. [University of California, San Francisco, Institute for Health Policy Studies] The costs and risks of medical care. An annotated bibliography for clinicians and educators. West J Med 1982;137(2):145-161.

UF7 Showstack JA, Schroeder SA, Matsumoto MF. [University of California, San Francisco, Institute for Health Policy Studies] Changes in the use of medical technologies, 1972-1977. A study of 10 in-patient diagnoses. N Engl J Med 1982;306:706-712.

UF8 Simborg DW, Whiting-O'Keefe QE. [University of California, San Francisco, Institute for Health Policy Studies] Evaluation methodology for ambulatory care information systems. Med Care 1982;20:255-265.

UF9 Myers LP, Schroeder SA. [University of California, San Francisco, Institute for Health Policy Studies] Physician use of services for the hospitalized patient: a review, with implications for cost containment. Milbank Mem Fund Q 1981;59(4):481-507.

UF10 Showstack JA, Schroeder SA, Steinberg HR. [University of California, San Francisco, Institute for Health Policy Studies] Evaluating the costs and benefits of a diagnostic technology: the case of upper gastrointestinal endoscopy. Med Care 1981;19:498-508.

University of Lausanne

Institute of Social and Preventive Medicine
Evaluation of the Efficacy and Safety of Chorionic Villi Sampling
17 r. Bugnon
1005 Lausanne, Switzerland
(41-21) 41-28-66

Contact: R. Chrzanowski, M.D., M.PH; or G. Pesia, Professor, Department of Human Genetics, University Hospital (CHUV) 1011 Lausanne, Switzerland.

Overview: The Evaluation of the Efficacy and Safety of Chorionic Villi Sampling (CVS) is a randomized clinical trial sponsored by the Institute of Social and Preventive Medicine, University of Lausanne. The CVS registry and trial began January 20, 1986. By October 1, 1986, the pilot stage of the study had ended and a 3-year grant was awarded.

Purpose: To evaluate the efficacy and safety of prenatal diagnostic tests for genetic disease.

Primary intended users: Patients, physicians, health/medical professional associations, consumer associations, third party payers, government regulators.

Technologies: Medical or surgical procedure.

Specifically, chorionic villi sampling (CVS) and amniotic liquid sampling (ALS) are assessed.

Intervention: *Diagnosis.*

Stage: *New,* established or widespread practice.

Properties: *Efficacy;* safety; effectiveness; cost-benefit; cost-effectiveness; acceptance/adoption level; system impact; ethical, legal, social implications.

Selection process: Physicians, health/medical associations, third party payers, and government regulators can request that an assessment be conducted. An interdisciplinary research group at the direction of the Institute sets assessment topic priorities.

Methods: *Clinical trials,* expert opinion, modeling, cost analyses, epidemiological and other observational methods.

The assessment project consists of a questionnaire, registry (computerized database), followup, intermediary analysis and report, and a final statistical analysis and report. Project presentations are made to the Directory Committee, the Ethical Committee, and the Expert Committee. The CVS assessment will be completed in 1989.

Assessors: Assessors have expertise in the areas of community medicine, epidemiology, human genetics, gynecology, and biostatistics.

Assessment reports include: The purpose of the assessment; relationship of this assessment to prior or concurrent assessments of the technology or other technologies intended for similar purposes; who sponsored/commissioned/supported the assessment; who conducted the assessment; description of the technology; stage of life-cycle of technology when assessed; properties assessed; procedure used for the assessment; sources of data/information; methods for collecting data/information; methods for analyzing/synthesizing data/information; results; findings or conclusions; limitations of findings; implications of findings for practice; recommendations for practice, future assessments, technology development, research; how the technology works, including theory, principles.

Dissemination: *Printed reports,* journal articles, advisories to members/constituents.

Copies of publications and the final report are available from the Institute.

Budget: $60,000. Funding source: 100 percent parent organization.

Use: Third party payers and the federal insurance agency have asked to be informed about the project results.

Related activities: Project staff participate in international conference on CVS.

Completed Reports

UL1 Gutzwiller F, Grob PJ, Boppart I, Marguerat PH, eds. [University of Lausanne, Institute of Social and Preventive Medicine] Swiss alpha-foetoprotein screening working group: results of the collaborative study of early detection of neural tube defects. 1985. [Epidemiological and other observational methods]

Ongoing Assessments

UL2 [University of Lausanne, Institute of Social and Preventive Medicine] Evaluation of efficacy and safety of chorionic villi sampling (CVS). Ongoing. [Clinical trials]

University of Pennsylvania

Leonard Davis Institute of Health Economics
3641 Locust Walk
Philadelphia, PA 19104
215-898-6011

Contact: Joanne Levy, Assistant Director.

Overview: The Leonard Davis Institute of Health Economics is a not-for-profit research institute that emphasizes an interdisciplinary approach to health services research. Allied principally with the Wharton School and the University of Pennsylvania's medical school, the Institute is perhaps the earliest effort to build formal partnerships within the same university among the clinical, management, and social sciences.

The Institute assesses impact and cost-effectiveness of various health policy practices. Projects in the area of medical technology examine patterns of technology adoption, diffusion, and use, particularly as they relate to management decision-making.

Purpose: To promote an interdisciplinary approach to health services research and education in the organization, financing, and delivery of health care.

Primary intended users: Providers, generally; physicians; acute facility administrators; long- term care facility administrators; health product manufacturers; health industry associations; government regulators; public policy-makers, legislators.

Technologies: *Organizational or administrative system,* device, medical or surgical procedure, support system.

Intervention: Prevention, diagnosis, rehabilitation.

Stage: *New,* emerging, established or widespread practice.

The Institute focuses on health policies that are just coming into practice.

Properties: *Cost-effectiveness, economic implications,* efficacy, effectiveness, cost, cost-benefit, acceptance/adoption level, system impact.

Selection process: Assessments are initiated by senior fellows of the Institute, individually or jointly, based on their interests, the availability of data, and availability of funding. Investigators respond to requests for proposals or submit unsolicited grant proposals to government agencies, foundations, corporations, university funding sources, and providers.

Assessment topic priorities are set by the Institute's national advisory council, its governing board, and its executive committee. Followup studies are undertaken when interest persists and funding is available.

Methods: *Cost analyses, modeling,* information syntheses, expert opinion, group judgment, epidemiological and other observational methods.

Specifically, methods include interviews, on-site observations, and computer modeling and simulation. Medical management models are developed to improve the screening, diagnostic, and treatment decisions of clinicians and to understand resource allocation decisions at a societal level. Descriptive studies examine the actual decision processes used by clinicians when recommending the use of alternative technologies, procedures, and pharmaceuticals.

The average project is completed in 18 months although the range is from 4 months to 5 years.

Assessors: The Institute draws upon health services researchers in the university community and faculty from a variety of disciplines, including management, insurance, medicine, economics, decision sciences, dentistry, law, psychology, nursing, and sociology.

Assessment reports include: Abstract; the assessment's intended audience; the purpose of the assessment; relationship of this assessment to prior or concurrent assessments of the technology or other technologies intended for similar purposes; who sponsored/commissioned/supported the assessment; who conducted the assessment; description of the technology; stage of life-cycle of technology when assessed; properties assessed; procedure used for the assessment; sources of data/information; methods for collecting data/information; methods for analyzing/synthesizing data/information; results; findings or conclusions; limitations of findings; implications of findings for practice; recommendations for practice, future assessments, technology development, research; how much the assessment cost; how the technology works, including theory, principles; coverage/reimbursement status of the technology.

Dissemination: *Journal articles;* printed reports; advisories to members/constituents; press conferences/news releases, TV/radio broadcasts, video products.

Research results are disseminated through published articles in the academic, professional, and popular press; press releases; books; and book chapters. In addition, senior fellows are frequent lecturers at universities, professional conferences, and association meetings. The Institute also has its own publication series. To obtain publications, contact Jennifer Conway, Editor and Manager of Information Services, Leonard Davis Institute of Health Economics, 215-898-4750.

Budget: $1,723,300. Funding for current and recent projects has ranged from $3,000 to $612,000 with scope and length of the project being the determining factors. Funding sources: 2 percent parent organization; 42 percent government grants/contracts; 56 percent foundations, other private grants.

Use: The Institute's studies are used primarily by policy-makers, researchers, and practitioners judging from citations in the literature, speaking invitations, and followup work.

Related activities: The Institute conducted a two-part conference on Medicare research and policy in 1986 and 1987. Two books will contain the conference papers and presentations. In addition, the Institute sponsors advanced education programs and a seminar series on health services research topics.

Completed Reports

UP1 University of Pennsylvania, Leonard Davis Institute of Health Economics. A study of voluntary hospital governance. 1986 Sep. (Study for the Robert Wood Johnson Foundation)

UP2 ______. Antecedents and consequences of contract management. 1986 Feb. (Final report to National Center for Health Services Research, DHHS)

UP3 ______. Cost of generic vs. branded ethical drugs. 1986 Jun. (Final report to Ayerst Laboratories)

UP4 ______. Financing options for health care for uninsured poor. 1986 Dec. (Study for North Carolina Hospital Foundation, Inc)

UP5 ______. Hospital contract management: structure, process, and outcome. 1986 Apr. (Final report to the Hospital Corporation of America)

UP6 ______. Magnetic resonance imaging. 1986 Dec. (Pilot study for University of Pennsylvania)

UP7 ______. Designing and evaluating incentives for ambulatory surgery: a nationwide study. 1986 Dec. (Study for Robert Wood Johnson Foundation)

UP8 ______. Adjustment artifacts in DRG-based Medicare reimbursement. 1985 Aug. (Final report to the National Center for Health Services Research, DHHS)

UP9 ______. DRG's disease staging, and variance reduction. 1985 Jul. (Final Report to the National Center for Health Services Research, DHHS)

UP10 ______. The effect of telemetry on advanced life support care. 1984 Apr. (Final Report to the National Center for Health Services Research, DHHS)

UP11 ______. Vertically-integrated systems: a preliminary study. 1984 Jul. (Final report to the Center for the Study of Aging, University of Pennsylvania)

UP12 ______. Cost benefit, cost effectiveness, and other decision making techniques in health care resource allocation. 1983. (Proceedings of a Regional Symposium, November 4-6, 1982, funded by Smith Kline and French Laboratories)

UP13 ______. Cost of medical education in West Virginia: policy research and analysis. 1983 Dec. (Final report to the Claude Worthington Benedum Foundation)

UP14 ______. The spatial distribution of hospital utilization. 1983 May. (Final report submitted to the National Center for Health Services Research, DHHS)

UP15 ______. A review of the economic benefits of selected health education and promotion activities. 1982 May. (Interim report submitted to Johnson and Johnson Live for Life Program)

UP16 ______. Cost-benefit and cost-effectiveness analysis in policymaking: cimetidine as an example. 1982. (Proceedings of an International Symposium, November 22-24, 1981, funded by Smith Kline and French Laboratories)

UP17 ______. Hospital services coordination: a comparative case study of triad and care program management systems. 1982 May. (A final report to the National Center for Health Services Research, DHHS)

UP18 ______. Methodological limitations of hospital case-mix measures (Task III). 1982 Aug. (Final report to the Hospital Research and Educational Trust of New Jersey)

UP19 ______. Indentifying hospital variables that might improve the incentives in New Jersey's prospective hospital reimbursement program (Task II). 1981 Oct. (Final report to the Hospital Research and Educational Trust of New Jersey)

UP20 ______. National conference monograph: evaluating the performance of multi institutional systems. 1981 Sep. (Final report to the National Center for Health Services Research, DHHS)

UP21 ______. The causes and signifigance of clinically inappropriate patient assignments. 1981 Oct. (Final report to the Hospital Research and Educational Trust of New Jersey)

UP22 ______. Vertical integration of care for cancer patients: a Markovian approach. 1981 May. (Final report to the Cancer Center, Hospitals of the University of Pennsylvania)

Ongoing Assessments

UP23 ______. Adoption and diffusion of magnetic resonance imaging under DRGs. Ongoing. (Study for the National Center for Health Services Research, DHHS)

UP24 ______. Adverse selection in multiple-option group insurance. Ongoing. (Study for National Center for Health Services Research, DHHS)

UP25 ______. Evaluation of the DEW National Dental Education Program. Ongoing. (Study for the Glenmede Trust Co)

UP26 ______. Heuristics and biases in diagnostic decisions. Ongoing. (Study for the National Science Foundation and the National Library of Medicine)

UP27 ______. Policy implications of hospital contract management. Ongoing. (Project for the Commonwealth Fund)

Planned Assessments

UP28 ______. Evaluation of magnetic resonance imaging. Planned. (Submitted to Riverside Methodist Hospital, Columbus, OH).

UP29 ______. Full Medicare capitation for ESRD beneficiaries: design, implementation, and evaluation of a controlled nationwide demonstration. Planned. (Submitted to the Health Care Financing Administration).

UP30 ______. The cost-quality tradeoff for trauma patients treated in a non-designated trauma hospital. Planned. (Submitted to University of Pennsylvania)

Veterans Administration Cooperative Studies Program (151 I)

Veterans Administration Medical Center
150 South Huntington Avenue
Boston, MA 02130
617-739-3479

Contact: Daniel Deykin, M.D., Chief; or Ping C. Huang, Ph.D., Staff Assistant, Cooperative Studies Program, Veterans Administration, 810 Vermont Ave. NW, Washington, DC 20420, 202-872-1151.

Overview: The Veterans Administration (VA) extends to eligible veterans free or highly subsidized health care services, including hospital, ambulatory, and nursing home care. Most of these services are provided at its 172 hospital centers. The VA annually assists about 3 million veteran patients, including about 1.4 million inpatients.

The VA also has three major research and development services: the Medical Research Service, the Rehabilitation Research and Development Service, and the Health Services Research and Development Service. The Cooperative Studies Program is in the Medical Research Service. The Program in its present form was instituted in 1972 in recognition of the growing number of multi-hospital studies in the VA medical system. The VA is an especially useful environment for multicenter study because it has a relatively uniform and large patient base under one management.

Purpose: To provide coordination and support for multiple medical centers to study collectively a selected medical problem in a uniform manner, using a common protocol.

Primary intended users: Providers, generally; physicians; acute facility administrators; long-term facility administrators; other care givers; regulators; biomedical researchers; public policy-makers.

Technologies: Drug, device, medical or surgical procedure, support system.

If drugs or devices used in a study require approval from the Food and Drug Administration, an investigational new drug application or investigational device exemption must be filed with the FDA before the study can begin.

Intervention: Diagnosis, treatment, rehabilitation.

Stage: Emerging, new, established or widespread practice.

Properties: *Safety, efficacy,* effectiveness, cost-benefit, cost-effectiveness.

Selection process: Any eligible (more than 5/8 time) researcher-physician or medical investigator in the VA system can request the support to undertake a cooperative study, by sending a proposal to the Chief of the Program. The Chief may encourage studies in certain areas of special interest to the VA. Proposals are reviewed by experts in the area of the study and then either assigned to a coordinating center for planning, returned to the requester for revision, or rejected. This process culminates in the development of a final protocol that is reviewed by the Cooperative Studies Evaluation Committee, a group of medical and biostatistical experts who serve 3-year terms. The Committee's recommendations are reviewed by the Director of the Medical Research Service. Reassessments are initiated in the same way.

Methods: *Clinical trials,* cost analyses, epidemiological and other observational methods.

The majority of VA cooperative studies are randomized clinical trials. A few have been nonrandomized trials and observational studies. Cost analyses are included when appropriate.

Five groups share the responsibility for conducting or monitoring a cooperative study: a study group, an executive committee, an operations committee, the cooperative studies coordinating center human rights committee, and the cooperative studies evaluation committee. In general, the study group, executive committee, and operations committee meet prior to patient intake for organizational, information, and training purposes; again 9 months after patient intake; and annually for the duration of the study. The human rights committee meets with the operations committee at least once a year for the course of the study. All cooperative studies undergo an in-depth review by the cooperative studies evaluation committee at 3-year intervals during their active phase.

The approximate turnaround time from selection of assessment topic to reporting of findings may range from 1 to 7 years.

Assessors: Assessors include physicians and other health care providers, biostatisticians, clinical pharmacists, and other experts in the subject matter of the study.

Assessment reports include: Abstract; the purpose of the assessment; relationship of the assessment to prior or concurrent assessments of the technology or other technologies intended for similar purposes; who sponsored/commissioned/supported the assessment; who conducted the assessment; description of the technology; properties assessed; procedure used for the assessment; sources of data/information; methods for collecting data/information; methods for analyzing/synthesizing data/information; results; findings or conclusions; limitations of findings; implications of findings for practice; recommendations for practice, future assessments, technology development, research.

Dissemination: Journal articles; press conferences/news releases, TV/radio broadcasts, video products.

All VA medical centers conducting medical research report regularly to the VA Medical Research Service which maintains an R&D Information System database. An annual report to Congress on medical research in the VA includes summaries of cooperative studies. Results are also presented at scientific meetings and published in refereed journals. Reprints of articles may be requested from the author or through the Program office.

Budget: $14,000,000. The average cost for a clinical trial is $2-2.5 million. Funding sources: 86 percent parent organization; 7 percent government grants/contracts (interagency agreements); 7 percent foundations, other private grants.

Use: Citations in the published literature to the Program include the following:

Institute of Medicine, Committee on Evaluating Medical Technologies in Clinical Use. *Assessing medical technologies*. Washington, DC: National Academy Press, 1985.

James KE. A model for the development, conduct, and monitoring of multicenter clinical trials in the Veterans Administration. *Controlled Clin Trials* 1980;1:193-207.

Henderson WG. Some operational aspects of the Veterans Administration Cooperative Studies Program from 1972 to 1979. *Controlled Clin Trials* 1980;1:209-226.

Kathe BA, et al. Patients rights and welfare in the VA Cooperative Studies Program. *Controlled Clin Trials* 1981;4:267-274.

Program evaluation: To review the progress and future direction of certain aspects of the Program, evaluations have been made from time to time, as requested by the Director of the Medical Research Service and the Chief of the Program. Congress also has asked the Government Accounting Office to evaluate VA medical research, including the Cooperative Studies Program.

In 1983, evaluations were performed for the Program as a whole and for its cost-effectiveness analysis activities. An ad hoc advisory committee of experts was appointed to conduct site visits, interviews, and group discussions. The committee's recommendations were adopted whenever feasible.

Completed Reports

VC1 Veterans Administration, Cooperative Studies Program. A randomized clinical trial of total parenteral nutrition in malnourished surgical patients. Pending. [Clinical trials]

VC2 ______. Anticoagulants in the Rx of CA (RA-233). Pending. [Clinical trials]

VC3 ______. Bactrim in leukopenia with non-lymphocytic leukemia. Pending. [Clinical trials]

VC4 ______. Effects of reduction in drugs or dosage after long term control of hypertension. Pending. [Clinical trials]

VC5 ______. Evaluations of corticosteroid therapy in gram negative sepsis. Pending. [Clinical trials]

VC6 ______. Surgical shunt vs. medical treatment in alcoholic cirrhosis ascites. Pending. [Clinical trials]

VC7 ______. Treatment of mild hypertension in the aged. Antihypertensive effectiveness and patients' toleration of different regimens. Pending. [Clinical trials]

VC8 ______. A comparison of hospital and home treatment programs for aphasic patients. [1980] [Clinical trials]

VC9 ______. Alcoholic hepatitis (steroid therapy). [1980] [Clinical trials]

VC10 ______. Antabuse in the treatment of alcoholics on methadone maintenance. [1980] [Clinical trials]

VC11 ______. Anticoagulants in RX of CA (warfarin). [1980] [Clinical trials]

VC12 ______. Clinical studies on captopril: evaluation of low doses, twice daily doses and addition of hydrochlorothiazide. [1980] [Clinical trials]

VC13 ______. Community vs. VA nursing home care vs. hospitalization in psychiatric patients. [1980] [Clinical trials]

VC14 ______. Comparison of propranolol with hydrochlorothiazide for the "step 1" treatment of hypertension. [1980] [Clinical trials]

VC15 ______. Disulfiram (antabuse) in the treatment of alcoholism. [1980] [Clinical trials]

VC16 ______. Efficacy of low doses of reserpine plus chlorthalidone in comparison with standard dosage of reserpine plus chlorthalidone in hypertension. [1980] [Clinical trials]

VC17 ______. Evaluation of anti-epileptic drugs (phenobarb vs. phenytoin vs. primidone vs. carbamazepine). [1980] [Clinical trials]

VC18 ______. Evaluation of nadolol in treatment of hypertension. [1980]. [Clinical trials]

VC19 ______. Hepatitis and dentistry. [1980]. [Clinical trials]

VC20 ______. Nafcillin therapy of staphylococcal bacteremia. [1980]. [Clinical trials]

VC21 ______. Oxprenolol vs. propranolol in hypertension. [1980]. [Clinical trials]

VC22 ______. Platelet aggregation in diabetes (use of ASA & persantine). [1980]. [Clinical trials]

VC23 ______. Pneumococcal capsular vaccine immunity in high risk patients. [1980]. [Clinical trials]

VC24 ______. Prazosin vs. hydralazine in hypertension. [1980] [Clinical trials]

VC25 ______. Renal failure self-care dialysis (hemo vs. peritoneal dialysis). [1980]. [Clinical trials]

VC26 ______. Treatment and prevention of infection-induced urinary stones in spinal cord injuries. [1980]. [Clinical trials]

VC27 ______. Vasodilators used in chronic heart failure (CSP 153). [1980]. [Clinical trials]

VC28 ______. Vasodilators used in chronic heart failure (CSP 19). [1980]. [Clinical trials]

Ongoing Assessments

VC29 ______. A five year clinical evaluation of alternative crown and bridge systems (NIDR). Ongoing. [Clinical trials]

VC30 ______. A new strategy to preserve the larynx in treatment of advanced laryngeal cancer. Ongoing. [Clinical trials]

VC31 ______. A prospective randomized cooperative study of cochlear implants. Ongoing. [Clinical trials]

VC32 ______. A prospective randomized trial of medical and surgical therapies for gastroesophageal reflux disease. Ongoing. [Clinical trials]

VC33 ______. A randomized study of prostatic surgery for moderately symptomatic benign prostatic hyperplasia in elderly men. Ongoing. [Clinical trials]

VC34 ______. Antiplatelet therapy after coronary artery by-pass graft (CABG) surgery-I. Ongoing. [Clinical trials]

VC35 ______. Antiplatelet therapy after coronary artery bypass graft (CABG) surgery-II. Ongoing. [Clinical trials]

VC36 ______. Asymptomatic carotoid stenosis etiological importance in development of stroke. Ongoing. [Clinical trials]

VC37 ______. Clinical comparison of base metal alloys vs. a gold alloy used in the fabrication of fixed (crown and bridge) restorations. Ongoing. [Clinical trials]

VC38 ______. Clinical studies of biphasic calcium phosphate ceramic in peridontal osseous defects. [Clinical trials]

VC39 ______. Comparative efficacy of vascular by-pass graft materials in lower extremity revascularization. Ongoing. [Clinical trials]

VC40 ______. Cooperative clinical trial of sclerotherapy for esophageal varices in alcoholic liver disease. Ongoing. [Clinical trials]

VC41 ______. Coronary artery surgery I: stable angina (vein by-pass). Ongoing. [Clinical trials]

VC42 ______. Coronary artery surgery II: unstable angina (vein by-pass). Ongoing. [Clinical trials]

VC43 ______. Dental implants (removable vs. permanent dentures). Ongoing. [Clinical trials]

VC44 ______. Detection and treatment of influenza A infections in high risk ambulatory care patients. Ongoing. [Clinical trials]

VC45 ______. Efficacy and toxicity of carbamazepine vs. valproic acid for partial seizures. Ongoing. [Clinical trials]

VC46 ______. Evaluations of corticosteroid therapy in severe sepsis. Ongoing. [Clinical trials]

VC47 ______. Lithium treatment in alcohol dependence. [Clinical trials]

VC48 ______. Monotherapy of hypertension. Ongoing. [Clinical trials]

VC49 ______. Percutaneous transluminal angioplasty in the lower extremity. Ongoing. [Clinical trials]

VC50 ______. Percutaneous transluminal coronary angioplasty (PTCA). Ongoing. [Clinical trials]

VC51 ______. Prognosis and outcome following heart valve replacement (non-biological vs. tissue). Ongoing. [Clinical trials]

VC52 ______. Prospective evaluation of the efficacy & tolerance of oral trimethoprim sulfamethoxazole prophylaxis in granulocytopenic patients with acute non-lymphocytic leukemia. Ongoing. [Clinical trials]

VC53 ______. Protein-calorie therapy in combination with anabolic steroids in alcoholic hepatitis. Ongoing. [Clinical trials]

VC54 ______. Randomized clinical trial of total parenteral nutrition in malnourished surgical patients. Ongoing. [Clinical trials]

VC55 ______. Spontaneous pneumothorax. Ongoing. [Clinical trials]

VC56 ______. Stroke prevention in non-valvular atrial fibrillation. Ongoing. [Clinical trials]

VC57 ______. Treatment of AIDS and AIDS related complex. Ongoing. [Clinical trials]

VC58 ______. Treatment of multiple myeloma directed by in vitro chemosensitivity testing. Ongoing. [Clinical trials]

VC59 ______. Vasodilators used in chronic heart failure-II. Ongoing. [Clinical trials]

Veterans Administration
Health Services Research and Development Service (152)

810 Vermont Avenue NW
Washington, DC 20420

In collaboration with:
Special Projects Office
VA Medical Center (152)
Perry Point, MD 21902
301-642-2411

Contact: Prakash L. Grover, Ph.D., Chief, Special Projects Office.

Overview: The Veterans Administration Health Services Research and Development Service (VA-HSR&D) works to improve the health care of veterans by supporting research on the planning, organization, management, delivery, utilization, and evaluation of health care. The overall purpose is to generate information and to improve understanding of how health services may be provided more effectively, efficiently, and at lower cost without compromising quality of care.

The Special Projects Office (SPO) was created in August 1984 to provide scientific, educational, and administrative support to the VA-HSR&D system through the VA Central Office, Washington, DC. The SPO was fully staffed in March 1985, plans for a technology assessment system were developed during the spring 1985, and activities began in June 1985.

Purpose: To monitor and evaluate emerging and new health care technologies and to provide information needed by policy-makers and managers regarding adoption and acquisition of such technologies in the VA health care system; and to identify emerging or new technologies that may be useful for improving the health care of veterans.

Primary intended users: Physicians, acute facility administrators, long-term care facility administrators, government regulators, public policy-makers, legislators.

Technologies: *Device,* medical or surgical procedure, support system, organizational or administrative system.

The SPO assesses any discrete and identifiable regimen or modality used to diagnose and treat illness, prevent disease, maintain patient health and quality of life, or facilitate the provision of health care services. It examines processes of health care delivery aimed at achieving outcomes such as improved health, improved quality of life, optimal use of resources, lower costs, and rational use of health services.

Intervention: *Diagnosis,* prevention, treatment, rehabilitation.

Stage: *New,* emerging.

Properties: *Cost-effectiveness,* safety, efficacy, effectiveness, cost, service requirements, economic implications.

Assessments primarily focus on the technical characteristics, established and potential clinical applications, cost-effectiveness, and capital costs of a medical technology. There is some attention to the safety, efficacy, service requirements, and system impact (i.e.,on the VA health care system). When appropriate, modeling is conducted to determine levels of potential utilization and application in veteran populations.

Selection process: System level managers in the VA Central Office request that an assessment be conducted. Requests are made to the SPO through the HSR&D in the Office of the Assistant Chief Medical Director, Research and Development.

Senior managers in the VA Central Office set assessment topic priorities depending on the projected needs of the VA health care system and financial considerations. Highest priority is given to the assessment of tangible technologies (e.g., diagnostic imaging equipment) that have costs expected to (1) exceed $100,000 per unit, (2) in the aggregate exceed $1,000,000 per year, or (3) result in annual use costs that in the aggregate exceed $10,000,000.

Methods: *Information syntheses,* expert opinion, modeling, cost analyses, epidemiological and other observational methods.

The SPO normally synthesizes existing knowledge from the medical, health services, and health policy literature with the assistance of expert consultants. The staff identifies and works with an expert panel of consultants, identifies and reviews published and unpublished literature, solicits expert opinion, analyzes and synthesizes this information, and develops a draft final report. The draft report is reviewed by VA Central Office managers and expert VA and non-VA consultants. No consensus of expert opinion is developed for the content or findings of the report. The final report generally concerns the technical attributes of the technology, clinical effectiveness, capital acquisition, operational costs, cost-effectiveness, and a summary of findings.

The average turnaround time from selection of assessment topic to reporting of findings is 9 months with a range from 6 to 15 months. The amount of time and the resources needed to conduct an assessment vary, depending on the amount of available information and whether it is necessary to collect and analyze primary data.

Assessors: The SPO has a staff of three permanent health science specialists that spend some portion of their time in technology assessment activity. Areas of expertise include health care, social science, statistics, public health, and evaluation. Outside consultants are contracted to conduct review and draft reports. Consultants are recruited from universities, private research organizations, and the government.

Assessment reports include: Abstract; the purpose of the assessment; relationship of this assessment to prior or concurrent assessments of the technology or other technologies intended for similar purposes; who conducted the assessment; description of the technology; stage of life-cycle of technology when assessed; properties assessed; procedure used for the assessment; sources of data/information; methods for collecting data/information; methods for analyzing/synthesizing data/information; results; findings or conclusions; limitations of findings; implications of findings for practice; recommendations for practice, future assessments, technology development, research.

Two types of reports have been developed: a technology assessment information synthesis and a technology assessment. The information synthesis reports are more narrowly focused on new and emerging medical technologies or specific issues in technology assessment. A technology assessment involves a more comprehensive evaluation of the performance standards; safety; efficacy; clinical effectiveness; cost-effectiveness; the immediate and long-term social, economic, and organizational consequences of the new medical technology; and guidance on policy questions regarding its acquisition and use. The information synthesis report usually covers one or more of the issues within a technology assessment.

Dissemination: Printed reports, journal articles.

Following approval by the VA Central Office, the SPO disseminates reports to the VA Central Office managers and VA medical center clinicians and administrators. On request, the reports are transmitted to other government agencies, universities, professional associations, and private organizations. Copies of the reports may be obtained by contacting the SPO at 301-642-2411 Ext. 5442 or the Director, HSR&D, VA Central Office (152), 810 Vermont Ave. NW, Washington, DC 20420, 202-233-2666.

Budget: $100,000. The approximate cost per assessment is $30,000 to $50,000. Funding source: 100 percent parent organization.

Use: The Chief Medical Director of the VA recently commissioned a task force to develop policy options on technology assessment, including those focusing on formalizing ways to use the products of assessment in planning the acquisition and location of new medical technology for the VA.

Completed Reports

VH1 Health Systems Research and Development Division. [Veterans Administration] Management of technology assessment. Perry Point, MD: Special Projects Office, Health Systems Research and Development Division, Veterans Administration, in preparation, expected 1987.

VH2 Health Systems Research and Development Division. [Veterans Administration] Technology assessment of magnetoencephalography (MEG). Perry Point, MD: Special Projects Office, Health Systems Research and Development Division, Veterans Administration, in preparation, expected August 1987.

VH3 Goldschmidt PG. [Veterans Administration] Health services research and development: the Veterans Administration program. Health Serv Res 1986;20(6):Part II 789-824.

VH4 Health Services Research and Development Service. [Veterans Administration] Nuclear magnetic resonance imaging: information synthesis on clinical applications and cost considerations. Perry Point, MD: Special Projects Office, Health Services Research and Development, Veterans Administration, April 1986.

VH5 Health Services Research and Development Service. [Veterans Administration] Technology assessment of extracorporeal shock wave lithotripsy (ESWL). Perry Point, MD: Special Projects Office, Health Services Research and Development, Veterans Administration, 1986.

VH6 Health Services Research and Development Service. [Veterans Administration] The cost-effectiveness of lithotripsy: an information synthesis. Perry Point, MD: Special Projects Office, Health Services Research and Development, Veterans Administration, 1986.

ASSESSMENT REPORT CODE PREFIXES

The assessment report citations listed in Part 1 are grouped by sponsoring assessment program. Each citation has been assigned a unique code consisting of a prefix designating the sponsoring program and a sequential report number. This list contains all the report code prefixes and the corresponding program. The prefixes are arranged alphabetically; the first letter of the prefix is the first initial of a program's name. The Index to Assessment Report Citations guides the user to a specific report code.

Prefix	Program Name
AA	- American Academy of Neurology, Practice Committee
AB	- American Academy of Ophthalmology, Ophthalmic Procedures Assessment Program
AC	- American Academy of Pediatrics
AD	- American College of Cardiology/American Heart Association Task Force on Assessment of Diagnostic and Therapeutic Cardiovascular Procedures
AE	- American College of Obstetricians and Gynecologists, Committee Opinions
AF	- American College of Obstetricians and Gynecologists, Committee on Technical Bulletins
AG	- American College of Physicians, Clinical Efficacy Assessment Project
AH	- American College of Radiology, Task Force on Breast Cancer
AJ	- American Dental Association, Council on Dental Materials, Instruments, and Equipment
AK	- American Dental Association, Council on Dental Therapeutics
AL	- American Diabetes Association
AM	- American Gastroenterological Association, Patient Care Committee
AN	- American Hospital Association, Hospital Technology Series Program
AO	- American Medical Association, Council on Scientific Affairs
AP	- American Medical Association, Diagnostic and Therapeutic Technology Assessment
AQ	- American Medical Association, Drug Evaluations
AS	- American Society for Gastrointestinal Endoscopy
BA	- Battelle Memorial Institute
BC	- Blue Cross and Blue Shield Association, Medical Necessity Program
BS	- Blue Cross and Blue Shield Association, Technology Evaluation and Coverage Program
BU	- Brandeis University Health Policy Center
CA	- California Medical Association
CB	- Centraal Begeleidingsorgaan voor de Intercollegiale Toetsing, National Organization for Quality Assurance in Hospitals
CP	- College of American Pathologists
CU	- Congress of the United States, Office of Technology Assessment
DC	- Duke University, Center for Health Policy Research and Educating
EH	- ECRI Health Devices Program
ET	- ECRI Technology Assessment Program
FA	- Food and Drug Administration, Center for Devices and Radiological Health
FD	- Food and Drug Administration, Center for Drugs and Biologics

Prefix	Program Name
GU	- Georgetown University Medical Center, Institute for Health Policy Analysis
HA	- Harvard School of Public Health, Institute for Health Research
HC	- Hastings Center
HF	- Health Care Financing Administration, Office of Research and Demonstrations
HN	- Health Council of The Netherlands
HW	- Health and Welfare Canada
JH	- Johns Hopkins Program for Medical Technology and Practice Assessment
KF	- Kings Fund Centre for Service Development
LE	- Lewin and Associates, Inc.
LU	- Linköping University, Center for Medical Technology Assessment
MG	- McGill University, Department of Epidemiology and Biostatistics
MM	- McMaster University, Department of Clinical Epidemiology and Biostatistics
MR	- Medical Research Council, Canada
MT	- Medical Technology and Practice Patterns Institute
NA	- National Center for Health Services Research and Health Care Technology Assessment, Division of Extramural Research
NC	- National Center for Health Services Research and Health Care Technology, Office of Health Technology Assessment
ND	- National Health Research and Development Program (Canada)
NH	- National Heart, Lung, and Blood Institute
NK	- National Institute of Child Health and Human Development
NL	- National Institutes of Health, Consensus Development Program
NM	- National Library of Medicine
NS	- Netherlands Organization for Applied Scientific Research
PA	- Policy Analysis, Inc.
PH	- Project HOPE
PP	- Prospective Payment Assessment Commission
SC	- Steering Committee on Future Health Scenarios
SP	- Swedish Planning and Rationalization Institute of the Health Services
UA	- United Kingdom Department of Health and Social Security
UB	- U.S. Administrators, Inc.
UF	- University of California, San Francisco, Institute for Health Policy Studies
UL	- University of Lausanne, Institute of Social and Preventive Medicine
UP	- University of Pennsylvania, Leonard Davis Institute of Health Economics
VC	- Veterans Administration, Cooperative Studies Program
VH	- Veterans Administration, Health Services Research and Development Service

INDEX TO REPORT CITATIONS

Part 2
Technology Thesaurus and Assessment Report Citations

Part 2: Assessment Report Citations Listed by Technology

This part has two major sections: a 1,200-term technology thesaurus beginning on page 313, and a listing of assessment report citations by technology beginning on page 361. The listing of assessment report citations is arranged according to the terminology set forth in the technology thesaurus. Referring to the technology thesaurus first is the best way to search for assessment report citations by technology.

To enhance searching, the thesaurus includes many synonyms, acronyms, and cross-references, and indicates broader and narrower terms to lead users to desired citations. The thesaurus uses the following reference terms:

BT	indicates to the user a broader term under which additional citations may be listed. Most, but not all, **BTs** have additional citations. Some terms have more than one **BT.** This is the complementary reference to **NT.**
NT	indicates to the user a narrower term under which additional citations are listed. This is the complementary reference to **BT.**
SEE	refers the user to a searchable term, i.e. a synonym or closely related term under which citations are listed, from a non-searchable term. This is the complementary reference to **x.**
x	indicates a non-searchable term, i.e. a synonym or closely related term, from which the user may have been referred to the present searchable term. This is the complementary reference to **SEE.**
SEE ALSO	refers the user to a related, though not necessarily synonymous, searchable term.

TECHNOLOGY THESAURUS

Absorptiometry
x Radiographic absorptiometry
BT Bone mineral studies

—Dual photon

—Single photon

Acetaminophen
BT Analgesics
Antipyretics

Acetohydroxamic acid
BT Antiurolithics

Acidulated phosphate fluoride
x APF
BT Dental materials

Acoustic impedance tests
x Tympanometry
BT Audiometry tests

Activated prothrombin-complex concentrate
SEE Anti-inhibitor coagulant complex

Acupuncture
BT Alternative medicine
Pain therapy

Acute Physiology and Chronic Health Evaluation
SEE APACHE

Acyclovir
BT Antivirals

Adenoidectomy
BT Surgery

Adhesives
NT Bone cements
Cyanoacrylates

Adjuvant chemotherapy, Breast cancer
SEE Chemotherapy—Cancer

Admission testing, Routine
SEE ALSO specific diagnostic tests, procedures, e.g. Radiography

Adrenal cortex hormones
x Adrenocorticoids
Corticosteroids
BT Hormones
Steroids
NT Androgens
Estrogens
Glucocorticoids
Progestins

Adrenergic beta receptor blockaders
SEE Beta blockers

Adrenocorticoids
SEE Adrenal cortex hormones

Aerosol therapy
BT Respiratory therapy
SEE ALSO Nebulizers

AFP monitoring
SEE Alpha fetoprotein assays
Maternal serum alpha fetoprotein monitoring

AIDS tests
SEE HIV detection assays

Albuterol
BT Bronchodilators

Alclometasone diproprionate
BT Anti-inflammatory agents
Glucocorticoids

Alcohol-abuse deterrents
NT Disulfiram

Alcoholism screening

Allergy-immunology tests
BT Diagnostic tests
NT Challenge food testing
Cytotoxic food testing
ELISA
Immunoradiometric assays
Intracutaneous titration
Migration inhibition test
Patch tests
SEE ALSO Immunoassay systems, Fluorescence

Allogenic bone marrow transplantation
SEE Transplantation—Bone marrow, Allogenic

Allopurinol
BT Antigout agents
Antihyperuricemics
Antiurolithics

Alpha fetoprotein assays
x AFP monitoring
Alpha fetoprotein monitoring
BT Maternal serum alpha fetoprotein monitoring
Oncology tests
SEE ALSO Tumor markers

Alpha fetoprotein monitoring
SEE Alpha fetoprotein assays
Maternal serum alpha fetoprotein monitoring

Alpha receptor blocking agents
NT Dihydroergotamine
Yohimbine

Alprazolam
BT Antianxiety agents

Alprostadil
BT Ductus arteriosus patency adjuncts
Prostaglandins

Alternative medicine
NT Acupuncture

Amantadine
BT Antivirals

Ambulances
SEE ALSO Intensive care systems, Mobile

Ambulatory surgery
SEE Surgery—Ambulatory

Amcinonide
BT Glucocorticoids

Amiloride
BT Diuretics

Amino acids
BT Metabolic and nutrient agents

Aminocaproic acids
BT Antihemorrhagics

Aminoglutethimide
BT Antiadrenals

Aminophylline
BT Bronchodilators
Diuretics
SEE ALSO Theophylline

Amoxicillin
BT Antibiotics

Anabolic steroids
SEE Protein-calorie therapy with anabolic steroids

Analgesia
SEE Pain therapy

Analgesics
NT Acetaminophen
Aspirin
Benoxaprofen
Buprenophine
Narcotic analgesics

Nonsteroidal anti-inflammatory analgesics
Zomepirac sodium
SEE ALSO Pain therapy

Androgens
BT Adrenal cortex hormones
Sex hormones
SEE ALSO Protein-calorie therapy with anabolic steroids

Anesthesia
NT Dental anesthesia
Gas scavengers
SEE ALSO Anesthetics

—Epidural

—Inhalation

Anesthetics
NT Bupivacaine
Etomidate
Lidocaine
SEE ALSO Anesthesia

Angiographic injectors
SEE ALSO Angiography

Angiography
NT Arteriography
Digital subtraction angiography
Lymphangiography
Radionuclide angiography
SEE ALSO Angiographic injectors
Cardiac catheterization
Coronary artery disease diagnosis

Angioplasty
BT Surgery
NT Laser angioplasty
Percutaneous transluminal angioplasty
SEE ALSO Balloon dilatation catheters

Antabuse
SEE Disulfiram

Anthelmintics
BT Antiparasitics
NT Niclosamide
Praziquantel

Antiacne agents
NT Isotretinoin

Antiadrenals
NT Aminoglutethimide

Antiallergic agents
NT Disodium cromoglycate

Antianxiety agents
x Tranquilizers
BT Psychoactive drugs
NT Alprazolam
Clorazepate
Diazepam
Halazepam
Lactates
Lithium
Temazepam
Triazolam

Anti-arrhythmics
NT Digitalis
Digoxin
Disopyramide

Antiarthritics
NT Benoxaprofen
Esterine
Methotrexate
Metronidazole
Penicillamine

Antibacterials
BT Antibiotics
NT Cephalosporins
Chlorhexidine
Hexachlorophene
Sulfamethoxazole
Trimethoprim

Antibiotics
NT Amoxicillin
Antibacterials
Antifungal agents
Antiparasitics
Antiprotozoals
Antivirals
Azlocillin
Bacampicillin
Erythromycin
Mezlocillin

Metronidazole
Nafcillin
Piperacillin
Silver sulfadiazine
Sisomicin
Tobramycin
Trimethoprim

—Intravenous

—Prophylactic

Antibodies
SEE Monoclonal antibodies

Antibody tests
SEE DNA antibody test
HIV detection assays
Rubella tests

Anticholinergics

Anticoagulants
NT Heparin
Warfarin

Anticonvulsants
NT Carbamazepine
Magnesium sulfate
Phenobarbital
Phenytoin
Primadone
Valproate

Antidepressants
BT Psychoactive drugs
NT Trazodone
Tryptophan

Antidyskinetics
NT Levodopa

Antifungal agents
BT Antibiotics
NT Ciclopirox
Clotrimazole
Econazole
Ketoconazole
Miconazole nitrate
Selenium sulfide
Sporicidin
Tioconazole

Antiglaucoma agents
NT Timolol

Antigout agents
NT Allopurinol
Sulfinpyrazone

Antihemorrhagics
x Hemostatic drugs
NT Aminocaproic acids
SEE ALSO Hemostatic materials

Antihistamines
NT Azatadine
Chlorpheniramine

Antihyperlipidemics
NT Cholestryamine
Gemfibrozil

Antihyperprolactinemics
NT Bromocriptine

Antihypertensives
NT Bethanidine sulfate
Captopril
Captopril with hydrochlorothiazide
Clonidine
Enalapril
Guanabenz
Guanadrel sulfate
Hydralazine
Methyldopa
Metolazone
Nitroprusside
Prazosin
Reserpine
Reserpine with chlorthalidone
Saralasin

Antihyperuricemics
NT Allopurinol
Sulfinpyrazone

Anti-inflammatory agents
NT Alclometasone dipropionate
Aspirin
Benoxaprofen
Dimethyl sulfoxide

Anti-inhibitor coagulant complex
x Activated prothrombin-complex concentrate
Prothrombin-complex concentrate

Antilymphocyte serum
BT Immunosuppressants

Antimanics
NT Lithium

Antineoplastics
NT Carmustine
Cyclophosphamide
Dacarbazine
Estramustine
Interferons
Methotrexate
Streptozocin
Tamoxiphen
SEE ALSO Antineoplastics handling
Chemotherapy—Cancer

Antineoplastics handling
SEE ALSO Antineoplastics

Antiparasitics
BT Antibiotics
NT Anthelmintics
Insecticides

Antiplatelet therapy

Antiprotozoal agents
BT Antibiotics
NT Pyrimethamine
Sulfadoxine

Antipruritics
NT Camphor

Antipsoriatics
NT Methotrexate
Methoxsalen
SEE ALSO PUVA therapy

Antipsychotics
BT Psychoactive drugs
NT Rubidium

Antipyresis
SEE ALSO Antipyretics

Antipyretics
NT Acetaminophen
Aspirin
Benoxaprofen
Ibuprofen
SEE ALSO Antipyresis

Antiseborrheic agents
NT Selenium sulfide

Antispasmodics
NT Oxybutynin chloride with metoclopramide

Antithymocyte serum
BT Immunosuppressants

Antitussives
NT Dextromethorphan

Antiulcer agents
NT Gastric acid secretion inhibitors
Sucralfate

Antiurolithics
NT Acetohydroxamic acid
Allopurinol
Penicillamine

Antivirals
BT Antibiotics
NT Acyclovir
Amantadine
Interferons
Vidarabine

Aortocoronary bypass
SEE Coronary artery bypass grafting

APACHE
x Acute Physiology and Chronic Health Evaluation

APF
SEE Acidulated phosphate fluoride

Apheresis
NT Plasma exchange
Plasma perfusion
Plasmapheresis
SEE ALSO Plasma separation systems

Apnea monitoring
SEE ALSO Apnea monitors

Apnea monitors
SEE ALSO Apnea monitoring
Physiologic monitoring systems

Appetite suppressants
NT Diethylpropion
Phenylpropranolamine

Appointment reminders
SEE Reminder systems

Appropriateness Evaluation Protocol

Arrhythmia monitoring
BT Electrocardiography
SEE ALSO Arrhythmia monitors

Arrhythmia monitors
SEE ALSO Arrhythmia monitoring

Arteriography
BT Angiography
NT Ultrasound—Arteries

Arthritis tests
SEE Rheumatology tests

Arthroscopy
BT Endoscopy

Artificial heart
BT Circulatory assistance

Artificial hip
SEE Hip joint replacement
Hip prothesis

Artificial intelligence
SEE Expert systems

Artificial pancreas

Artificial procreation
NT In vitro fertilization

Artificial sweeteners
BT Metabolic and nutrient agents
NT Aspartame
Saccharin
Sorbitol
Xylitol

Aspartame
BT Artificial sweeteners

Aspirin
BT Analgesics
Antipyretics
Anti-inflammatory agents

Assertiveness training

Assessment methods
NT Clinical trials
Cost benefit/effectiveness analysis
Double blinding
Postmarketing surveillance

Asthma prophylactics
NT Disodium cromoglycate

Atenolol
BT Beta blockers

Attention deficit disorder therapy
SEE Methylphenidate

Audiometry tests
BT Diagnostic tests
NT Acoustic impedance test

Autologous blood transfusion
SEE Blood transfusion—Autologous

Autologous bone marrow transplantation
SEE Transplantation—Bone marrow, Autologous

Automated microbiology systems

Automobile passenger restraints
x Car seats
Seat belts (Automobile)

Autopsy

Autotransfusion units
BT Blood transfusion systems

Aversion therapy

Azatadine
BT Antihistamines

Azathioprine
BT Immunosuppressants

Azlocillin
BT Antibiotics

B-mode scanning
SEE Ultrasonography

Bacampicillin
BT Antibiotics

Bacterial antigens

Balance training devices

Balloon angioplasty
SEE Percutaneous transluminal angioplasty

Balloon dilatation catheters
x Dilatation catheters
SEE ALSO Angioplasty
Percutaneous balloon valvuloplasty

Bar codes

Barbiturates
BT Sedatives

Barium enema with sigmoidoscopy
SEE ALSO Cancer screening, Colorectal
Sigmoidoscopy

Batteries, Electric

BCG immunotherapy
BT Immunotherapy—Cancer

BCG vaccine
BT Vaccines

BCNU
SEE Carmustine

BEAM
SEE Brain electrical activity mapping

Beclomethasone
BT Glucocorticoids

Beds, Electric

Behavioral disorders screening

Behavioral therapy

Bendien's test
BT Oncology tests

Benoxaprofen
BT Analgesics
Antiarthritics
Anti-inflammatory agents
Antipyretics

Bentonite flocculation test
x DNA-bentonite flocculation test
BT Rheumatology tests

Benzyl alcohol

Beta blockers
x Adrenergic beta receptor blockaders
NT Atenolol
Labetalol
Metoprolol
Nadolol
Oxprenolol
Pindolol
Propranolol

Beta-carotene
SEE ALSO Vitamin A

Betamethasone
BT Glucocorticoids

Bethanidine sulfate
BT Antihypertensives

Bibliographic information bases
x Computer databases
Databases
BT Information systems
NT CHEMLINE
HISTLINE
MEDLINE
TOXLINE
SEE ALSO Computer-assisted instruction
Computer-assisted patient care
Data banks

—Training

Bicap probe treatment
SEE Endoscopy and electrocoagulation

Bilio-pancreatic bypass
BT Surgery—Morbid obesity

Bilirubinometers

Biochemical analyzers
SEE ALSO Biochemical profiles

Biochemical profiles
BT Diagnostic tests
SEE ALSO Biochemical analyzers

Biofeedback
x Electromyographic biofeedback

Biopsy
BT Diagnostic tests
Surgery

—Endometrial

—Fetal blood

—Renal

Blood banks
SEE ALSO Blood transfusion

Blood cell count
BT Cell counts
Hematology tests

Blood chemistry analyzers
SEE ALSO Blood gas monitors
Blood glucose monitors

Blood cultures
BT Infectious disease tests

Blood gas monitoring
BT Cardiopulmonary tests
SEE ALSO Blood gas monitors

Blood gas monitors
x Carbon dioxide monitors
NT Oximeters
SEE ALSO Blood chemistry analyzers
Blood gas monitoring
Oxygen analyzers

Blood glucose control devices
SEE ALSO Blood glucose monitors

Blood glucose monitoring
BT Endocrinology-metabolism tests
SEE ALSO Blood glucose monitors

Blood glucose monitors
SEE ALSO Blood chemistry analyzers
Blood glucose control devices
Blood glucose monitoring

Blood pressure monitoring
x Sphygmomanometry
SEE ALSO Blood pressure monitors

Blood pressure monitors
x Sphygmomanometers
SEE ALSO Blood pressure monitoring
Physiologic monitoring systems

Blood substitutes

Blood transfusion
BT Transfusion
SEE ALSO Blood banks
Blood transfusion systems
Infectious disease tests

—Autologous

Blood transfusion systems
NT Autotransfusion units
SEE ALSO Blood transfusion
Granulocyte transfusion

Blood urea concentration
BT Kidney function tests

Blood warmers

Bolen's test
BT Oncology tests

Bone cements
BT Adhesives
SEE ALSO Bone prosthesis
Joint prosthesis

Bone densitometry
SEE Bone mineral studies

Bone growth stimulation
x Electrical stimulation—Bone growth
SEE ALSO Bone growth stimulators

Bone growth stimulators
SEE ALSO Bone growth stimulation

Bone marrow transplantation
SEE Transplantation—Bone marrow

Bone mineral studies
x Bone densitometry
Densitometry
Photodensitometry
Radiogrammetry
BT Endocrinology-metabolism tests
NT Absorptiometry
Computed tomography—Bone mineral

Bone prosthesis
SEE ALSO Bone cements
Joint prosthesis

Boston elbow
SEE Elbow prosthesis

Botulinum toxin
BT Neurotoxins

Brain electrical activity mapping
x BEAM
SEE ALSO Electroencephalography
Evoked potentials

Breast cancer screening
SEE Cancer screening—Breast

Breast feeding

Breast imaging
NT Mammography
Thermography—Breast
Transillumination—Breast
Ultrasonography—Breast
SEE ALSO Breast physical examination
Cancer screening—Breast

Breast physical examination
SEE ALSO Breast imaging
Cancer screening—Breast

Breath tests
BT Gastroenterology tests

Bromocriptine
BT Antihyperprolactinemics

Bronchodilators
NT Albuterol
Aminophylline
Ephedrine
Iodide therapy
Theophylline

Bumetanide
BT Diuretics

Bupivacaine
BT Anesthetics

Buprenorphine
BT Analgesics

Burn units
SEE ALSO Supportive care

Bypass graft materials

CABG
SEE Coronary artery bypass grafting

CAD
SEE Computer-aided design

Caerulein
x Ceruletide
BT Diagnostic agents

CAI
SEE Computer-assisted instruction

Calcium channel blockers
NT Diltiazem
Nifedipine
Verapamil

Calcium chloride
BT Metabolic and nutrient agents

Camphor
BT Antipruritics

Cancer screening
SEE ALSO Oncology tests

—Breast
SEE ALSO Breast imaging
Breast physical examination

—Cervical
SEE ALSO Pap smear

—Colorectal
SEE ALSO Barium enema with sigmoidoscopy
Colonoscopy
Sigmoidoscopy
Stool guaiac

—Lung

Cannabis
x Marijuana

CAPD
SEE Continuous ambulatory peritoneal dialysis

Capitation payment
x Prepayment
SEE ALSO Competition
Health maintenance organizations
Incentive payment
Prospective payment systems

Capsule method

Captopril
BT Antihypertensives

Captopril with hydrochlorthiazide
BT Antihypertensives
SEE ALSO Hydrochlorthiazide

Car seats
SEE Automobile passenger restraints

Carbamazepine
BT Anticonvulsants

Carbon dioxide laser surgery
SEE Laser surgery—Carbon dioxide

Carbon dioxide lasers
SEE Lasers—Carbon dioxide

Carbon dioxide monitors
SEE Blood gas monitors

Carcinoembryonic antigen assays
x CEA
BT Oncology tests
SEE ALSO Tumor markers

Cardiac catheterization
x Heart catheterization
BT Surgery—Heart
SEE ALSO Angiography
Catheters

Cardiac enzyme assays
BT Cardiopulmonary tests

Cardiac monitors
x Heart monitors
NT Electrocardiographs

Cardiac pacemakers
SEE ALSO Circulatory assistance

Cardiac rehabilitation
BT Rehabilitation

Cardiointegram
BT Coronary artery disease dignosis
SEE ALSO Electrocardiography

Cardiokymography
x Electrokymography
SEE ALSO Coronary artery disease diagnosis

Cardiopulmonary tests
BT Diagnostic tests
NT Blood gas monitoring
Cardiac enzyme assays
Ergonovine provocative testing
Lipoprotein evaluation

Carmustine
x BCNU
BT Antineoplastics

Carotid body resection
BT Surgery

Carotid endarterectomy
BT Surgery

Case management

CAT scanners
SEE Computed tomography scanners

CAT scans
SEE Computed tomography

Cataract extraction
BT Surgery—Eye
SEE ALSO Corneal endothelial cell microscopy

Catheters
NT Dilatation catheters
SEE ALSO Cardiac catheterization

CEA
SEE Carcinoembryonic antigen assays

Cefotaxime
BT Cephalasporins

Cell counters
NT Leukocyte differential counters
SEE ALSO Cell counts

Cell counts
BT Diagnostic tests
NT Blood cell count
SEE ALSO Cell counters

Centrifuges

Cephalosporins
BT Antibacterials
NT Cefotaxime
Cephradine
Moxalactam

Cephradine
BT Cephalasporins

Cerebral artery anastomosis
BT Surgery
SEE ALSO Extracranial-intracranial arterial bypass

Cerebrospinal fluid shunt valves

Ceruletide
SEE Caerulein

Cervical cancer screening
SEE Cancer screening—Cervical

Cervical cap
BT Contraception

Cervical dilators

Cesarean section
BT Surgery

Challenge food testing
x Provocation tests
BT Allergy-immunology tests
SEE ALSO Cytotoxic food testing

Chelation therapy

—Deferoxamine
x Hemoperfusion with deferoxamine

—EDTA

—Penicillamine
SEE ALSO Penicillamine

Chemical Dictionary Online
SEE CHEMLINE

CHEMLINE
x Chemical Dictionary Online
BT Bibliographic information bases
MEDLARS

Chemonucleolysis
x Enzyme therapy
SEE ALSO Chymopapain

Chemonucleolytics
NT Chymopapain

Chemotherapy—Cancer
x Adjuvant chemotherapy, Breast cancer
SEE ALSO Antineoplastics
In vitro chemosensitivity testing

Chlorhexidine
BT Antibacterials

Chlorpheniramine
BT Antihistamines

Chlorthalidone
BT Diuretics
SEE ALSO Reserpine with chlorthalidone

Cholangiography
SEE ALSO Cholangiopancreatography
Cholecystography

Cholangiopancreatography
x Endoscopic retrograde cholangiopancreatography
ERCP
BT Gastroenterology tests
SEE ALSO Cholangiography
Cholecystography

Cholecystectomy
BT Surgery

Cholecystography
SEE ALSO Cholangiography
Cholangiopancreatography

Cholestryamine
BT Antihyperlipidemics

Chorionic villi sampling
BT Genetic screening

Chromatogenesis assist devices

Chymopapain
BT Chemonucleolytics
SEE ALSO Chemonucleolysis

Ciclopirox
BT Antifungal agents

Cimetidine
BT Histamine H2-receptor antagonists

Cine-CT
BT Computed tomography

Cingulotomy
BT Surgery

Circulatory assistance
NT Artificial heart
External counterpulsation
Intra-aortic balloon pumps
Ventricular assist devices
SEE ALSO Cardiac pacemakers

Circumcision
BT Surgery

Citrates
SEE Potassium citrate

Clinical ecology

Clinical trials
BT Assessment methods

—Randomized

Clonidine
BT Antihypertensives

Clorazepate
BT Antianxiety agent

Clotrimazole
BT Antifungal agents

Coagulation assays
BT Hematology tests
NT Partial thromboplastin time
Prothrombin time

Cochlear implantation
BT Surgery
SEE ALSO Cochlear implants

Cochlear implants
SEE ALSO Cochlear implantation
Hearing aids

Cochleostomy
BT Surgery

Codeine
NT Narcotic analgesics

Cognitive therapy

Collagen implants
BT Surgery

Colonoscopy
BT Gastrointestinal endoscopy
SEE ALSO Cancer screening—Colorectal

Colorectal cancer screening
SEE Cancer screening—Colorectal

Communication aids for the handicapped

Communication systems
NT Emergency communications systems
Satellite communication
Telemetry
SEE ALSO Information systems

Community health centers

Competition
NT Competitive bidding
SEE ALSO Capitation payment
Prospective payment systems

Competitive bidding
BT Competition

Computed tomography
x CAT scans
CT scans
Tomography, X-ray computed
BT Radiography
NT Cine-CT
Dual-energy scanned projection radiography
SEE ALSO Computed tomography scanners
SPECT imaging
Stereotactic neurosurgery, Computed tomography-assisted

—Bone mineral assessments
BT Bone mineral studies

—Head

—Liver and spleen

—Pancreas

—Spine

Computed tomography scanners
x CAT scanners
CT scanners
Tomographic scanners
BT Radiographic equipment
SEE ALSO Computed tomography

Computer-aided design
x CAD

Computer-assisted instruction
x CAI
BT Information systems
SEE ALSO Bibliographic information bases
Computer-assisted patient care
Computer equipment
Computer software

Computer-assisted patient care
NT Decision support systems
Expert systems
SEE ALSO Bibliographic information bases
Computer-assisted education
Computer equipment
Data banks
Medical record systems

Computer databases
SEE Bibliographic information bases
Data banks

Computer equipment
x Decision support systems
SEE ALSO Computer-assisted education
Computer-assisted patient care
Computer software
Expert systems
MEDLINE—Optical disks

Computer software
SEE ALSO Computer equipment

Contact lens cleaners
SEE ALSO Contact lenses

Contact lens lubricants
SEE ALSO Contact lenses

Contact lens markers
SEE ALSO Contact lenses

Contact lenses
NT Contact lenses, Hydrophilic
SEE ALSO Contact lens cleaners
Contact lens lubricants
Contact lens markers

Contact lenses, Hydrophilic
BT Contact lenses

Continuing medical education
SEE Physician education

Continuous ambulatory peritoneal dialysis
x CAPD
BT Peritoneal dialysis

Continuous arteriovenous hemofiltration
SEE Hemofiltration

Continuous passive motion devices
SEE ALSO Continuous passive motion therapy

Continuous passive motion therapy
BT Exercise therapy
SEE ALSO Continuous passive motion devices

Continuous positive airway pressure
x CPAP
BT Respiratory therapy

Contraception
NT Cervical cap
Oral contraceptives
Tubal ligation
SEE ALSO Estrogens

Contralateral breast surgery
BT Surgery—Breast

Contrast media
SEE Radiographic contrast dyes

Cornea transplantation
SEE Transplantation—Cornea

Corneal endothelial cell microscopy
SEE ALSO Cataract extraction

Corneal grafts
BT Surgery—Eye

Coronary artery bypass grafting
x Aortocoronary bypass
CABG
Coronary artery surgery
BT Surgery—Heart

Coronary artery disease diagnosis
SEE ALSO Angiography
Cardiointegram
Cardiokymography
Echocardiography
Electrocardiography
Exercise tests
Photokymography
Ultrasound—Cardiac output

Coronary artery jeopardy score

Coronary artery surgery
SEE Coronary artery bypass grafting
Percutaneous transluminal coronary angioplasty

Coronary care units

Coronary care units, Mobile
SEE Intensive care systems, Mobile

Corticosteroids
SEE Adrenal cortex hormones

Cost benefit/effectiveness analysis
BT Assessment methods

Counseling
NT Genetic counseling
Nutritional counseling
Peer group counseling

CPAP
SEE Continuous positive airway pressure

CPT-4 codes
x Current Procedural Terminology

Creatinine concentration, Serum
x Serum creatinine concentration
BT Kidney function tests

Cromolyn sodium
SEE Disodium cromoglycate

Cryometers
SEE ALSO Cryopreservation

Cryopreservation
SEE ALSO Cryometers

Cryosurgery
BT Surgery

—Arrhythmias

CT scanners
SEE Computed tomography scanners

CT scans
SEE Computed tomography

Current Procedural Terminology
SEE CPT-4 codes

Cushions

Cyanoacrylates
BT Adhesives

Cyclophosphamide
x Cytoxan
BT Antineoplastics

Cyclothiazide
BT Diuretics

Cytotoxic food testing
BT Allergy-immunology tests

Cytotoxic tests
SEE ALSO Challenge food testing

Cytotoxic tests
BT Diagnostic tests
NT Cytotoxic food testing
Hair analysis
Micronucleus test

Cytoxan
SEE Cyclophosphamide

Dacarbazine
x DTIC
BT Antineoplastics

DAF
SEE Discretionary adjustment factor

Darkrooms
SEE Radiographic darkrooms

Data banks
x Computer databases
Databases
SEE ALSO Bibliographic information bases
Computer-assisted patient care
Information systems
Registries

Databases
SEE Bibliographic information bases
Data banks

Day care

Debridement
BT Surgery

Decision support systems
SEE Computer-assisted patient care
Computer equipment
Information systems

Decubitus surgery
BT Surgery

Deferoxamine
SEE Chelation therapy—Deferoxamine

Defibrillation
SEE ALSO Defibrillators

Defibrillators
SEE ALSO Defibrillation

Densitometry
SEE Bone mineral studies

Dental alloys
BT Dental materials

Dental amalgam
BT Dental materials
SEE ALSO Dental amalgamators

Dental amalgamators
x Dental equipment
SEE ALSO Dental amalgam

Dental anesthesia
BT Anesthesia

Dental bonding
SEE ALSO Dental resins

Dental bridges

Dental caries removal systems

Dental ceramics
BT Dental materials

Dental crowns

Dental equipment
SEE Dental amalgamators
Dental scaling and stain-removal devices
Dental sterilization devices
Dental visible light-curing units

Dental implants
x Osseointegrated implants

Dental materials
NT Acidulated phosphate fluoride
Dental alloys
Dental amalgam
Dental ceramics
Dental resins
Dental sealants
Fluoride varnishes
Toothpaste

Dental radiography
x Radiography, Dental
X-rays, Dental
NT Radiopaque plastics

Dental resins
BT Dental materials
SEE ALSO Dental bonding

Dental scaling and stain-removal devices
x Dental equipment

Dental sealants
BT Dental materials

Dental sterilization devices
x Dental equipment

Dental visible light-curing units
x Dental equipment

Denture cleansers

Dentures

Depo-Provera
SEE Medroxyprogesterone

Desoximetasone
BT Glucocorticoids

Detoxification
NT Hubbard method

Developmental disabilities screening

Dexamethasone
BT Glucocorticoids
SEE ALSO Dexamethasone suppression test

Dexamethasone suppression test
BT Endocrinology-metabolism tests
SEE ALSO Dexamethasone

Dextromethorphan
BT Antitussives

Dextrose
BT Metabolic and nutrient agents

Dextrose with saline solution
BT Metabolic and nutrient agents

Diagnosis related groups
SEE DRGs

Diagnostic agents
NT Caerulein
Isosulfan blue
Secretin
SEE ALSO Radiographic contrast dyes
Radiopharmaceuticals

Diagnostic imaging
NT Magnetic resonance imaging
Positron emission tomography
Radionuclide imaging
Radiography
Thermography
Transillumination
Ultrasonography
SEE ALSO specific anatomical sites, e.g.
Angiography;
Breast imaging

Diagnostic tests
NT Allergy-immunology tests
Audiometry tests
Biochemical profiles
Biopsy
Cardiopulmonary tests
Cell counts
Cytotoxic tests
Endocrinology-metabolism tests
Fertility tests
Gastroenterology tests
Genetic tests
Hematology tests
Infectious disease tests
Kidney function tests
Microbiological testing systems
Oncology tests
Rheumatology tests
Seromucoid assays

Dialysis
NT Hemodialysis
Peritoneal dialysis

Diaphanography
SEE Transillumination

Diathermy

Diazepam
BT Antianxiety agents

Diet therapy
NT Sodium restriction
Protein-calorie therapy with anabolic steroids
SEE ALSO Food diaries
Ileal bypass with diet therapy
Infant foods
Nutritional counseling

Diethylpropion
BT Appetite suppressants

Diflunisal
BT Nonsteroidal anti-inflammatory analgesics

Digital imaging
x Digital radiography
NT Digital subtraction angiography
Dual-energy scanned projection radiography
SEE ALSO Picture archiving and communication systems
Radiography

Digital radiography
SEE Digital imaging

Digital subtraction angiography
x DSA
BT Angiography
Digital imaging

Digitalis
BT Anti-arrhythmics

Digoxin
BT Anti-arrhythmics

Dihydroergotamine
BT Alpha receptor blocking agents
Vascular headache suppressants

Dilatation and curettage
BT Surgery

Dilatation catheters
SEE Balloon dilatation catheters

Diltiazem
BT Calcium channel blockers

Dimethyl sulfoxide
x DMSO
BT Anti-inflammatory agents

Dipyridamole
x Persantine
BT Vasodilators

Discography
BT Radiography

Discretionary adjustment factor
x DAF
BT Prospective payment systems
SEE ALSO DRGs

Disodium cromoglycate
x Cromolyn sodium
BT Antiallergic agents
Asthma prophylactics

Disopyramide
BT Anti-arrhythmics

Disposables reuse
SEE Reuse of disposables

Disulfiram
x Antabuse
BT Alcohol-abuse deterrents

Diuretics
NT Amiloride
Aminophylline
Bumetanide
Chlorthalidone
Cyclothiazide
Furosemide
Hydrochlorthiazide
Metolazone
Triamterene

DMSO
SEE Dimethyl sulfoxide

DNA antibody test
x Antibody tests
BT Rheumatology tests

DNA-bentonite flocculation test
SEE Bentonite flocculation test

Doman-Delacato treatment
BT Physical therapy

Dopamine
BT Vasopressors

Doppler ultrasound
SEE Ultrasound

Dosimetry
SEE Radiation measurement

Double blinding
BT Assessment methods

DRGs
x Diagnosis related groups
SEE ALSO Discretionary adjustment factor
Prospective payment systems

Drug costs

Drug labeling

Drug monitoring
SEE Therapeutic drug monitoring

Drug ordering
x Drug prescribing
Prescribing

Drug preparation
NT Ethanol

Drug prescribing
SEE Drug ordering

Drug regulation

DSA
SEE Digital subtraction angiography

DTIC
  SEE Dacarbazine

Dual-energy scanned projection radiography
  BT Computed tomography
    Digital imaging

Ductus arteriosus patency adjuncts
  NT Alprostadil

ECG
  SEE Electrocardiography

Echocardiography
  BT Ultrasonography
  SEE ALSO Coronary artery disease diagnosis

Echocine
  SEE Ultrasonography

ECMO
  SEE Extracorporeal membrane oxygenation

Econazole
  BT Antifungal agents

ECT
  SEE Electroconvulsive therapy

Edinburgh masker

EDTA
  SEE Chelation therapy—EDTA

EEG
  SEE Electroencephalography

EKG
  SEE Electrocardiography

Elbow prosthesis
  x Boston elbow
  BT Joint prosthesis

Electrical stimulation
  NT Transcutaneous electrical nerve stimulation
  SEE ALSO Electrical stimulators

  —Bone growth
  SEE Bone growth stimulation

  —Cardiac

  —Cerebellar

  —Cerebral palsy

  —Cranial

  —Facial nerve palsy

  —Muscular

  —Neural

  —Neuromuscular

  —Scoliosis

  —Spinal

Electrical stimulators
  SEE ALSO Bone growth stimulators
    Electrical stimulation

Electrocardiographs
  NT Cardiac monitors
  SEE ALSO Electrocardiography
    Physiologic monitoring systems

Electrocardiography
  x ECG
    EKG
  NT Arrhythmia monitoring
    Holter monitoring
    Minnesota Q-Q codes
    Ventricular mapping, Intraoperative
  SEE ALSO Coronary artery disease diagnosis
    Cardiointegram
    Electrocardiographs

Electrocoagulation
  BT Surgery
  SEE ALSO Laser photocoagulation

Electroconvulsive therapy
  x ECT

Electroencephalographs
SEE ALSO Electroencephalography

Electroencephalography
x EEG
SEE ALSO Brain electrical activity mapping
Electroencephalographs
Evoked potentials
Stereotaxic depth electrode implantation
Topographic brain mapping

Electrokymography
SEE Cardiokymography

Electrolyte injection
BT Metabolic and nutrient agents

Electromyographic biofeedback
SEE Biofeedback

Electronystagmography

Electrosurgery
BT Surgery
SEE ALSO Electrosurgical devices

Electrosurgical devices
SEE ALSO Electrosurgery

Electroversion therapy

ELISA
x Enzyme-linked immunosorbent assay
BT Allergy-immunolgy tests

Embolotherapy
SEE Therapeutic embolization

Emergency communication systems
BT Communication systems

Emergency kits
SEE ALSO Emergency services
First aid

Emergency services
SEE ALSO Emergency kits

Enalapril
BT Antihypertensives

Endocrinology-metabolism tests
BT Diagnostic tests
NT Blood glucose monitoring
Bone mineral studies
Dexamethasone suppression test
Hydroxycholecalciferol level
Thyroxine assays
Vitamin B12 assay

Endoscopes
SEE ALSO Endoscopy

Endoscopic retrograde cholangiopancreatography
SEE Cholangiopancreatography

Endoscopic retrograde sphincterotomy
SEE Sphincterotomy

Endoscopy
BT Surgery
NT Arthroscopy
Esophagoscopy
Fetoscopy
Gastrointestinal endoscopy
Hysteroscopy
Ureteroscopy

Endoscopy and electrocoagulation
x Bicap probe treatment

Endothelial cell photography
x Specular microscopy

Enteral nutrition
SEE ALSO Enteral nutrition pumps

Enteral nutrition pumps
SEE ALSO Enteral nutrition
Metabolic and nutrient agents

Enzyme-albumin polymers
x Enzyme therapy

Enzyme-linked immunosorbent assay
SEE ELISA

Enzyme therapy
SEE Chemonucleolysis
Enzyme-albumin polymers
Hyaluronidase

Ephedrine
BT Bronchodilators

Epikeratophakia
BT Keratoplasty

ERCP
SEE Cholangiopancreatography

Ergonovine provocative testing
BT Cardiopulmonary tests

Ericsson sex selection method
x Sex selection

ERS
SEE Sphincterotomy

Erythrocyte sedimentation rate
BT Hematology tests

Erythromycin
BT Antibiotics

Esophageal pH monitoring
BT Gastroenterology tests

Esophageal reflux surgery
SEE Surgery—Esophageal reflux

Esophagoscopy
BT Endoscopy

Esterine
x Antiarthritics

Estramustine
BT Antineoplastics

Estrogen replacement therapy
BT Hormone therapy
SEE ALSO Estrogens

Estrogens
BT Adrenal cortex hormones
Sex hormones
SEE ALSO Estrogen replacement therapy
Oral contraceptives

ESWL
SEE Lithotripsy—Extracorporeal shock wave

Ethanol
BT Drug preparation

Ethynodiol diacetate with ethinyl estradiol
BT Oral contraceptives

Etomidate
BT Anesthetics

Evoked potentials
x Visual evoked potentials
SEE ALSO Brain electrical activity mapping
Electroencephalography

Exercise tests
x Stress tests
SEE ALSO Coronary artery disease diagnosis

Exercise therapy
BT Physical therapy
NT Continuous passive motion
SEE ALSO Physical therapy with home exercise

Expert system evaluation
SEE ALSO Expert systems

Expert systems
x Artificial intelligence
BT Computer-assisted patient care
SEE ALSO Computer equipment
Expert system evaluation
Information systems
Medical record systems

External counterpulsation
BT Circulatory assistance

Extracorporeal membrane oxygenation
x ECMO

Extracorporeal shock wave lithotripsy
SEE Lithotripsy—Extracorporeal shock wave

Extracranial-intracranial arterial bypass
BT Surgery
SEE ALSO Cerebral artery anastomosis

Eye surgery
SEE Surgery—Eye

Eyeglasses
BT Vision aids

Fat emulsions
SEE Intravenous fat emulsions

Fertility tests
BT Diagnostic tests
NT Sperm penetration assay

Fertilization in vitro
SEE In vitro fertilization

Fetal monitoring
SEE ALSO Fetal monitors

Fetal monitors
SEE ALSO Fetal monitoring

Fetal shunts
SEE ALSO Surgery—Fetal

Fetal surgery
SEE Surgery—Fetal

Fetoscopy
BT Endoscopy
SEE ALSO Genetic screening

Fibrinogen scanning

First aid
SEE ALSO Emergency kits
Heimlich maneuver

Fish oils
x Omega-3 fatty acids

Flagyl
SEE Metronidazole

Flexible sigmoidoscopy
SEE Sigmoidoscopy

Fluid therapy
SEE Oral rehydration therapy

Fluoride varnishes
BT Dental materials

Fluoroscopy
BT Radiography
SEE ALSO Fluoroscopy units

Fluoroscopy units
BT Radiographic equipment
SEE ALSO Fluoroscopy

Food diaries
SEE ALSO Diet therapy

Food irradiation

Fructose
BT Metabolic and nutrient agents

Functional tests

Furosemide
BT Diuretics

Gait assessment

Gamma cameras
BT Radionuclide imaging

Gammaglobulin, Total serum
SEE Kunkel test

Garren gastric bubble
SEE Gastric bubble

Gas scavengers
BT Anesthesia

Gastric acid secretion inhibitors
BT Antiulcer agents
NT Histamine H2-receptor antagonists
Secretin

Gastric balloon dilatation

Gastric bubble
x Garren gastric bubble

Gastric freezing

Gastric restrictive surgery
BT Surgery—Morbid obesity

Gastroenterology tests
BT Diagnostic tests
NT Breath tests
Cholangiopancreatography
Esophageal pH monitoring
Rehfuss test

Gastroesophageal antireflux prosthesis
BT Prostheses

Gastro-ileal bypass
BT Surgery—Morbid obesity

Gastrointestinal endoscopy
BT Endoscopy
NT Colonoscopy
Sigmoidoscopy

Gemfibrozil
BT Antihyperlipidemics

Generators, Electric

Genetic complementation test
BT Genetic tests

Genetic counseling
BT Counseling
SEE ALSO Genetic screening

Genetic engineering
SEE ALSO Interferons
Monoclonal antibodies

Genetic screening
BT Genetic tests
NT Chorionic villi sampling
Hemoglobinopathies screening
Maternal serum alpha fetoprotein monitoring
Hypothyroidism screening, Neonatal
Phenylketonuria screening
SEE ALSO Fetoscopy
Genetic counseling

Genetic tests
BT Diagnostic tests
NT Genetic complementation tests
Genetic screening
Genetic toxicology tests
Somatic cell mutation tests

Genetic toxicology tests
BT Genetic tests

Glaucoma screening
BT Vision screening
SEE ALSO Perimetry
Tonometry

Glucocorticoids
BT Adrenal cortex hormones
NT Alclometasone dipropionate
Amcinonide
Beclomethasone
Betamethasone
Desoximetasone
Dexamethasone
Hydrocortisone

Glutathione disulfides
BT Metabolic and nutrient agents

Glyceryl trinitrate
x Nitroglycerin
BT Vasodilators

Gonadorelin hydrochloride
BT Pituitary and hypothalmic hormones

Granulocyte transfusion
BT Transfusion

Growth hormone
SEE Human growth hormone

Guanabenz
BT Antihypertensives

Guanadrel sulfate
BT Antihypertensives

Hair analysis
BT Cytotoxic tests

Halazepam
BT Antianxiety agents

Health examination
x Medical evaluation
Physical examination

Health insurance
NT Unbundling

Health maintenance organizations
x HMOs
SEE ALSO Capitation payment

Health promotion
x Disease prevention

Hearing aids
SEE ALSO Cochlear implants

—Use

Heart catheterization
SEE Cardiac catheterization

Heart-lung transplantation
SEE Transplantation—Heart-lung

Heart monitors
SEE Cardiac monitors

Heart surgery
SEE Surgery—Heart

Heart transplantation
SEE Transplantation—Heart

Heart valve implantation
SEE ALSO Heart valve prosthesis

Heart valve prosthesis
SEE ALSO Heart valve implantation

Heavy-ion irradiation
SEE Radiation therapy

Heimlich maneuver
SEE ALSO First aid

Hematology tests
BT Diagnostic tests
NT Blood cell count
Coagulation assays
Erythrocyte sedimentation rate
Hemoglobin A1C measurements
Hemoglobinopathies screening

Hemodialysis
BT Dialysis
SEE ALSO Chelation therapy—Deferoxamine
Hemofiltration

Hemofiltration
x Continuous arteriovenous hemofiltration
SEE ALSO Hemodialysis

Hemoglobin A1C measurements
BT Hematology tests

Hemoglobinopathies screening
x Sickle cell screening
BT Genetic screening
Hematology tests

Hemoperfusion with deferoxamine
SEE Chelation therapy—Deferoxamine

Hemophilus influenza type B vaccine
x HiB vaccine
BT Vaccines

Hemostatic drugs
SEE Antihemorrhagics

Hemostatic materials
SEE ALSO Antihemorrhagics

Heparin
BT Anticoagulants

Hepatitis B tests
BT Infectious disease tests

Hepatitis B vaccine
SEE Viral hepatitis vaccine

Herpes simplex infection screening, Neonatal

Hexachlorophene
BT Antibacterials

HGH
SEE Human growth hormone

HiB vaccine
SEE Hemophilus influenza type B vaccine

Hip joint replacement
x Artificial hip
Total hip joint replacement
BT Surgery
SEE ALSO Hip prosthesis

Hip prosthesis
x Artificial hip
BT Joint prosthesis
SEE ALSO Hip joint replacement

Histamine H2-receptor antagonists
BT Gastric acid secretion inhibitors
NT Cimetidine
Ranitidine

Histamine therapy

HISTLINE
x History of Medicine Online
BT Bibliographic information bases
MEDLARS

History of Medicine Online
SEE HISTLINE

HIV detection assays
x AIDS tests
Antibody tests
HTLV III antigen detection assays
BT Infectious disease tests

HMOs
SEE Health maintenance organizations

Holter monitoring
BT Electrocardiography

Home care

Hormone therapy
NT Estrogen replacement therapy
SEE ALSO Hormones

Hormones
NT Adrenal cortex hormones
Pituitary and hypothalmic hormones
Secretin
Sex hormones
SEE ALSO Hormone therapy

Hospice

Hostel

HTLV III antigen detection assays
SEE HIV detection assays

Hubbard method
BT Detoxification

Human growth hormone
x Growth hormone
HGH
Somatotropin
BT Pituitary and hypothalmic hormones

Human milk banking

Humidifiers

Hyaluronidase
BT Enzyme therapy

Hybridomas
SEE ALSO Monoclonal antibodies

Hydralazine
BT Antihypertensives

Hydrochlorothiazide
BT Diuretics
SEE ALSO Captopril with hydrochlorothiazide

Hydrocortisone
BT Glucocorticoids

Hydromorphone
BT Narcotic analgesics

Hydrotherapy
x Whirlpool baths

Hydroxycholecalciferol level
x 25 hydroxyvitamin D level
BT Endocrinology-metabolism tests

Hyperbaric oxygen therapy
BT Oxygen therapy

Hyperthermia systems
SEE ALSO Hyperthermia therapy

Hyperthermia therapy
SEE ALSO Hyperthermia systems

Hypnosis
SEE ALSO Hypnotic drugs

Hypnotic drugs
BT Psychoactive drugs
NT Methaqualone
Phenobarbital
SEE ALSO Hypnosis

Hypothyroidism screening, Neonatal

Hysterectomy
BT Surgery

Hysteroscopy
BT Endoscopy

Ibuprofen
BT Antipyretics
Nonsteroidal anti-inflammatory analgesics

Ileal bypass
BT Surgery—Morbid obesity
SEE ALSO Ileal bypass and diet therapy

Ileal bypass and diet therapy
SEE ALSO Diet therapy
Ileal bypass

Imaging centers
SEE ALSO Radiography

Immunoassay systems, Fluorescence
SEE ALSO Allergy-immunology tests

Immunologic diagnostic tests
SEE Allergy-immunology tests

Immunoradiometric assay with monoclonal antibodies
BT Immunoradiometric assays
SEE ALSO Monoclonal antibodies

Immunoradiometric assays
x Radioimmunoassays
BT Allergy-immunology tests
NT Immunoradiometric assay with monoclonal antibodies
Radioallergosorbent test

Immunosuppressants
NT Antilymphocyte serum
Antithymocyte serum
Azathioprine

Immunotherapy

—Cancer
NT BCG immunotherapy

Impedance plethysmography
SEE Plethysmography

Impotence diagnosis
NT Papaverine
SEE ALSO Plethysmography

Impotence surgery
SEE Surgery—Impotence

Impotence treatment
NT Papaverine
Yohimbine

In vitro chemosensitivity testing
SEE ALSO Chemotherapy
Oncology testing

In vitro fertilization
x Fertilization in vitro
BT Artificial procreation

Incentive payment
SEE ALSO Capitation payment

Incentive spirometry
BT Respiratory therapy

Incontinent pads

Incubator therapy
SEE ALSO Incubators

Incubators
SEE ALSO Incubator therapy
Radiant warmers

Indomethacin
BT Nonsteroidal anti-inflammatory analgesics

Induction of labor

Infant foods
BT Metabolic and nutrient agents
SEE ALSO Diet therapy

Infectious disease tests
BT Diagnostic tests
NT Blood cultures
Hepatitis B tests

HIV detection assays
Rubella tests
Syphilis tests
Throat cultures
Urinalysis

Influenza vaccine
BT Vaccines

Information systems
x Decision support systems
Online information systems
NT Bibliographic information bases
Computer-assisted instruction
Medical record systems
MEDLARS
Reminder systems
SEE ALSO Communication systems
Data banks
Expert systems

Infusion controllers
SEE Infusion pumps

Infusion pumps
x Infusion controllers
Insulin delivery devices
Insulin pumps

—External

—Implantable

Injury severity scales

Insecticides
BT Antiparasitics
NT Malathion

Insulin

Insulin delivery devices
SEE Infusion pumps

Insulin injection

Insulin pumps
SEE Infusion pumps

Intensive care
NT Neonatal intensive care
SEE ALSO Intensive care systems, Mobile
Physiologic monitoring systems

Intensive care systems, Mobile
x Coronary care units, Mobile
Mobile intensive care systems
SEE ALSO Ambulances
Intensive care

Interferons
BT Antineoplastics
Antivirals
SEE ALSO Genetic engineering

Intermittent positive pressure breathing
x IPPB
BT Respiratory therapy

Intra-aortic balloon pumps
BT Circulatory assistance

Intracranial pressure monitoring
SEE ALSO Intracranial pressure monitors

Intracranial pressure monitors
SEE ALSO Intracranial pressure monitoring

Intracutaneous titration
x Rinkel serial intracutaneous titration
BT Allergy-immunology tests

Intraocular lens implantation
BT Surgery—Eye
SEE ALSO Intraocular lenses

Intraocular lenses
SEE ALSO Intraocular lens implantation

Intraosseous pressure measurement

Intravenous fat emulsions
x Fat emulsions

Iodide therapy
BT Bronchodilators

Iodoxamate meglumine
BT Radiographic contrast dyes

Iontophoresis

IPPB
SEE Intermittent positive pressure breathing

Iridology

Iron-dextran complex
BT Metabolic and nutrient agents

Isosulfan blue
BT Diagnostic agents

Isotretinoin
BT Antiacne agents

Joint prosthesis
x Orthopedic joint implants
BT Prostheses
NT Elbow prosthesis
Hip prosthesis
Knee prosthesis
SEE ALSO Bone cements
Bone prosthesis

Joint scanning using Technetium Tc-99m
SEE Scintiphotography—Joint

Keratomileusis
BT Keratoplasty

Keratophakia
BT Keratoplasty

Keratoplasty
NT Epikeratophakia
Keratomileusis
Keratophakia
Radial keratotomy

Ketoconazole
BT Antifungal agents

Keyes technique

Kidney function tests
BT Diagnostic tests
NT Blood urea concentration
Creatinine concentration, Serum

Kidney transplantation
SEE Transplantation—Kidney

Kinetic therapy
BT Physical therapy

Knee prosthesis
x New Jersey integrated knee replacement system
BT Joint prosthesis

Kunkel test
x Gammaglobulin, Total serum
BT Rheumatology tests

Kyphoscoliosis surgery
SEE Surgery—Scoliosis

L-Dopa
SEE Levodopa

Labetalol
BT Beta blockers

Lactates
BT Anti-anxiety agents

Laparotomy
BT Surgery

Laser angioplasty
BT Angioplasty
Laser surgery

Laser iridotomy
BT Laser surgery
Surgery—Eye

Laser photocoagulation
x Photocoagulation
BT Laser surgery
SEE ALSO Electrocoagulation

Laser radiation therapy
x Photoradiation therapy

Laser surgery
BT Surgery
NT Laser angioplasty
Laser iridotomy
Laser photocoagulation
Laser trabeculoplasty
SEE ALSO Lasers

—Carbon dioxide

—Nd:YAG

Laser trabeculoplasty
x Trabeculoplasty
BT Laser surgery

Lasers
SEE ALSO Laser surgery

—Carbon dioxide

—Nd:YAG

x Neodymium:Yttrium-aluminum garnet lasers

Laxatives
NT Sodium cellulose phosphate
Sodium phosphate

Lead screening

Leisure skills training

Leukocyte differential counters
BT Cell counters

Levodopa
x L-Dopa
BT Antidyskinetics

Lidocaine
BT Anesthetics

Ligament prosthesis
BT Prostheses

Limb perfusion

Linear pumps

Lipectomy
SEE Suction lipectomy

Lipoprotein evaluation
BT Cardiopulmonary tests

Lithium
BT Anti-anxiety agents
Antimanics

Lithotripsy
—Extracorporeal shock wave
x ESWL
Extracorporeal shock wave lithotripsy
SEE ALSO Lithotripters, Extracorporeal shock wave

—Percutaneous

—Transurethral
SEE ALSO Nephrolithotomy

Lithotripters, Extracorporeal shock wave
BT Ultrasound equipment—Therapeutic
SEE ALSO Lithotripsy—Extracorporeal shock wave

Liver transplantation
SEE Transplantation—Liver

Lixiscope
BT Radiographic equipment

Long term care
x Nursing homes

Lung cancer screening
SEE Cancer screening—Lung

Lymphangiography
BT Angiography

Magnesium chloride
BT Metabolic and nutrient agents

Magnesium sulfate
BT Anticonvulsants

Magnetic resonance imaging
x MRI
NMR
Nuclear magnetic resonance
BT Diagnostic imaging
SEE ALSO Magnetic resonance imaging systems

—Brain and spine

—Lung injury

—Multiple sclerosis

—Neoplasms

Magnetic resonance imaging systems
SEE ALSO Magnetic resonance imaging

Magnetic resonance spectroscopy

Magnetoencephalography
x MEG

Malathion
BT Insecticides

Mammographic devices
SEE ALSO Mammography

Mammography
BT Breast imaging
SEE ALSO Mammographic devices

Maple syrup urine disease screening

Marijuana
SEE Cannabis

Mass spectroscopy

Mastectomy
BT Surgery—Breast

Maternal serum alpha fetoprotein monitoring
x AFP monitoring
Alpha fetoprotein monitoring
BT Genetic screening
NT Alpha fetoprotein assays

Measles-mumps-rubella vaccine
x MMR vaccine
BT Vaccines

Medical evaluation
SEE Health examination

Medical Literature Analysis and Retrieval System
SEE MEDLARS

Medical record systems
BT Information systems
NT Registries
SEE ALSO Computer-assisted patient care
Expert systems
Reminder systems

Medicare Prospective Payment System
SEE Prospective payment systems

MEDLARS
x Medical Literature Analysis and Retrieval System
BT Information systems
NT CHEMLINE
HISTLINE
MEDLINE
TOXLINE

MEDLARS Online
SEE MEDLINE

MEDLINE
x MEDLARS Online
BT Bibliographic information bases
MEDLARS
—Optical disks
SEE ALSO Computer equipment

Medroxyprogesterone
x Depo-Provera
BT Progestins

MEG
SEE Magnetoencephalography

Melodic intonation therapy

Metabolic and nutrient agents
x Minerals
NT Amino acids
Artificial sweeteners
Calcium chloride
Dextrose
Dextrose with saline solution
Electrolyte injection
Fructose
Glutathione disulfides
Infant foods
Magnesium chloride

Polydextrose
Potassium chloride
Potassium citrate
Potassium phosphate
Vitamins
SEE ALSO Enteral nutrition
Oral rehydration therapy
Parenteral nutrition
Protein-calorie therapy with anabolic steroids

Methaqualone
BT Hypnotic drugs
Sedatives

Methotrexate
BT Antiarthritics
Antineoplastics
Antipsoriatics

Methoxsalen
BT Antipsoriatics
Repigmenting agents

Methyldopa
BT Antihypertensives

Methylethylketone
BT Solvents

Methylphenidate
x Attention deficit disorder therapy

Metoclopramide
SEE Oxybutynin chloride with metoclopramide

Metolazone
BT Antihypertensives
Diuretics

Metoprolol
BT Beta-blockers

Metronidazole
BT Antiarthritics
Antibiotics

Mezlocillin
BT Antibiotics

Miconazole
BT Antifungal agents

Microbiological testing systems
BT Diagnostic tests
NT Automated microbiology systems

Microbiology equipment

Micronucleus test
BT Cytotoxic tests

Microsurgery
BT Surgery

Migration inhibition test
BT Allergy-immunology tests

Minerals
BT Metabolic and nutrient agents

Minnesota Q-Qs codes
BT Electrocardiography

MMR vaccine
SEE Measles-mumps-rubella vaccine

Mobile intensive care systems
SEE Intensive care systems, Mobile

Mobility aids

Moire topography
x Photogrammetry
Shadow moire contourography

Monoclonal antibodies
x Antibodies
SEE ALSO Genetic engineering
Hybridomas
Immunoradiometric assay with monoclonal antibodies

Mouth protectors

Moxalactam
BT Cephalosporins

MRI
SEE Magnetic resonance imaging

Mycoplasma complement fixation test
BT Rheumatology tests

Myoelectric prostheses
BT Prostheses

Nadolol
BT Beta blockers

Nafcillin
BT Antibiotics

Nail bed transplantation
SEE Transplantation—Nail bed

Naloxone
BT Narcotic antagonists

Narcotic analgesics
BT Analgesics
NT Codeine
Hydromorphone
Pentazocine

Narcotic antagonists
NT Naloxone

Nd:YAG laser surgery
SEE Laser surgery—Nd:YAG

Nd:YAG lasers
SEE Lasers—Nd:YAG

Nebulizers
SEE ALSO Aerosol therapy

Needle aspiration cytology

Negative pressure respirators
BT Respirators

Neodymium:Yttrium-aluminum garnet lasers
SEE Nd:YAG lasers

Neonatal intensive care
BT Intensive care
SEE ALSO Neonatal monitors

Neonatal monitors
SEE ALSO Neonatal intensive care

Nephrolithotomy
BT Surgery
SEE ALSO Lithotripsy—Transurethral

Nephrostomy
BT Surgery

Neurosonology
SEE Ultrasound

Neurotoxins
NT Botulinum toxin

Neutralization therapy

—Food allergies
SEE ALSO Challenge food testing

New Jersey integrated knee replacement system
SEE Knee prosthesis

Niclosamide
BT Anthelmintics

Nicotine gum

Nifedipine
BT Calcium channel blockers

Nissen fundoplication
BT Surgery—Morbid obesity

Nitroglycerin
SEE Glyceryl trinitrate

Nitroprusside
BT Antihypertensives

NMR
SEE Magnetic resonance imaging

Noncardiac pain diagnosis

Nonionizing radiation measurement devices
BT Radiation measurement devices

Nonsteroidal anti-inflammatory analgesics
NT Diflunisal
Ibuprofen
Indomethacin
Piroxicam

Norethindrone with ethinyl estradiol
BT Oral contraceptives

Normaline kit

Nuclear magnetic resonance imaging
SEE Magnetic resonance imaging

Nursing homes
SEE Long term care

Nutritional counseling
BT Counseling
SEE ALSO Diet therapy

Obesity surgery
SEE Surgery—Morbid obesity

Omega-3 fatty acids
SEE Fish oils

Oncology tests
BT Diagnostic tests
NT Alpha fetoprotein assays
Bendien's test
Bolen's test
Carcinoembryonic antigen assays
In vitro chemosensitivity testing
Pap smear
Prostatic acid phosphatase kits
Stool guaiac
Tumor stem cell assays
SEE ALSO Cancer screening

Online information bases
SEE Information systems

Optical disk
SEE MEDLINE—Optical disks

Oral contraceptives
BT Contraception
NT Ethynodiol diacetate with ethinyl estradiol
Norethindrone with ethinyl estradiol
SEE ALSO Estrogens
Progestins

Oral rehydration therapy
x Fluid therapy
ORT
Rehydration therapy
SEE ALSO Metabolic and nutrient agents

Organ preservation
SEE ALSO Organ procurement
Transplantation

Organ procurement
SEE ALSO Organ preservation
Transplantation

Organ transplantation
SEE Transplantation

Orphan devices

ORT
SEE Oral rehydration therapy

Orthodontic appliances
x Orthodontic wires

Orthodontic wires
SEE Orthodontic appliances

Orthopedic joint implants
SEE Joint prosthesis

Orthotic devices
NT Posture control devices
Shoe insoles

Osseointegrated implants
SEE Dental implants

Osteoporosis screening

Osteotomy
SEE Tibial osteotomy

Outpatient surgery
SEE Surgery, Ambulatory

Oximeters
BT Blood gas monitors
SEE ALSO Oximetry

Oximetry
SEE ALSO Oximeters

Oxprenolol
BT Beta blockers

Oxybutynin chloride with metoclopramide
x Antispasmodics
Metoclopramide

Oxygen-air proportioners

Oxygen analyzers
SEE ALSO Blood gas monitors

Oxygen therapy
NT Hyperbaric oxygen therapy

—Inhalation

—Topical

PACS
SEE Picture archiving and communication systems

Pain assessment

Pain therapy
x Analgesia
NT Acupuncture
Transcutaneous electrical nerve stimulation
SEE ALSO Analgesics

Palatopharyngoplasty
BT Surgery

Pancreas transplantation
SEE Transplantation—Pancreas

Pap smear
BT Oncology tests
SEE ALSO Cancer screening—Cervical

Papaverine
BT Impotence diagnosis
Impotence treatment
Vasodilators

Parenteral nutrition
x Total parenteral nutrition
TPN
SEE ALSO Metabolic and nutrient agents

Partial thromboplastin time
BT Coagulation assays

Patch tests
BT Allergy-immunology tests

PEEP valves
x Positive end expiratory pressures valves

Peer group counseling
BT Counseling

Penicillamine
BT Antiarthritics
Antiurolithics
SEE ALSO Chelation therapy—Pencillamine

Penile artery bypass
BT Surgery—Impotence

Penile prosthesis
BT Prostheses

Pentazocine
BT Narcotic analgesics

Pentetate indium disodium
BT Radiopharmaceuticals

Percutaneous balloon valvuloplasty
BT Surgery
SEE ALSO Balloon dilatation catheters

Percutaneous transluminal angioplasty
x Balloon angioplasty
PTA
BT Angioplasty
NT Percutaneous transluminal coronary angioplasty

Percutaneous transluminal coronary angioplasty
x Coronary artery surgery
PTCA
BT Percutaneous transluminal angioplasty
Surgery—Heart

Perimetry
BT Vision screening

Periodontal ligament injection

Peritoneal dialysis
BT Dialysis
NT Continuous ambulatory peritoneal dialysis
SEE ALSO Peritoneal dialysis cyclers
Peritoneal dialysis solutions

Peritoneal dialysis cyclers
SEE ALSO Peritoneal dialysis
Peritoneal dialysis solutions

Peritoneal dialysis solutions
SEE ALSO Peritoneal dialysis
Peritoneal dialysis cyclers

Permanent eyeliner
BT Surgery

Persantine
SEE Dipyridamole

Pertussis vaccine
BT Vaccines

PET scan
SEE Positron emission tomography

Phenobarbital
BT Anticonvulsants
Hypnotic drugs
Sedatives

Phenylketonuria screening
BT Genetic screening

Phenylpropanolamine
BT Appetite suppressants

Phenytoin
BT Anticonvulsants

Phlebography
x Venography

Phonocardiography

Photocoagulation
SEE Laser photocoagulation

Photodensitometry
SEE Bone mineral studies

Photogrammetry
SEE Moire topography

Photokymography
SEE ALSO Coronary artery disease diagnosis

Photoplethysmography
SEE Plethysmography

Photoradiation therapy
SEE Laser radiation therapy

Phototherapy
NT Ultraviolet therapy
SEE ALSO Laser radiation therapy

Phyllocontin
SEE Aminophylline

Physical examination
SEE Health examination

Physical therapy
x Physiotherapy
NT Doman-Delacato treatment
Exercise therapy
Kinetic therapy

Physical therapy with home exercise
SEE ALSO Exercise therapy

Physician education
x Continuing medical education
SEE ALSO Computer-assisted instruction

Physiologic monitoring systems
SEE ALSO Apnea monitors
Blood pressure monitors
Electrocardiographs
Intensive care

Physiotherapy
SEE Physical therapy

Picture archiving and communication systems
x PACS
SEE ALSO Digital imaging

Pindolol
BT Beta blockers

Piperacillin
BT Antibiotics

Piroxicam
BT Nonsteroidal anti-inflammatory analgesics

Pituitary and hypothalmic hormones
BT Hormones
NT Gonadorelin hydrochloride
Human growth hormone

Plasma exchange
x Therapeutic plasma exchange
TPE
BT Apheresis
SEE ALSO Plasma exchange devices
Plasma, Frozen
Plasma infusion
Plasmapheresis

Plasma exchange devices
SEE ALSO Plasma exchange

Plasma filters
SEE ALSO Plasma perfusion
Plasma separation systems

Plasma, Frozen
SEE ALSO Plasma exchange
Plasma infusion

Plasma infusion
SEE ALSO Plasma exchange
Plasma, Frozen

Plasma perfusion
BT Apheresis
SEE ALSO Plasma filters

Plasma separation systems
SEE ALSO Apheresis
Plasma filters

Plasmapheresis
BT Apheresis
SEE ALSO Plasma exchange

Plasminogen activators
SEE Tissue plasminogen activators

Plasticizers

Platelet transfusion
x Thrombocyte transfusion
BT Transfusion

Plethysmography
x Impedance plethysmography
Photoplethysmography
SEE ALSO Impotence diagnosis

Pneumococcal vaccine
BT Vaccines

Polydextrose
BT Metabolic and nutrient agents

Polypectomy
BT Surgery

Polyurethane tubing

Positive end expiratory pressure valves
SEE PEEP valves

Positron emission tomography
x PET scan
Tomography, Emission computed
Tomography, Positron emission
SEE ALSO SPECT imaging

Postmarketing surveillance
BT Assessment methods

Postural drainage
BT Respiratory therapy

Posture control devices
BT Orthotics

Potassium chloride
BT Metabolic and nutrient agents

Potassium citrate
x Citrates
BT Metabolic and nutrient agents

Potassium phosphate
BT Metabolic and nutrient agents

PPS
SEE Prospective payment systems

Praziquantel
BT Anthelmintics

Prazosin
BT Antihypertensives

Prenatal care

Prenatal education

Prepayment
SEE Capitation payment

Prescribing
SEE Drug ordering

Pressure transducers

Primadone
BT Anticonvulsants

Progestin receptor assays

Progestins
BT Adrenal cortex hormones
Sex hormones
NT Medroxyprogesterone
SEE ALSO Oral contraceptives
Progestin receptor assays

Prolotherapy
SEE ALSO Sclerotherapy

Propranolol
BT Beta blockers

Prospective payment systems
x Medicare Prospective Payment System
PPS
NT Discretionary adjustment factor
SEE ALSO Capitation payment
Competition
DRGs

Prostaglandins
NT Alprostadil

Prostate surgery
SEE Surgery—Prostate

Prostatic acid phosphatase kits
BT Oncology tests
SEE ALSO Tumor markers

Prostheses
NT Gastroesophageal antireflux prosthesis
Joint prosthesis
Ligament prosthesis
Myoelectric prostheses
Penile prosthesis
Socket prosthesis

Protein-calorie therapy with anabolic steroids
x Anabolic steroids
BT Diet therapy
SEE ALSO Metabolic and nutrient agents

Prothrombin-complex concentrate
SEE Anti-inhibitor coagulant complex

Prothrombin time
BT Coagulation assays

Provocation tests—Food allergies
SEE Challenge food testing

Psoralens and ultraviolet A therapy
SEE PUVA therapy

Psychoactive drugs
BT Psychotherapy
NT Antianxiety agents
Antidepressants
Antipsychotics
Hypnotic drugs
Sedatives

Psychosurgery
BT Psychotherapy
Surgery

Psychotherapy
NT Psychoactive drugs
Psychosurgery

PTA
SEE Percutaneous transluminal angioplasty

PTCA
SEE Percutaneous transluminal coronary angioplasty

Pulmonary function tests
SEE ALSO Respiratory therapy

Punctal occlusion
BT Surgery—Eye

PUVA therapy
x Psoralens and ultraviolet A therapy
BT Ultraviolet therapy

Pyelography
BT Radiography

Pyrimethamine
BT Antiprotozoal agents

Quality assurance programs

Radial keratotomy
BT Keratoplasty

Radiant warmers
SEE ALSO Incubators

Radiation measurement
x Dosimetry
NT Nonionizing radiation measurement devices
SEE ALSO Radiation protection

Radiation protection
SEE ALSO Radiation measurement

Radiation therapy
x Heavy-ion irradiation

Radioactive materials
NT Radiopharmaceuticals

Radioallergosorbent test
x RAST
BT Immunoradiometric assays

Radiogrammetry
SEE Bone mineral studies

Radiographic absorptiometry
SEE Absorptiometry

Radiographic contrast dyes
x Contrast media
BT Radiographic materials
NT Iodoxemate meglumine
SEE ALSO Radiopharmaceuticals

Radiographic darkrooms
x Darkrooms

Radiographic equipment
x X-ray equipment
NT Computed tomography scanners
Fluoroscopy units
Lixiscope
Radiographic film processors
SEE ALSO Radiography

Radiographic film
x X-ray film
BT Radiographic materials

Radiographic film processors
x X-ray film processors
BT Radiographic equipment

Radiographic materials
NT Radiographic contrast dyes
Radiographic film

Radiography
x Roentgenography
X-rays
BT Diagnostic imaging
NT Cholangiography
Cholangiopancreatography
Cholecystography
Computed tomography
Discography
Fluoroscopy
Pyelography
Urography
SEE ALSO Digital imaging
Imaging centers
Radiation protection
Radiographic equipment
Radiographic materials

Radiography, Dental
SEE Dental radiography

Radioimmunoassays
SEE Immunoradiometric assays

Radionuclide angiography
BT Angiography
Radionuclide imaging

Radionuclide imaging
BT Diagnostic imaging
NT Gamma cameras
Radionuclide angiography

Scintiphotography
SPECT
Thallium imaging
Ventilation-perfusion lung scans
SEE ALSO Radionuclide laboratories
Radiopharmaceuticals

Radionuclide laboratories
SEE ALSO Radionuclide imaging

Radiopaque plastics
BT Dental radiography

Radiopharmaceuticals
BT Radioactive materials
NT Pentetate indium sodium
Technetium Tc-99m kits
Xenon
SEE ALSO Radiographic contrast dyes
Radionuclide imaging

Randomized clinical trials
SEE Clinical trials—Randomized

Ranitidine
BT Histamine H2-receptor antagonists

RAST
SEE Radioallergosorbent test

Rectal mucosal replacement

Registries
BT Medical record systems
SEE ALSO Data banks

Rehabilitation
NT Cardiac rehabilitation
Pain rehabilitation
SEE ALSO Rehabilitation programs

Rehabilitation programs
SEE ALSO Rehabilitation

—Spinal cord injury

—Stroke

Rehfuss test
BT Gastroenterology tests

Rehydration therapy
SEE Oral rehydration therapy

Relative value scales

Relaxation therapy

Reminder systems
x Appointment reminders
BT Information systems
SEE ALSO Medical record systems

Repigmenting agents
NT Methoxsalen

Reserpine
BT Antihypertensives

Reserpine with chlorthalidone
BT Antihypertensives
SEE ALSO Chlorthalidone

Respirators
NT Negative pressure repirators
SEE ALSO Respiratory therapy
Ventilators

Respiratory therapy
NT Aerosol therapy
Continuous positive airway pressure
Incentive spirometry
Intermittent positive pressure breathing
Postural drainage
SEE ALSO Pulmonary function tests
Respirators

Resuscitation
SEE ALSO Resuscitators

—Mouth-to-mouth

Resuscitators
SEE ALSO Resuscitation

Reuse of disposables
x Disposables reuse

Rheumatology tests
x Arthritis tests
BT Diagnostic tests
NT Bentonite flocculation test
DNA-antibody test
Kunkel test
Mycoplasma complement fixation test

Rhinoplasty
BT Surgery

Ringer's irrigation

Rinkel serial intracutaneous titration
SEE Intracutaneous titration

Roentgenography
SEE Radiography

Routine admission testing
SEE Admission testing, Routine

Rubella tests
x Antibody tests
BT Infectious disease tests

Rubidium
BT Antipsychotics

Saccharin
BT Artificial sweeteners

Saralasin
BT Antihypertensives

Satellite communication
BT Communication systems

Scales, Patient

Schizophrenia screening

Scintiphotography
BT Radionuclide imaging
SEE ALSO Technetium Tc-99m kits

—Heart

—Joint

Sclerotherapy
SEE ALSO Prolotherapy

Scoliosometry

Screening
SEE specific diseases or disorders, e.g. Cancer screening

Seat belts (Automobile)
SEE Automobile passenger restraints

Second opinions

Secretin
BT Diagnostic agents
Gastric acid secretion inhibitors
Hormones

Sedatives
BT Psychoactive drugs
NT Barbiturates
Methaqualone
Phenobarbital

Selenium sulfide
BT Antifungal agents
Antiseborrheic agents

Sensory integrative therapy

Seromucoid assay
BT Diagnostic tests

Serum creatinine concentration
SEE Creatinine concentration, Serum

Sex hormones
BT Hormones
Steroids
NT Androgens
Estrogens
Progestins

Sex selection
SEE Ericsson sex selection method

Shadow moire contourography
SEE Moire topography

Shape sensor

Shoe insoles
BT Orthotic devices

SI units
SEE Systeme International units

Sickle cell screening
SEE Hemoglobinopathies screening

Sigmoidoscopy
x Flexible sigmoidoscopy
BT Gastrointestinal endoscopy

SEE ALSO Barium enema with sigmoidoscopy
Cancer screening—Colorectal

Silver sulfadiazine
BT Antibiotics

Singer-Blom valve operation
BT Surgery

Single photon emission computed tomography
SEE SPECT imaging

Sisomicin
BT Antibiotics

Smoke detectors

Socket prosthesis
BT Prostheses

Sodium cellulose phosphate
BT Laxatives

Sodium chloride
BT Metabolic and nutrient agents

Sodium phosphate
BT Laxatives

Sodium restriction
BT Diet therapy

Solvents
NT Methylethylketone

Somatic cell mutation tests
BT Genetic tests

Somatotropin
SEE Human growth hormone

Sorbitol
BT Artificial sweeteners

SPECT imaging
x Single photon emission computed tomography
Tomography, Single photon emission computed
BT Radionuclide imaging
SEE ALSO Computed tomography
Positron emission tomography

Specular microscopy
SEE Endothelial cell photography

Sperm penetration assay
BT Fertility tests

Sphincterotomy
x Endoscopic retrograde sphincterotomy
ERS
BT Surgery

Sphygmomanometers
SEE Blood pressure monitors

Sphygmomanometry
SEE Blood pressure monitoring

Spinal injury programs
SEE Rehabilitation programs—Spinal cord injury

Spinal puncture
BT Surgery

Sporicidin
BT Antifungal agents

Sprinklers

Standardized Medreview Instrument

Stapedectomy
BT Surgery

Stapling
SEE Surgical stapling

Stereotaxic depth electrode implantation
BT Surgery
SEE ALSO Electroencephalography

Stereotaxic neurosurgery, Computed tomography-assisted
BT Surgery

Sterile water for injection

Sterilization equipment
SEE ALSO Sterilizers

Sterilizers
SEE ALSO Sterilization equipment

Steroids
NT Adrenal cortex hormones
Sex hormones
SEE ALSO Hydroxycholecalciferol level
Protein-calorie therapy with anabolic steroids

Stool guaiac
BT Oncology tests
SEE ALSO Cancer screening—Colorectal

Streptokinase
x Thrombolytic therapy

Streptozocin
BT Antineoplastics

Stress tests
SEE Exercise tests

Stroke programs
SEE Rehabilitation programs—Stroke

Sucralfate
BT Antiulcer agents

Suction equipment

Suction lipectomy
x Lipectomy
BT Surgery—Morbid obesity

Sulfadoxine
BT Antiprotozoal agents

Sulfamethoxazole
x Sulfonamides
BT Antibacterials

Sulfinpyrazone
BT Antigout agents
Antihyperuricemics

Sulfonamides
SEE Sulfamethoxazole

Suloctidil
BT Vasodilators

Sunlamps
SEE ALSO Phototherapy

Supportive care
SEE ALSO Burn units

Surgery
NT Adenoidectomy
Angioplasty
Biopsy
Carotid body resection
Carotid endarterectomy
Cerebral artery anastomosis
Cesarean section
Cholecystectomy
Cingulotomy
Circumcision
Cochlear implantation
Cochleostomy
Collagen implants
Cryosurgery
Debridement
Decubitus surgery
Dilatation and curettage
Electrocoagulation
Electrosurgery
Endoscopy
Extracranial-intracranial arterial bypass
Hip joint replacement
Hysterectomy
Laparotomy
Laser surgery
Mastectomy
Microsurgery
Nephrolithotomy
Nephrostomy
Palatopharyngoplasty
Percutaneous balloon valvuloplasty
Permanent eyeliner
Polypectomy
Psychosurgery
Rhinoplasty
Singer-Blom valve operation
Sphincterotomy
Spinal puncture
Stapedectomy
Stereotaxic depth electrode implantation
Stereotaxic neurosurgery, Computed tomography-assisted
Surgical stapling
Temporomandibular joint procedure
Thoracentesis

Tibial osteotomy
Tibial tubercle elevation
Tonsillectomy
Tooth extraction
Transplantation
Transsexual surgery
Tubal ligation
Vertebral artery surgery

—Ambulatory
x Outpatient surgery

—Breast
NT Contralateral breast surgery
Mastectomy

—Esophageal reflux

—Eye
NT Cataract extraction
Corneal grafts
Intraocular lens implantation
Keratoplasty
Laser iridotomy
Punctal occlusion
SEE ALSO Surgical aids—Ophthalmic

—Fetal
SEE ALSO Fetal shunts

—Heart
NT Cardiac catheterization
Coronary artery bypass grafting
Percutaneous transluminal coronary angioplasty
SEE ALSO Cryosurgery—Arrhythmias
Percutaneous transluminal valvuloplasty

—Impotence
NT Penile artery bypass

—Morbid obesity
NT Bilio-pancreatic bypass
Gastric restrictive surgery
Gastro-ileal bypass
Ileal bypass
Nissen fundoplication
Suction lipectomy

—Prostate

—Scoliosis

Surgical aids

—Ophthalmic

Surgical case carts

Surgical drapes

Surgical gloves

Surgical shunt

Surgical stapling
x Stapling
BT Surgery

Sutures

Syphylis tests
BT Infectious disease tests

Syringe pumps

Systeme International units
x SI units

Tamoxifen
BT Antineoplastics

Team care

Technetium Tc 99m kits
BT Radiopharmaceuticals
SEE ALSO Scintiphotography

Telemetry
BT Communication systems

Temazepam
BT Antianxiety agents

Temporomandibular joint procedure
x TMJ procedure
BT Surgery

TENS
SEE Transcutaneous electrical nerve stimulation

Thallium imaging
BT Radionuclide imaging

Theo-Dur
SEE Theophylline

Theophylline
x Theo-Dur
BT Bronchodilators
SEE ALSO Aminophylline

Therapeutic drug monitoring
x Drug monitoring

Therapeutic embolization
x Embolotherapy

Therapeutic plasma exchange
SEE Plasma exchange

Thermography
BT Diagnostic imaging

—Breast
BT Breast imaging

Thermometers

Thiamine
SEE Vitamin B1

Thoracentesis
BT Surgery

Throat cultures
BT Infectious disease tests

Thrombocyte transfusion
SEE Platelet transfusion

Thrombolytic therapy
NT Streptokinase
Tissue plasminogen activators

Thymoxamine
BT Vasodilators

Thyroxine assays
BT Endocrinology-metabolism tests

Tibial osteotomy
x Osteotomy
BT Surgery

Tibial tubercle elevation
BT Surgery

Timolol
BT Antiglaucoma agents

Tinnitus maskers

Tioconazole
BT Antifungal agents

Tissue banks
SEE ALSO Tissue preservation technics

Tissue plasminogen activators
x Plasminogen activators
TPA
BT Thrombolytic therapy

Tissue preservation technics
SEE ALSO Tissue banks

TMJ procedure
SEE Temporomandibular joint procedure

Tobramycin
BT Antibiotics

Tocodynamometry
x Uterine monitoring

Tomographic scanners
SEE Computed tomographic scanners

Tomography, Emission computed
SEE Positron emission tomography

Tomography, Positron emission
SEE Positron emission tomography

Tomography, Single photon emission computed
SEE SPECT imaging

Tomography, Standard

Tomography, X-ray computed
SEE Computed tomography

Tonometry
BT Vision screening

Tonsillectomy
BT Surgery

Tooth extraction
BT Surgery

Toothpaste
BT Dental materials

Topical oxygen therapy
SEE Oxygen therapy—Topical

Topographic brain mapping
SEE ALSO Electroencephalography

Total hip joint replacement
SEE Hip joint replacement

Total parenteral nutrition
SEE Parenteral nutrition

Tourniquets

Toxicology Information Online
SEE TOXLINE

TOXLINE
x Toxicology Information Online
BT Bibliographic information bases
MEDLARS

TPA
SEE Tissue plasminogen activators

TPE
SEE Plasma exchange

TPN
SEE Parenteral nutrition

Trabeculoplasty
SEE Laser trabeculoplasty

Tranquilizers
SEE Antianxiety agents

Transcutaneous electrical nerve stimulation
x TENS
BT Electrical stimulation
Pain therapy

Transfer factor therapy

Transfusion
NT Blood transfusion
Granulocyte transfusion
Platelet transfusion

Transillumination

—Breast
x Diaphanography
BT Breast imaging
Diagnostic imaging

Transplantation
BT Surgery
SEE ALSO Organ preservation
Organ procurement

—Bone marrow

—Bone marrow, Allogenic

—Bone marrow, Autologous

—Cornea

—Heart

—Heart-lung

—Kidney

—Liver

—Nail bed

—Pancreas

Transsexual surgery
BT Surgery

Trazodone
BT Antidepressants

Triamterene
BT Diuretics

Triazolam
BT Antianxiety agents

Trimethoprim
BT Antibiotics

Tryptophan
BT Antidepressants

Tubal ligation
BT Contraception
Surgery

Tuberculosis screening

Tumor markers
SEE ALSO Alpha fetoprotein assays
Carcinoembryonic antigen assays
Prostatic acid phosphatase kits

Tumor stem cell assay
BT Oncology tests

Tympanometry
SEE Acoustic impedance test

Type A score

Ultrasonography
x B-mode scanning
Echocine
BT Diagnostic imaging
Ultrasound
NT Echocardiography

—Arteries
BT Arteriography
SEE ALSO Echocardiography

—Breast

—Follicular growth
SEE ALSO Ultrasound—Obstetrics and gynecology

—Head

—Pancreas

—Pregnancy
SEE ALSO Ultrasound—Obstetrics and gynecology

—Prostate

—Sinuses

Ultrasound
x Doppler ultrasound
Neurosonology
NT Ultrasonography
SEE ALSO Lithotripsy, Extracorporeal shock wave
Lithotripsy, Percutaneous
Ultrasound equipment—Therapeutic

—Cardiac output
SEE ALSO Coronary artery disease diagnosis

—Intraoperative

—Obstetrics and gynecology
SEE ALSO Ultrasonography—Follicular growth

—Pelvimetry

Ultrasound equipment
SEE ALSO Ultrasound

—Diagnostic

—Therapeutic
NT Lithotripters, Extracorporeal shockwave

Ultraviolet therapy
BT Phototherapy
NT PUVA therapy

Unbundling
BT Health insurance

Ureteroscopy
BT Endoscopy

Urinalysis
x Urine culture
BT Infectious disease tests
SEE ALSO Urologic disease screening

Urinary sphincter, Artificial

Urine autoinjection

Urine culture
SEE Urinalysis

Urography
BT Radiography

Urologic disease screening
SEE ALSO Urinalysis

Uterine monitoring
SEE Tocodynamometry

Vaccination policy

Vaccines
NT BCG vaccine
Hemophilus influenza type B vaccine
Influenza vaccine
Measles-mumps-rubella vaccine
Pertussis vaccine
Pneumococcal vaccine
Viral hepatitis vaccine

Valproate
x Valproic acid
BT Anticonvulsants

Valproic acid
SEE Valproate

Vascular access ports

Vascular headache suppressants
NT Dihydroergotamine

Vasodilators
NT Dipyridamole
Glyceryl trinitrate
Papaverine
Suloctidil
Thymoxamine

Vasopressors
NT Dopamine

Venography
SEE Phlebography

Ventilation-perfusion lung scans
BT Radionuclide imaging

Ventilators
SEE ALSO Respirators

Ventricular assist devices
BT Circulatory assistance

Ventricular mapping, Intraoperative
BT Electrocardiography

Verapamil
BT Calcium channel blockers

Vertebral artery surgery
BT Surgery

Vidarabine
BT Antivirals

Viral hepatitis vaccine
x Hepatitis B vaccine
BT Vaccines

Vision aids
NT Eyeglasses

Vision screening
NT Glaucoma screening
Perimetry
Tonometry

Visual evoked potentials
SEE Evoked potentials

Vitamin A
SEE ALSO Beta-carotene

Vitamin B1
x Thiamine

Vitamin B12 assay
BT Endocrinology-metabolism tests
Vitamins

Vitamin E
BT Vitamins

Vitamins
BT Metabolic and nutrient agents
NT Vitamin A
Vitamin B1
Vitamin B12 assay
Vitamin E
SEE ALSO Hydroxycholecalciferol level

Warfarin
BT Anticoagulants

Wheelchair tray systems

Wheelchairs

Whirlpool baths
SEE Hydrotherapy

X-ray equipment
SEE Radiographic equipment

X-ray film
SEE Radiographic film

X-ray film processors
SEE Radiographic film processors

X-rays
SEE Radiography

X-rays, Dental
SEE Radiography, Dental

Xenon
BT Radiopharmaceuticals

Xylitol
BT Artificial sweeteners

Yohimbine
BT Alpha receptor blocking agents
Impotency treatment

Zomepirac sodium
BT Analgesics

25 hydroxyvitamin D level
SEE Hydroxycholecalciferol level

ASSESSMENT REPORT CITATIONS BY TECHNOLOGY

Absorptiometry

National Center for Health Servicés Research and Health Care Technology Assessment, Office of Health Technology Assessment. Bone mineral density studies: radiographic absorptiometry. Ongoing.

Absorptiometry—Dual photon

Blue Cross and Blue Shield Association, Technology Evaluation and Coverage Program. Absorptiometry, dual photon for osteoporosis monitoring. 1986. [Information syntheses]

Blue Cross and Blue Shield Association, Technology Evaluation and Coverage Program. Absorptiometry, single and dual photon. 1986. [Information syntheses]

ECRI Technology Assessment Program. Bone mineral assessment, noninvasive (dual photon absorptiometry and quantitative computed tomography). J Health Care Technol 1986;2:183-200. [Information syntheses]

National Center for Health Services Research and Health Care Technology Assessment, Office of Health Technology Assessment. Dual photon absorptiometry for measuring bone mineral density. 1986.

ECRI Technology Assessment Program. Dual-photon absorptiometry for bone mineral content. Issues Health Care Technol 1984;sec.5.A.3. [Information syntheses]

Absorptiometry—Single photon

Blue Cross and Blue Shield Association, Technology Evaluation and Coverage Program. Absorptiometry, single and dual photon. 1986. [Information syntheses]

National Center for Health Services Research and Health Care Technology Assessment, Office of Health Technology Assessment. Single photon absorptiometry for measuring bone mineral density. 1986.

Acetaminophen

Racz WJ. [Department Pharmacology, Queens University] [Medical Research Council - Canada] Acetaminophen induced hepatotoxicity. (Grant period 1983-1985).

Food and Drug Administration, Center for Drugs and Biologics. Pentazocine hydrochloride and acetaminophen. 1982. (NTIS order no. PB82-915904). [Information syntheses, Expert opinion, epidemiological and other observational methods, Clinical trials, Bench testing]

Acetohydroxamic acid

Food and Drug Administration, Center for Drugs and Biologics. Acetohydroxamic acid. 1987. (Summary basis of approval, NDA # 18-749). [Information syntheses, Expert opinion, Epidemiological and other observational methods, Clinical trials, Bench testing]

Acidulated phosphate fluoride

Clark DC, Hanley JA, Stamm JW, Weinstein PL. [McGill University, Department of Epidemiology and Biostatistics] An empirically based system to estimate the effectiveness of caries-preventive agents: a comparison of the effectiveness estimates of APF gels and solutions and fluoride varnishes. Caries Res 1985;19:83-95.

Acoustic impedance tests

California Medical Association, Medical Practice Opinion Program. Acoustic impedance testing in school screening. 1985 Sep. (Medical Practice Opinion #325) [Group judgment]

Acupuncture

American Academy of Neurology, Practice Committee. Acupuncture. 1981 Jul. [Expert opinion, Group judgment]

American Medical Association, Council on Scientific Affairs. Acupuncture. 1981. [Group judgment]

Acyclovir

Food and Drug Administration, Center for Drugs and Biologics. Acyclovir. 1982. (NTIS order no. PB82-915902). [Information syntheses, Expert opinion, Epidemiological and other observational methods, Clinical trials, Bench testing]

Adenoidectomy

National Institutes of Health, Consensus Development Program. Indications for tonsillectomy and adenoidectomy: phase I. (Consensus Development Conference Statement, Jul 20 1978). [Group judgment]

Adhesives

American Dental Association, Council on Dental Materials, Instruments and Equipment. Council update on "adhesion" and "adhesive" materials. J Am Dent Assoc 1981;103:252-253.

Admission testing, Routine

U.S. Administrators, Professional Policy Committee. Admission screening - hospital. [7/86] [Group judgment]

U.S. Administrators, Professional Policy Committee. Preadmission/presurgical screening. [7/86] [Group judgment]

Kaplan EB, et al. [National Center for Health Services Research and Health Care Technology Assessment, Division of Extramural Research] The usefulness of preoperative laboratory screening. JAMA 1985 Jun;253(24):3576-3589.

Blue Cross and Blue Shield Association, Medical Necessity Program. Routine admission testing - medical admissions. 1983. [Information syntheses]

Blue Cross and Blue Shield Association, Medical Necessity Program. Routine admission testing - surgical admissions. 1983. [Information syntheses]

Adrenal cortex hormones

Veterans Administration, Cooperative Studies Program. Evaluations of corticosteroid therapy in gram negative sepsis. Pending. [Clinical trials]

Keogh BA, Bernardo J, Hunninghake GW, et al. [National Heart, Lung, and Blood Institute] Effect of intermittent high dose parenteral corticosteroids on the alveolitis of idiopathic pulmonary fibrosis. Am Rev Respir Dis 1983;127:18-27.

Veterans Administration, Cooperative Studies Program. Evaluations of corticosteroid therapy in severe sepsis. Ongoing. [Clinical trials]

Aerosol therapy

Blue Cross and Blue Shield Association, Medical Necessity Program. Respiratory therapy: aerosol therapy. 1982. [Information syntheses]

Albuterol

Food and Drug Administration, Center for Drugs and Biologics. Albuterol sulfate. 1982. (NTIS order no. PB82-915903). [Information syntheses, Expert opinion, Epidemiological and other observational methods, Clinical trials, Bench testing]

Alclometasone dipropionate

Food and Drug Administration, Center for Drugs and Biologics. Alclometasone dipropionate. 1983. (NTIS order no. PB83-915901). [Information syntheses, Expert opinion, Epidemiological and other observational methods, Clinical trials, Bench testing]

Alcoholism screening

Hirst M. [National Health Research and Development Program - Canada] Toward a non-invasive screen for susceptibility to alcoholism. 1986. (Grant No. 6606-2676-52).

Allergy-immunology tests

American College of Physicians, Clinical Efficacy Assessment Project. Allergy testing, expected completion 1988. [Information syntheses]

Allopurinol

Food and Drug Administration, Center for Drugs and Biologics. Allopurinol 100 mg. 1987. (Summary basis of approval, NDA # 18-832). [Information syntheses, Expert opinion, Epidemiological and other observational methods, Clinical trials, Bench testing]

Food and Drug Administration, Center for Drugs and Biologics. Allopurinol 300 mg. 1987. (Summary basis of approval, NDA # 18-832). [Information syntheses, Expert opinion, Epidemiological and other observational methods, Clinical trials, Bench testing]

Alpha fetoprotein assays

Travenol Labs, Inc. [Food and Drug Administration, Center for Devices and Radiological Health] Gamma dab (1251) AFP RIA kit: summary of safety and effectiveness. 1986 Jun 17. (PMA no. P790032-000).

Centers for Disease Control. [Food and Drug Administration, Center for Devices and Radiological Health] AFP mid-pregnancy reference preparation: summary of safety and effectiveness. 1985 Jan 3 (PMA no. P820077-000).

Hybritech, Inc. [Food and Drug Administration, Center for Devices and Radiological Health] Tandem (R)-E AFP: summary of safety and effectiveness. 1985 May 23. (PMA no. P840035-000).

Kallestad Labs, Inc. [Food and Drug Administration, Center for Devices and Radiological Health] Quantitope 1251 AFP kit and control serum: summary of safety and effectiveness. 1985 Feb 17. (PMA no. PB00025-000).

Abbott. [Food and Drug Administration, Center for Devices and Radiological Health] Abbott AFP: summary of safety and effectiveness. 1984 Jul 25. (PMA no. P780005-000).

Amersham Corporation. [Food and Drug Administration, Center for Devices and Radiological Health] Amersham AFP: summary of safety and effectiveness. 1984 Jul 6 (PMA no. P78006-000).

Wampole Labs. [Food and Drug Administration, Center for Devices and Radiological Health] AFP RIA kit: summary of safety and effectiveness. 1984 Feb 17. (PMA no.P76001-000).

Abbott Labs. [Food and Drug Administration, Center for Devices and Radiological Health] Abbott AF-P-EIA diagnostic kit for cancer: summary of safety and effectiveness. 1983 Jul 19. (PMA no. P820060).

Alprazolam

Food and Drug Administration, Center for Drugs and Biologics. Alprazolam. 1982. (NTIS order no. PB82-915901). [Information syntheses, Expert opinion, Epidemiological and other observational methods, Clinical trials, Bench testing]

Alprostadil

Food and Drug Administration, Center for Drugs and Biologics. Alprostadil (PGE1). 1982. (NTIS order no. PB82-915901). [Information syntheses, Expert opinion, Epidemiological and other observational methods, Clinical trials, Bench testing]

Alternative medicine

Office of Technology Assessment, U.S. Congress. Nontraditional methods of cancer management. Washington, D.C.: U.S. Government Printing Office (to be completed in Summer 1988).

Health Council of the Netherlands. Alternative medicine. Ongoing assessment.

Amantadine

National Institutes of Health, Consensus Development Program. Amantadine: does it have a role in the prevention and treatment of influenza? (Consensus Development Conference Statement, Oct 15-16 1979). [Group judgment]

Ambulances

American Academy of Pediatrics, Committee on Hospital Care. Guidelines for air and ground transportation. Pediatrics (To be published).

Amcinonide

Food and Drug Administration, Center for Drugs and Biologics. Amcinonide. 1982. (NTIS order no. PB82-915901). [Information syntheses, Expert opinion, Epidemiological and other observational methods, Clinical trials, Bench testing]

Amiloride

Food and Drug Administration, Center for Drugs and Biologics. Amiloride HCl. 1982. (NTIS order no. PB82-915901). [Information syntheses, Expert opinion, Epidemiological and other observational methods, Clinical trials, Bench testing]

Food and Drug Administration, Center for Drugs and Biologics. Amiloride HCl/hydrochlorothiazide. 1982. (NTIS order no. PB82-915901). [Information syntheses, Expert opinion, Epidemiological and other observational methods, Clinical trials, Bench testing]

Amino acids

Food and Drug Administration, Center for Drugs and Biologics. 8% amion [sic] acid injection. 1982. (NTIS order no. PB82-915904). [Information syntheses, Expert opinion, Epidemiological and other observational methods, Clinical trials, Bench testing]

Aminocaproic acids

Food and Drug Administration, Center for Drugs and Biologics. 8% amino acid injection. 1982. (NTIS order no.PB82-915904). [Information syntheses, Expert opinion, Epidemiological and other observational methods, Clinical trials, Bench testing]

Aminoglutethimide

Food and Drug Administration, Center for Drugs and Biologics. Aminoglutethimide. 1981. (NTIS order no. PB81-915901). [Information syntheses, Expert opinion, Epidemiological and other observational methods, Clinical trials, Bench testing]

Aminophylline

Food and Drug Administration, Center for Drugs and Biologics. Aminophylline, USP. 1982/ (NTIS order no. PB82-915903). [Information syntheses, Expert opinion, Epidemiological and other observational methods, Clinical trials, Bench testing]

Amoxicillin

Food and Drug Administration, Center for Drugs and Biologics. Amoxicillin. 1981. (NTIS order no. PB81-915901). [Information syntheses, Expert opinion, Epidemiological and other observational methods, Clinical trials, Bench testing]

Analgesics

National Institutes of Health, Consensus Development Program. Analgesic-associated kidney disease. (Consensus Development Conference Statement, Feb 27-29, 1984).

Androgens

Sherwin BB [Sir Mortimer B. Davis-Jewish General Hospital, Montreal] [Medical Research Council- Canada] Long-term effects of androgen and/or estrogen on psychosexual functioning, hormone levels, and lipid metabolism in surgically menopausal women. (Grant period 1984-1985)

Anesthesia

Cohen C. [The Hastings Center] Ethical problems in the clinical practice of anesthesia. In: Dekornfeld T, ed. Textbook of anesthesia. 1986.

Duncan PG. [National Health Research and Development Program - Canada] The influence of anesthesia and surgery on the outcome of pregnancy - pilot analysis. 1986. (Grant No. 6607-1289-53).

American Academy of Pediatrics, Committee on Drugs. Guidelines for the elective use or conscious use of sedation, deep sedation, and general anesthesia in pediatric patients. Pediatrics 1985 Aug.

ECRI Technology Assessment Program. Deaths during general anesthesia. J Health Care Technol 1985;1:155-75. [Information syntheses]

ECRI Technology Assessment Program. Monitoring of exhaled CO2 levels during anesthesia. Issues Health Care Technol 1985;sec.5.M.4. [Information syntheses]

American College of Obstetricians and Gynecologists, Committee on Technical Bulletins. Anesthesia for cesarean section. 1982 May. (Technical bulletin no. 65). [Expert opinion]

Health Council of the Netherlands. Recent developments in anesthesiology. 1978.

Anesthesia—Epidural

Blue Cross and Blue Shield Association, Technology Evaluation and Coverage Program. Epidural analgesia therapy. 1986. [Information syntheses]

Anesthesia—Inhalation

Health Council of the Netherlands. Inhalation sedation in dentistry. 1986. [English summary only].

Angiographic injectors

Food and Drug Administration, Center for Devices and Radiological Health. Safety and performance of angiographic and lymphographic injectors. 1984. (NTIS Order No. PB84-195544).

Angiography

United Kingdom Department of Health and Social Security, Medical Devices Evaluation Programme. Assessment of IGE L/U arm angiograph unit. 1986 Feb. (Report no. STB/86/7) [Epidemiological and other observational methods, Bench testing]

Blue Cross and Blue Shield Association, Medical Necessity Program. Coronary angiography and cardiac catheterization. 1985. [Information syntheses]

American College of Cardiology/American Heart Association Task Force on Assessment of Cardiovascular Procedures. Guidelines for coronary angiography. Ongoing. [Group judgment]

Angioplasty

U.S. Administrators, Professional Policy Committee. Coronary artery angioplasty. [7/86] [Group judgment]

Anthelmintics

American Academy of Pediatrics, Committee on Drugs. Commentary on anthelmintics. Pediatrics 1978 Aug.

Antianxiety agents

American Medical Association, Council on Scientific Affairs. Prescription of tranquilizers and antidepressants for women (Board of Trustees report X, I-80). 1981. [Group judgment]

Anti-arrhythmics

Nattel S. [Department Pharmacology and Therapeutics, McGill University] [Medical Research Council - Canada] Effects of antiarrhythmic drugs on arrhythmias related myocardial infarction. (Grant period 1981-1985).

Antibiotics

American College of Obstetricians and Gynecologists, Committee on Technical Bulletins. Antimicrobial therapy for gynecologic infections. 1986 Oct. (Technical bulletin no. 97). [Expert opinion]

Health Council of the Netherlands. Use of antibiotics. 1977.

Antibiotics—Intravenous

[Lewin and Associates, Inc.] The safety, efficacy, and cost effectiveness of home intravenous antibiotics. 1986 Feb. [Information syntheses, Modeling, Cost analyses]

Antibiotics—Prophylactic

American College of Obstetricians and Gynecologists, Committee Opinion. Prophylactic use of antibiotics with abdominal hysterectomy. [Information syntheses]

American Academy of Pediatrics, Committee on Drugs. Antimicrobial prophylaxis in pediatric surgical patients. Pediatrics 1984 Sep.

American Academy of Pediatrics, Committee on Infectious Diseases. Antimicrobial prophylaxis in pediatric surgical patients. Pediatrics 1984 Sep.

Anticholinergics

California Medical Association, Medical Practice Opinion Program. Anticholinergic drugs for nicotine addiction. 1985 May. (Medical Practice Opinion #322) [Group judgment]

Blazer DG, et al. [National Center for Health Services Research and Health Care Technology Assessment, Division of Extramural Research] The risk of anticholinergic toxicity in the elderly: a study of prescribing practices in two populations. J Cardiol 1983 Jan;38(1):31-35.

Anticoagulants

Veterans Administration, Cooperative Studies Program. Anticoagulants in the Rx of CA (RA-233). Pending. [Clinical trials]

Blue Cross and Blue Shield Association, Medical Necessity Program. Anticoagulant therapy in the myocardial infarction patient. 1985. [Information syntheses]

Anticonvulsants

American Academy of Pediatrics, Committee on Drugs. Behavioral and cognitive effects of anticonvulsant therapy. Pediatrics 1985 Oct.

American College of Obstetricians and Gynecologists, Committee Opinion. Anticonvulsants and pregnancy. Revised 1984 Jul. [Information syntheses]

American Academy of Pediatrics, Committee on Drugs. Anticonvulsants and pregnancy. Pediatrics 1980 Feb.

Antidepressants

American Medical Association, Council on Scientific Affairs. Prescription of tranquilizers and antidepressants for women (Board of Trustees report X, I-80). 1981. [Group judgment]

Antihypertensives

Curb JD, Borhani NO, Blaszkowski TP, et al. [National Heart, Lung, and Blood Institute] Patient perceived side effects to antihypertensive drugs. J Community Health, accepted for publication.

Curb DJ, Borhani NO, et al. [National Heart, Lung, and Blood Institute] Long-term surveillance for adverse effects of antihypertensive drugs. JAMA 1985;253:3263-3268.

Hypertension Detection and Follow-up Program Cooperative Group. [National Heart, Lung, and Blood Institute] Five-year findings of the Hypertension Detection and Follow-up Program. Prevention and reversal of left ventricular hypertrophy with antihypertensive drug therapy. Hypertension 1985;7:105-112.

Multiple Risk Factor Intervention Trial Research Group. [National Heart, Lung, and Blood Institute] Baseline rest electrocardiographic abnormalities, antihypertensive treatment, and mortality in the Multiple Risk Factor Intervention Trial. Am J Cardiol 1985;55:1-15.

Hypertension Detection and Follow-up Program Cooperative Research Group. [National Heart, Lung, and Blood Institute] The effect of antihypertensive drug treatment on mortality in the presence of testing electrocardiographic abnormalities at baseline: the HDFP experience. Circulation 1984;70:996-1003.

Lasser N, Grandits G, Caggiula A, et al. [National Heart, Lung, and Blood Institute] Effects of antihypertensive therapy on plasma lipids and lipoproteins in the Multiple Risk Factor Intervention Trial. Am J Med 1984;76:52-66.

Hardy RJ, Hawkins CM. [National Heart, Lung, and Blood Institute] The impact of selected indices of anti-hypertensive treatment on all-cause mortality. Am J Epidemiol 1983;117:566-574.

Wassertheil-Smoller S, Langford HG, Blaufox MD et al. [National Heart, Lung, and Blood Institute] Rate of hypertension return after withdrawal of prolonged antihypertensive therapy. Clin Sci 1982;63(Suppl 8):4235-4255.

Anti-inhibitor coagulant complex

National Center for Health Services Research and Health Care Technology Assessment, Office of Health Technology Assessment. The use of anti-inhibitor coagulant complex (activated prothrombin--complex concentrate) in the treatment of patients with hemophilia A and antibodies to factor VIII. 1981.

Antilymphocyte serum

American College of Physicians, Clinical Efficacy Assessment Project. Antilymphocyte (ALG) and antithymocyte (ATG) globulin in renal transplantation. 1982. [Information syntheses]

Antineoplastics handling

American Medical Association, Council on Scientific Affairs. Guidelines for handling parenteral antineoplastics. JAMA 1985 Mar 15;253:1590-1592. [Group judgment]

Antiplatelet therapy

Veterans Administration, Cooperative Studies Program. Antiplatelet therapy after coronary artery by--pass graft (CABG) surgery-I. Ongoing. [Clinical trials]

Veterans Administration, Cooperative Studies Program. Antiplatelet therapy after coronary artery bypass graft (CABG) surgery-II. Ongoing. [Clinical trials]

Antipyresis

Kramer MS, Naimark LE, Leduc DG. [McGill University, Department of Epidemiology and Biostatistics] Is antipyresis harmful? Proceedings of the Ambulatory Pediatric Association 1984 annual meeting, San Francisco. 1984:88.

APACHE

Wagner DP, Draper EA. [National Center for Health Services Research and Health Care Technology Assessment, Division of Extramural Research] Acute Physiology and Chronic Health Examination (APACHE II) and Medicare reimbursement. Health Care Finance Rev 1984 Nov;annual suppl:91-105.

Apheresis

Health Council of the Netherlands. Therapeutic hemapheresis. 1986. [English summary only].

National Center for Health Services Research and Health Care Technology Assessment, Office of Health Technology Assessment. Apheresis in the treatment of systemic lupus erythematosus (SLE). 1986.

U.S. Administrators, Professional Policy Committee. Therapeutic apheresis (plasmapheresis). [7/86] [Group judgment]

American Academy of Neurology, Practice Committee. Apheresis (therapeutic) in the treatment of Guillain-Barré syndrome. 1985 Jun. [Expert opinion, Group judgment]

American Academy of Neurology, Practice Committee. Apheresis in treatment of systemic lupus erythematosus. 1985 Jun. [Expert opinion, Group judgment]

American College of Physicians, Clinical Efficacy Assessment Project. Apheresis in chronic inflammatory demyelinating polyneuropathy and in renal transplantation. Ann Inter Med 1985;103:630-3. [Information syntheses]

ECRI Technology Assessment Program. Therapeutic apheresis. J Health Care Technol 1985;1:279-98. [Information syntheses]

National Center for Health Services Research and Health Care Technology Assessment. Apheresis in the treatment of Guillain-Barré syndrome. 1985.

American Academy of Neurology, Practice Committee. Apheresis in treatment of chronic relapsing polyneuropathy. 1984 Feb. [Expert opinion, Group judgment]

American College of Physicians, Clinical Efficacy Assessment Project. Apheresis in chronic severe rheumatoid arthritis. 1984. [Information syntheses]

National Center for Health Services Research and Health Care Technology Assessment, Office of Health Technology Assessment. Apheresis in the treatment of chronic relapsing polyneuropathy. 1984.

National Center for Health Services Research and Health Care Technology Assessment, Office of Health Technology Assessment. Apheresis used in preparation for kidney transplant. 1984.

National Center for Health Services Research and Health Care Technology Assessment, Office of Health Technology Assessment. Apheresis for the treatment of Goodpasture's syndrome and membranous proliferative glomerulonephritides. 1983.

Office of Technology Assessment, U.S. Congress. The safety, efficacy, and cost effectiveness of therapeutic apheresis. Washington, D.C.: U.S. Government Printing Office, July 1983. (Health technology case study series #23).

National Center for Health Services Research and Health Care Technology Assessment, Office of Health Technology Assessment. Apheresis for multiple sclerosis. 1982.

National Center for Health Services Research and Health Care Technology Assessment, Office of Health Technology Assessment. Rheumatoid vasculitis therapeutic apheresis. 1982.

American Academy of Neurology, Practice Committee. Apheresis for multiple sclerosis. 1981 Jul. [Expert opinion, Group judgment]

National Center for Health Services Research and Health Care Technology Assessment, Office of Health Technology Assessment. Therapeutic apheresis for rheumatoid arthritis. 1981.

Apnea monitoring

National Institute of Child Health and Human Development. Infantile apnea and home monitoring. Bethesda, MD: National Institute of Child Health and Human Development, 1987 (in press). [Group judgment, Expert opinion]

Blue Cross and Blue Shield Association, Technology Evaluation and Coverage Program. SIDS (home apnea monitoring of siblings). 1986. [Information syntheses]

National Institutes of Health, Consensus Development Program. Infantile apnea and home monitoring. (Consensus Development Conference Statement, Sep 29-Oct 1 1986). [Group judgment]

American Medical Association, Diagnostic and Therapeutic Technology Assessment. Apnea monitoring for 24-hour surveillance of newborns at risk for sudden infant death syndrome. JAMA 1984 Jan 27. [Expert opinion, Information syntheses]

Apnea monitors

Teledyne, Inc. [Food and Drug Administration, Center for Devices and Radiological Health] Sleep sentry (TM): summary of safety and effectiveness. 1982 Sep 17. (PMA no. P81004-000).

Appropriateness Evaluation Protocol

Appropriateness of hospitalization: a comparative analysis of reliability and validity of the Appropriateness Evaluation Protocol and the Standardized Medreview Instrument. In: Office of Research and Demonstrations, Health Care Financing Administration. Health care financing status report: research and demonstrations in health care financing. Jan 1986. (HCFA Pub. No. 03219).

Reducing inappropriate use of inpatient medical, surgical, and pediatric services—extension of the Appropriateness Evaluation Protocol. In: Office of Research and Demonstrations, Health Care Financing Administration. Health care financing status report: research and demonstrations in health care financing. Jan 1986. (HCFA Pub. No. 03219).

Arrhythmia monitors

ECRI Health Devices Program. Arrhythmia monitoring systems, computerized. Health Devices 1985;14:287-319.

American Hospital Association, Hospital Technology Series Program. Computerized arrhythmia monitoring systems. 1982. (Guideline report) [Information syntheses, Expert opinion, Cost analyses]

ECRI Health Devices Program. Arrhythmia monitoring systems, computerized. Health Devices 1982;11:211-247.

Arteriography

U.S. Administrators, Professional Policy Committee. Coronary arteriography. [7/86] [Group judgment]

Gersh BJ, Kronmal RA, Frye RL, et al. [National Heart, Lung, and Blood Institute] Coronary arteriography and coronary artery bypass surgery: morbidity and mortality in patients ages 65 years or older: a report from the Coronary Artery Surgery Study. Circulation 1983;67:483-490.

Arthroscopy

U.S. Administrators, Professional Policy Committee. Arthroscopy of joints other than the knee. [7/86] [Group judgment]

U.S. Administrators, Professional Policy Committee. Arthroscopy of knee. [7/86] [Group judgment]

California Medical Association, Medical Practice Opinion Program. Assistant surgeon for arthroscopic procedures. 1984 Apr. (Medical Practice Opinion #239) [Group judgment]

ECRI Technology Assessment Program. Diagnostic and operative arthroscopy. Issues Health Care Technol 1982;sec.5.A.1. [Information syntheses]

Artificial heart

Office of Technology Assessment, U.S. Congress. The artificial heart: cost, risks, and benefits. Washington, D.C.: U.S. Government Printing Office, May 1982. (Health technology case study series #9).

Artificial pancreas

Albisser AM. [Hospital for Sick Children, Toronto] [Medical Research Council - Canada] Clinical applications of an artificial pancreas. (Grant period 1975-1985).

Artificial procreation

Health Council of the Netherlands. Artificial procreation. 1986. (English summary only).

Artificial sweeteners

American Diabetes Association, Task Force of the Council on Nutrition Sciences and Metabolism. Position statment on use of noncaloric sweeteners. 1987. [Expert opinion, Group judgment]

Aspartame

American Medical Association, Council on Scientific Affairs. Aspartame: review of safety issues. JAMA 1985 Jul 18;254:400-402. [Group judgment]

Aspirin

Hennekens C, Eberlein K. [National Heart, Lung, and Blood Institute] A randomized trial of aspirin and beta-carotene among U.S. physicians. Prev Med 1985:Appendix VI.

American Academy of Pediatrics, Committee on Infectious Diseases. Aspirin and Reye syndrome. Pediatrics 1982 Jun.

Aspirin Myocardial Infarction Research Group. [National Heart, Lung, and Blood Institute] Aspirin Myocardial Infarction Study: design, methods and baseline results. DHEW Pub. No. (NIH) 80-2106, 1980.

Aspirin Myocardial Infarction Research Group. [National Heart, Lung, and Blood Institute] A randomized controlled trial of aspirin in persons recovered from myocardial infarction. JAMA 1980;243:661-669.

Aspirin Myocardial Infarction Study Research Group. [National Heart, Lung, and Blood Institute] The Aspirin Myocardial Infarction Study: final results. Circulation 1980;60(Suppl V)V79-V84.

Coronary Drug Research Group. [National Heart, Lung, and Blood Institute] Aspirin in coronary heart disease. Circulation 1980;62(Suppl V):V59-V62.

Gent M, Barnett HJM, Sackett DL, Taylor DW. [McMaster University, Department of Clinical Epidemiology and Biostatistics] A randomized trial of aspirin and sulfinpyrazone in patients with threatened stroke: results and methodologic issues. Circulation 1980;62(Suppl V):V-97.

Assertiveness training

Glueckauf RL. [National Health Research and Development Program - Canada] Assertion training for disabled persons in wheelchairs. 1986. (Grant No. 6606-2255-01).

Assessment methods

Griffith BD, White HD, Drott MC, Saye JD. [National Library of Medicine] Tests of methods for evaluating bibliographic databases—an analysis of the National Library of Medicine's handling of literatures in the medical behavioral sciences. J Am Soc Info Sci 1986;37:261-70.

Atenolol

Food and Drug Administration, Center for Drugs and Biologics. Atenolol. 1981. (NTIS order no. PB81-915911). [Information syntheses, Expert opinion, Epidemiological and other observational methods, Clinical trials, Bench testing]

Audiometry tests

Smith A, MacMurray SB, Goodman JT. [National Health Research and Development Program - Canada] A comparison of crib-o-gram and brainstem electric response audiometry in the screening of hearing loss in high risk neonates. 1986. (Grant No. 6606-1924-43).

Automated microbiology systems

Roche Diagnostic Systems. [Food and Drug Administration, Center for Devices and Radiological Health] Cobas bact: summary of safety and effectiveness. 1986 Jul 7. (PMA no. P840065-000).

ECRI Technology Assessment Program. Automated microbiology systems. Issues Health Care Technol 1985;sec.5.M.5. [Information syntheses]

ECRI Technology Assessment Program. Automated microbiology systems. J Health Care Technol 1985;1:213-30. [Information syntheses]

Automobile passenger restraints

American College of Obstetricians and Gynecologists, Committee on Technical Bulletins. Automobile passenger restraints for children and pregnant women. 1983 Dec. (Technical bulletin no. 74). [Expert opinion]

Office of Technology Assessment, U.S. Congress. Mandatory passive restraint systems in automobiles. Washington, D.C.: U.S. Government Printing Office, September 1982. (Health technology case study series #20).

Autopsy

American Medical Association, Council on Scientific Affairs. Autopsies: interim report (Substitute Resolution 11, A-84). 1985. [Group judgment]

American Academy of Neurology, Practice Committee. Autopsies on patients with slow virus diseases. 1984 Nov. [Expert opinion, Group judgment]

Autotransfusion units

American Hospital Association, Hospital Technology Series Program. Autotransfusion units. 1982. (Guideline report) [Information syntheses, Expert opinion, Cost analyses]

Aversion therapy

American College of Physicians, Clinical Efficacy Assessment Project. Chemical aversion therapy in the treatment of alcoholism, expected completion 1988. [Information syntheses]

California Medical Association, Medical Practice Opinion Program. Aversion therapy for alcoholism. 1984 Feb. (Medical Practice Opinion #311) [Group judgment]

National Center for Health Services Research and Health Care Technology Assessment, Office of Health Technology Assessment. Alcohol aversion therapy. 1981.

National Center for Health Services Research and Health Care Technology Assessment, Office of Health Technology Assessment. Chemical aversion therapy for treatment of alcoholism. Ongoing.

Azatadine

Food and Drug Administration, Center for Drugs and Biologics. Azatadine maleate & pseud. sulfate. 1982. (NTIS order no. PB82-915902). [Information syntheses, Expert opinion, Epidemiological and other observational methods, Clinical trials, Bench testing]

Azathioprine

Parfrey PS, Hutchinson TA, Lowry RP, Knaack J, Guttman RD. [McGill University, Department of Epidemiology and Biostatistics] Causes of late allograft failure and the role of azathioprine reduction. Transplant Proc 1984;16:1100-1102.

Food and Drug Administration, Center for Drugs and Biologics. Azathioprine. 1981. (NTIS order no. PB81-915907). [Information syntheses, Expert opinion, Epidemiological and other observational methods, Clinical trials, Bench testing]

Azlocillin

Food and Drug Administration, Center for Drugs and Biologics. Azlocillin sodium. 1982. (NTIS order no. PB82-915904). [Information syntheses, Expert opinion, Epidemiological and other observational methods, Clinical trials, Bench testing]

Bacampicillin

Food and Drug Administration, Center for Drugs and Biologics. Bacampicillin hydrochloride. 1982. (NTIS order no. PB82-915902). [Information syntheses, Expert opinion, Epidemiological and other observational methods, Clinical trials, Bench testing]

Bacterial antigens

California Medical Association, Medical Practice Opinion Program. Injections of universal bacterial antigen. 1980 Jan. (Medical Practice Opinion #210) [Group judgment]

Balance training devices

Fernie GR. [National Health Research and Development Program - Canada] Balance training device for stroke rehabilitation. 1986. (Grant No. 6606-3023-45).

Balloon dilatation catheters

Scimed Life Systems, Inc. [Food and Drug Administration, Center for Devices and Radiological Health] Scimed PTCA dilatation catheter: summary of safety and effectiveness. 1987 Jan 16. (PMA no. P860019-000).

Medi-tech. [Food and Drug Administration, Center for Devices and Radiological Health] Med-tech coronary balloon dilatation catheter system: summary of safety and effectiveness. 1986 Feb 10. (PMA no. P840040-000).

Advanced Catheter Systems. [Food and Drug Administration, Center for Devices and Radiological Health] Simpson-Robert coronary balloon dilatation catheter: summary of safety and effectiveness. 1982 Mar 26. (PMA no. P810046-000).

Bar codes

American Hospital Association, Hospital Technology Series Program. Bar coding technology - applications in health care. 1984. (Guideline report)

Barbiturates

California Medical Association, Medical Practice Opinion Program. Barbiturate coma. 1983 Feb. (Medical Practice Opinion #280) [Group judgment]

Barium enema with sigmoidoscopy

Irvine EJ. [National Health Research and Development Program - Canada] A prospective study to compare diagnostic agreement and cost-effectiveness of air contrast barium enema plus flexible sigmoidoscopy with colonoscopy in rectal bleeding. 1986. (Grant No. 6606-2974-42).

Batteries, Electric

ECRI Health Devices Program. Batteries, zinc air. Health Devices 1985;14:209-211.

BCG immunotherapy

American Medical Association, Diagnostic and Therapeutic Technology Assessment. BCG immunotherapy in bladder cancer. Mar 31, 1986. [Expert opinion, Information syntheses]

BCG vaccine

Pabst HF. [National Health Research and Development Program - Canada] BCG vaccine take in babies with and without maternal PPD sensitization. 1986. (Grant No. 6609-1205-54).

Beclomethasone

Food and Drug Administration, Center for Drugs and Biologics. Beclomethasone dipropionate. 1981. (NTIS order no. PB81-915912). [Information syntheses, Expert opinion, Epidemiological and other observational methods, Clinical trials, Bench testing]

Beds, Electric

ECRI Health Devices Program. Electric beds. Health Devices 1986;15-299-316.

Behavioral disorders screening

Byles JA. [National Health Research and Development Program - Canada] An assessment of a survey instrument designed to diagnose children's behavioural disorders. 1986. (Grant No. 6606-2245-04).

Behavioral therapy

Cunningham AJ. [National Health Research and Development Program - Canada] A randomized control trial of a brief behavioural training group programme for alleviating psychological distress in cancer patients. 1986. (Grant No. 6606-2884-44).

D'Arcy C. [National Health Research and Development Program - Canada] Phobia, anxiety and alcoholism: evaluating a behavioural treatment program. 1986. (Grant No. 6608-1182-43).

White DR. [National Health Research and Development Program - Canada] Evaluation of a behavioral--development treatment for childhood obesity. 1986. (Grant No. 6605-1876-42).

Bendien's test

National Center for Health Services Research and Health Care Technology Assessment, Office of Health Technology Assessment. Bendien's test for cancer and tuberculosis. 1982.

Benoxaprofen

Food and Drug Administration, Center for Drugs and Biologics. Benoxaprofen. 1982. (NTIS order no. PB82-915903). [Information syntheses, Expert opinion, Epidemiological and other observational methods, Clinical trials, Bench testing]

Bentonite flocculation test

American College of Physicians, Clinical Efficacy Assessment Project. Bentonite flocculation test. 1982. [Information syntheses]

National Center for Health Services Research and Health Care Technology Assessment, Office of Health Technology Assessment. Desoxyribonucleic acid-bentonite flocculation for the diagnosis of rheumatoid arthritis. 1981.

National Center for Health Services Research and Health Care Technology Assessment, Office of Health Technology Assessment. The use of the bentonite flocculation test in the diagnosis of rheumatoid arthritis. 1981.

Benzyl alcohol

American Academy of Pediatrics, Committee on Drugs. Benzyl alcohol: toxic agent in neonatal units. Pediatrics 1983 Sep.

American Academy of Pediatrics, Committee on Fetus and Newborn. Benzyl alcohol: toxic agent in neonatal units. Pediatrics 1983 Sep.

Beta blockers

Beta-Blocker Heart Attack Study Group. [National Heart, Lung, and Blood Institute] The Beta-Blocker Heart Attack Trial: cooperative trial-preliminary report. JAMA 1986;246:2073-2074.

Byington RP for the Beta-Blocker Heart Attack Trial Research Group. [National Heart, Lung, and Blood Institute] Beta-Blocker Heart Attack Trial - design, methods and baseline results. Controlled Clin Trials 1984;4:382-437.

Korenbrot CC, Aalto LH, Laros RK. [University of California, San Francisco, Institute for Health Policy Studies] The cost effectiveness of stopping preterm labor with beta-adrenergic treatment. N Engl J Med 1984;310:691-696.

Furberg CD, Byington RP for the BHAT Research Group. [National Heart, Lung, and Blood Institute] What do subgroup analyses reveal about differential response to beta-blocker therapy? The Beta-Blocker Heart Attack Trial experience. Proceedings of the Workshop on Implications of Recent Beta-Blocker Trials for Post-Myocardial Infarction Patients. Circulation 1983;67(Supplement I):I-98.

Beta-Blocker Heart Attack Trial Research Group. [National Heart, Lung, and Blood Institute] Beta-Blocker heart attack trial - design features. Controlled Clin Trials 1981;2:275-285.

Beta-carotene

Hennekens C, Eberlein K. [National Heart, Lung, and Blood Institute] A randomized trial of aspirin and beta-carotene among U.S. physicians. Prev Med 1985:Appendix VI.

Willett WC, Polk BF, Underwood BA, et al. [National Heart, Lung, and Blood Institute] Relation of serum vitamins A and E and carotenoids to the risk of cancer. N Engl J Med 1984;310:410-434.

Betamethasone

Food and Drug Administration, Center for Drugs and Biologics. Betamethasone dipropionate. 1987. (Summary basis of approval, NDA #19-136). [Information syntheses, Expert opinion, Epidemiological and other observational methods, Clinical trials, Bench testing]

Food and Drug Administration, Center for Drugs and Biologics. Betamethasone dipropionate. 1987. (Summary basis of approval, NDA #19-137). [Information syntheses, Expert opinion, Epidemiological and other observational methods, Clinical trials, Bench testing]

Food and Drug Administration, Center for Drugs and Biologics. Betamethasone dipropionate. 1987. (Summary basis of approval, NDA #19-138). [Information syntheses, Expert opinion, Epidemiological and other observational methods, Clinical trials, Bench testing]

Food and Drug Administration, Center for Drugs and Biologics. Betamethasone valerate. 1983. (NTIS order no. PB83-915902). [Information syntheses, Expert opinion, Epidemiological and other observational methods, Clinical trials, Bench testing]

Bethanidine sulfate

Food and Drug Administration, Center for Drugs and Biologics. Bethanidine sulfate. 1981. (NTIS order no. PB81-915908). [Information syntheses, Expert opinion, Epidemiological and other observational methods, Clinical trials, Bench testing]

Bibliographic information bases

[National Library of Medicine] An analysis of the National Library of Medicine's (NLM) handling of the medical behavioral sciences' (MBS) literatures. Final report. (Five volumes plus executive summary). Bethesda, MD: National Library of Medicine, 1984. [Epidemiological and other observational methods]

Siegel ER, Kameen K, Sinn SK, Weise FO. [National Library of Medicine] A comparative evaluation of the technical performance and user acceptance of two prototype online catalog systems. Info Technol Libr 1984;3:35-46. [Epidemiological and other observational methods]

Bibliographic information bases—Training

[National Library of Medicine] Evaluation of PC-oriented training packages for the NLM chemical and toxicological online files. Bethesda, MD: National Library of Medicine. Ongoing. [Epidemiological and other observational methods]

Bilio-pancreatic bypass

California Medical Association, Medical Practice Opinion Program. Bilio-pancreatic bypass surgery for obesity. 1983 Mar. (Medical Practice Opinion #284) [Group judgment]

Bilirubinometers

ECRI Technology Assessment Program. Noninvasive bilirubinometers. Issues Health Care Technol 1983;sec.5.B.4. [Information syntheses]

Biochemical analyzers

United Kingdom Department of Health and Social Security, Medical Devices Evaluation Programme. An evaluation of the Beckman Astra 8 with enzymes. 1985 Jul. (Report no. STB3A/85/32) [Epidemiological and other observational methods, Bench testing]

United Kingdom Department of Health and Social Security, Medical Devices Evaluation Programme. Evaluation of Analogue LM3 analyser. 1985 May. (Report no. STB3/85/25) [Epidemiological and other observational methods, Bench testing]

United Kingdom Department of Health and Social Security, Medical Devices Evaluation Programme. Evaluation of the IQ Bio Microlite Floteskan system. 1985 Oct. (Report No. STB3A/85/43) [Epidemiological and other observational methods, Bench testing]

Biochemical profiles

Blue Cross and Blue Shield Association, Medical Necessity Program. Biochemical profiles in ambulatory screening and preadmission testing of adults. 1987. [Information syntheses]

Biofeedback

Milner M, Levison H. [National Health Research and Development Program - Canada] Evaluation of relaxed breathing and its augmentation with biofeedback upon bronchospasm induced by methacholine in paediatric patients with chronic asthma. 1986. (Grant No. 6606-2113-53).

Sullivan SJ. [National Health Research and Development Program - Canada] Electromyographic biofeedback and the learning process in the treatment of hemiplegia. 1986. (Grant No. 6605-2415-45).

U.S. Administrators, Professional Policy Committee. Biofeedback. [7/86] [Group judgment]

American College of Physicians, Clinical Efficacy Assessment Project. Biofeedback for gastrointestinal disorders. Ann Intern Med 1985;103:291-3,240-44. [Information syntheses]

American College of Physicians, Clinical Efficacy Assessment Project. Biofeedback for headaches. Ann Intern Med 1985;102:128-31. [Information syntheses]

American College of Physicians, Clinical Efficacy Assessment Project. Biofeedback for hypertension. Ann Intern Med 1985;102:709-15. [Information syntheses]

American College of Physicians, Clinical Efficacy Assessment Project. Biofeedback for neuromuscular disorders. Ann Intern Med 1985;102:854-8. [Information syntheses]

American Academy of Neurology, Practice Committee. Electromyographic biofeedback in treatment of hyperactivity. 1984 Feb. [Expert opinion, Group judgment]

American Medical Association, Diagnostic and Therapeutic Technology Assessment. Biofeedback for managing vascular and tension headaches. JAMA 1983 Nov 14. [Expert opinion, Information syntheses]

California Medical Association, Medical Practice Opinion Program. Biofeedback. 1983 Aug. (Medical Practice Opinion #240) [Group judgment]

American Academy of Neurology, Practice Committee. Biofeedback for headaches. 1982 Jun. [Expert opinion, Group judgment]

American Academy of Neurology, Practice Committee. Biofeedback treatment for migraine headache. 1980 Apr. [Expert opinion, Group judgment]

Biopsy—Endometrial

American College of Obstetricians and Gynecologists, Committee Opinion. Endometrial sampling. 1985 Jun. [Information syntheses]

Biopsy—Fetal blood

American College of Obstetricians and Gynecologists, Committee on Technical Bulletins. Fetal blood sampling. 1976 Oct. (Technical bulletin no. 42). [Expert opinion]

Biopsy—Renal

Parfrey PS, et al. [McGill University, Department of Epidemiology and Biostatistics] The diagnostic and prognostic value of renal allograft biopsy. Transplantation 1984;38(6):586-590.

Blood banks

Office of Technology Assessment, U.S. Congress. Blood policy and technology. Washington, D.C.: U.S. Government Printing Office, January 1985.

Blood cell count

Blue Cross and Blue Shield Association, Medical Necessity Program. Complete blood count and leukocyte differential count. 1987. [Information syntheses]

Koepke JA, ed. Differential leukocyte counting. CAP Conference/Aspen 1977. Skokie, IL: College of American Pathologists, 1978. [Expert opinion, Bench testing]

Blood chemistry analyzers

United Kingdom Department of Health and Social Security, Medical Devices Evaluation Programme. An evaluation of the Kone Process selective chemistry analyser. 1985 Jul. (Report no. STB3A/85/31) [Epidemiological and other observational methods, Bench testing]

Office of Technology Assessment, U.S. Congress. Cost-effectiveness of automated multichannel chemistry analyzers. Washington, D.C.: U.S. Government Printing Office, April 1981. (Health technology case study series #4).

Weinstein MC, Pearlman LA. [Harvard School of Public Health, Institute for Health Research] Case study on cost-effectiveness of automated multichannel chemistry analyzers. The implications of cost-effectiveness analysis of medical technology background paper #2: case studies of medical technologies. Office of Technology Assessment, U.S. Congress. Washington, D.C.: U.S. Government Printing Office, 1981. [Epidemiological methods]

Blood cultures

Blue Cross and Blue Shield Association, Medical Necessity Program. Blood cultures. 1987. [Information syntheses]

Blood gas monitoring

Blue Cross and Blue Shield Association, Medical Necessity Program. Arterial blood gas analysis. 1987. [Information syntheses]

Medical Technology and Practice Patterns Institute. End tidal carbon dioxide monitoring. 1987.

Blue Cross and Blue Shield Association, Medical Necessity Program. Diagnostic studies for respiratory patients: arterial blood gas analysis. 1982. [Information syntheses]

Blood gas monitors

ECRI Health Devices Program. Carbon dioxide monitors. Health Devices 1986;15:255-85.

Litton Datamedix. [Food and Drug Administration, Center for Devices and Radiological Health] Litton transcutaneous C02 system: summary of safety and effectiveness. 1986 Sep 26. (PMA no. P850087-000).

Radiometer! America. [Food and Drug Administration, Center for Devices and Radiological Health] Radiometer TCM-10 transcutaneous carbon dioxide monitor: summary of safety and effectiveness. 1984 Apr 13. (PMA no. P800043-002).

ECRI Health Devices Program. Blood gas/pH analyzers. Health Devices 1983;12:59-78.

ECRI Health Devices Program. Oxygen monitors, transcutaneous. Health Devices 1983;12:213-51.

ECRI Technology Assessment Program. Transcutaneous CO2 monitors. Issues Health Care Technol 1983;sec.5.M.3. [Information syntheses]

Narco Scientific. [Food and Drug Administration, Center for Devices and Radiological Health] Monitoring system TCPC02: summary of safety and effectiveness. 1983 Feb 15. (PMA no. P820025-000).

Sensormedics. [Food and Drug Administration, Center for Devices and Radiological Health] Cutaneous gas monitor: summary of safety and effectiveness. 1983 Sep 16. (PMA no. P830008-000).

Biochem International Inc. [Food and Drug Administration, Center for Devices and Radiological Health] Lifespan (TM) 100 TCPC02 monitor: summary of safety and effectiveness. 1982 Oct 1. (PMA no. P820019-000).

Hewlett-Packard Co. [Food and Drug Administration, Center for Devices and Radiological Health] H-P capnometer model 47210A, option A10 cutaneous: summary of safety and effectiveness. 1982 Apr 13. (PMA no. P810043-000).

Kontron Cardiovascular Inc. [Food and Drug Administration, Center for Devices and Radiological Health] Kontron cutaneous PC02 monitor: summary of safety and effectiveness. 1982 Jun 18. (PMA no. P810037-000).

Orange Medical Instruments. [Food and Drug Administration, Center for Devices and Radiological Health] Transconjunctival oxygen monitor: summary of safety and effectiveness. 1982 Nov 19. (PMA no. P820011-000).

ECRI Technology Assessment Program. Noninvasive blood gas oxygen monitors. Issues Health Care Technol 1981;sec.5.M.1. [Information syntheses]

Blood glucose control devices

National Center for Health Services Research and Health Care Technology Assessment, Office of Health Technology Assessment. Closed-loop blood glucose control device. 1983.

Blood glucose monitoring

American Diabetes Association, Consensus Development Panel. Consensus statement on self-monitoring of blood glucose. Diabetes Care 1987;10:95-99. [Expert opinion, Group judgment]

American Diabetes Association. Bedside blood glucose monitoring in hospitals. Diabetes Care 1986;9:89. [Expert opinion, Group judgment]

American College of Physicians, Clinical Efficacy Assessment Project. Home blood glucose monitoring. Ann Intern Med 1983;99:272-4. [Information syntheses]

Blood glucose monitors

National Center for Health Services Research and Health Care Technology Assessment, Office of Health Technology Assessment. Home blood glucose monitors. 1982.

California Medical Association, Medical Practice Opinion Program. Stat-tek glucose analyzer for diabetes. 1981 Aug. (Medical Practice Opinion #260) [Group judgment]

Blood pressure monitoring

Medical Technology and Practice Patterns Institute. Ambulatory blood pressure monitoring. 1987.

American College of Physicians, Clinical Efficacy Assessment Project. Automated ambulatory blood pressure monitoring. Ann Intern Med 1986;104:275-8. [Information syntheses]

Blue Cross and Blue Shield Association, Technology Evaluation and Coverage Program. Automated and semi-automated ambulatory blood pressure monitoring. 1986. [Information syntheses]

Georgetown University Medical Center, Institute for Health Policy Analysis. National Health Services and Practice Patterns Survey. Report on fully automated blood pressure monitoring: current and future applications. Washington, DC: Institute for Health Policy Analysis, 1986. [Information syntheses, Expert opinion, Group judgment, Cost analyses]

National Center for Health Services Research and Health Care Technology Assessment, Office of Health Technology Assessment. Fully automated blood pressure monitoring of hypertension. 1986.

Barnett GO, et al. [National Center for Health Services Research and Health Care Technology Assessment, Division of Extramural Research] A computer-based monitoring system for follow-up of elevated blood pressure. Med Care 1983 Apr;21(4):400-409.

National Center for Health Services Research and Health Care Technology Assessment, Office of Health Technology Assessment. Fully automated ambulatory blood pressure monitoring of hypertension. 1983.

California Medical Association, Medical Practice Opinion Program. Constant blood pressure monitoring. 1982 Aug. (Medical Practice Opinion #275) [Group judgment]

National Center for Health Services Research and Health Care Technology Assessment, Office of Health Technology Assessment. Ambulatory blood pressure monitoring in hypertensives using semiautomatic, patient-activated portable devices. 1982.

American College of Physicians, Clinical Efficacy Assessment Project. 24-hour sphygmomanometry. 1981. [Information syntheses]

National Institutes of Health, Consensus Development Program. Improving clinical and consumer use of blood pressure measuring devices. (Consensus Development Conference Statement, Apr 26-27 1979). [Group judgment]

Johns Hopkins Program for Medical Technology and Practice Assessment. An assessment of automatic blood pressure monitoring. Planned.

Blood pressure monitors

ECRI Health Devices Program. Sphygmomanometers, automatic. Health Devices 1986;15:187-208.

American Hospital Association, Hospital Technology Series Program. Automated indirect blood pressure measurement devices. 1982. (Guideline report) [Information syntheses, Expert opinion, Cost analyses]

ECRI Technology Assessment Program. Automatic indirect blood pressure monitors. Issues Health Care Technol 1982;sec.5.B.2. [Information syntheses]

Netherlands Organization for Applied Scientific Research, Medical Technology Unit (TNO). Sphygmomanometers. 1978.

Blood substitutes

ECRI Technology Assessment Program. Blood substitute. Issues Health Care Technol 1982;sec.5.B.3. [Information syntheses]

Blood transfusion

U.S. Administrators, Professional Policy Committee. Transfusion - preparation of blood. [7/86] [Group judgment]

CBO (Centraal Begeleidingsorgaan voor de Intercollegiale Toetsing) Consensus Development Program. Blood transfusion therapy. 1982. [Dutch language only] [Group judgment, Expert opinion]

Polesky HF, Walker RH, eds. Safety in transfusion practices. CAP Conference/Aspen 1980. Skokie, IL: College of American Pathologists, 1981. [Expert opinion, Bench testing]

National Institutes of Health, Consensus Development Program. Transfusion therapy in pregnant sickle cell disease patients. (Consensus Development Conference Statement, Apr 23-24 1979). [Group judgment]

Blood transfusion—Autologous

U.S. Administrators, Professional Policy Committee. Autologous blood transfusions. Ongoing. [Group judgment]

Blood urea concentration

Blue Cross and Blue Shield Association, Medical Necessity Program. Blood urea nitrogen concentration and serum creatinine concentration. 1987. [Information syntheses]

Blood warmers

ECRI Health Devices Program. Blood warmers. Health Devices 1984;13:191-219.

Netherlands Organization for Applied Scientific Research, Medical Technology Unit (TNO). Bloodwarmers for use during transfusion. 1981.

Bolen's test

National Center for Health Services Research and Health Care Technology Assessment, Office of Health Technology Assessment. Bolen's test for cancer. 1982.

Bone cements

Food and Drug Administration, Center for Devices and Radiological Health. To cement or not to cement? or has the FDA approved the use of this device? 1986. (FDA Pub No. FDA86-4202).

Miller JE. [Montreal General Hospital Research Institute] [Medical Research Council - Canada] Optimization of fixation of artificial joint components to bone - the prevention of loosening in total joint arthroplasty. (Grant period 1974-1985).

Dow Corning Wright [Food and Drug Administration, Center for Devices and Radiological Health] CMW bone cement: summary of safety and effectiveness. 1984 Apr 24. (PMA no. N18466-000).

EM Labs. [Food and Drug Administration, Center for Devices and Radiological Health] Palacos R bone cement: summary of safety and effectiveness. 1984 Feb 28. (PMA no. P810020-000).

Bone growth stimulation

Blue Cross and Blue Shield Association, Technology Evaluation and Coverage Program. Electrical bone growth stimulation. 1986. [Information syntheses]

U.S. Administrators, Professional Policy Committee. Bone healing/electromagnetic stimulation. Ongoing. [Group judgment]

Bone growth stimulators

Advanced Biosearch Assn. [Food and Drug Administration, Center for Devices and Radiological Health] Orthopak (R) bone growth stimulator: summary of safety and effectiveness. 1986 Apr 9. (PMA no. P850022-000).

American Medical Electronics, Inc. [Food and Drug Administration, Center for Devices and Radiological Health] Physio-stim (TM) I & II Model 6000 & 7000: summary of safety and effectiveness. 1986 Apr 18. (PMA no. P850007-000).

ECRI Technology Assessment Program. Bone growth stimulators. Issues Health Care Technol 1981;sec.5.B.1. [Information syntheses]

Bone mineral studies

American College of Physicians,Clinical Efficacy Assessment Project. Bone mineral densitometry, 1987. [Information syntheses]

American College of Physicians, Clinical Efficacy Assessment Project. Radiologic methods to evaluate bone mineral content. Ann Intern Med 1984;100:108-11. [Information syntheses]

California Medical Association, Medical Practice Opinion Program. Bone densitometry. 1982 Nov. (Medical Practice Opinion #254) [Group judgment]

National Center for Health Services Research and Health Care Technology Assessment, Office of Health Technology Assessment. Bone mineral studies. 1982.

Bone prosthesis

Unilab, Inc. [Food and Drug Administration, Center for Devices and Radiological Health] Kiel Surgibone: summary of safety and effectiveness. 1982 Jun 18. (PMA no. P800044-000).

Botulinum toxin

American Academy of Ophthalmology. Botulinum toxin therapy of eye muscle disorders: safety and effectiveness. San Francisco, CA: American Academy of Ophthalmology, 1984. [Information syntheses, Expert opinion]

Brain electrical activity mapping

U.S. Administrators, Professional Policy Committee. B.E.A.M. [7/86] [Group judgment]

Breast feeding

American Academy of Pediatrics, Committee on Nutrition. Promotion of breast feeding. 1982.

American Academy of Pediatrics, Committee on Nutrition. Breast feeding and contraception. 1981.

American College of Obstetricians and Gynecologists, Committee Opinion. Breast-feeding and contraception. 1981 May. [Information syntheses]

American Academy of Pediatrics, Committee on Nutrition. Encouraging breast-feeding. Pediatrics 1980 Mar.

American Academy of Pediatrics, Committee on Nutrition. Breast-feeding. Pediatrics 1978 Oct.

American Academy of Pediatrics, Committee on Nutrition. Commentary on breast-feeding and infant formulas, including proposed standards for formulas. Pediatrics 1976 Feb.

Health Council of the Netherlands. Breast feeding (contamination of milk). Ongoing assessment.

Breast imaging

U.S. Administrators, Professional Policy Committee. Breast imaging. [7/86] [Group judgment]

Blue Cross and Blue Shield Association, Medical Necessity Program. Diagnostic imaging in the evaluation of breast disease. 1984. [Information syntheses]

Breast physical examination

Eddy DM. [Duke University, Center for Health Policy Research and Education] The effectiveness, cost, & cost-effectiveness of breast cancer screening with annual mammography & breast physical exam. for women over 65. Report prepared for Committee on Ways & Means, Subcommittee on Health, U.S. House of Representatives. 1986 Jan 7. [Information syntheses]

Breath tests

National Center for Health Services Research and Health Care Technology Assessment, Office of Health Technology Assessment. 13CO2 breath test for diagnosing bile acid malabsorption. 1984.

National Center for Health Services Research and Health Care Technology Assessment, Office of Health Technology Assessment. 13CO2 breath test for diagnosing fat malabsorption. 1984.

American College of Physicians, Clinical Efficacy Assessment Project. 13C and 14C glycocholate tests. 1983. [Information syntheses]

American College of Physicians, Clinical Efficacy Assessment Project. 13C and 14C glycocholate, H2 breath, 13C trioctanoin, and 14C triolein breath tests. 1983.[Information syntheses]

American College of Physicians, Clinical Efficacy Assessment Project. 14C xylose breath test. 1983. [Information syntheses]

American College of Physicians, Clinical Efficacy Assessment Project. Lactulose H2 breath test. 1983. [Information syntheses]

American College of Physicians, Clinical Efficacy Assessment Project. The H2 breath test. 1983. [Information syntheses]

National Center for Health Services Research and Health Care Technology Assessment, Office of Health Technology Assessment. Lactose breath hydrogen test for the diagnosis of lactose malabsorption.

National Center for Health Services Research and Health Care Technology Assessment, Office of Health Technology Assessment. Lactulose breath hydrogen test for small bowel bacterial overgrowth and small bowel transit time. 1983.

Bromocriptine

American College of Obstetricians and Gynecologists, Committee Opinion. Clinical use of bromocriptine. Pending. [Information syntheses]

Food and Drug Administration, Center for Drugs and Biologics. Bromocriptine mesylate. 1981. (NTIS order no. PB81-915912). [Information syntheses, Expert opinion, Epidemiological and other observational methods, Clinical trials, Bench testing]

Bumetanide

Food and Drug Administration, Center for Drugs and Biologics. Bumetanide injectable. 1987. (Summary basis of approval, NDA #18-226). [Information syntheses, Expert opinion, Epidemiological and other observational methods, Clinical trials, Bench testing]

Food and Drug Administration, Center for Drugs and Biologics. Bumetanide tablets. 1987. (Summary basis of approval, NDA #18-225). [Information syntheses, Expert opinion, Epidemiological and other observational methods, Clinical trials, Bench testing]

Bupivacaine

Food and Drug Administration, Center for Drugs and Biologics. Bupivacaine hydrochloride. 1982. (NTIS order no. PB82-915901). [Information syntheses, Expert opinion, Epidemiological and other observational methods, Clinical trials, Bench testing]

Buprenorphine

Food and Drug Administration, Center for Drugs and Biologics. Buprenorphine HCl. 1982. (NTIS order no. PB82-915901). [Information syntheses, Expert opinion, Epidemiological and other observational methods, Clinical trials, Bench testing]

Burn units

Subcommittee on Institutional Program Guidelines. [Health and Welfare Canada, Health Services and Promotion Branch, Institutional and Professional Services Division] Burn unit guidelines. Revised 1985. [Information syntheses, Expert opinion, Group judgment]

Payne BC. [National Center for Health Services Research and Health Care Technology Assessment, Division of Extramural Research] Burn care facility study. 1984. (NTIS order no. PB84-240688)

Bypass graft materials

Veterans Administration, Cooperative Studies Program. Comparative efficacy of vascular by-pass graft materials in lower extremity revascularization. Ongoing. [Clinical trials]

Caerulein

Food and Drug Administration, Center for Drugs and Biologics. Ceruletide diethylamine. 1982. (NTIS order no. PB82-915901). [Information syntheses, Expert opinion, Epidemiological and other observational methods, Clinical trials, Bench testing]

Calcium channel blockers

American Medical Association, Council on Scientific Affairs. Calcium channel blocking agents. JAMA 1983 Nov 11;250:2522-2524. [Group judgment]

Calcium chloride

Food and Drug Administration, Center for Drugs and Biologics. CaCl2, MgCl, Kcl, & NaCl. 1982. (NTIS order no. PB82-915902). [Information syntheses, Expert opinion, Epidemiological and other observational methods, Clinical trials, Bench testing]

Camphor

American Academy of Pediatrics, Committee on Drugs. Camphor: who needs it? Pediatrics 1978 Sep.

Cancer screening

American College of Obstetricians and Gynecologists, Committee Opinion. ACOG statement on periodic cancer screening for women. 1980 Jun. [Information syntheses]

Cancer screening—Breast

Eddy DM. [Duke University, Center for Health Policy Research and Education] Screening for breast cancer, reassessment. (Expected publication 1988) [Information syntheses].

Miller AB. [National Health Research and Development Program - Canada] National study of screening for breast cancer. 1986. (Grant No. 6613-1149-X).

American College of Physicians, Clinical Efficacy Assessment Project. Screening for breast cancer. Ann Intern Med 1985;103:143-6,79-85. [Information syntheses]

American College of Radiology, Task Force on Breast Cancer. Policy statement: breast cancer screening centers. 1985. [Group judgment]

American College of Obstetricians and Gynecologists, Committee on Technical Bulletins. Epidemiology and diagnosis of breast disease. 1983 Sep. (Technical bulletin no. 71). [Expert opinion]

National Institutes of Health, Consensus Development Program. Breast cancer screening. (Consensus Development Conference Statement, Sep 14-16 1977). [Group judgment]

Health Council of the Netherlands. Screening for breast cancer. Ongoing assessment.

Cancer screening—Cervical

Eddy DM. [Duke University, Center for Health Policy Research and Education] Screening for cervical cancer, reassessment. (Expected publication 1988). [Information syntheses]

Cohen MM. [National Health Research and Development Program - Canada] A population-based study of cervical screening in Manitoba. 1986. (Grant No. 6607-1401-53).

American College of Obstetricians and Gynecologists, Committee on Technical Bulletins. Cervical cytology: evaluation and management of abnormalities. 1984 Oct. (Technical bulletin no. 81). [Expert opinion]

American College of Obstetricians and Gynecologists, Committee on Technical Bulletins. Diagnosis and management of invasive cervical carcinomas. 1983 May. (Technical bulletin no. 69). [Expert opinion]

Eddy DM. [Duke University, Center for Health Policy Research and Education] Appropriateness of cervical cancer screening. Gynecol Oncol 1981;12:S168-187. [Information syntheses]

Office of Technology Assessment, U.S. Congress. Allocating costs and benefits in disease prevention: an application to cervical cancer screening. Washington, D.C.: U.S. Government Printing Office, May 1981. (Health technology case study series #7)

Cancer screening—Colorectal

Eddy DM. [Duke University, Center for Health Policy Research and Education] Screening for colorectal cancer, reassessment. (Expected publication 1988). [Information syntheses]

Brandeau ML, Eddy DM. [Duke University, Center for Health Policy Research and Education] The workup of the asymptomatic patient with a positive fecal occult blood test. Med Decis Making 1987;7:32-46. [Information syntheses]

Eddy DM, Nugent FW, Eddy JF, et al. [Duke University, Center for Health Policy Research and Education] Screening for colorectal cancer in a high-risk population: results of a mathematical model. Gastroenterology 1987;92:682-692. [Information syntheses]

Wiens E, Kumpula VW, Hill GB. [National Health Research and Development Program -Canada] Early detection of colorectal cancer in Northern Alberta. 1986. (Grant No. 6609-1243-53).

Eddy DM. [Duke University, Center for Health Policy Research and Education] Screening for colon cancer: a technology assessment. 1981. (Office of Technology Assessment background paper #2: case studies of medical technologies) [Information syntheses]

Office of Technology Assessment, U.S. Congress. Screening for colon cancer. Washington, D.C.: U.S. Government Printing Office, April 1981. (Health technology case study series #3).

National Institutes of Health, Consensus Development Program. Mass screening for colo-rectal cancer. (Consensus Development Conference Statement, June 26-28 1978). [Group judgment]

Cancer screening—Lung

Eddy DM. [Duke University, Center for Health Policy Research and Education] Screening for lung cancer, reassessment. (Expected publication, 1988) [Information syntheses]

Chretien M, M'Bikay M. [National Health Research and Development Program - Canada] Screening of bronchogenic adenocarcinoma: development of a model to use tumour markers. 1986. (Grant No. 6605-2299-52).

California Medical Association, Medical Practice Opinion Program. Early detection of lung cancer. 1985 Dec. (Medical Practice Opinion #337) [Group judgment]

National Institutes of Health, Consensus Development Program. Mass screening for lung cancer. (Consensus Development Conference Statement, Sep 18-20 1978). [Group judgment]

Cannabis

American Medical Association, Council on Scientific Affairs. Marijuana, its health hazards and therapeutic potentials. JAMA 1981 Oct 16;246:1823. [Group judgment]

American Medical Association, Council on Scientific Affairs. Marijuana in the 80's. 1980. [Group judgment]

Capitation payment

Alternate models for prepaid capitation of health care services for Medicare beneficiaries—Oregon. In: Office of Research and Demonstrations, Health Care Financing Administration. Health care financing status report: research and demonstrations in health care financing. Jan 1986. (HCFA Pub. No. 03219).

Analysis of long-term care payment systems. In: Office of Research and Demonstrations, Health Care Financing Administration. Health care financing status report: research and demonstrations in health care financing. Jan 1986. (HCFA Pub. No. 03219).

Capitation payment system for all end-stage renal disease services. In: Office of Research and Demonstrations, Health Care Financing Administration. Health care financing status report: research and demonstrations in health care financing. Jan 1986. (HCFA Pub. No. 03219).

Determination of health maintenance organization capitation rates for Medicare beneficiaries. In: Office of Research and Demonstrations, Health Care Financing Administration. Health care financing status report: research and demonstrations in health care financing. Jan 1986. (HCFA Pub. No. 03219).

Evaluation of health maintenance organization (HMO) capitation demonstrations. In: Office of Research and Demonstrations, Health Care Financing Administration. Health care financing status report: research and demonstrations in health care financing. Jan 1986. (HCFA Pub. No. 03219).

Evaluation of prepaid managed health care demonstration. In: Office of Research and Demonstrations, Health Care Financing Administration. Health care financing status report: research and demonstrations in health care financing. Jan 1986. (HCFA Pub. No. 03219).

Evaluation of prepaid risk-bearing care organization. In: Office of Research and Demonstrations, Health Care Financing Administration. Health care financing status report: research and demonstrations in health care financing. Jan 1986. (HCFA Pub. No. 03219).

Health Care Plus: the Lutheran Medical Center program for prepaid managed health care. In: Office of Research and Demonstrations, Health Care Financing Administration. Health care financing status report: research and demonstrations in health care financing. Jan 1986. (HCFA Pub. No. 03219).

Medicare Prospective Capitation Demonstration Project. In: Office of Research and Demonstrations, Health Care Financing Administration. Health care financing status report: research and demonstrations in health care financing. Jan 1986. (HCFA Pub. No. 03219).

Missouri Medicaid Prepaid Health Demonstration Project. In: Office of Research and Demonstrations, Health Care Financing Administration. Health care financing status report: research and demonstrations in health care financing. Jan 1986. (HCFA Pub. No. 03219).

Program for prepaid managed health care. In: Office of Research and Demonstrations, Health Care Financing Administration. Health care financing status report: research and demonstrations in health care financing. Jan 1986. (HCFA Pub. No. 03219).

Project HOPE, Center for Health Affairs. Access to technology and quality of care in capitated plans. Ongoing.

University of Pennsylvania, Leonard Davis Institute of Health Economics. Full Medicare capitation for ESRD beneficiaries: design, implementation, and evaluation of a controlled nationwide demonstration. Planned. (Submitted to the Health Care Financing Administration).

Capsule method

American College of Physicians, Clinical Efficacy Assessment Project. Gastric analysis by the capsule method (Heidelberg). 1981. [Information syntheses]

Captopril

Food and Drug Administration, Center for Drugs and Biologics. Captopril. 1981. (NTIS order no. PB81-915907). [Information syntheses, Expert opinion, Epidemiological and other observational methods, Clinical trials, Bench testing]

Veterans Administration, Cooperative Studies Program. Clinical studies on captopril: evaluation of low doses, twice daily doses and addition of hydrochlorothiazide. [1980] [Clinical trials]

Captopril with hydrochlorothiazide

Veterans Administration, Cooperative Studies Program. Clinical studies on captopril: evaluation of low doses, twice daily doses and addition of hydrochlorothiazide. [1980] [Clinical trials]

Carbamazepine

Garfinkel PE. [Department Psychiatry, University Toronto] [Medical Research Council - Canada] Bulimia: neuroendocrine evaluation, relationship to effective disorder and treatment with carbamazepine. (Grant period 1983-1985).

Food and Drug Administration, Center for Drugs and Biologics. Carbamazepine. 1982. (NTIS order no. PB82-915901). [Information syntheses, Expert opinion, Epidemiological and other observational methods, Clinical trials, Bench testing]

Veterans Administration, Cooperative Studies Program. Evaluation of anti-epileptic drugs (phenobarb vs. phenytoin vs. primidone vs. carbamazepine). [1980] [Clinical trials]

Veterans Administration, Cooperative Studies Program. Efficacy and toxicity of carbamazepine vs. valproic acid for partial seizures. Ongoing. [Clinical trials]

Carcinoembryonic antigen assays

Blue Cross and Blue Shield Association, Medical Necessity Program. Carcinoembryonic antigen. 1987. [Information syntheses]

Hybritech Inc. [Food and Drug Administration, Center for Devices and Radiological Health] Tandem (R)-R carcinoembryonic antigen assay: summary of safety and effectiveness. 1986 Jul 1. (PMA no. P840019-000).

Hoffman-LaRoche Inc. [Food and Drug Administration, Center for Devices and Radiological Health] CEA-Roche (R) EIA: summary of safety and effectiveness. 1985 Jun 12. (PMA no. P840027-000).

Abbott Laboratories. [Food and Drug Administration, Center for Devices and Radiological Health] Abbott CEA-EIA kit: summary of safety and effectiveness. 1984 Aug 21. (PMA no. P830066-000).

National Institutes of Health, Consensus Development Program. CEA as a cancer marker. (Consensus Development Conference Statement, Sep 29-Oct 1 1980). [Group judgment]

U.S. Administrators, Professional Policy Committee. CEA testing. Ongoing. [Group judgment]

Cardiac catheterization

Miller RS. [National Health Research and Development Program - Canada] Psychological preparation for stressful medical procedures: heart catheterization. 1986. (Grant No. 6606-2640-44).

American College of Physicians, Clinical Efficacy Assessment Project. The safety and efficacy of ambulatory cardiac catheterization in the hospital and free standing setting. Ann Intern Med 1985:103;294-8. [Information syntheses]

Blue Cross and Blue Shield Association, Medical Necessity Program. Coronary angiography and cardiac catheterization. 1985. [Information syntheses]

National Center for Health Services Research and Health Care Technology Assessment, Office of Health Technology Assessment. Cardiac catheterization in a freestanding setting. Ongoing.

Cardiac enzyme assays

Blue Cross and Blue Shield Association, Medical Necessity Program. Cardiac enzyme assays in the diagnosis of myocardial infarction. 1987. [Information syntheses]

Cardiac monitors

Food and Drug Administration, Center for Devices and Radiological Health. Development of test methods and draft standard for cardiac monitors. 1984. (NTIS Order No. PB84-187756).

Food and Drug Administration, Center for Devices and Radiological Health. Standard for cardiac monitors, heart rate meters, and alarms. 1984. (NTIS Order No. PB84-188812).

Netherlands Organization for Applied Scientific Research, Medical Technology Unit (TNO). Heart monitors. 1981.

National Center for Health Services Research and Health Care Technology Assessment, Office of Health Technology Assessment. Real time cardiac monitors. Ongoing.

Cardiac pacemakers

Cardiac pacemakers. In: Prospective Payment Assessment Commission. Technical appendixes to the report and recommendations to the Secretary, U.S. Department of Health and Human Services, April 1, 1986. Washington, DC: Government Printing Office, 1986:99-101. [Information syntheses, Cost analyses]

Cardiac Pacemakers, Inc. [Food and Drug Administration, Center for Devices and Radiological Health] Models 925, 2040, 2041, 6564: summary of safety and effectiveness. 1986 Jan 24. (PMA no. P840068-000).

ECRI Technology Assessment Program. Temporary external noninvasive pacemakers. Issues Health Care Technol 1986;sec.5.P.11. [Information syntheses]

Georgetown University Medical Center, Institute for Health Policy Analysis. New medical technologies in a cost containment environment: implantable antitachyarrhythmia devices. Washington, DC: Institute for Health Policy Analysis, 1986. [Information syntheses, Expert opinion, Group judgment, Cost analyses]

Medtronic, Inc. [Food and Drug Administration, Center for Devices and Radiological Health] Activitrax models 8400, 8402, 8403: summary of safety and effectiveness. 1986 Jul 11. (PMA no. P850051-000).

Medtronic, Inc. [Food and Drug Administration, Center for Devices and Radiological Health] Steroid tip (TM) model 4503 & 4003 transvenous pacing: summary of safety and effectiveness. 1986 Aug 22. (PMA no. P830061-000).

Medtronic. [Food and Drug Administration, Center for Devices and Radiological Health] Model 5525 transvenous atrial & Model 5025 ventrical: summary of safety and effectiveness. 1986 Aug 22. (PMA no. P850089-000).

Pacemaker Systems, Inc. a Siemens Co. [Food and Drug Administration, Center for Devices and Radiological Health] DDD pulse generator 674: summary of safety and effectiveness. 1986 Sep 8. (PMA no. P840014-000).

Seecor, Inc. [Food and Drug Administration, Center for Devices and Radiological Health] Stat-Pace II: summary of safety and effectiveness. 1986 Jul 1. (PMA no.P840002-000).

Telectronics LTD. [Food and Drug Administration, Center for Devices and Radiological Health] Telectronics pasar model 4171 PG: summary of safety and effectiveness. 1986 Nov 10. (PMA no. P850027-000).

American Medical Association, Council on Scientific Affairs. The use of cardiac pacemakers in medical practice. JAMA 1985 Oct 11;254 (14) 1952-1954. [Group judgment]

Blue Cross and Blue Shield Association, Medical Necessity Program. Permanent cardiac pacemakers. 1985. [Information syntheses]

Biotronik Sales, Inc. [Food and Drug Administration, Center for Devices and Radiological Health] Diplos model 03: summary of safety and effectiveness. 1984 Apr 6. (PMA no. P820076-000).

California Medical Association, Medical Practice Opinion Program. Cardiac pacemakers. 1984 Mar. (Medical Practice Opinion #291) [Group judgment]

Frye RL, Collins JJ, DeSanctis RW, et al. [American College of Cardiology/American Heart Association Task Force on Assessment of Cardiovascular Procedures] Guidelines for permanent cardiac pacemaker implantation. J Am Coll Cardiology 1984;4:434-42. [Group judgment]

Intermedics Inc. [Food and Drug Administration, Center for Devices and Radiological Health] Cosmos (TM) system: summary of safety and effectiveness. 1984 Apr 25. (PMA no. P830026-000).

Intermedics, Inc. [Food and Drug Administration, Center for Devices and Radiological Health] Cybertach (TM) 60 pulse generator & programmer: summary of safety and effectiveness. 1984 Dec 12. (PMA no. P820022-000).

Pacesetter Systems Inc. [Food and Drug Administration, Center for Devices and Radiological Health] Model 283 pulse generator & model 370/375 supports: summary of safety and effectiveness. 1984 Apr 20. (PMA no. P830045-000).

Cordis Corp. [Food and Drug Administration, Center for Devices and Radiological Health] Gemini (R) theta model 415A cardiac pacer: summary of safety and effectiveness. 1983 Dec 7. (PMA no. P830007-000).

ECRI Health Devices Program. External transcutanaeous pacemakers, Pace*Aid Model 50C. Health Devices 1983;13:3-13.

Medtronic, Inc. [Food and Drug Administration, Center for Devices and Radiological Health] Versatrax model 7000 universal A-V pulse generator: summary of safety and effectiveness. 1983 Jan 7. (PMA no. P820003-000).

Pacesetter Systems, Inc. [Food and Drug Administration, Center for Devices and Radiological Health] Programalith (TM) model 223 pulse generator 398 P: summary of safety and effectiveness. 1983 Feb 25. (PMA no. P820023-000).

Telectronics, Inc. [Food and Drug Administration, Center for Devices and Radiological Health] Autima (TM) model 2251 & model 2600: summary of safety and effectiveness. 1983 Mar 11. (PMA no. P820018-000).

Cordis Corp. [Food and Drug Administration, Center for Devices and Radiological Health] Cordis sequicor theta models 233D & 233E: summary of safety and effectiveness. 1982 Dec 10. (PMA no. P820014-000).

ECRI Technology Assessment Program. Multiprogrammable pacemakers. Issues Health Care Technol 1982;sec.5.P.3. [Information syntheses]

ECRI Technology Assessment Program. Multiprogrammable pacemakers. Issues Health Care Technol 1982;sec.5.P.3. [Information syntheses]

Siemens-Elema Pacmaker Div. [Food and Drug Administration, Center for Devices and Radiological Health] Endocardial pacemaker lead w/carbon tip: summary of safety and effectiveness. 1982 Sep 24. (PMA no. P800041-000).

Netherlands Organization for Applied Scientific Research, Medical Technology Unit (TNO). External pacemakers. 1978.

Cardiac rehabilitation

American College of Physicians, Clinical Efficacy Assessment Project. Rehabilitation of the myocardial infarction patient, expected completion 1988. [Information syntheses]

American Medical Association, Diagnostic and Therapeutic Technology Assessment. Cardiac rehabilitation services. Jul 16, 1986. [Expert opinion, Information syntheses]

Oldridge NB. [National Health Research and Development Program - Canada] Comprehensive early rehabilitation after myocardial infarction (MI). 1986. (Grant No. 6606-2724-44).

U.S. Administrators, Professional Policy Committee. Cardiac rehabilitation programs. [7/86] [Group judgment]

Blue Cross and Blue Shield Association, Medical Necessity Program. Outpatient cardiac rehabilitation. 1985. [Information syntheses]

National Center for Health Services Research and Health Care Technology Assessment, Office of Health Technology Assessment. Cardiac rehabilitation program services. Ongoing.

Cardiointegram

National Center for Health Services Research and Health Care Technology Assessment, Office of Health Technology Assessment. Cardiointegram as an alternative to stress test or thallium stress test. Ongoing.

Cardiokymography

American College of Physicians, Clinical Efficacy Assessment Project. Cardiokymography. ACP Observer 1986 Jan:8,10. [Information syntheses]

ECRI Technology Assessment Program. Cardiokymography. Issues Health Care Technol 1986;sec.5.C.8. [Information syntheses]

Blue Cross and Blue Shield Association, Medical Necessity Program. Cardiokymography. 1985. [Information syntheses]

National Center for Health Services Research and Health Care Technology Assessment, Office of Health Technology Assessment. Reassessment of cardiokymography. 1985.

American Medical Association, Diagnostic and Therapeutic Technology Assessment. Cardiokymography for (non-invasive) cardiological diagnosis. JAMA 1984 Feb 24. [Expert opinion, Information syntheses]

National Center for Health Services Research and Health Care Technology Assessment, Office of Health Technology Assessment. Cardiokymography. 1983.

National Center for Health Services Research and Health Care Technology Assessment, Office of Health Technology Assessment. Cardiokymography. Ongoing.

Carmustine

American Academy of Neurology, Practice Committee. Carotid infusion of BCNU for glioblastoma multiforme. 1982 Jun. [Expert opinion, Group judgment]

California Medical Association, Medical Practice Opinion Program. Intraarterial BCNU chemotherapy. 1982 Oct. (Medical Practice Opinion #276) [Group judgment]

Carotid body resection

National Center for Health Services Research and Health Care Technology Assessment, Office of Health Technology Assessment. Bilateral carotid body resection. 1985.

Carotid endarterectomy

National Center for Health Services Research and Health Care Technology Assessment, Office of Health Technology Assessment. Carotid endarterectomy. Ongoing.

U.S. Administrators, Professional Policy Committee. Carotid endarterectomy. Ongoing. [Group judgment]

Case management

Case-managed medical care for nursing home patients. In: Office of Research and Demonstrations, Health Care Financing Administration. Health care financing status report: research and demonstrations in health care financing. Jan 1986. (HCFA Pub. No. 03219).

Evaluation of Massachusetts case-managed medical care for nursing home patients. In: Office of Research and Demonstrations, Health Care Financing Administration. Health care financing status report: research and demonstrations in health care financing. Jan 1986. (HCFA Pub. No. 03219).

Cataract extraction

American Academy of Ophthalmology. Cataract surgery in the 1980's. San Francisco, CA: American Academy of Ophthalmology, 1987. [Information syntheses, Expert opinion]

California Medical Association, Medical Practice Opinion Program. Assistant surgeon at cataract surgery. 1985 May. (Medical Practice Opinion #324) [Group judgment]

Project HOPE, Center for Health Affairs. Background paper on cataract surgery and physician payment under the Medicare program. (for U.S. Congress, Office of Technology Assessment). 1985 Oct. [Information syntheses. Cost analyses]

Catheters

U.S. Administrators, Professional Policy Committee. Swan Ganz. [7/86] [Group judgment]

Food and Drug Administration, Center for Devices and Radiological Health. Vascular catheter devices: a study of safety and performance - volume 1. 1983. (NTIS Order No. PB83-144659).

Food and Drug Administration, Center for Devices and Radiological Health. Vascular catheter devices: a study of safety and performance - volume 2. 1983. (NTIS Order No. 83-144667).

Storz Instrument Co. [Food and Drug Administration, Center for Devices and Radiological Health] Lincoff--design scleral buckling balloon catheter: summary of safety and effectiveness. 1983 Nov 21. (PMA no. P820009-000).

Cefotaxime

Food and Drug Administration, Center for Drugs and Biologics. Sterile cefotaxime sodium. 1981. (NTIS order no. PB81-915906). [Information syntheses, Expert opinion, Epidemiological and other observational methods, Clinical trials, Bench testing]

Cell counters

Food and Drug Administration, Center for Devices and Radiological Health. Evaluation of automated differential cell counting devices - Volume I: review of literature and labeling. 1984. (NTIS Order No. PB84-189356).

Cell counts

California Medical Association, Medical Practice Opinion Program. Endothelial cell counts. 1983 Sep. (Medical Practice Opinion #303) [Group judgment]

Centrifuges

United Kingdom Department of Health and Social Security, Medical Devices Evaluation Programme. Survey of bench top centrifuges. 1985 May. (Report no. STB3A/85/20) [Epidemiological and other observational methods, Bench testing]

Cephradine

Food and Drug Administration, Center for Drugs and Biologics. Cephradine. 1982. (NTIS order no. PB82-915901). [Information syntheses, Expert opinion, Epidemiological and other observational methods, Clinical trials, Bench testing]

Cerebral artery anastomosis

U.S. Administrators, Professional Policy Committee. Cerebral artery anastomosis, superficial temporal--middle. [Group judgment]

U.S. Administrators, Professional Policy Committee. Cerebral artery anastomosis, superficial temporal--middle. [7/86] [Group judgment]

Cerebrospinal fluid shunt valves

Food and Drug Administration, Center for Devices and Radiological Health. An investigation of cerebrospinal fluid shunt valves - test results for twenty-five valves: final report - Phase III.

Cervical cap

Love E, Cruickshank B. [National Health Research and Development Program - Canada] A study in Canadian women of the clinical efficacy and acceptability of the cervical cap as a method of reversible contraception. 1986. (Grant No. 6613-1232-X).

Cervical dilators

Gynotech, Inc. [Food and Drug Administration, Center for Devices and Radiological Health] Dilapan (TM): summary of safety and effectiveness. 1986 Jun 11. (PMA no. P840045-000).

Cabot Medical Corp. [Food and Drug Administration, Center for Devices and Radiological Health] Lamicel (TM): summary of safety and effectiveness. 1983 Jul 19. (PMA no. P820075-000).

Cesarean section

American College of Obstetricians and Gynecologists, Committee on Technical Bulletins. Anesthesia for cesarean section. 1982 May. (Technical bulletin no. 65). [Expert opinion]

National Institute of Child Health and Human Development. Cesarean childbirth. Bethesda, MD: National Institute of Child Health and Human Development, 1981. (NIH publication no. 82-2067) [Group judgment, Expert opinion]

National Institutes of Health, Consensus Development Program. Cesarean childbirth. (Consensus Development Conference Statement, Sep 22-24 1980). [Group judgment]

Challenge food testing

California Medical Association, Medical Practice Opinion Program. Intradermal provocative titration/diagnosis of food allergy. 1984 Feb. (Medical Practice Opinion #293) [Group judgment]

California Medical Association, Medical Practice Opinion Program. Sublingual challenge technique/diagnosis of food allergy. 1984 Feb. (Medical Practice Opinion #294) [Group judgment]

California Medical Association, Medical Practice Opinion Program. Challenge food testing for depression. 1982 Feb. (Medical Practice Opinion #257b) [Group judgment]

California Medical Association, Medical Practice Opinion Program. Challenge food testing for respiratory disorders. 1982 Feb. (Medical Practice Opinion #257c) [Group judgment]

California Medical Association, Medical Practice Opinion Program. Challenge food testing for rheumatoid arthritis. 1982 Feb. (Medical Practice Opinion #257a) [Group judgment]

National Center for Health Services Research and Health Care Technology Assessment, Office of Health Technology Assessment. Intracutaneous (intradermal) and subcutaneous provocative and neutralization testing and neutralization therapy for food allergies. 1981.

National Center for Health Services Research and Health Care Technology Assessment, Office of Health Technology Assessment. Sublingual provocative testing and neutralization therapy for food allergies. 1981

Chelation therapy

McLachlan DR, Dalton AJ. [National Health Research and Development Program - Canada] Aluminum chelation in Alzheimer's disease: a therapeutic proposal. 1986. (Grant No. 6606-2330-08).

American Medical Association, Council on Scientific Affairs. Chelation therapy. 1984. [Group judgment]

Chelation therapy—Deferoxamine

National Center for Health Services Research and Health Care Technology Assessment, Office of Health Technology Assessment. Hemoperfusion in conjunction with deferoxamine for the treatment of aluminum toxicity or iron overload in ESRD patients. 1986.

Chelation therapy—EDTA

American Medical Association, Diagnostic and Therapeutic Technology Assessment. Chelation therapy (with EDTA) for atherosclerosis. JAMA 1983 Aug 5. [Expert opinion, Information syntheses]

National Center for Health Services Research and Health Care Technology Assessment, Office of Health Technology Assessment. Ethylenediamine-tetra-acetic acid (EDTA) chelation therapy for atherosclerosis. 1981.

Chelation therapy—Penicillamine

Crawhall, J. [National Health Research and Development Program - Canada] Effect of D-penicillamine on circulating immune complexes and rheumatoid factor. What is the mechanism of its therapeutic action? 1986. (Grant No. 6605-1758-52).

CHEMLINE

Siegel ER, Spann M, Collins KA, Hazard G, Woodsmall RM. [National Library of Medicine] Report on the CHEMLINE evaluation study. Bethesda, MD: National Library of Medicine, 1985. [Epidemiological and other observational methods]

Woelfel JC, Tesorero J. [National Library of Medicine] An evaluation of CHEMLINE: the results of a survey of users by the National Library of Medicine. Vienna, VA: Market Dynamics, Inc, 1985. [Epidemiological and other observational methods]

Chemonucleolysis

ECRI Technology Assessment Program. Chemonucleolysis of herniated lumbar disks. Issues Health Care Technol 1983;sec.5.C.3. [Information syntheses]

Chemotherapy—Cancer

Lymphomas, leukemia, and chemotherapy. In: Prospective Payment Assessment Commission. Technical appendixes to the report and recommendations to the Secretary, U.S. Department of Health and Human Services, April 1, 1986. Washington, DC: Government Printing Office, 1986:121-123. [Information syntheses, Cost analyses]

U.S. Administrators, Professional Policy Committee. Adjuvant chemotherapy for breast cancer. [7/86]. [Group judgment]

U.S. Administrators, Professional Policy Committee. Chemotherapy. [7/86]. [Group judgment]

National Institutes of Health, Consensus Development Program. Adjuvant chemotherapy for breast cancer. (Consensus Development Conference Statement, Sep 9-11 1985). [Group judgment]

Pritchard KI. [Department Medicine, University of Toronto] [Medical Research Council - Canada] A trial of adjuvant therapy in post menopausal women with axillary node positive breast cancer. (Grant period 1984-1985).

National Institutes of Health, Consensus Development Program. Adjuvant chemotherapy of breast cancer. (Consensus Development Conference Statement, Jul 14-16 1980). [Group judgment]

Chlorhexidine

Food and Drug Administration, Center for Drugs and Biologics. Chlorhexidine gluconate. 1981. (NTIS order no. PB81-915911). [Information syntheses, Expert opinion, Epidemiological and other observational methods, Clinical trials, Bench testing]

Chlorpheniramine

Food and Drug Administration, Center for Drugs and Biologics. Chlorpheniramine maleate pseudoephedrine sulfate. 1981. (NTIS order no.PB81-915906). [Information syntheses, Expert opinion, Epidemiological and other observational methods, Clinical trials, Bench testing]

Food and Drug Administration, Center for Drugs and Biologics. Phenylpropanolamine hydrochloride chlorpheniramine maleate. 1981. (NTIS order no. PB81-915910). [Information syntheses, expert opinion, Epidemiological and other observational methods, Clinical trials, Bench testing]

Chlorthalidone

Grimm RH, Neaton JD, McDonald M, et al for the Multiple Risk Factor Intervention Trial Research Group. [National Heart, Lung, and Blood Institute] Beneficial effects from systematic dosage reduction of the diuretic chlorthalidone: a randomized study within a clinical trial. Am Heart J 1985;109:858-864.

Hulley SB, Furberg CD, Gurland BJ, et al for the SHEP Research Group. [National Heart, Lung, and Blood Institute] The Systolic Hypertension in the Elderly Program (SHEP): antihypertensive efficacy of chlorthalidone. Am J Cardiol 1985;56:913-920.

Cholangiography

U.S. Administrators, Professional Policy Committee. Cholangiography, routine operative. [7/86] [Group judgment]

Kreek MJ, Balint JA. [American Gastroenterological Association, Patient Care Committee] "Skinny needle" cholangiography: results of a pilot study of a voluntary prospective method for gathering risk data on new procedures. Gastroenterology 1980;78:598-604. [Information syntheses]

Cholangiopancreatography

American College of Physicians, Clinical Efficacy Assessment Project. Efficacy of endoscopic retrograde cholangiopancreatography (ERCP) and endoscopic retrograde sphincterotomy (ERS). 1984. [Information syntheses]

Cholecystectomy

U.S. Administrators, Professional Policy Committee. Cholecystectomy. [7/86] [Group judgment]

Cholecystography

Food and Drug Administration, Center for Devices and Radiological Health. Assessment and modification of clinical utility in diagnostic radiology: the oral cholecystogram and the upper gastrointestinal examinations. 1985. (NTIS Order No. PB85-246916/AS)

Cholestryamine

Oster G, Epstein AM. [Policy Analysis, Inc.] The cost-effectiveness of cholestyramine in the prevention of coronary heart disease: whom should we treat? JAMA (submitted for publication)

Brensike JF, Levy RI, Kelsey SF, et al. [National Heart, Lung, and Blood Institute] Effects of therapy with cholestyramine on progression of coronary arteriosclerosis: results of the NHLBI Type II Coronary Intervention Study. Circulation 1984:69;313-324.

Levy RI, Brensike JF, Epstein SF, et al. [National Heart, Lung, and Blood Institute] The influence of changes in lipid values induced by cholestyramine and diet on progression of coronary artery disease: results of the NHLBI Type II Coronary Intervention Study. Circulation 1984;69:325-337.

Chorionic villi sampling

Blue Cross and Blue Shield Association, Technology Evaluation and Coverage Program. Chorionic villi sampling. 1986. [Information syntheses]

ECRI Technology Assessment Program. Chorionic villus sampling (CVS). Issues Health Care Technol 1986;sec.5.C.6. [Information syntheses]

Hunter A. [National Health Research and Development Program - Canada] The use of chorionic villi biopsy for the first trimester diagnosis of genetic diseases. 1986. (Grant No. 6606-2681-52).

California Medical Association, Medical Practice Opinion Program. Chorionic villus biopsy. 1985 Sep. (Medical Practice Opinion #328) [Group judgment]

[University of Lausanne, Institute of Social and Preventive Medicine] Evaluation of efficacy and safety of chorionic villi sampling (CVS). Ongoing. [Clinical trials]

Chromatogenesis assist devices

Repro-Med System, Inc. [Food and Drug Administration, Center for Devices and Radiological Health] Repro-Med-THD: summary of safety and effectiveness. 1985 Jan 25. (PMA no. P820034-000).

Chymopapain

Food and Drug Administration, Center for Drugs and Biologics. Chymopapain. 1983. (NTIS order no. PB83-915901). [Information syntheses, Expert opinion, Epidemiological and other observational methods, Clinical trials, Bench testing]

Health Council of the Netherlands. Chymopapain. Ongoing.

Ciclopirox

Food and Drug Administration, Center for Drugs and Biologics. Ciclopirox olamine. 1983. (NTIS order no. PB83-915901). [Information syntheses, Expert opinion, Epidemiological and other observational methods, Clinical trials, Bench testing]

Cimetidine

Carlsson P, Jonsson. [Linköping University, Center for Medical Technology Assessment] Medical technology assessment in a macroeconomic perspective—a study of the introduction of cimetidine for treatment of ulcers. 1986. (Discussion series paper #1) [Swedish language only] [Cost analyses, Epidemiological methods]

University of Pennsylvania, Leonard Davis Institute of Health Economics. Cost-benefit and cost-effectiveness analysis in policymaking: cimetidine as an example. 1982. (Proceedings of an International Symposium. November 22-24, 1981, funded by Smith Kline and French Laboratories).

Fineberg HV, Pearlman LA. [Harvard School of Public Health, Institute for Health Research] Benefit-and--cost analysis of medical interventions: the case of cimetidine and peptic ulcer disease. In: The implications of cost-effectiveness analysis of medical technology/background paper #2: case studies of medical technologies. Office of Technology Assessment, U.S. Congress. Washington, D.C.: U.S. Government Printing Office, 1981. [Information syntheses]

Office of Technology Assessment, U.S. Congress. Benefit and cost analysis of medical interventions: the case of cimetidine and peptic ulcer disease. Washington, D.C.: U.S. Government Printing Office, September 1981. (Health technology case study series #11).

Cine-CT

American Hospital Association, Hospital Technology Series Program. Cine-CT: progress and opportunities. 1986. (Guideline report) [Information syntheses, Expert opinion, Cost analyses]

Cingulotomy

American Medical Association, Diagnostic and Therapeutic Technology Assessment. Sterotactic cingulotomy treatment for psychiatric disorders. JAMA 1985 Nov 15. [Expert opinion, Information syntheses]

National Center for Health Services Research and Health Care Technology Assessment, Office of Health Technology Assessment. Stereotactic cingulotomy as a means of psychosurgery. 1985.

American Academy of Neurology, Practice Committee. Sterotactic cingulotomy. 1984 Nov. [Expert opinion, Group judgment]

Circumcision

American Academy of Pediatrics, Committee on Fetus and Newborn. Report of the Ad Hoc Task Force on Circumcision. Pediatrics 1975 Oct.

Clinical ecology

American College of Physicians, Clinical Efficacy Assessment Project. Clinical ecology, expected completion 1988. [Information syntheses]

Clinical trials

Mattson M, Curb JD, McArdle R and the AMIS and BHAT Research Group. [National Heart, Lung, and Blood Institute] Participation in a clinical trial: the patient's point of view. Controlled Clin Trial 1985;6:156-167.

Thomson ME, Kramer MS. [McGill University, Department of Epidemiology and Biostatistics] Methodological standards for controlled clinical trials of perinatal contact: studies of early contact and maternal-infant behavior. Pediatrics 1983;73:294-300.

Lipid Research Clinics Program. [National Heart, Lung, and Blood Institute] Recruitment for clinical trials: the Lipid Research Clinics Coronary Primary Prevention Trial experience. Its implications for future trials. (AHA Monograph No. 93) Circulation 1982;66:IV1-IV78.

Mosteller F. [National Center for Health Services Research and Health Care Technology Assessment, Division of Extramural Research] Improving the precision of clinical trials. Am J Public Health 1982 May;72(5):430.

Howard JM, DeMets D, and the BHAT Research Group. [National Heart, Lung, and Blood Institute] How informed is informed consent? The BHAT experience. Controlled Clin Trials 1981;2:287-303.

Clinical trials—Randomized

Antczak AA, Tang J, Chalmers TC. [National Center for Health Services Research and Health Care Technology Assessment, Division of Extramural Research] Quality assessment of randomized control trials in dental research. I. Methods. J Periodont Dis 1986;21:305-314.

Antczak AA, Tang J, Chalmers TC. [National Center for Health Services Research and Health Care Technology Assessment, Division of Extramural Research] Quality assessment of randomized control trials in dental research. II Results. J Periodent Res 1986;21:315-321.

Office of Technology Assessment, U.S. Congress. The impact of randomized clinical trials on health policy and medical practice. Washington, D.C.: U.S. Government Printing Office, August 1983.

Clonidine

Food and Drug Administration, Center for Drugs and Biologics. Clonidine. 1987. (Summary basis of approval, NDA # 18-891). [Information syntheses, Expert opinion, Epidemiological and other observational methods, Clincial trials, Bench testing]

Clorazepate

Food and Drug Administration, Center for Drugs and Biologics. Clorazepate dipotassium. 1981. (NTIS order no. PB81-915904). [Information syntheses, Expert opinion, Epidemiological and other observational methods, Clinical trials, Bench testing]

Clotrimazole

Food and Drug Administration, Center for Drugs and Biologics. Clotrimazole. 1987. (Summary basis of approval, NDA #18-827). [Information syntheses, Expert opinion, Epidemiological and other observational methods, Clinical trials, Bench testing]

Coagulation assays

Triplett DA, ed. Advances in coagulation testing: interpretation and application. Skokie, IL: College of American Pathologists. (expected 1987) [Expert opinion, Bench testing]

Triplett DA, ed. Standardization of coagulation assays: an overview. CAP Conference/Aspen 1980. Skokie, IL: College of American Pathologists, 1981. [Expert opinion, Bench testing]

Cochlear implantation

Medical Technology and Practice Patterns Institute. Cochlear implantation. 1987.

Cochlear implants

Medical Technology and Practice Patterns Institute. Cochlear implants outpatient training. 1987.

ECRI Technology Assessment Program. Multichannel cochlear implants for profound deafness. Issues Health Care Technol 1986;sec.5.C.7. [Information syntheses]

National Center for Health Services Research and Health Care Technology Assessment, Office of Health Technology Assessment. Cochlear implants. 1986.

U.S. Administrators, Professional Policy Committee. Cochlear implants. [7/86] [Group judgment]

3M. [Food and Drug Administration, Center for Devices and Radiological Health] 3M brand cochlear implant system/house design: summary of safety and effectiveness. 1984 Dec 24. (PMA no. P830069-000).

American Medical Association, Council on Scientific Affairs. Cochlear implants. JAMA 1983 Jul 15;250:391-392. [Group judgment]

ECRI Technology Assessment Program. Single-channel cochlear implants for profound deafness. Issues Health Care Technol 1983;sec.5.C.1. [Information syntheses]

California Medical Association, Medical Practice Opinion Program. Cochlear implant for deafness. 1981 Aug. (Medical Practice Opinion Program #178) [Group judgment]

Veterans Administration, Cooperative Studies Program. A prospective randomized cooperative study of cochlear implants. Ongoing. [Clinical trials]

Cochleostomy

American Academy of Neurology, Practice Committee. Cochleostomy with neurovascular transplant in treatment of Ménière's Disease. 1982 Oct. [Expert opinion, Group judgment]

Codeine

American Academy of Pediatrics, Committee on Drugs. Use of codeine- and dextromethorphan-containing cough syrups in pediatrics. Pediatrics 1978 Jul.

Cognitive therapy

Cott A. [National Health Research and Development Program - Canada] Intervention in disability and chest pain associated with (a) mitral valve prolapse and (b) no known cardiac disease: a cognitive-behavioral approach. (Grant No. 6606-2250-05).

Garner DM. [National Health Research and Development Program - Canada] Cognitive therapy for anorexia nervosa and bulimia. 1986. (Grant No. 6606-2666-46).

Collagen implants

Blue Cross and Blue Shield Association, Technology Evaluation and Coverage Program. Collagen implants. 1986. [Information syntheses]

California Medical Association, Medical Practice Opinion Program. Collagen implant. 1983 Apr. (Medical Practice Opinion #283) [Group judgment]

ECRI Technology Assessment Program. Collagen implants for smoothing skin. Issues Health Care Technol 1983;sec.5.C.2. [Information syntheses]

Colonoscopy

Mellow MH. Endoscopic laser treatment of colon cancer. In: American Society for Gastrointestinal Endoscopy, Committee on Technology Assessment. Therapeutic gastrointestinal endoscopy: an information resource manual. 1987. [Information syntheses, Expert opinion, Group judgment, Cost analyses]

American Society for Gastrointestinal Endoscopy. The role of colonoscopy in the management of patients with colonic polyps. Revised 1986 May.

American Society for Gastrointestinal Endoscopy. The role of colonoscopy in the patients with inflammatory bowel diseases. Revised 1986 May.

Irvine EJ. [National Health Research and Development Program - Canada] A prospective study to compare diagnostic agreement and cost-effectiveness of air contrast barium enema plus flexible sigmoidoscopy with colonoscopy in rectal bleeding. 1986. (Grant No. 6606-2974-42).

American College of Physicians, Clinical Efficacy Assessment Project. Colonoscopy: management of colorectal neoplasia. 1985. [Information syntheses]

Communication aids for the handicapped

Parnes PH. [National Health Research and Development Program - Canada] Towards development of a modular universal wheelchair tray system for communication control and ADL. 1986. (Grant No. 6605-3006-51).

Office of Technology Assessment, U.S. Congress. Assistive devices for severe speech impairments. Washington, D.C.: U.S. Government Printing Office, December 1983. (Health technology case study series #26)

Office of Technology Assessment, U.S. Congress. Selected telecommunications devices for hearing-impaired persons. Washington, D.C.: U.S. Government Printing Office, December 1982. (Health technology case study series #21)

Communication systems

Darnell JC, et al. [National Center for Health Services Research and Health Care Technology Assessment, Division of Extramural Research] After hours telephone access to physicians with access to computerized medical records. Med Care 1985 Jan;23(1):20-26.

Simborg DW, et al. [National Center for Health Services Research and Health Care Technology Assessment, Division of Extramural Research] A hospital local area communication network: the first year's experience. IEEE 1982:479-481.

Community health centers

Grossman M, et al. [National Center for Health Services Research and Health Care Technology Assessment, Division of Extramural Research] An economic analysis of community health centers. 1984. (NTIS order no. PB84-159185)

Competition

Competitive managed health plans for AFDC Medicaid recipients. In: Office of Research and Demonstrations, Health Care Financing Administration. Health care financing status report: research and demonstrations in health care financing. Jan 1986. (HCFA Pub. No. 03219).

Costs, outcomes, and competition in the End-Stage Renal Disease Program. In: Office of Research and Demonstrations, Health Care Financing Administration. Health care financing status report: research and demonstrations in health care financing. Jan 1986. (HCFA Pub. No. 03219).

Enrollment of Medicare beneficiaries under a unique intra-health maintenance organization competition model. In: Office of Research and Demonstrations, Health Care Financing Administration. Health care financing status report: research and demonstrations in health care financing. Jan 1986. (HCFA Pub. No. 03219).

Evaluation of Medicaid competition demonstrations. In: Office of Research and Demonstrations, Health Care Financing Administration. Health care financing status report: research and demonstrations in health care financing. Jan 1986. (HCFA Pub. No. 03219).

Evaluation of the Medicare competition demonstrations. In: Office of Research and Demonstrations, Health Care Financing Administration. Health care financing status report: research and demonstrations in health care financing. Jan 1986. (HCFA Pub. No. 03219).

Independent broker: coordinating open enrollment for Medicare health maintenance organizations and competitive medical plans. In: Office of Research and Demonstrations, Health Care Financing Admimistration. Health care financing status report: reseaarch and demonstrations in health care financing. Jan 1986. (HCFA Pub. No. 03219).

Medicaid voucher demonstration. In: Office of Research and Demonstrations, Health Care Financing Administration. Health care financing status report: research and demonstrations in health care financing. Jan 1986. (HCFA Pub. No. 03219).

Medicare competition demonstrations. In: Office of Research and Demonstrations, Health Care Finanicng Administration. Health care financing status report: research and demonstrations in health care financing. Jan 1986. (HCFA Pub. No. 03219).

Research on competitive forces driving Medicare utilization. In: Office of Research and Demonstrations, Health Care Financing Administration. Health care financing status report: research and demonstrations in health care financing. Jan 1986. (HCFA Pub. No. 03219).

Senior Group Health Plan Waiver-Only Medicare Competition Demonstration Program. In: Office of Research and Demonstrations, Health Care Financing Administration. Health care financing status report: research and demonstrations in health care financing. Jan 1986. (HCFA Pub. No. 03219).

Statewide Medicaid competition demonstration. In: Office of Research and Demonstrations, Health Care Financing Administration. Health care financing status report: research and demonstrations in health care financing. Jan 1986. (HCFA Pub. No. 03219).

Waiver-Only Competition Project for Southern California, Illinois, Indiana, and Texas. In: Office of Research and Demonstrations, Health Care Financing Administration. Health care financing status report: research and demonstrations in health care financing. Jan 1986. (HCFA Pub. No. 03219).

American Medical Association, Council on Scientific Affairs. Effects of competition in medicine. JAMA 1983 Apr 8;249:1864-1868. [Group judgment]

Office of Technology Assessment, U.S. Congress. Medical technology under proposals to increase competition in health care. Washington, D.C.: U.S. Government Printing Office, October 1982.

Competitive bidding

Demonstration and evaluation of competitive bidding as a method of purchasing durable medical equipment. In: Office of Research and Demonstrations, Health Care Financing Administration. Health care financing status report: research and demonstrations in health care financing. Jan 1986. (HCFA Pub. No. 03219).

Demonstration and evaluation of competitive bidding as a method to purchase clinical laboratory services. In: Office of Research and Demonstrations, Health Care Financing Administration. Health care financing status report: research and demonstrations in health care financing. Jan 1986. (HCFA Pub. No. 03219).

End-stage renal disease competitive bidding demonstration. In: Office of Research and Demonstrations, Health Care Financing Administration. Health care financing status report: research and demonstrations in health care financing. Jan 1986. (HCFA Pub. No. 03219).

Computed tomography

Hussain S, Belidegrun A, Seltzer SE, Feldstein ML, et al. [Harvard School of Public Health, Institute for Health Research] CT differentiation of malignant from benign adrenal masses. Am J Roentgenol, in press [Epidemiological methods]

American College of Physicians, Clinical Efficacy Assessment Project. A comparative assessment of standard and computed tomography in the evaluation of neoplasms of the chest. 1986. [Information syntheses]

ECRI Technology Assessment Program. Three-dimensional computed tomography. Issues Health Care Technol 1986;sec.5.T.6. [Information syntheses]

California Medical Association, Medical Practice Opinion Program. Computed tomography - multiplanar reconstruction. 1984 Nov. (Medical Practice Opinion #310) [Group judgment]

Fineberg HV, Wittenberg J , Ferrucci J, Meuller P, Simeone J, Goldman J. [Harvard School of Public Health, Institute for Health Research] The clinical value of body computed tomography over time and technologic change. Am J Roentgenol 1983;141:1067-1072. [Epidemiological methods]

Office of Technology Assessment, U.S. Congress. The feasibility of economic evaluation of diagnostic procedures: the case of CT scanning. Washington, D.C.: U.S. Government Printing Office, April 1981. (Health technology case study series #2)

Swedish Planning and Rationalization Institute of the Health Services. Spri technology report 2: CT scanning in Sweden - costs and effectiveness. 1981. (Spri report 73) [Cost analyses, Epidemiological and other observational methods]

American Medical Association, Council on Scientific Affairs. Importance of diagnostic computerized tomographic scanning. 1980. [Group judgment]

Subcommittee on Institutional Program Guidelines. [Health and Welfare Canada, Health Services and Promotion Branch, Institutional and Professional Services Division] Computed tomography guidelines. 1980. [Information syntheses, Expert opinion, Group judgment]

Wittenberg J, Fineberg HV, Ferrucci JT Jr, Simeone JF, Mueller PR, van Sonnenberg E, Kirkpatrick RH. [Harvard School of Public Health, Institute for Health Research] The clinical efficacy of computed body tomography. II. Am J Roentgenol 1980;134:1111-1120. [Epidemiological methods]

Fineberg HV, Wittenberg J, Ferruci JT, Jr. [Harvard School of Public Health, Institute for Health Research] The clinical value of diagnostic tests: CT as a prototype. IN: Margulis A, Burhenne HJ, eds. Alimentary tract radiology: abdominal imaging, v. 3. St. Louis, Missouri: C.V. Mosby, 1979. [Epidemiological methods]

Fineberg HV. [Harvard School of Public Health, Institute for Health Research] Medical technology policies and computed tomography. Ann Intern Med 1979;90:114-115. [Information syntheses]

Wittenberg J, Fineberg HV, Black EB, Kirkpatrick RH, Schaffer DL, Ikeda MK, Ferrucci JT Jr. [Harvard Medical School, Institute for Health Research] The clinical efficacy of computerized body tomography. Am J Roentgenol 1978;131:5-14. [Epidemiological methods]

Computed tomography—Bone mineral assessments

ECRI Technology Assessment Program. Bone mineral assessment, noninvasive (dual photon absorptiometry and quantitative computed tomography). J Health Care Technol 1986;2:183-200. [Information syntheses]

National Center for Health Services Research and Health Care Technology Assessment, Office of Health Technology Assessment. Bone mineral density studies: computed tomography. Ongoing.

Computed tomography—Head

U.S. Administrators, Professional Policy Committee. CT scans - head. [7/86] [Group judgment]

American Medical Association, Diagnostic and Therapeutic Technology Assessment. Enhanced computed tomography in head trauma. JAMA 1985 Dec 20. [Expert opinion, Information syntheses]

Blue Cross and Blue Shield Association, Medical Necessity Program. CT scan in the evaluation of headaches, cerebrovascular disease and dementia. 1984. [Information syntheses]

Blue Cross and Blue Shield Association, Medical Necessity Program. Head CT scan and ultrasound in the pediatric patient. 1984. [Information syntheses]

McNeil BJ, Hanley JA. [McGill University, Department of Epidemiology and Biostatistics] Critical questions regarding a new diagnostic technology: a case study using computed tomography (CT) of the head. In: Culyer AJ, Horisberger, eds. Economic and medical evaluation of health care technologies, proceedings of Wolfsberg Conference. 1983.

National Institutes of Health, Consensus Development Program. Computed tomographic scanning of the brain. (Consensus Development Conference Statement, Nov 4-6 1981). [Group judgment]

Fineberg HV, Bauman K, Sossman M. [Harvard School of Public Health, Institute for Health Research] Computerized cranial tomography: effect on diagnostic and therapeutic plans. JAMA 1977;238:224-227. [Epidemiological methods]

Computed tomography—Liver and spleen

U.S. Administrators, Professional Policy Committee. Liver/spleen scans. Ongoing. [Group judgment]

Computed tomography—Pancreas

Fineberg HV, Wittenberg J. [Harvard School of Public Health, Institute for Health Research] Evaluation of computed tomography in pancreatic cancer. Bull Cancer (Paris) 1980;67:390-394. [Epidemiological methods]

Fineberg HV. [Harvard School of Public Health, Institute for Health Research] Assessing the diagnostic contribution of imaging tests: computed tomography and ultrasound of the pancreas. In: Alperovitch A, de Dombal FT, Gremy F, eds. Evaluation of efficacy of medical action. New York: Elsevier-North Holland, 1979. [Epidemiological methods]

Computed tomography—Spine

U.S. Administrators, Professional Policy Committee. CT scans cervical and lumbar spine. [7/86] [Group judgment]

California Medical Association, Medical Practice Opinion Program. Computerized tomography for lumbar spine. Feb 1983. (Medical Practice Opinion #282) [Group judgment]

Computed tomography scanners

United Kingdom Department of Health and Social Security, Medical Devices Evaluation Programme. Comparison of imaging performance of CT scanners (Issue four). 1986 Mar. (Report no. STB/86/10) [Epidemiological and other observational methods, Bench testing]

ECRI Technology Assessment Program. Imatron high--speed CT scanner. Issues Health Care Technol 1985;sec.5.C.5. [Information synthesis]

United Kingdom Department of Health and Social Security, Medical Devices Evaluation Programme. Assessment of Picker Modulex T for radiography, tomography and occasional peripheral angiography. 1985 Dec. (Report no. STB6E/85/45) [Epidemiological and other observational methods, Bench testing]

American Hospital Association, Hospital Technology Series Program. Computerized tomographic scanners. 1984. (Guideline report) [Information syntheses, Expert opinion, Cost analyses]

Office of Technology Assessment, U.S. Congress. Policy implications of computed tomography (CT) scanners: an update. Washington, D.C.: U.S. Government Printing Office, January 1981.

Office of Technology Assessment, U.S. Congress. Policy implications of computed tomography (CT) scanners. Washington, D.C.: U.S. Government Printing Office, August 1978.

Fineberg HV, Parker GS, Pearlman LA. [Harvard School of Public Health, Institute for Health Research] CT scanners: distribution and planning status in the United States. N Eng J Med 1977;297:216-218. [Epidemiological methods]

Johns Hopkins Program for Medical Technology and Practice Assessment. An evaluation of patterns of utilization of CT scanners, with particular attention to variations in practice patterns. Planned.

Computer-aided design

Fernie GR. [National Health Research and Development Program - Canada] An evaluation of computer--aided design of trans-tibial prosthetic sockets. 1986. (Grant No. 6606-3024-51).

Computer-assisted instruction

Office of Technology Assessment, U.S. Congress. Computer technology in medical education and assessment. Washington, D.C.: U.S. Government Printing Office, September 1979.

[National Library of Medicine] Evaluation of the Technological Innovations in Medical Education (TIME) Project. Bethesda, MD: Lister Hill Center, National Library of Medicine. Ongoing. [Epidemiological and other observational methods]

Computer-assisted patient care

McDonald CJ, Tierney WM. [National Center for Health Services Research and Health Care Technology Assessment, Division of Extramural Research] The medical gopher: a microcomputer system to help find, organize, and decide about patient data. West J Med (in press)

Self-care home computer program to reduce health care costs. In: Office of Research and Demonstrations, Health Care Financing Administration. Health care financing status report: research and demonstrations in health care financing. Jan 1986. (HCFA Pub. No. 03219).

ECRI Health Devices Program. Patient care management system, SpaceLabs. Health Devices 1986;15:286-94.

American Academy of Pediatrics, Committee on Practice and Ambulatory Medicine. Computers in your practice. Pediatrics 1985 Jul.

Bleich HC. [National Center for Health Services Research and Health Care Technology Assessment, Division of Extramural Research] Clinical computing in a teaching hospital. N Engl J Med 1985 Mar 31(12):756-764.

Computer equipment

American Hospital Association, Hospital Technology Series Program. Microcomputers in hospitals. 1984. (Guideline report) [Information syntheses, Expert opinion, Cost analyses]

Computer software

Self-care home computer program to reduce health care costs. In: Office of Research and Demonstrations, Health Care Financing Administration. Health care financing status report: research and demonstrations in health care financing. Jan 1986. (HCFA Pub. No. 03219).

Contact lens cleaners

Stericon Laboratories. [Food and Drug Administration, Center for Devices and Radiological Health] Stericon saline solution: summary of safety and effectiveness. 1987 Jan16. (PMA no. P850070-000).

Allergan Pharmaceuticals, Inc. [Food and Drug Administration, Center for Devices and Radiological Health] Oxysept system: summary of safety and effectiveness. 1986 Nov 20. (PMA no. P850088-000).

Barnes-Hind Inc. [Food and Drug Administration, Center for Devices and Radiological Health] Softmate (R) hydrogen peroxide disinfection system: summary of safety and effectiveness. 1986 Oct 6. (PMA no. P840066-000).

Bausch & Lomb (R). [Food and Drug Administration, Center for Devices and Radiological Health] B & L sterile all purpose solution & contact cleaner: summary of safety and effectiveness. 1986 Dec 16. (PMA no. P830002-000).

Bausch & Lomb. [Food and Drug Administration, Center for Devices and Radiological Health] B & L Sensitive Eyes (TM) saline/cleaning solution: summary of safety and effectiveness. 1986 Jul 7. (PMA no. 850036-000).

Bausch & Lomb. [Food and Drug Administration, Center for Devices and Radiological Health] B & L Therma-zyne, Fizziclean: summary of safety and effectiveness. 1986 Nov 5. (PMA no. P850093-000).

Bausch & Lomb. [Food and Drug Administration, Center for Devices and Radiological Health] Sensitive eyes chemical disinfectant: summary of safety and effectiveness. 1986 Jan 2. (PMA no. P840020-000).

Blairex Laboratories, Inc. [Food and Drug Administration, Center for Devices and Radiological Health] Blairex sterile saline solution: summary of safety and effectiveness. 1986 Mar 6. (PMA no. P850045-000).

Coopervision, Inc. [Food and Drug Administration, Center for Devices and Radiological Health] Coopervision peroxide system: summary of safety and effectiveness. 1986 Mar 12. (PMA no. P830023-000).

Coopervision, Inc. [Food and Drug Administration, Center for Devices and Radiological Health] Mirasoak (TM) rinsing, disinfecting & storage solution: summary of safety and effectiveness. 1986 Aug 18. (PMA no. P810038-000).

Coopervision. [Food and Drug Administration, Center for Devices and Radiological Health] Miraflow extra strength cleaner: summary of safety and effectiveness. 1986 Nov 5. (PMA no. P850055-000).

Dey Laboratories, Inc. [Food and Drug Administration, Center for Devices and Radiological Health] Dey-vial (R): summary of safety and effectiveness. 1986 Apr 1. (PMA no.P840061-000).

Ocumed Inc. [Food and Drug Administration, Center for Devices and Radiological Health] Sodium chloride tablets 250 MG: summary of safety and effectiveness. 1986 Mar 12. (PMA no. P850016-000).

Paco Pharmaceutical Services, Inc. [Food and Drug Administration, Center for Devices and Radiological Health] Non-preserved saline solution: summary of safety and effectiveness. 1986 Sep 23. (PMA no. P850025-000).

Paco Pharmaceutical Services, Inc. [Food and Drug Administration, Center for Devices and Radiological Health] Sorbic acid preserved daily cleaner: summary of safety and effectiveness. 1986 Nov 10. (PMA no. P850076-000).

Paco Research Corp. [Food and Drug Administration, Center for Devices and Radiological Health] Charter Labs saline solution: summary of safety and effectiveness. 1986 Dec 17. (PMA no. P840069-000).

Stericon Laboratories. [Food and Drug Administration, Center for Devices and Radiological Health] Crystalens saline spray: summary of safety and effectiveness. 1986 Mar 24. (PMA no. P850065-000).

Alcon Labs., Inc. [Food and Drug Administration, Center for Devices and Radiological Health] Polquat disinfection system: summary of safety and effectiveness. 1985 Sep 18. (PMA no. P830034-000).

Allergan. [Food and Drug Administration, Center for Devices and Radiological Health] Model no. ALS-IV heat disinfection unit: summary of safety and effectiveness. 1985 May 20. (PMA no. P840054-000).

Bausch & Lomb. [Food and Drug Administration, Center for Devices and Radiological Health] B & L Sensitive Eyes (TM) daily cleaner: summary of safety and effectiveness. 1985 Jul 9. (PMA no. P830013-000).

Pharmafair, Inc. [Food and Drug Administration, Center for Devices and Radiological Health] Saltair tablets (250MG): summary of safety and effectiveness. 1985 Jun 5. (PMA no. P840034-000).

Allergan Optical. [Food and Drug Administration, Center for Devices and Radiological Health] The soft lens thermal disinfecting unit: summary of safety and effectiveness. 1984 Jan 4. (PMA no. P820082-000).

Alcon Laboratories, Inc. [Food and Drug Administration, Center for Devices and Radiological Health] Micro-therm disinfectant unit: summary of safety and effectiveness. 1983 Jan 25. (PMA no. P820041-000).

Alcon Laboratories, Inc. [Food and Drug Administration, Center for Devices and Radiological Health] Opti-clean (TM) LC 1323: summary of safety and effectiveness. 1983 May 13. (PMA no. P820036-000).

Alcon Labs, Inc. [Food and Drug Administration, Center for Devices and Radiological Health] Alcon enzyme cleaner: summary of safety and effectiveness. 1983 Jan 25.(PMA no. P820001-000).

Allergan Pharmaceuticals, Inc. [Food and Drug Administration, Center for Devices and Radiological Health] Lens Plus (TM): summary of safety and effectiveness. 1983 Jul 19. (PMA no. P820050-000).

Amcon Inc. [Food and Drug Administration, Center for Devices and Radiological Health] The Amcon Way Plus: summary of safety and effectiveness. 1983 Feb 22. (PMA no. P800069-002).

Barnes-Hind/Hydrocurve, Inc. [Food and Drug Administration, Center for Devices and Radiological Health] Soft lens salt tablets: summary of safety and effectiveness. 1983 Jul 29. (PMA no. P800067-000).

Bausch & Lomb Optics Center. [Food and Drug Administration, Center for Devices and Radiological Health] Sensitive Eyes (TM) saline & cleaning solution: summary of safety and effectiveness. 1983 Sep 16. (PMA no. P820031-000).

Blairex Laboratories, Inc. [Food and Drug Administration, Center for Devices and Radiological Health] The Blairex system: summary of safety and effectiveness. 1983 Feb 18. (PMA no. PB00028-003).

C.C. Kelly Enterprises. [Food and Drug Administration, Center for Devices and Radiological Health] Eyerisol (R): summary of safety and effectiveness. 1983 May 31. (PMA no. P810034-000).

CIBA Vision Care [Food and Drug Administration, Center for Devices and Radiological Health] Salt tablets: summary of safety and effectiveness. 1983 Feb 18. (PMA no. P810015-001).

CIBA Vision Care Corporation. [Food and Drug Administration, Center for Devices and Radiological Health] Septicon (TM) disinfection regimen for use with . . . : summary of safety and effectiveness. 1983 Apr 8. (PMA no. P820040-000).

Coopervision, Inc. [Food and Drug Administration, Center for Devices and Radiological Health] Heatcase (TM): summary of safety and effectiveness. 1983 Jul 19. (PMA no. P830001-000).

Eaton Medical Corporation. [Food and Drug Administration, Center for Devices and Radiological Health] Easy Eyes (TM): summary of safety and effectiveness. 1983 Jul 19. (PMA no. P830009-000).

Horizon Pharmacal, Inc. [Food and Drug Administration, Center for Devices and Radiological Health] The Horizon system: summary of safety and effectiveness. 1983 Feb 18. (PMA no. P810009-002).

Kestrel. [Food and Drug Administration, Center for Devices and Radiological Health] Kestrel no. 695 heater: summary of safety and effectiveness. 1983 Jun 10. (PMA no. P820087-000).

Marlin Industries. [Food and Drug Administration, Center for Devices and Radiological Health] Marlin squeeze bottle & Marlin salt tablets: summary of safety and effectiveness. 1983 Feb 18. (PMA no. P800038-001).

National Patent Development Corporation. [Food and Drug Administration, Center for Devices and Radiological Health] Hydron (TM) saline system (135 & 250 mg): summary of safety and effectiveness. 1983 Feb 25. (PMA no. P810047-002).

Professional Supplies. [Food and Drug Administration, Center for Devices and Radiological Health] The soft rinse system: summary of safety and effectiveness. 1983 Feb 18. (PMA no. P800060-003).

Amcon Inc. [Food and Drug Administration, Center for Devices and Radiological Health] Nor-Sa-Tab: summary of safety and effectiveness. 1982 Feb 19. (PMA no. P800069-000).

Barnes-Hind Pharmaceuticals, Inc. [Food and Drug Administration, Center for Devices and Radiological Health] Softmate weekly cleaning solution: summary of safety and effectiveness. 1982 Mar 26. (PMA no. P810017-000).

Bausch & Lomb. [Food and Drug Administration, Center for Devices and Radiological Health] Sensitive eyes (TM) saline solution: summary of safety and effectiveness. 1982 Nov 11. (PMA no. P810039-000).

Central Pharmaceuticals, Inc. [Food and Drug Administration, Center for Devices and Radiological Health] Central's pharm. salt tablets for disinfection: summary of safety and effectiveness. 1982 Jan 15. (PMA no. P810030-000).

Coopervision, Inc. [Food and Drug Administration, Center for Devices and Radiological Health] Mirasol (TM): summary of safety and effectiveness. 1982 Jan 12. (PMA no. P810008-000).

Horizon Pharmacal, Inc. [Food and Drug Administration, Center for Devices and Radiological Health] The Horizon system: summary of safety and effectiveness. 1982 Jan 12. (PMA no. P810009-000).

International Hydron Corporation. [Food and Drug Administration, Center for Devices and Radiological Health Hydron (TM) saline system (135 & 250 mg): summary of safety and effectiveness. 1982 Apr 9. (PMA no. P810047-000).

International Hydron Corporation. [Food and Drug Administration, Center for Devices and Radiological Health] Hydron (R) lens care unit: summary of safety and effectiveness. 1982 Oct 9. (PMA no. P820007-000).

Professional Pharmaceal Co. [Food and Drug Administration, Center for Devices and Radiological Health] Salt tablets: summary of safety and effectiveness. 1982 Jan 5. (PMA no.P810003-000).

Professional Supplies. [Food and Drug Administration, Center for Devices and Radiological Health] The soft rinse system: summary of safety and effectiveness. 1982 Jan 1. (PMA no. P800060-000).

Sherman Labs, Inc. [Food and Drug Administration, Center for Devices and Radiological Health] Sof! Pro--clean contact lens cleaner: summary of safety and effectivness. 1982 Jul 23. (PMA no. P810041-000).

Standard Pharmacal Corp. [Food and Drug Administration, Center for Devices and Radiological Health] Lens-sol: summary of safety and effectiveness. 1982 Mar 26. (PMA no. P810012-000).

Contact lens lubricants

Paco Pharmaceutical Services, Inc. [Food and Drug Administration, Center for Devices and Radiological Health] Sorbic acid preserved lens lubricant: summary of safety and effectiveness. 1986 Oct 9. (PMA no. P850075-000).

Allergan Pharmaceuticals. [Food and Drug Administration, Center for Devices and Radiological Health] Lens-wet (TM): summary of safety and effectiveness. 1982 May 14. (PMA no. P800065-000).

Cooper Labs, Inc. [Food and Drug Administration, Center for Devices and Radiological Health] Clerz lubricating & rewetting eye drops: summary of safety and effectiveness. 1982 Jul 13. (PMA no. PB00034-000).

Contact lens markers

Frigitronics, Inc. [Food and Drug Administration, Center for Devices and Radiological Health] Softmark: summary of safety and effectiveness. 1983 Jul 19. (PMA no. P820027-000).

Contact lenses

Alcon Laboratories, Inc. [Food and Drug Administration, Center for Devices and Radiological Health] Scanlens (Scafilcon A contact lens): summary of safety and effectiveness. 1987 Jan 16. (PMA no. P850033-000).

Paragon Optical Inc. [Food and Drug Administration, Center for Devices and Radiological Health] Paraperm E.W. blue rigid gas permeable contact lens: summary of safety and effectiveness. 1987 Feb 18. (PMA no. P850038-000).

CTL, Inc. [Food and Drug Administration, Center for Devices and Radiological Health] Customeyes (TM) 45L & 55L (Bufilcon A): summary of safety and effectiveness. 1986 Jul 1. (PMA no. P850057-000).

CTL, Inc. [Food and Drug Administration, Center for Devices and Radiological Health] Customeyes 70L & 79L (Lidofilcon A & B): summary of safety and efectiveness. 1986 Jul 1. (PMA no. P850058-000).

Custom Tint Lab., Inc. [Food and Drug Administration, Center for Devices and Radiological Health] Permatint (R): summary of safety and effectiveness. 1986 Mar 14. (PMA no. P820059-000).

Custom Tint Lab., Inc. [Food and Drug Administration, Center for Devices and Radiological Health] Permatint (R): summary of safety and effectiveness. 1986 Mar 26. (PMA no. P820059-000).

Oculus Contact Lens Company. [Food and Drug Administration, Center for Devices and Radiological Health] Ocusil (TM) contact lens: summary of safety and effectiveness. 1986 Jan 2. (PMA no. P840050-000).

Syntex Opthalmics Inc. [Food and Drug Administration, Center for Devices and Radiological Health] Polycon contact lens: summary of safety and effectiveness. 1986 Feb 10.(PMA no. N18120-015).

University Optical Products Co. [Food and Drug Administration, Center for Devices and Radiological Health] The Boston lens II Alges (R) bifocal contact lens: summary of safety and effectiveness. 1986 Jan 24. (PMA no. P850008-000).

University Optical Products Company. [Food and Drug Administration, Center for Devices and Radiological Health] Alges (TM) (Hefilcon A) contact lens: summary of safety and effectiveness. 1986 Apr 28. (PMA no. P850002-000).

Bausch & Lomb. [Food and Drug Administration, Center for Devices and Radiological Health] B & L 58 (TM) (Etafilcona) contact lens: summary of safety and effectiveness. 1985 Sep 23. (PMA no. P850039-000).

Frigitronics, Inc. [Food and Drug Administration, Center for Devices and Radiological Health] Saturn II (TM) (Synergicon A) contact lens: summary of safety and effectiveness. 1985 Mar 22 (PMA no. P840004-000).

Heyer Schulte Corp. [Food and Drug Administration, Center for Devices and Radiological Health] Sauflon (R) PW (Lidofilcon B): summary of safety and effectiveness. 1985 May 10. (PMA no. P790020-008).

Heyer Schulte Corp. [Food and Drug Administration, Center for Devices and Radiological Health] Sauflon (r) 70 (Lidofilcon A): summary of safety and effectiveness. 1985 May 10 (PMA no. P790020-002).

Hydracon. [Food and Drug Administration, Center for Devices and Radiological Health] Hydracon (R) contact lenses: summary of safety and effectiveness. 1985 Nov 19. (PMA no. P820017-001).

University Optical Products Company. [Food and Drug Administration, Center for Devices and Radiological Health] Alges (TM) (Hefilcon A) contact lens: summary of safety and effectiveness. 1985 Dec 4. (PMA no. 850002-000).

Visiontech, Inc. [Food and Drug Administration, Center for Devices and Radiological Health] Sauflon PW-70 A & B: summary of safety and effectiveness. 1985 Jun 19. (PMA no. P840031-000).

Wesley Jessen. [Food and Drug Administration, Center for Devices and Radiological Health] Airlens (R) (Airfocon A) lens blue & clear: summary of safety and effectiveness. 1985 Jan 18. (PMA no. P830070-000).

Advanced Optical Inc. [Food and Drug Administration, Center for Devices and Radiological Health] Softics (TM) (polymacon): summary of safety and effectiveness. 1984 Jul3. (PMA no. P830012-000).

Barnes-Hind Pharmaceuticals. [Food and Drug Administration, Center for Devices and Radiological Health] Gas permeable regimen: summary of safety and effectiveness. 1984 Apr 25. (PMA no. P820053-000).

CIBA Vision Care Corporation. [Food and Drug Administration, Center for Devices and Radiological Health] Cibatint (TM) tinting process: summary of safety and effectiveness. 1984 Apr 10. (PMA no. P820086-000).

Committee on Ophthalmic Procedures Assessment. [American Academy of Ophthalmology] Therapeutic contact lenses for recurrent corneal erosion. San Francisco, CA: American Academy of Ophthalmology, 1984. [Information syntheses, Expert opinion]

Hydracon. [Food and Drug Administration, Center for Devices and Radiological Health] Hydracon (R) contact lenses: summary of safety and effectiveness. 1984 Aug 7. (PMA no. P820017-002).

Office of Technology Assessment, U.S. Congress. The contact lens industry. Washington, D.C.: U.S. Government Printing Office, December 1984 (Health technology case study series #31)

Polymer Technology Corporation. [Food and Drug Administration, Center for Devices and Radiological Health] Boston lens (R) lens-clear: summary of safety and effectiveness. 1984 Jan 27. (PMA no. P820065-000).

Salvatori Ophthalmics, Inc. [Food and Drug Administration, Center for Devices and Radiological Health] Paraperm 02 clear & blue lens: summary of safety and effectiveness. 1984 Apr 25. (PMA no. 820062-000).

Bausch and Lomb. [Food and Drug Administration, Center for Devices and Radiological Health] 03/04 (TM) lens series: summary of safety and effectiveness. 1983 Aug 16. (PMA no. N16895-025).

Con-cise. [Food and Drug Administration, Center for Devices and Radiological Health] Paraperm O2 contact lens clear & blue: summary of safety and effectiveness. 1983 Dec 8. (PMA no. P820061-000).

Custom Tint Lab., Inc. [Food and Drug Administration, Center for Devices and Radiological Health] Perma-tint (R): summary of safety and effectiveness. 1983 Nov 9. (PMA no. P820059-000).

Frigitronics, Inc. [Food and Drug Administration, Center for Devices and Radiological Health] Opus-III contact lenses: summary of safety and effectiveness. 1983 Sep 2. (PMA no. P820074-000).

Hydracon. [Food and Drug Administration, Center for Devices and Radiological Health] Hydracon (R) contact lenses: summary of safety and effectiveness. 1983 Mar 25. (PMA no. P820017-000).

Optacryl Inc. [Food and Drug Administration, Center for Devices and Radiological Health] Optacryl 60-clear: summary of safety and effectiveness. 1983 Dec 8. (PMA no. P820056-000).

Paragon Optical Inc. [Food and Drug Administration, Center for Devices and Radiological Health] Paraperm O2 contact lens: summary of safety and effectiveness. 1983 Dec 8. (PMA no. P820063-000).

Johnson and Johnson Co. [Food and Drug Administration, Center for Devices and Radiological Health] Chamber lens models 101, 101B, 101T: summary of safety and effectiveness. 1982 Mar 26. (PMA no. P790027-000).

Salvatori Ophthalmics, Inc. [Food and Drug Administration, Center for Devices and Radiological Health] (Polymacon) contact lenses: summary of safety and effectiveness. 1982 Sep 17. (PMA no. P820005-000).

Syntex Ophthalmics Inc. [Food and Drug Administration, Center for Devices and Radiological Health] Polycon contact lens: summary of safety and effectiveness. 1982 Sep 21 (PMA no. N18120-008).

Georgetown University Medical Center, Institute for Health Policy Analysis. Extended wear contact lenses. (Planned).

Contact lenses, Hydrophilic

Bausch & Lomb (R). [Food and Drug Administration, Center for Devices and Radiological Health] B & L (R) (Amefocon A) oxygen permeable lens: summary of safety and effectiveness. 1986 Aug 7. (PMA no. P830050-000).

Bausch & Lomb. [Food and Drug Administration, Center for Devices and Radiological Health] Silsoft (Elastofilcon A) contact lenses: summary of safety and effectiveness. 1986 Feb 2. (PMA no. P850068-000).

Briggs Ophthalmics Corp. [Food and Drug Administration, Center for Devices and Radiological Health] Sunsoft (Methafilcon A) hydrophilic contact lens: summary of safety and effectiveness. 1986 Aug 7. (PMA no. P850077-001).

Briggs Ophthalmics Corporation. [Food and Drug Administration, Center for Devices and Radiological Health] Sunsoft (Methafilcon A) hydrophilic contact lens: summary of safety and effectiveness. 1986 Mar 28. (PMA no. P850077-000).

Coast Contact Lens, Inc. [Food and Drug Administration, Center for Devices and Radiological Health] Hydra (Methafilcon A) contact lens: summary of safety and effectiveness. 1986 Aug 7. (PMA no. P850079-001).

Coast Contact Lens, Inc. [Food and Drug Administration, Center for Devices and Radiological Health] Hydrasoft (Methafilcon A) contact lens: summary of safety and effectiveness. 1986 Mar 28. (PMA no. P850079-000).

Kontur Kontact Lens Co. Inc. [Food and Drug Administration, Center for Devices and Radiological Health] Kontur soft (Methafilcon A) contact lens: summary of safety and effectiveness. 1986 Aug 7. (PMA no. P850078-000).

Kontur Kontact Lens Co. Inc. [Food and Drug Administration, Center for Devices and Radiological Health] Kontur soft (Methafilcon A) contact lens: summary of safety and effectiveness. 1986 Mar 28. (PMA no. P850078-000).

N & N Menicon Inc. [Food and Drug Administration, Center for Devices and Radiological Health] (Mafilcon) soft contact lenses: summary of safety and effectiveness. 1986 Dec 17. (PMA no. PB00031-000).

Permeable Contact Lenses, Inc. [Food and Drug Administration, Center for Devices and Radiological Health] SGP lens (TM): summary of safety and effectiveness. 1986 Jan 21. (PMA no. P840055-000).

Toray Industries Inc. [Food and Drug Administration, Center for Devices and Radiological Health] Toray soft contact lenses: summary of safety and effectiveness. 1986 Mar 5. (PMA no. P840044-000).

UCO Optics, Inc. [Food and Drug Administration, Center for Devices and Radiological Health] Aquasept II: summary of safety and effectiveness. 1986 Feb 14. (PMA no. N17679-008).

Wesley-Jessen. [Food and Drug Administration, Center for Devices and Radiological Health] Durasoft 4 (ofilcon A) spherical hydrophilic lens: summary of safety and effectiveness. 1986 Aug 14. (PMA no. P85).

International Hydron Corp. [Food and Drug Administration, Center for Devices and Radiological Health] X-70 soft contact lens: summary of safety and effectiveness. 1985 May 10. (PMA no. P830047-000).

National Patent Development Corporation. [Food and Drug Administration, Center for Devices and Radiological Health] Hydron hydrophilic contact lens: summary of safety and effectiveness. 1985 Nov 18. (PMA no. P78007-016).

Optical Plastic Research. [Food and Drug Administration, Center for Devices and Radiological Health] Softview spherical & toric contact lens: summary of safety and effectiveness. 1985 Feb 20. (PMA no. P830003-000).

Paris Contact Lens Lab. [Food and Drug Administration, Center for Devices and Radiological Health] Softsite (Hefilcon A) contact lens: summary of safety and effectiveness. 1985 Nov 21. (PMA no. N17793-006).

Product Development Corp. [Food and Drug Administration, Center for Devices and Radiological Health] Soft hydrophilic contact lens: summary of safety and effectiveness. 1985 Nov 21. (PMA no. P850041-000).

Salvatori Ophthalmics, Inc. [Food and Drug Administration, Center for Devices and Radiological Health] Synsoft (TM) (polymacon) bifocal contact lens: summary of safety and effectiveness. 1985 Mar 22. (PMA no. P840006-000).

Soft Lense Inc. [Food and Drug Administration, Center for Devices and Radiological Health] Hydrocurve II bifocal lens: summary of safety and effectiveness. 1985 Mar 22. (PMA no. N17752-016).

Wesley-Jessen. [Food and Drug Administration, Center for Devices and Radiological Health] Durasoft (R) 3 for extended wear: summary of safety and effectiveness. 1985 Sep 11. (PMA no. P830039-000).

Alden Optical Labs., Inc. [Food and Drug Administration, Center for Devices and Radiological Health] AL-47 soft contact lens: summary of safety and effectiveness. 1984 Mar 9. (PMA no. P820078-000).

Comfort Flex Hydrophilics Inc. [Food and Drug Administration, Center for Devices and Radiological Health] TRI POL 43 contact lens: summary of safety and effectiveness. 1984 Apr 17. (PMA no. P780013-004).

Frontier Contact Lense. [Food and Drug Administration, Center for Devices and Radiological Health] Hydro marc lenses (hydrophilic): summary of safety and effectiveness. 1984 Sep 17. (PMA no. N18033-006).

Metrosoft, Inc. [Food and Drug Administration, Center for Devices and Radiological Health] Metro 55 (Methafilcon A): summary of safety and effectiveness. 1984 Jul 3. (PMA no. P830077-000).

Ocu-Ease Optical Products, Inc. [Food and Drug Administration, Center for Devices and Radiological Health] Ocu-flex: summary of safety and effectiveness. 1984 Apr 25. (PMA no. P820051-000).

Syntex Ophthalmics Inc. [Food and Drug Administration, Center for Devices and Radiological Health] Soft contact lens: summary of safety and effectiveness. 1984 Jan 17. (PMA no. N17987-007).

Vision Ease Contact Lens Co. [Food and Drug Administration, Center for Devices and Radiological Health] VE soft hydrophilic contact lens: summary of safety and effectiveness. 1984 Mar 9. (PMA no. P830049-000).

CIBA Vision Care Corporation. [Food and Drug Administration, Center for Devices and Radiological Health] Softcon (Vifilcon A) soft contact extended wear lens: summary of safety and effectiveness. 1983 Apr 29. (PMA no. P820021-000).

Contact Lens Corporation of America. [Food and Drug Administration, Center for Devices and Radiological Health] Softact II (polymacon): summary of safety and effectiveness. 1983 Aug 5. (PMA no. P830006-000).

Dow Corning Corporation. [Food and Drug Administration, Center for Devices and Radiological Health] Silicon(R) (silafilcon A) contact lens daily wear: summary of safety and effectiveness. 1983 Dec 12. (PMA no. P800054-004).

Optech, Inc, [Food and Drug Administration, Center for Devices and Radiological Health] Optech fre-flex soft contact lens: summary of safety and effectiveness.1983 Feb 15. (PMA no. P810050-000).

Wesley Jesson Inc. [Food and Drug Administration, Center for Devices and Radiological Health] Durasoft (R) Trufocal (TM): summary of safety and effectiveness. 1983 Jun 3. (PMA no. N17852-008).

Bausch and Lomb. [Food and Drug Administration, Center for Devices and Radiological Health] Soflens (r) polymacon P.A.1 series: summary of safety and effectiveness. 1982 Dec 17. (PMA no. N16895 019).

CIBA Vision Care. [Food and Drug Administration, Center for Devices and Radiological Health] Weicon (R) (Tefilicon) hydrophilic contact lens: summary of safety and effectiveness. 1982 Jul 27. (PMA no. P810005-002).

Coopervision, Inc. [Food and Drug Administration, Center for Devices and Radiological Health] Cooper (TM) 38 (polymacon) hydrophilic contact lens: summary of safety and effectiveness. 1982 May 21. (PMA no. P810057-000).

Danker and Wohlk, Inc. [Food and Drug Administration, Center for Devices and Radiological Health] Danker silicone lens (Dimefocon-A): summary of safety and effectiveness. 1982 Jun 13. (PMA no. P790010-000).

Metrosoft, Inc. [Food and Drug Administration, Center for Devices and Radiological Health] Metrosoft (TM) II (polymacon) hydrophilic contact: summary of safety and effectiveness. 1982 Sep 24. (PMA no. P820026-000).

Soft Lense Inc. [Food and Drug Administration, Center for Devices and Radiological Health] Hydrocurve: summary of safety and effectiveness. 1980 Jan 11. (PMA no.N17752-000).

Soft Lense Inc. [Food and Drug Administration, Center for Devices and Radiological Health] Hydrocurve: summary of safety and effectiveness. 1980 Mar 14. (PMA no. N17752-001).

Continuous ambulatory peritoneal dialysis

Office of Technology Assessment, U.S. Congress. The effectiveness and costs of continuous ambulatory peritoneal dialysis. Washington, D.C.: U.S. Government Printing Office, September 1985. (Health technology case study series #35)

Stason WB, Barnes BA. [Harvard School of Public Health, Institute for Health Research] Effectiveness and costs of continuous ambulatory peritoneal dialysis (CAPD). Washington, D.C.: U.S. Congress, Office of Technology Assessment, July 1985. (Health Technology Case Study 35, OTA-HCS-35) [Information syntheses]

American Medical Association, Council on Scientific Affairs. Continuous ambulatory peritoneal dialysis. JAMA 1982 Nov 12;248:2340. [Group judgment]

Hutchinson TA, Cole CH, Kaye M. [McGill University, Department of Epidemiology and Biostatistics] Chronic ambulatory peritoneal dialysis versus other dialysis therapy - a matched cohort study. Clin Res 1982;30:431A.

Continuous passive motion devices

Blue Cross and Blue Shield Association, Technology Evaluation and Coverage Program. Continuous passive motion device. 1986.

ECRI Health Devices Program. Continuous passive motion (CPM) leg exercisers. Health Devices 1986;15:3-22.

ECRI Technology Assessment Program. Continuous passive motion (CPM) devices. Issues Health Care Technol 1985;sec.5.C.4. [Information syntheses]

Continuous passive motion therapy

California Medical Association, Medical Practice Opinion Program. Continuous passive motion for stiffening conditions. 1983 Mar. (Medical Practice Opinion #306) [Group judgment]

Continuous positive airway pressure

Blue Cross and Blue Shield Association, Technology Evaluation and Coverage Program. Nasal continuous positive airway pressure. 1986. [Information syntheses]

National Center for Health Services Research and Health Care Technology Assessment, Office of Health Technology Assessment. Continuous positive airway pressure (CPAP) for the treatment of obstructive sleep apnea. 1986.

Contraception

American College of Obstetricians and Gynecologists, Committee Opinion. Contraception for women in their later reproductive years. 1985 Dec. [Information syntheses]

American Academy of Pediatrics, Committee on Nutrition. Breast feeding and contraception. 1981

American Academy of Pediatrics, Committee on Adolescence. Contraception for the adolescent. Pediatrics 1980 Mar.

Contralateral breast surgery

California Medical Association, Medical Practice Opinion Program. Contralateral breast surgery following mastectomy. 1986 Feb. (Medical Practice Opinion #338) [Group judgment]

Corneal endothelial cell microscopy

Blue Cross and Blue Shield Association, Technology Evaluation and Coverage Program. Corneal endothelial cell microscopy. 1986. [Information syntheses]

Eddy JF, Eddy, DM. [Duke University, Center for Health Policy Research and Education] The value of corneal endothelial cell microscopy for cataract surgery. Report prepared for the Blue Cross and Blue Shield Association. 1986. [Information syntheses]

Corneal grafts

Chipman ML. [National Health Research and Development Program - Canada] Population-based studies of corneal graft outcome. 1986. (Grant No. 6606-2671-46).

Coronary artery bypass grafting

American College of Physicians, Clinical Efficacy Assessment Project. A comparative assessment of coronary artery bypass surgery and percutaneous transluminal coronary angioplasty, expected completion 1988. [Information syntheses]

Frasure-Smith N. [National Health Research and Development Program - Canada] The psychosocial outcomes of coronary bypass surgery: a study of patient and spouse adjustment during the first post-surgical year. 1986. (Grant No. 6605-2021-44).

Gersh BJ, Kronmal RA, Schaff HV, et al. [National Heart, Lung, and Blood Institute] Comparison of coronary artery bypass surgery and medical therapy in patients 65 years of age or older: a nonrandomized study from the Coronary Artery Surgery Study (CASS) registry. N Engl J Med 1985;313:217-224.

Passamani E, David B, Gillespie MJ, et al. [National Heart, Lung, and Blood Institute] A randomized trial of coronary artery bypass surgery: survival of patients with a low ejection fraction. N Engl J Med 1985;312:1655-1671.

Wortman PM, Yeaton WH. [National Center for Health Services Research and Health Care Technology Assessment, Division of Extramural Research] Cumulating quality of life results in controlled clinical trials of coronary artery bypass graft surgery. Controlled Clin Trials 1985 Dec;6(4):289-305.

Yeaton WH and Wortman PM. [National Center for Health Services Research and Health Care Technology Assessment, Division of Extramural Research] Medical technology assessment: the evaluation of coronary artery bypass graft surgery using data synthesis techniques. Int J Technol Assessment Health Care 1985 Jan; 1(1):125-1416.

CASS Principal Investigators and Their Associates. [National Heart, Lung, and Blood Institute] Coronary Artery Surgery Study (CASS): a randomized trial of coronary artery bypass surgery: myocardial infarction and mortality in the randomized trial. N Engl J Med 1984;310:750-758.

King's Fund. [King's Fund Centre for Service Development. King's Fund Forum Consensus and Controversies in Medicine] Coronary artery bypass surgery: the First UK Consensus Development Conference. 1984.

CASS Principal Investigators and Their Associates. [National Heart, Lung, and Blood Institute] Coronary Artery Surgery Study (CASS): a randomized trial of coronary artery bypass surgery: quality of life in patients randomly assigned to treatment groups. Circulation 1983;68:951-960.

CASS Principal Investigators and Their Associates. [National Heart, Lung, and Blood Institute] Coronary Artery Surgery Study (CASS): randomized trial of coronary artery bypass surgery: survival data. Circulation 1983;68:939-950.

CASS Principal Investigators and Their Associates. [National Heart, Lung, and Blood Institute] Coronary Artery Surgery Study (CASS): a randomized trial of coronary artery bypass surgery: comparability of entry characteristics and survival in randomized patients and nonrandomized patients meeting randomization criteria. J Am Coll Card 1983;3:114-128.

Davis KB, Chatman BR, Killip T, et al. [National Heart, Lung, and Blood Institute] Effect of coronary bypass surgery on operative mortality and survival patterns in subsets of patients with left main coronary artery disease. In: Hammermeister KE, ed. Coronary bypass surgery. New York: Praeger Scientific, 1983:99-127.

Davis KB, Kennedy JW, Berger RL, et al. [National Heart, Lung, and Blood Institute] Operative mortality in the CASS registry. In: Hammermeister KE ed. Coronary bypass surgery. New York: Praeger Scientific, 1983:99-127.

Frommer PL, Fisher LD, Moek MB, et al. [National Heart, Lung, and Blood Institute] The Coronary Artery Surgery Study: a randomized trial in the context of the registry. In: Hammermeister KE, ed. Coronary bypass surgery. New York: Praeger Scientific, 1983:57-82.

Gersh BJ, Kronmal RA, Frye RL, et al. [National Heart, Lung, and Blood Institute] Coronary arteriography and coronary artery bypass surgery: morbidity and mortality in patients ages 65 years or older: a report from the Coronary Artery Surgery Study. Circulation 1983;67:483-490.

Ryan TJ, Bailey KR, McCabe CH, et al. [National Heart, Lung, and Blood Institute] The effects of digitalis on survival in high-risk patients with coronary artery disease: the Coronary Artery Surgery Study (CASS). Circulation 1983;67:735-742.

Mock MB, Ringvist I, Fisher LD, et al. [National Heart, Lung, and Blood Institute] Survival of medically treated patients in the Coronary Artery Surgery Study (CASS) registry. Circulation 1982;66:562-568.

Weinstein MC, Stason WB. [Harvard School of Public Health, Institute for Health Research] Cost-effectiveness of coronary artery bypass surgery. Circulation 1982;66(Suppl III):III56-III66. [Information syntheses]

Berger RL, Davis KB, Kaiser GC, et al. [National Heart, Lung, and Blood Institute] Preservation of the myocardium during coronary artery bypass grafting. Circulation 1981;64 (Supplement II):II61-II66.

Chaitman BR, Fisher LD, Bourassa MG, et al. [National Heart, Lung, and Blood Institute] Effect of coronary bypass surgery on survival patterns in subsets of patients with left main coronary artery disease. Report of the collaborative study in Coronary Artery Surgery (CASS). Am J Cardiol 1981;48:765-777.

Kennedy JW, Kaiser GC, Fisher LD, et al. [National Heart, Lung, and Blood Institute] Clinical and angiographic predictors of operative mortality from the collaborative study in Coronary Artery Surgery (CASS). Circulation 1981;63;793-802.

Principal Investigators of CASS and Their Associates. [National Heart, Lung, and Blood Institute] National Heart, Lung, and Blood Institute Coronary Artery Surgery Study. Circulation 1981;63 (AHA Monograph No. 79):I1-I81.

Kennedy JW, Kaiser GC, Fisher LD, et al. [National Heart, Lung, and Blood Institute] Multivariate discriminant analysis of the clinical and angiographic predictors of operative mortality from the Collaborative Study in Coronary Artery Surgery (CASS). J Thorac Cardiovasc Surg 1980;80:876.

National Institutes of Health, Consensus Development Program. Coronary artery bypass surgery: scientific and clinical aspects. (Consensus Development Conference Statement, Dec 3-5 1980). [Group judgment]

Russell RO, Wayne JB, Kronenfeld J, et al. [National Heart, Lung, and Blood Institute] Surgical versus medical therapy for treatment of unstable angina: changes in work status and family income. Am J Cardiology 1980;45:134-140.

Unstable Angina Pectoris Study Group. [National Heart, Lung, and Blood Institute] Unstable Angina Pectoris Study National Cooperative Study Group to compare medical and surgical therapy. III. Results in patients with S-T segment elevation during pain. Am J Cardiology 1980;45:819-824.

Unstable Angina Pectoris Study Group. [National Heart, Lung, and Blood Institute] Unstable Angina Pectoris National Cooperative Study Group to compare medical and surgical therapy. II. In-hospital experience and initial follow-up results in patients with one, two and three vessel disease. Am J Cardiol 1978;42:839-848.

Neuhauser D, Jonsson E. [Harvard School of Public Health, Institute for Health Research] Managerial response to new health care technology: coronary artery bypass surgery. In: Abernathy WJ, Sheldon A, Prahalad CK, eds. The management of health care. Cambridge: Ballinger Press, 1975. [Information syntheses]

Veterans Administration, Cooperative Studies Program. Coronary artery surgery I: stable angina (vein by-pass). Ongoing. [Clinical trials]

Veterans Administration, Cooperative Studies Program. Coronary artery surgery II: unstable angina (vein by-pass). Ongoing. [Clinical trials]

Coronary artery disease diagnosis

Fineberg HV, Stason WB. [Harvard School of Public Health, Institute for Health Research] Cost-effectiveness of alternative diagnostic strategies for coronary artery disease. Circulation 1982;66(III):80-86. [Information syntheses]

Coronary artery jeopardy score

Califf RM, et al. [National Center for Health Services Research and Health Care Technology Assessment, Division of Extramural Research] Prognostic value of a coronary artery jeopardy score. J Am Coll Cardiol May 1985;5(5):1055-1063.

Coronary care units

U.S. Administrators, Professional Policy Committee. Coronary care units, admission to. [7/86] [Group judgment]

Blue Cross and Blue Shield Association, Medical Necessity Program. Intensive cardiac care unit. 1985. [Information syntheses]

Cost benefit/effectiveness analysis

Health Industry Manufacturers Association. [Battelle Medical Technology Assessment Program] A guide to cost-effectiveness analysis for medical device and diagnostic manufacturers. Washington, D.C.: Health Industry Manufacturers Association, 1985. (HIMA Report Number B5-2, HIMA Research Reports Series Number 3) [Cost analyses]

Avorn JL. [National Center for Health Services Research and Health Care Technology Assessment, Division of Extramural Research] Benefit and cost analysis in geriatric care: turning age discrimination into health policy. N Engl J Med 1984 May;310(20):1294-1301.

University of Pennsylvania, Leonard Davis Institute of Health Economics. Cost benefit, cost effectiveness, and other decision making techniques in health care resource allocation. 1983. (Proceedings of a Regional Symposium, November 4-6, 1982, funded by Smith Kline and French Laboratories).

Lubeck D. [National Center for Health Services Research and Health Care Technology Assessment, Division of Extramural Research] Cost-benefit analysis of heart disease research. 1982. (NTIS order no. PB82-194556)

Swedish Planning and Rationalization Institute of the Health Services. Spri technology report 3: cost effectiveness analysis in health care. 1981. [Cost analyses, Epidemiological and other observational methods]

Office of Technology Assessment, U.S. Congress. The implications of cost-effectiveness analysis of medical technology. Washington, D.C.: U.S. Government Printing Office, August 1980.

Linköping University, Center for Medical Technology Assessment . Development of simulation models for use in cost-effectiveness studies. Planned.

Counseling

Pless IB. [National Health Research and Development Program - Canada] Social support & counselling in the prevention of psychosocial maladjustment in children with chronic illness. 1986. (Grant No. 6605-2060-43).

American Academy of Pediatrics, Committee on Adolescence. Pregnancy and abortion counseling. Pediatrics 1979 Jun.

CPT-4 codes

Feasibility of incorporating CPT-4 codes for physician billing into the diagnosis-related groups system for in-hospital Medicare surgical patients. In: Office of Research and Demonstrations, Health Care Financing Administration. Health care financing status report: research and demonstrations in health care financing. Jan 1986. (HCFA Pub. No. 03219).

Creatinine concentration, Serum

Blue Cross and Blue Shield Association, Medical Necessity Program. Blood urea nitrogen concentration and serum creatinine concentration. 1987. [Information syntheses]

Cryometers

Food and Drug Administration, Center for Devices and Radiological Health. Hypodermic thermocouple tissue cryometers. 1984. (NTIS Order No. PB84-190776).

Cryopreservation

Martin RH. [National Health Research and Development Program - Canada] The effect of cryopreservation on the frequency of chromosome abnormalities in human sperm. 1986. (Grant No. 6609-1319-52).

Schachar NS. [Department Surgery, University Calgary] [Medical Research Council - Canada] Investigation of optimal methods of cryopreservation of osteoarticular allografts for transplantation. (Grant period 1984-1985).

Cryosurgery

American College of Obstetricians and Gynecologists, Committee Opinion. The use of cryosurgery in the treatment of CIN. Revised 1986 Nov. [Information syntheses]

Cryosurgery—Arrhythmias

American Medical Association, Diagnostic and Therapeutic Technology Assessment. Ablation of accessory pathways in Wolff-Parkinson-White Syndrome. Mar 31, 1986. [Expert opinion, Information syntheses]

Cushions

Conine TA. [National Health Research and Development Program - Canada] A controlled randomized trial of two seat cushions in the prevention of decubitus ulcers in institutionalized elderly persons. 1986. (Grant No. 6610-1493-55).

Cyanoacrylates

Committee on Ophthalmic Procedures Assessment. [American Academy of Ophthalmology] Cyanoacrylate tissue adhesive. San Francisco, CA: American Academy of Ophthalmology, 1984. [Information syntheses, Expert opinion]

Cyclophosphamide

California Medical Association, Medical Practice Opinion Program. Cytoxan therapy for multiple sclerosis. 1985 Oct. (Medical Practice Opinion #329) [Group judgment]

Cyclothiazide

Food and Drug Administration, Center for Drugs and Biologics. Cyclothiazide. 1981. (NTIS order no. PB81-915905). [Information syntheses, Expert opinion, Epidemiological and other observational methods, Clinical trials, Bench testing]

Cytotoxic food testing

California Medical Association, Medical Practice Opinion Program. Cytotoxic testing for food allergy. 1984 Feb. (Medical Practice Opinion #265) [Group judgment]

American College of Physicians, Clinical Efficacy Assessment Project. Cytotoxic food testing. 1981. [Information syntheses]

National Center for Health Services Research and Health Care Technology Assessment, Office of Health Technology Assessment. Cytotoxic leukocyte test for the diagnois of food allergy. 1981.

Dacarbazine

Food and Drug Administration, Center for Drugs and Biologics. DTIC (Dome). 1981. (NTIS order no. PB81-15907). [Information syntheses, Expert opinion, Epidemiological and other observational methods, Clinical trials, Bench testing]

Data banks

Medicare automated data retrieval system. In: Office of Research and Demonstrations, Health Care Financing Administration. Health care financing status report: research and demonstrations in health care financing. Jan 1986. (HCFA Pub. No. 03219).

Seshia SS, Shwedyk E. [National Health Research and Development Program - Canada] Computerized EEG data base from prolonged ambulatory 4 channel (cassette) recordings in children. 1986. (Grant No. 6607-1257-42).

Pryor DB, et al. [National Center for Health Services Research and Health Care Technology Assessment, Division of Extramural Research] Clinical databases—accomplishments and unrealized potential. Med Care 1985 May 23(5):648-662.

Tugwell P. [Department Medicine, McMaster University] [Medical Research Council - Canada] Clinical trials computer network. (Grant period 1984-1985).

Fries JF. [National Center for Health Services Research and Health Care Technology Assessment, Division of Extramural Research] The chronic disease data bank: first principles to future directions. J Med and Philos 1984 May;9(2):161-180.

Li Tem, Sherman H, Cook EF, et al. [Harvard School of Public Health, Institute for Health Research] The selective impact of a cardiology data bank on physician's therapeutic recommendations. Medical Decision Making 1984;4(2):165-177. [Epidemiological methods]

Stead EA. [National Center for Health Services Research and Health Care Technology Assessment, Division of Extramural Research] A medical database approach to evaluate technology. 1984. (NTIS order no. PB84-200559)

Brian EW. [National Center for Health Services Research and Health Care Technology Assessment, Division of Extramural Research] Evaluation of automated hospital data management systems in 100-300 bed hospitals. 1983. (NTIS order no. PB83-153437).

Loeser J, Zvagulis I, Hercz L, Pless IB. [McGill University, Department of Epidemiology and Biostatistics] The organization and evaluation of a computer-assisted centralized immunization registry. Am J Public Health 1983;73(11):1298-1301.

Lundberg ED, McBride R, Rawson TE, et al. [National Heart, Lung, and Blood Institute] A data base management system developed for the Coronary Artery Surgery Study (CASS) and other clinical studies. In: Riddle K, Thurber P, Keen P, et al. eds. Proc of the 15th Hawaii Internat Conf on Systems Sciences, 1982, Vol II, Software, Hardware, Decision Support Systems, Special Topics, North Hollywood, CA: Western Periodicals Co, 1982:484-500.

Wiederhold GC, Blum RL. [National Center for Health Services Research and Health Care Technology Assessment, Division of Extramural Research] Integrating medical knowledge and clinical data banks. 1981. (NTIS order no. PB81-227233)

Day care

Subcommittee on Special Services in Hospitals. [Health and Welfare Canada, Health Services and Promotion Branch, Institutional and Professional Services Division] Hospital day medicine unit guidelines. 1984. [Information syntheses, Expert opinion, Group judgment]

Subcommittee on Special Services in Hospitals. [Health and Welfare Canada, Health Services and Promotion Branch, Institutional and Professional Services Division] Geriatric units in hospitals, geriatric day hospital guidelines. 1979. [Information syntheses, Expert opinion, Group judgment]

Subcommittee on Special Services in Hospitals. [Health and Welfare Canada, Health Services and Promotion Branch, Institutional and Professional Services Division] Diabetic day care unit guidelines. 1978. [Information syntheses, Expert opinion, Group judgment]

Debridement

National Center for Health Services Research and Health Care Technology Assessment, Office of Health Technology Assessment. Debridement and other treatment of mycotic toenails. 1985.

Decubitus surgery

U.S. Administrators, Professional Policy Committee. Decubitus surgery. [7/86] [Group judgment]

Defibrillation

Eisenberg MS, Hallstrom A, Bergner LG. [National Center for Health Services Research and Health Care Technology Assessment, Division of Extramural Research] Defibrillation by emergency medical technicians. 1983 May. (NTIS order no. PB85-163632/AS).

Eisenberg MS, et al. [National Center for Health Services Research and Health Care Technology Assessment, Division of Extramural Research] Treatment of ventricular fibrillation: emergency medical technician defibrillation and paramedic services. JAMA 1984 Apr;251(13):1723-26.

Defibrillators

Blue Cross and Blue Shield Association, Technology Evaluation and Coverage Program. Automatic implantable cardioverter defibrillator. 1986. [Information syntheses]

ECRI Technology Assessment Program. Automatic implantable cardioverter/defibrillator. Issues Health Care Technol 1986;sec.5.D.3. [Information syntheses]

Implantable defibrillator. In: Prospective Payment Assessment Commission. Technical appendixes to the report and recommendations to the Secretary, U.S. Department of Health and Human Services, April 1, 1986. Washington, DC: Government Printing Office, 1986:103. [Information syntheses, Cost analyses]

U.S. Administrators, Professional Policy Committee. Cardioverter defibrillator, implantable. [7/86] [Group judgment]

Cardiac Pacemakers, Inc. [Food and Drug Administration, Center for Devices and Radiological Health] AID-B automatic implantable cardiovertor defibrillator: summary of safety and effectiveness. 1985 Nov 15. (PMA no. P830060-000).

National Center for Health Services Research and Health Care Technology Assessment, Office of Health Technology Assessment. Implantable automatic cardioverter-defibrillators. 1985.

Food and Drug Administration, Center for Devices and Radiological Health. A study of DC defibrillator safety and performance - performance and safety standard - volume II. 1984. (NTIS Order No. PB84-188838).

ECRI Health Devices Program. Defibrillators, line-powered. Health Devices 1983;12:291-314.

Netherlands Organization for Applied Scientific Research, Medical Technology Unit (TNO). Defibrillators. 1983.

Netherlands Organization for Applied Scientific Research, Medical Technology Unit (TNO). Portable defibrillators. 1983.

Battelle Medical Technology Assessment Program. Cost-effectiveness of the implantable cardiac defibrillator. Ongoing.

Johns Hopkins Program for Medical Technology and Practice Assessment. An analysis of automatic implantable cardiac defibrillators (AICDs). Planned.

Dental alloys

American Dental Association, Council on Dental Materials, Instruments and Equipment. Report on base metal alloys for crown and bridge applications: benefits and risks. J Am Dent Assoc 1985;111:479-483.

American Dental Association, Council on Dental Materials, Instruments and Equipment. Classification system for cast alloys. J Am Dent Assoc 1984;109:766.

American Dental Association, Council on Dental Materials, Instruments and Equipment. Biological effects of nickel-containing dental alloys. J Am Dent Assoc 1982;104:501-505.

American Dental Association, Council on Dental Materials, Instruments and Equipment. Classification and definition of alloys used for casting substrates for porcelain veneering. J Am Dent Assoc 1981;103:755-757.

American Dental Association, Council on Dental Materials, Instruments and Equipment. Porcelain-metal alloy compatibility: criteria and test methods. J Am Dent Assoc 1981;102:71-72.

American Dental Association, Council on Dental Materials, Instruments and Equipment. Status report on low-gold-content alloys for fixed prostheses. J Am Dent Assoc 1980;100:237-240.

Veterans Administration, Cooperative Studies Program. Clinical comparison of base metal alloys vs. a gold alloy used in the fabrication of fixed (crown and bridge) restorations. Ongoing. [Clinical trials]

Dental amalgam

American Dental Association, Council on Dental Materials, Instruments and Equipment. Safety of dental amalgam. J Am Dent Assoc 1983;106:519-520.

American Dental Association, Council on Dental Materials, Instruments and Equipment. High copper-content amalgam alloys. J Am Dent Assoc 1982;105:1077-1080.

Dental amalgamators

American Dental Association, Council on Dental Materials, Instruments and Equipment. Status report on amalgamators. J Am Dent Assoc 1983;107:639-640.

Dental anesthesia

National Institutes of Health, Consensus Development Program. Anesthesia and sedation in the dental office. (Consensus Development Conference Statement, Apr 22-24 1985). [Group judgment]

Dental bonding

American Dental Association, Council on Dental Materials, Instruments and Equipment. Dentin bonding systems: an update. J Am Dent Assoc 1987;114:91-95.

American Dental Association, Council on Dental Materials, Instruments and Equipment. Resin dental bonding systems. J Am Dent Assoc 1984;108:240-241.

American Dental Association, Council on Dental Materials, Instruments and Equipment. Status report on enamel bonding of composites, preformed laminate, and laboratory fabricated resin veneers. J Am Dent Assoc 1984;109:762-764.

American Dental Association, Council on Dental Materials, Instruments and Equipment. State of the art and science of bonding in orthodontic treatment. J Am Dent Assoc 1982;105:844-850.

Dental bridges

Veterans Administration, Cooperative Studies Program. A five year clinical evaluation of alternative crown and bridge systems (NIDR). Ongoing. [Clinical trials]

Dental caries removal systems

National Patent Development Corp. [Food and Drug Administration, Center for Devices and Radiological Health] GE-101E caries removal agent/system: summary of safety and effectiveness. 1986 May 2. (PMA no. P830035-000).

Dental ceramics

Veterans Administration, Cooperative Studies Program. Clinical studies of biphasic calcium phosphate ceramic in peridontal osseous defects. [Clinical trials]

Dental crowns

American Dental Association, Council on Dental Materials, Instruments and Equipment. Recent developments in materials and process for ceramic crowns. J Am Dent Assoc 1985;110:548-549.

Veterans Administration, Cooperative Studies Program. A five year clinical evaluation of alternative crown and bridge systems (NIDR). Ongoing. [Clinical trials]

Dental implants

American Dental Association, Council on Dental Materials, Instruments and Equipment. Dental endosseous implants. J Am Dent Assoc 1986;113:949-950.

Karlsson CT. [Linköping University, Center for Medical Technology Assessment] Economics of osseointegrated implants—a prestudy. 1986. (Discussion series paper #8) [Swedish language only] [Cost analyses, Epidemiological methods]

American Dental Association, Council on Dental Materials, Instruments and Equipment, Council on Dental Research, and Council on Dental Therapeutics. Hydroxylapatite, beta tricalcium phosphate, and autogenous and allogenic bone for filling periodontal defects, alveolar ridge augmentation, and pulp capping. J Am Dent Assoc 1984;108:822-831.

American Dental Association, Council on Dental Materials, Instruments and Equipment. Council reevaluates position on dental endosseous implants. J Am Dent Assoc 1980;100:247.

National Institutes of Health, Consensus Development Program. Dental implants: benefit and risk. (Consensus Development Conference Statement, Jun 13-14 1978). [Group judgment]

Linköping University, Center for Medical Technology Assessment. Economics of ossointegrated implants. Ongoing.

Veterans Administration, Cooperative Studies Program. Dental implants (removable vs. permanent dentures). Ongoing. [Clinical trials]

Dental materials

American Dental Association, Council on Dental Therapeutics, Council on Dental Materials, Instruments, and Equipment. The use of root canal filling materials containing paraformaldehyde: a status report. J Am Dent Assoc 1987 Jan;114:95.

Helitrex, Inc. [Food and Drug Administration, Center for Devices and Radiological Health] Collacote (TM): summary of safety and effectiveness. 1986 Jan 2. (PMA no. P840062-000).

American Dental Association, Council on Dental Materials, Instruments and Equipment. Recommendations in dental mercury hygiene, 1984. J Am Dent Assoc 1984;109:617-619.

American Dental Association, Council on Dental Materials, Instruments and Equipment. Reported sensitivity to glass ionomer luting cements. J Am Dent Assoc 1984;109:617-619.

Osmed, Inc. [Food and Drug Administration, Center for Devices and Radiological Health] Drilac cubes (TM): summary of safety and effectiveness. 1983 Feb 25. (PMA no. P800012-000).

American Dental Association, Council on Dental Materials, Instruments and Equipment. Status report on precious metal scrap. J Am Dent Assoc 1982;105:1080-1081.

American Dental Association, Council on Dental Materials, Instruments and Equipment. A status report on resilient denture base materials. J Am Dent Assoc 1981;103:450-451.

American Dental Association, Council on Dental Materials, Instruments and Equipment. ADA Council issues updated mercury hygiene measures recommended. ADA News 1981 Sep 7.

Dental radiography

Food and Drug Administration, Center for Devices and Radiological Health. Basic concepts in the selection of patients for dental x-ray examinations. 1986. (GPO Stock No. 017-015-00230-6, NTIS Order No. PB86-126067/AS).

American Dental Association, Council on Dental Materials, Instruments and Equipment. Recommendations in radiographic practices, 1984. J Am Dent Assoc 1984;109:764-765.

American Dental Association, Council on Dental Materials, Instruments and Equipment. Biological effects of radiation from dental radiography. J Am Dent Assoc 1982;105:275-281.

American Dental Association, Council on Dental Materials, Instruments and Equipment. Recommendations in radiographic practices. J Am Dent Assoc 1981;103:103-104

Dental resins

American Dental Association, Council on Dental Materials, Instruments and Equipment. Posterior composite resins. J Am Dent Assoc 1986;112:717-709.

American Dental Association, Council on Dental Materials, Instruments and Equipment. Posterior composite resins: an update. J Am Dent Assoc 1986;113:950-952.

American Dental Association, Council on Dental Materials, Instruments and Equipment. Status report on enamel bonding of composites, preformed laminate, and laboratory fabricated resin veneers. J Am Dent Assoc 1984;109:762-764.

American Dental Association, Council on Dental Materials, Instruments and Equipment. Status report on posterior composites. J Am Dent Asso 1983;107:71-75.

American Dental Association, Council on Dental Materials, Instruments and Equipment. Status report on microfilled composite restorative resins. J Am Dent Assoc 1982-105:488-492.

Dental scaling and stain-removal devices

American Dental Association, Council on Dental Materials, Instruments and Equipment. Status report on professional scaling and stain-removal devices. J Am Dent Assoc 1985;111:801-802.

Dental sealants

American Dental Association, Council on Dental Materials, Instruments and Equipment. Pit and fissure sealants. J Am Dent Assoc 1983;107:465.

National Institutes of Health, Consensus Development Program. Dental sealants in the prevention of tooth decay. (Consensus Development Conference Statement, Dec 5-7 1983). [Group judgment]

Dental sterilization devices

American Dental Association, Council on Dental Materials, Instruments and Equipment. Current status of sterilization instruments, devices, and methods for the dental office. J Am Dent Assoc 1981;102:683-689.

Dental visible light-curing units

American Dental Association, Council on Dental Materials, Instruments and Equipment. Visible light-cured composites and activating units. J Am Dent Assoc 1985;110:100-103

American Dental Association, Council on Dental Materials, Instruments and Equipment. Status report: dental visible light-curing units. J Am Dent Assoc 1982;104:505.

Denture cleansers

American Dental Association, Council on Dental Materials, Instruments and Equipment. Denture cleansers. J Am Dent Assoc 1983;106:77-79.

Dentures

Veterans Administration, Cooperative Studies Program. Dental implants (removable vs. permanent dentures). Ongoing. [Clinical trials]

Desoximetasone

Food and Drug Administration, Center for Drugs and Biologics. Desoximetasone. 1982. (NTIS order no. Pb82-915902). [Information syntheses, Expert opinion, Epidemiological and other observational methods, Clinical trials, Bench testing]

Developmental disabilities screening

American Academy of Pediatrics, Committee on Disabilities. Screening for developmental disabilities. Pediatrics 1986 Sep.

Mowat DL. [National Health Research and Development Program - Canada] An outreach program to promote utilization of health and developmental screening for three-year-old children (Demonstration). 1985. (Grant No. 6601-1041-44).

Dexamethasone

Collaborative Group on Antenatal Steroid Therapy. [National Heart, Lung, and Blood Institute] Prevention of respiratory distress syndrome: effect of antenatal dexamethasone administration. Hospital and follow-up studies. 1985 [NIH Publication No. 85-2695]

Collaborative Group on Antenatal Steroid Therapy. [National Heart, Lung, and Blood Institute] Effects of antenatal dexamethasone administration in the infant: long-term follow-up. J Pediatr 1984;104:259-267.

Collaborative Group on Antenatal Steroid Therapy. [National Heart, Lung, and Blood Institute] Effect of antenatal dexamethasone administration on the prevention of respiratory distress syndrome. Am J Obstet Gynecol 1981;141:276-287.

Dexamethasone suppression test

American College of Physicians, Clinical Efficacy Assessment Project. The dexamethasone suppression test. Ann Intern Med 1983;100:307-8. [Information syntheses]

Dextromethorphan

Food and Drug Administration, Center for Drugs and Biologics. Dextromethorphan resin complex. 1983. (NTIS order no. PB83-915901). [Information syntheses, Expert opinion, Epidemiological and other observational methods, Clinical trials, Bench testing]

American Academy of Pediatrics, Committee on Drugs. Use of codeine- and dextromethorphan-containing cough syrups in pediatrics. Pediatrics 1978 Jul.

Dextrose

Food and Drug Administration, Center for Drugs and Biologics. Salts solution plus dextrose and glutathione disulfides. 1982. (NTIS order no. PB82-915901). [Information syntheses, Expert opinion, Epidemiological and other observational methods, Clinical trials, Bench testing]

Food and Drug Administration, Center for Drugs and Biologics. 10% Dextrose injection, USP. 1981. (NTIS order no. PB81-915909). [Information syntheses, Expert opinion, Epidemiological and other observational methods, Clinical trials, Bench testing]

Food and Drug Administration, Center for Drugs and Biologics. 5% Dextrose in lactated Ringer's injection in polyolefin bottle. 1981. [Information syntheses, Expert opinion, Epidemiological and other observational methods, Clinical trials, Bench testing]

Dextrose with saline solution

Food and Drug Administration, Center for Drugs and Biologics. 5% Dextrose & 0.3% NaCl Inj., USP. 1981. (NTIS order no. PB81-915909). [Information syntheses, Expert opinion, Epidemiological and other observational methods, Clinical trials, Bench testing]

Food and Drug Administration, Center for Drugs and Biologics. 5% Dextrose & 0.9% NaCl Inj., USP. 1981. (NTIS order no. PB81-915909). [Information syntheses, Expert opinion, Epidemiological and other observational methods, Clinical trials, Bench testing]

Dialysis

Medical Technology and Practice Patterns Institute. Dialysis treatment for end stage renal disease (inpatient). 1987.

Medical Technology and Practice Patterns Institute. Dialysis treatment for end stage renal disease (outpatient). 1987.

National Kidney Dialysis and Kidney Transplantation Study. In: Office of Research and Demonstrations, Health Care Financing Administration. Health care financing status report: research and demonstrations in health care financing. Jan 1986. (HCFA Pub. No. 03219).

Burton HJ. [National Health Research and Development Program - Canada] Factors influencing outcome of home and satellite care dialysis. 1986. (Grant No. 6606-2304-05).

Health Council of the Netherlands. Dialysis and kidney transplantation. 1986. [English summary only].

Hutchinson TA, Harvey CE. [McGill University, Department of Epidemiology and Biostatistics] Survival with different forms of dialysis treatment—a prognostically controlled comparison. J Am Soc Artif Inter Organs 1985;8:13-17.

Hutchinson TA, Michaud L, Thomas DC. [McGill University, Department of Epidemiology and Biostatistics] Comparison of survival with dialysis and renal transplantation - the effect of the method of statistical analysis on results. J Am Soc Artif Intern Organs 1985;8:18-21.

Parfrey PS, Hutchinson TA, Harvey C, Guttman RD. [McGill University, Department of Epidemiology and Biostatistics] Transplantation versus dialysis in diabetic patients with renal failure. Am J Kidney Dis 1985;5:112-116.

Hutchinson TA, Thomas DC, Lemieux JC, Harvey CF. [McGill University, Department of Epidemiology and Biostatistics] A prognostically controlled comparison of dialysis and renal transplantation. Kidney Int 1984;26:44-51.

Food and Drug Administration, Center for Devices and Radiological Health. Investigation of the risks & hazards with devices associated with peritoneal dialysis (including intermittent dialysis & continuous ambulatory peritoneal dialysis) & sorbent regenerated dialysate delivery systems. 1983. (NTIS Order No. PB83-175984).

Health Council of the Netherlands. Dialysis. Ongoing assessment.

Diathermy

Food and Drug Administration, Center for Devices and Radiological Health. Therapeutic microwave and shortwave diathermy: a review of thermal effectiveness, safe use, and state of the art: 1984. 1985. (GPO Stock No. 017-015-00226-8, NTIS Order No. PB85-170165/AS).

American Medical Association, Diagnostic and Therapeutic Technology Assessment. Diathermy for treating musculoskeletal conditions. JAMA 1983 Jul 22-29. [Expert opinion, Information syntheses]

National Center for Health Services Research and Health Care Technology Assessment, Office of Health Technology Assessment. Diathermy as a physical therapy modality. 1983.

National Center for Health Services Research and Health Care Technology Assessment, Office of Health Technology Assessment. Shortwave diathermy. 1981.

Diazepam

Ray WA, et al. [National Center for Health Services Research and Health Care Technology Assessment, Division of Extramural Research] Reducing long-term diazepam prescribing in office practice: a controlled trial of educational visits. JAMA 1986 Nov;256(18):2536-2539.

Food and Drug Administration, Center for Drugs and Biologics. Diazepam. 1981. (NTIS order no. PB81-915906). [Information syntheses, Expert opinion, Epidemiological and other observational methods, Clinical trials, Bench testing]

Diet therapy

American Diabetes Association. Nutritional recommendations and principles for individuals with diabetes mellitus. Diabetes Care 1987;10:126-132. [Expert opinion, Group judgment]

American Academy of Pediatrics, Committee on Nutrition. Prudent life-style for children: dietary fat and cholesterol. Pediatrics 1986 Sep.

Cameron R, Horlick L, Shepel L. [National Health Research and Development Program - Canada] Toward an economical, broadly accessible weight control program: the refinement and evaluation of a correspondence approach. 1986. (Grant No. 6606-2588-42).

End-Stage Renal Disease Nutritional Therapy Study. In: Office of Research and Demonstrations, Health Care Financing Administration. Health care financing status report: research and demonstrations in health care financing. Jan 1986. (HCFA Pub. No. 03219).

Haynes RB. [McMaster, Department of Clinical Epidemiology and Biostatistics] Is weight loss an effective treatment for hypertension? The evidence against. Can J Physiol Pharmacol 1986;64:825-830.

Health Council of the Netherlands. Very low energy diets. 1986. [English summary only].

Kramer MS. [National Health Research and Development Program - Canada] Infant determinants of childhood adiposity: the effectiveness of prophylactic nutrition. 1986. (Grant No. 6605-1693-43).

National Institutes of Health, Consensus Development Program. Diet and exercise in noninsulin-dependent diabetes mellitus. (Consensus Development Conference Statement, Dec 8-10 1986). [Group judgment]

Patrick J. [National Health Research and Development Program - Canada] The nutritional requirements for energy, potassium and zinc for rapid "catch-up" growth in children with cystic fibrosis. 1986. (Grant No. 6606-2303-07).

Langford HG, Blaufox MD, Oberman A, et al. [National Heart, Lung, and Blood Institute] Dietary therapy slows the return of hypertension after stopping prolonged medication. JAMA 1985;5:657-664.

Williams CN. [National Health Research and Development Program - Canada] Prevalence and pathogenesis of cholesterol gallstones in Halifax: prevention of recurrence by diet changes after medical dissolution therapy. 1985. (Grant No. 6603-1125-44).

Langford HG, Blaufox MD, Oberman A, et al. [National Heart, Lung, and Blood Institute] Effect of weight loss on the return of hypertension after withdrawal of prolonged antihypertensive therapy. In: Nutritional Prevention of Cardiovascular Disease. 1984:311-315.

Wing R, Caggiula A, Nowalk M, et al. [National Heart, Lung, and Blood Institute] Dietary approaches to the reduction of blood pressure: the independence of weight and sodium/potassium interventions. Prev Med 1984;13:233- 234.

American Academy of Pediatrics, Committee on Nutrition. Toward a prudent diet for children. Pediatrics 1983 Jan.

American Medical Association, Council on Scientific Affairs. Dietary and pharmacologic therapy for the lipid risk factors. JAMA 1983 Oct 14;250:1873-1879. [Group judgment]

National Center for Health Services Research and Health Care Technology Assessment, Office of Health Technology Assessment. Obesity and protein supplemented fasting. 1982.

National Institutes of Health, Consensus Development Program. Defined diets and childhood hyperactivity. (Consensus Development Conference Statement, Jan 13-15 1982). [Group judgment]

Remmell PS, Gorder DD, Hall Y, et al (for the MRFIT Group). [National Heart, Lung, and Blood Institute] Assessing dietary adherence in the Multiple Risk Factor Intervention Trial (MRFIT). I. Use of a dietary monitoring tool. J Am Dietetic Assn 1980;76:351-356.

Diethylpropion

Food and Drug Administration, Center for Drugs and Biologics. Diethylpropion hydrochloride. 1983. (NTIS order no. PB83-915901). [Information syntheses, Expert opinion, Epidemiological and other observational methods, Clinical trials, Bench testing]

Diflunisal

Food and Drug Administration, Center for Drugs and Biologics. Diflunisal. 1982. (NTIS order no. PB82-915904). [Information syntheses, Expert opinion, Epidemiological and other observational methods, Clinical trials, Bench testing]

Digital imaging

Steering Committee on Future Health Scenarios, Commission on Future Health Care Technology (Netherlands). Prospective assessment of future health care technology: digital imagery. 1987.

ECRI Technology Assessment Program. X-ray image digitizing systems. Issues Health Care Technol 1984;sec.5.D.4. [Information syntheses]

ECRI Technology Assessment Program. Digital radiography and fluoroscopy. Issues Health Care Technol 1983;sec.5.D.2. [Information syntheses]

Digital subtraction angiography

U.S. Administrators, Professional Policy Committee. Digital subtraction angiography - intravenous. [7/86] [Group judgment]

ECRI Technology Assessment Program. Digital subtraction angiography (DSA). J Health Care Technol 1985;1:177-212. [Information syntheses]

Office of Technology Assessment, U.S. Congress. The cost effectiveness of digital subtraction angiography in the detection of cerebrovascular disease. Washington, D.C.: U.S. Government Printing Office, May 1985. (Health technology case study series #34)

Swedish Planning and Rationalization Institute of the Health Services. Spri technology report 6: digital subtraction angiography—economical, medical, technical and planning aspects. 1985. [Swedish language only] [Cost analyses, Epidemiological and other observational methods]

American Hospital Association, Hospital Technology Series Program. Digital subtraction angiography. 1982. (Guideline report) [Information syntheses, Expert opinion, Cost analyses]

Digitalis

Byington R, Goldstein S, for the BHAT Research Group. [National Heart, Lung, and Blood Institute] Association of digitalis therapy with mortality in survivors of acute myocardial infarction: observation in the Beta-Blocker Heart Attack Trial. J Am Coll Cardiol 1985;6:976-982.

Digoxin

Muller JE, Turi ZG, Store PH, et al and the MILIS Study Group. [National Heart, Lung, and Blood Institute] Digoxin therapy and mortality after myocardial infarction. Experience in the MILIS Study. N Eng J Med 1986;314:265-271.

Food and Drug Administration, Center for Drugs and Biologics. Digoxin. 1982. (NTIS order no. PB82-915904). [Information syntheses, Expert opinion, Epidemiological and other observational methods, Clinical trials, Bench testing]

Dihydroergotamine

Food and Drug Administration, Center for Drugs and Biologics. Ergoloid mesylates. 1981. (NTIS order no. PB81-915904). [Information syntheses, Expert opinion, Epidemiological and other observational methods, Clinical trials, Bench testing]

Dilatation and curettage

U.S. Administrators, Professional Policy Committee. Dilatation and curettage. [7/86] [Group judgment]

Diltiazem

Food and Drug Administration, Center for Drugs and Biologics. Diltiazem hydrochloride. 1983. (NTIS order no. PB83-915901). [Information syntheses, Expert opinion, Epidemiological and other observational methods, Clinical trials, Bench testing]

Dimethyl sulfoxide

American Academy of Pediatrics, Committee on Drugs. Dimethyl sulfoxide (DMSO). Pediatrics 1983 Jan.

American Medical Association, Council on Scientific Affairs. Dimethyl sulfoxide. JAMA 1982 Sep 17;248:1369. [Group judgment]

California Medical Association, Medical Practice Opinion Program. DMSO. 1981 Jan. (Medical Practice Opinion #248) [Group judgment]

Dipyridamole

Veterans Administration, Cooperative Studies Program. Platelet aggregation in diabetes (use of ASA & persantine). [1980]. [Clinical trials]

Discography

California Medical Association, Medical Practice Opinion Program. Discography for cervical and lumbar disorders. 1985 Feb. (Medical Practice Opinion #317) [Group judgment]

Discretionary adjustment factor

Project HOPE, Center for Health Affairs. A technology-specific approach to estimating the scientific and technological component of the discretionary adjustment factor for excluded hospitals: options and issues.(for Prospective Payment Assessment Commissions). 1987 Feb. [Cost analyses]

Project HOPE, Center for Health Affairs. A technology-specific approach to estimating the scientific and technological component of the discretionary adjustment factor: options and issues. (for the Prospective Payment Assessment Commission). 1987 Feb. [Cost analyses]

Disodium cromoglycate

Food and Drug Administration, Center for Drugs and Biologics. Cromolyn sodium. 1982. (NTIS order no. PB82-915903). [Information syntheses, Expert opinion, Epidemiological and other observational methods, Clinical trials, Bench testing]

Disopyramide

Food and Drug Administration, Center for Drugs and Biologics. Disopyramide phosphate. 1982. (NTIS order no. PB82-915904). [Information syntheses, Expert opinion, Epidemiological and other observational methods, Clinical trials, Bench testing]

Disulfiram

Critchfield GC, Eddy DM. [Duke University, Center for Health Policy Research and Education] A confidence profile analysis of the effectiveness of disulfiram in the treatment of chronic alcoholism. Med Care (Submitted for publication) [Information syntheses]

Veterans Administration, Cooperative Studies Program. Antabuse in the treatment of alcoholics on methadone maintenance. [1980] [Clinical trials]

Veterans Administration, Cooperative Studies Program. Disulfiram (antabuse) in the treatment of alcoholism. [1980] [Clinical trials]

Diuretics

Kuller L, Farrier N, Borhani N, et al. [National Heart, Lung, and Blood Institute] Relationship of diuretic therapy and serum magnesium levels among participants in the Multiple Risk Factor Intervention Trial. Am J Epidemiol 1985;122:1045-1059.

Shekelle R. [National Heart, Lung, and Blood Institute] Diuretic treatment of hypertension and changes in plasma lipids over six years in the Multiple Risk Factor Intervention Trial. In: Paolette R et al. (eds). Endpoints for cardiovascular drug studies. New York: Raven, 1984:216.

Wassertheil-Smoller S, Langford HG, Blaaufox MD, et al. [National Heart, Lung, and Blood Institute] Diuretics and salt-restriction in blood pressure control. In: Winick M ed. Nutrition and drugs. New York: John Wiley and Sons Inc, 1983:175-189.

DNA antibody test

American College of Physicians, Clinical Efficacy Assessment Project. DNA antibody test. 1982. [Information syntheses]

Doman-Delacato treatment

American Academy of Pediatrics, Committee on Disabilities. The Doman-Delacato treatment of neurologically handicapped children. Pediatrics 1982 Nov.

Dopamine

Food and Drug Administration, Center for Drugs and Biologics. Dopamine HCl. 1987. (Summary basis of approval substitute, NDA # 19-099) [Information syntheses, Expert opinion, Epidemiological and other observational methods, Clinical trials, Bench testing]

Food and Drug Administration, Center for Drugs and Biologics. Dopamine HCl. 1987. (Summary basis of approval substitute, NDA # 19-099). [Information syntheses, Expert opinion, Epidemiological and other observational methods, Clinical trials, Bench testing]

Food and Drug Administration, Center for Drugs and Biologics. Dopamine hydrochloride injection. 1981. (NTIS order no. PB81-915908). [Information syntheses, Expert opinion, Epidemiological and other observational methods, Clinical trials, Bench testing]

Double blinding

Byington RP, Curb DJ, Mattson ME for the Beta Blocker Heart Attack Trial Research Group. [National Heart, Lung, and Blood Institute] Assessment of double-blindness at the conclusion of the Beta-Blocker Heart Attack Trial. JAMA 1985;253(12):1733-1766.

DRGs

Burn DRGs. In: Prospective Payment Assessment Commission. Technical appendixes to the report and recommendations to the Secretary, U.S. Department of Health and Human Services, April 1, 1986. Washington, DC: Government Printing Office, 1986:124-126. [Information syntheses, Cost analyses]

Creating diagnosis-related-group-based physician reimbursement schemes: a conceptual and empirical analysis. In: Office of Research and Demonstrations, Health Care Financing Administration. Health care financing status report: research and demonstrations in health care financing. Jan 1986. (HCFA Pub. No. 03219).

Development of staging for six rehabilitation conditions and a cross-reference system with their respective diagnois-related groups. In: Office of Research and Demonstrations, Health Care Financing Administration. Health care financing status report: research and demonstrations in health care financing. Jan 1986. (HCFA Pub. No. 03219).

Diagnosis-related groups and nursing resources. In: Office of Research and Demonstrations, Health Care Financing Administration. Health care financing status report: research and demonstrations in health care financing. Jan 1986. (HCFA Pub. No. 03219).

Diagnosis-related groups refinement for nursing care. In: Office of Research and Demonstrations, Health Care Financing Administration. Health care financing status report: research and demonstrations in health care financing. Jan 1986. (HCFA Pub. No. 03219).

Diagnosis-related groups refinement using measures of disease severity. In: Office of Research and Demonstrations, Health Care Financing Administration. Health care financing status report: research and demonstrations in health care financing. Jan 1986. (HCFA Pub. No. 03219).

Disease-specific severity adjustments to diagnosis-related groups. In: Office of Research and Demonstrations, Health Care Financing Administration. Health care financing status report: research and demonstrations in health care financing. Jan 1986. (HCFA Pub. No. 03219).

Economics of diagnosis-related-group-based physician reimbursement. In: Office of Research and Demonstrations, Health Care Financing Administration. Health care financing status report: research and demonstrations in health care financing. Jan 1986 (HCFA Pub. No. 03219).

Feasibility of incorporating CPT-4 codes for physician billing into the diagnosis-related groups system for in-hospital Medicare surgical patients. In: Office of Research and Demonstrations, Health Care Financing Administration. Health care financing status report: research and demonstrations in health care financing. Jan 1986. (HCFA Pub. No. 03219).

Further analysis of the medical doctor diagnosis-related groups algorithms. In: Office of Research and Demonstrations, Health Care Financing Administration. Health care financing status report: research and demonstrations in health care financing. Jan 1986. (HCFA Pub. No. 03219).

Learning from and improving diagnosis-related groups for end-stage renal disease patients. In: Office of Research and Demonstrations, Health Care Financing Administration. Health care financing status report: research and demonstrations in health care financing. Jan 1986. (HCFA Pub. No. 03219).

Lymphomas, leukemia, and chemotherapy. In: Prospective Payment Assessment Commission. Technical appendixes to the report and recommendations to the Secretary, U.S. Department of Health and Human Services, April 1, 1986. Washington, DC: Government Printing Office, 1986:121-123. [Information syntheses, Cost analyses]

Medical doctor diagnosis-related groups algorithms. In: Office of Research and Demonstrations, Health Care Financing Administration. Health care financing status report: research and demonstrations in health care financing. Jan 1986. (HCFA Pub. No. 03219).

PPS payments for expensive prosthetic and implantable devices and other medical supplies. In: Prospective Payment Assessment Commission. Technical appendixes to the report and recommendations to the Secretary, U.S. Department of Health and Human Services, April 1, 1986. Washington, DC: Government Printing Office, 1986:87-96 [Information syntheses, Cost analyses]

Project HOPE, Center for Health Affairs. Evaluating the heterogeneity of DRGs involving lymphomas, leukemias, and chemotherapy and developing alternative classifications of discharges. (for Prospective Payment Assessment Commission). 1986 Aug. [Information syntheses, Cost analyses]

Severity of illness and diagnosis-related groups in selected cancers. In: Office of Research and Demonstrations, Health Care Financing Administration. Health care financing status report: research and demonstrations in health care financing. Jan 1986. (HCFA Pub. No. 03219).

Upper extremity procedures. In: Prospective Payment Assessment Commission. Technical appendixes to the report and recommendations to the Secretary, U.S. Department of Health and Human Services, April 1, 1986. Washington, DC: Government Printing Office, 1986:115-117. [Information syntheses, Cost analyses]

University of Pennsylvania, Leonard Davis Institute of Health Economics. Adjustment artifacts in DRG-based Medicare reimbursement. 1985 Aug. (Final report to the National Center for Health Services Research, DHHS)

University of Pennsylvania, Leonard Davis Institute of Health Economics. DRG's disease staging, and variance reduction. 1985 Jul. (Final Report to the National Center for Health Services Research, DHHS)

Office of Technology Assessment, U.S. Congress. Diagnosis-related groups (DRGs) and the Medicare program: implications for medical technology, Washington, D.C.: U.S. Government Printing Office, July 1983.

Project HOPE, Center for Health Affairs, Evaluating the clinical and resource heterogeneity in DRG 468. (for Prospective Payment Assessment Commission). Ongoing; expected 1987. [Information syntheses]

Drug costs

Leonard Davis Institute of Health Economics. Cost of generic vs. branded ethical drugs. 1986 Jun. (Final report to Ayerst Laboratories)

Drug labeling

Office of Technology Assessment, U.S. Congress. Drug labeling in developing countries. Washington, D.C.: U.S. Government Printing Office (to be completed in Winter 1988/89).

American Academy of Pediatrics, Committee on Drugs. Unapproved uses of approved drugs: the physician, the package insert, and the FDA. Pediatrics 1978 Aug.

Drug ordering

Ray WA, Schaffner W, Federspiel CF. [National Center for Health Services Research and Health Care Technology Assessment, Division of Extramural Research] Persistence of improvement in antibiotic prescribing practice. JAMA 1985 Mar;253(12):1774-1776.

Ray WA, et al. [National Center for Health Services Research and Health Care Technology Assessment, Division of Extramural Research] Improving antibiotic prescribing in outpatient practice: nonassociation of outcome with prescriber characteristics and measures of receptivity. Med Care 1985 Nov;23(11):1307-1313.

Schaffner W, Ray WA, Federspiel CF. [National Center for Health Services Research and Health Care Technology Assessment, Division of Extramural Research] Improving prescribing in outpatient practice. 1985 Oct. (NTIS order no. PB86-218997/AS)

American Medical Association, Council on Scientific Affairs. Prescription Abuse Data Synthesis (PADS) Project and the AMA prescription drug abuse activity. 1984. [Group judgment]

Gehlbach SH, et al. [National Center for Health Services Research and Health Care Technology Assessment, Division of Extramural Research] Improving drug prescribing in a primary care practice. Med Care 1984 Mar;22(3):193-201.

Seigel. [National Center for Health Services Research and Health Care Technology Assessment, Division of Extramural Research] The effects of a computerized drug order review system. 1984. (NTIS order no. PB84-156199)

Soumerai SB, Avorn JL. [National Center for Health Services Research and Health Care Technology Assessment, Division of Extramural Research] Efficacy and cost-containment in hospital pharmacotherapy: state-of-the-art and future directions. Milbank Mem Fund Q 1984;63(3).

Blazer DG, et al. [National Center for Health Services Research and Health Care Technology Assessment, Division of Extramural Research] The risk of anticholinergic toxicity in the elderly: a study of prescribing practices in two populations. J Cardiol 1983 Jan;38(1):31-35.

Koespell TD, et al. [National Center for Health Services Research and Health Care Technology Assessment, Division of Extramural Research] The Seattle evaluation of computerized drug profiles: effect on provider activities. Med Care 1983 May 21(5):498-507.

Schaffner W, et al. [National Center for Health Services Research and Health Care Technology Assessment, Division of Extramural Research] Improving antibiotic prescribing in office practice. JAMA 1983 Oct;250(13):1728-1732.

Brand DA. [National Center for Health Services Research and Health Care Technology Assessment, Division of Extramural Research] A computer audit to improve ER drug prescribing. 1982. (NTIS order no. PB82-253188).

Tompkins RK, Koepsell TO. [National Center for Health Services Research and Health Care Technology Assessment, Division of Extramural Research] Experimental evaluation of computerized drug profiles. 1982. (NTIS no. PB82-265257)

American Academy of Pediatrics, Committee on Drugs. Generic prescribing. Pediatrics 1976 Feb.

Georgetown University Medical Center, Institute for Health Policy Analysis. Therapeutic drug substitution: legal liability. Ongoing.

Drug preparation

American Academy of Pediatrics, Committee on Drugs. "Inactive" ingredients in pharmaceutical products. Pediatrics 1985 Oct.

American Academy of Pediatrics, Committee on Drugs. "Look-alikes." Pediatrics 1983 Aug.

Drug regulation

Jonsson, B. [Linköping University, Center for Medical Technology Assessment] The economics of drug regulation. 1986. (Discussion series paper #5) [Information syntheses]

Dual-energy scanned projection radiography

ECRI Technology Assessment Program. Dual-energy scanned projection radiography. Issues Health Care Technol 1982;sec.5.D.1. [Information syntheses]

Echocardiography

ECRI Technology Assessment Program. Two-dimensional Doppler echocardiography. Issues Health Care Technol 1986;sec.5.E.5. [Information syntheses]

U.S. Administrators, Professional Policy Committee. Echocardiography in artherosclerotic coronary artery disease. [7/86]. [Group judgment]

Blue Cross and Blue Shield Association, Medical Necessity Program. Echocardiogram. 1985. [Information syntheses]

Blue Cross and Blue Shield Association, Medical Program. Doppler flow velocity study. 1985. [Information syntheses]

ECRI Technology Assessment Program. Two-dimensional Doppler echocardiography. J Health Care Technol 1985;2:129-50. [Information syntheses]

American Hospital Association, Hospital Technology Series Program. Echocardiography. 1984. (Guideline report) [Information syntheses, Expert opinion, Cost analyses]

U.S. Administrators, Professional Policy Committee. Echocardiography/re-evaluation. Ongoing. [Group judgment]

Econazole

Food and Drug Administration, Center for Drugs and Biologics. Econazole nitrate. 1983. (NTIS order no. PB83-915901). [Information syntheses, Expert opinion, Epidemiological and other observational methods, Clinical trials, Bench testing]

Edinburgh Masker

American Academy of Neurology, Practice Committee. Edinburgh Masker for stuttering. 1983 Jun. [Expert opinion, Group judgment]

Elbow prosthesis

Office of Technology Assessment, U.S. Congress. The Boston elbow. Washington, D.C.: U.S. Government Printing Office, November 1984. (Health technology case study series #29)

Electrical stimulation—Cardiac

Medical Technology and Practice Patterns Institute. Endocardial electrical stimulation. 1987.

American College of Physicians, Clinical Efficacy Assessment Project. Endocardial electrical stimulation. Ann Intern Med 1984;100:452-4. [Information syntheses]

National Center for Health Services Research and Health Care Technology Assessment, Office of Health Technology Assessment. Diagnostic endocardial electrical stimulation. 1984.

U.S. Administrators, Professional Policy Committee. Programmed electronic stimulation - post-myocardial infarct. Ongoing. [Group judgment]

Electrical stimulation—Cerebellar

American Academy of Neurology, Practice Committee. Cerebellar stimulator implantation for cerebral palsy. 1982 Oct. [Expert opinion, Group judgment]

American Academy of Neurology, Practice Committee. Cerebellar stimulator implantation. 1982 Jun. [Expert opinion, Group judgment]

Electrical stimulation—Cerebral palsy

Milner M. [Department Biomedical Engineering, University Toronto] [Medical Research Council - Canada] Therapeutic and orthotic aspects of electro-stimulation in paediatric cerebral palsy. (Grant period 1981-1985).

Electrical stimulation—Cranial

California Medical Association, Medical Practice Opinion Program. Cranial electrotherapy stimulation. 1984 Nov. (Medical Practice Opinion #315) [Group judgment]

American Medical Association, Diagnostic and Therapeutic Technology Assessment. Cranial electrostimulation for treatment of anxiety and/or depression. JAMA 1984 Feb 24. [Expert opinion, Information syntheses]

Electrical stimulation—Facial nerve palsy

National Center for Health Services Research and Health Care Technology Assessment, Office of Health Technology Assessment. Electrotherapy for treatment of facial nerve paralysis. 1984.

National Center for Health Services Research and Health Care Technology Assessment, Office of Health Technology Assessment. Electrotherapy for treatment of facial nerve paralysis (Bell's Palsy). 1982.

American Academy of Neurology, Practice Committee. Electrical stimulation for treatment of Bell's Palsy. 1981 Apr. [Expert opinion, Group judgment]

American Academy of Neurology, Practice Committee. Electrical stimulation for treatment of facial nerve palsy. 1981 May. [Expert opinion, Group judgment]

Electrical stimulation—Muscular

California Medical Association, Medical Practice Opinion Program. Noninvasive muscle stimulators for prevention of muscle atrophy. 1983 Jul. (Medical Practice Opinion #292) [Group judgment]

Electrical stimulation—Neural

Blue Cross and Blue Shield Association, Technology Evaluation and Coverage Program. Electrical nerve stimulation of the ear. 1986. [Information syntheses]

California Medical Association, Medical Practice Opinion Program. Neurostimulation for urethral sphincter spasticity. 1985 Dec. (Medical Practice Opinion #336) [Group judgment]

American Academy of Neurology, Practice Committee. Electrical nerve stimulation of post-surgical pain. 1981 Apr. [Expert opinion, Group judgment]

Electrical stimulation—Neuromuscular

National Center for Health Services Research and Health Care Technology Assessment, Office of Health Technology Assessment. Neuromuscular electrical stimulation in the treatment of disuse atrophy in the absence of nervous system involvement. 1984.

Electrical stimulation—Scoliosis

American Medical Association, Diagnostic and Therapeutic Technology Assessment. Implanted electrospinal stimulator for scoliosis. JAMA 1984 May 25. [Expert opinion, Information syntheses]

Electrical stimulation—Spinal

Blue Cross and Blue Shield Association, Technology Evaluation and Coverage Program. Electrical nerve stimulation (implantable spinal cord stimulator). 1986. [Information syntheses]

American Academy of Neurology, Practice Committee. Spinal cord stimulation for treatment of cerebral palsy. 1982 Jun. [Expert opinion, Group judgment]

American Academy of Neurology, Practice Committee. Spinal stimulation for multiple sclerosis. 1980 May. [Expert opinion, Group judgment]

Electrical stimulators

Medtronic, Inc. [Food and Drug Administration, Center for Devices and Radiological Health] Medtronic (R) scoliosis system, model 3100-2: summary of safety and effectiveness. 1986 Jan 2. (PMA no. P840022-000).

Medtronic, Inc. [Food and Drug Administration, Center for Devices and Radiological Health] Itrel (R) totally implantable spinal cord stimulation system: summary of safety and effectiveness. 1985 Jan 2. (PMA no. P840001-000).

Medtronic, Inc. [Food and Drug Administration, Center for Devices and Radiological Health] Isomed (R) electro-spinal orthosis single channel S: summary of safety and effectiveness. 1984 Jan 25. (PMA no. P810062-000).

Electro-Biology, Inc. [Food and Drug Administration, Center for Devices and Radiological Health] Scolitron (TM) stimulator: summary of safety and effectiveness. 1983 Feb 25. (PMA no .P820008-000).

Avery Labs, Inc. [Food and Drug Administration, Center for Devices and Radiological Health] Spinal epidural electrode for P.E.N.S. models E-355: summary of safety and effectiveness. 1982 Mar 2. (PMA no. P810033-000).

Electrocardiographs

Blue Cross and Blue Shield Association, Medical Necessity Program. Electrocardiogram. 1985. [Information syntheses]

ECRI Health Devices Program. Electrocardiographs, three-channel. Health Devices 1984;13:235-59.

Food and Drug Administration, Center for Devices and Radiological Health. Development of test methods for disposable ECG electrodes - Volume I. 1984. (NTIS Order No. PB84-193960).

ECRI Health Devices Program. Operating room ECG monitors. Health Devices 1982;11:155-74.

Netherlands Organization for Applied Scientific Research, Medical Technology Unit (TNO). Three channel (phono) electrocardiographs. 1977.

Netherlands Organization for Applied Scientific Research, Medical Technology Unit (TNO). One channel electrocardiographs. 1975.

Electrocardiography

Blue Cross and Blue Shield Association, Medical Necessity Program. Routine preoperative and general hospital admission electrocardiograms. 1987. [Information syntheses]

Blue Cross and Blue Shield Association, Technology Evaluation and Coverage Program. Signal averaged ECG. 1986. [Information syntheses]

Fancott T. [National Health Research and Development Program - Canada] A prototype ambulatory ECG tape analysis system. 1986. (Grant No. 6605-2052-51).

Blue Cross and Blue Shield Association, Medical Necessity Program. Vectorcardiogram. 1985. [Information syntheses]

Multiple Risk Factor Intervention Trial Research Group. [National Heart, Lung, and Blood Institute] Exercise electrocardiogram and coronary heart disease mortality in the Multiple Risk Factor Intervention Trial. Am J Cardiol 1985;55:16-24.

American Medical Association, Diagnostic and Therapeutic Technology Assessment. Mandatory EKG prior to elective surgery. JAMA 1983 Jul 29. [Expert opinion, Information syntheses]

ECRI Technology Assessment Program. Mobile computerized ECG interpretive systems. Issues Health Care Technol 1983;sec.5.E.2. [Information syntheses]

American College of Cardiology/American Heart Association Task Force on Assessment of Cardiovascular Procedures. Guidelines for ambulatory electrocardiographic monitoring. Ongoing. [Group judgment]

U.S. Administrators, Professional Policy Committee. Protocol for use of multiple EKG's and chest X-rays in CCUs and ICUs. Ongoing. [Group judgment]

Electrocoagulation

Johnston JH. Ulcer hemorrhage - heater probe treatment. In: American Society for Gastrointestinal Endoscopy, Committee on Technology Assessment. Therapeutic gastrointestinal endoscopy: an information resource manual. 1987. [Information syntheses, Expert opinion, Group judgment, Cost analyses]

Papp JP. Control of upper gastrointestinal bleeding by monopolar electrocoagulation. In: American Society for Gastrointestinal Endoscopy, Committee on Technology Assessment. Therapeutic gastrointestinal endoscopy: an information resource manual. 1987. [Information syntheses, Expert opinion, Group judgment, Cost analyses]

National Center for Health Services Research and Health Care Technology Assessment, Office of Health Technology Assessment. Endoscopic electrocoagulation of upper gastrointestinal bleeding. 1986.

American Medical Association, Diagnostic and Therapeutic Technology Assessment. Endoscopic electrocoagulation for gastrointestinal hemorrhage. JAMA 1985 May 11. [Expert opinion, Information syntheses]

Electroconvulsive therapy

Martin BA, Kedwood HB, Kramer PM. [National Health Research and Development Program - Canada] Electroconvulsive therapy for psychogeriatric patients: evaluation of new stimulus waveform technology. 1986. (Grant No. 6606-2460-44).

National Institutes of Health, Consensus Development Program. Electroconvulsive therapy. (Consensus Development Conference Statement, Jun 10-12 1985). [Group judgment]

Electroencephalographs

ECRI Health Devices Program. EEG monitors. Health Devices 1986;15:71-95.

Shwedyk E, Sesha S. [National Health Research and Development Program - Canada] Pattern recognition system for ambulatory electroencephalograms: design and evaluation. 1986. (Grant No. 6607-1352-51).

Netherlands Organization for Applied Scientific Research, Medical Technology Unit (TNO). Electro-encephalographs. 1981.

Electroencephalography

ECRI Technology Assessment Program. Computer--processed EEG monitoring during surgery. Issues Health Care Technol 1986;sec.5.E.4. [Information syntheses]

Seshia SS, Shwedyk E. [National Health Research and Development Program - Canada] Computerized EEG data base from prolonged ambulatory 4 channel (cassette) recordings in children. 1986. (Grant No. 6607-1257-42).

American Academy of Neurology, Practice Committee. EEG guidelines for epileptic mentally retarded. 1984 Nov. [Expert opinion, Group judgment]

California Medical Association, Medical Practice Opinion Program. Video electroencephalographic monitoring. 1984 Nov. (Medical Practice Opinion #314) [Group judgment]

National Center for Health Services Research and Health Care Technology Assessment, Office of Health Technology Assessment. Ambulatory electroencephalographic (EEG) monitoring. 1984.

American Academy of Neurology, Practice Committee. Twenty-four hour EEG ambulatory monitoring. 1983 Jun. [Expert opinion, Group judgment]

American Medical Association, Diagnostic and Therapeutic Technology Assessment. 24-hour ambulatory EEG monitoring for diagnosing seizure disorders. JAMA 1983 Dec 23. [Expert opinion, Information syntheses]

American Medical Association, Diagnostic and Therapeutic Technology Assessment. Quantitative EEG (fast Fourier transform analysis) operative monitoring of cerebrovascular status. JAMA 1983 Jul 15.[Expert opinion, Information syntheses]

National Center for Health Services Research and Health Care Technology Assessment, Office of Health Technology Assessment. EEG monitoring during open heart surgery. 1983.

American Academy of Neurology, Practice Committee. EEG monitoring - ambulatory. 1982 Apr. [Expert opinion, Group judgment]

American Academy of Neurology, Practice Committee. EEG monitoring during open-heart surgery and immediate post-operative period. 1982 Oct. [Expert opinion, Group judgment]

American Academy of Neurology, Practice Committee. EEG interpretation and brain stem evoked response. 1981 Jul. [Expert opinion, Group judgment]

American Academy of Neurology, Practice Committee. Continuous EEG monitoring during surgery. 1980 Apr. [Expert opinion, Group judgment]

Electrolyte injection

Food and Drug Administration, Center for Drugs and Biologics. Multiple electrolyte injection. 1981. (NTIS order no. PB81-915901). [Information syntheses, Expert opinion, Epidemiological and other observational methods, Clinical trials, Bench testing]

Electronystagmography

American Academy of Neurology, Practice Committee. Electronystagmography. 1984 Jun. [Expert opinion, Group judgment]

Electrosurgery

Food and Drug Administration, Center for Devices and Radiological Health. Investigation and studies in electrosurgery. 1984. (NTIS Order No. PB84-191634).

Electrosurgical devices

ECRI Health Devices Program. Electrosurgical active electrode pencils, hand controlled. Health Devices 1986;15:151-77.

ECRI Health Devices Program. Electrode monitoring systems, electrosurgical. Health Devices 1985;14:115-31.

Electroversion therapy

National Center for Health Services Research and Health Care Technology Assessment, Office of Health Technology Assessment. Electroversion therapy for the treatment of alcoholism. 1983.

ELISA

Spence L, Bishai FR, Sekla LH. [National Health Research and Development Program - Canada] Application of ELISA to monitoring for activity of western equine encephalitis. 1986. (Grant No. 6606-2368-54).

Emergency communication systems

ECRI Technology Assessment Program. Personal emergency response system (PERS). Issues Health Care Technol 1986;sec. 5.P.10. [Information syntheses]

Fine EG [National Center for Health Services Research and Health Care Technology Assessment, Division of Extramural Research] An evaluation of the 911 system. 1983 (NTIS order no. PB83-137968).

Dibner AS, Lowry L, Morris JN. [National Center for Health Services Research and Health Care Technology Assessment, Division of Extramural Research] Usage and acceptance of an emergency alarm system by the elderly. Gerontologist 1982;22(6):538-539.

Ruchlin HS, Morris JN. [National Center for Health Services Research and Health Care Technology Assessment, Division of Extramural Research] Cost-benefit analysis of an emergency alarm and response system: a case study of a long term care program. Health Serv Res 1981 Spring;16(1):65-80.

Sherwood S. [National Center for Health Services Research and Health Care Technology Assessment, Division of Extramural Research] Effects of an emergency alarm and response for the aged. 1981. (NTIS order no. PB81-137259)

Emergency kits

American Dental Association, Council on Dental Therapeutics. Office emergencies and emergency kits. J Am Dent Assoc 1980;101.

Emergency services

American Academy of Pediatrics, Committee on Hospital Care. Emergency services. Pediatrics (To be published).

U.S. Administrators, Professional Policy Committee. Emergency rooms. [7/86] [Group judgment]

Subcommittee on Institutional Program Guidelines. [Health and Welfare Canada, Health Services and Promotion Branch, Institutional and Professional Services Division] Prehospital emergency care services. 1985. [Information syntheses, Expert opinon, Group judgment]

Hallstrom A, Eisenberg MS, Bergner L. [National Center for Health Services Research and Health Care Technology Assessment, Division of Extramural Research] Modeling the effectiveness and cost-effectiveness of an emergency service system. Soc Sci Med 1981 Mar;15c(1):13-17.

Strauss J, et al. [National Center for Health Services Research and Health Care Technology Assessment, Division of Extramural Research] Evaluation of emergency room referral system. 1981. (NTIS order no. PB81-231755)

Eisenberg MS, Bergner L, Hallstrom A. [National Center for Health Services Research and Health Care Technology Assessment, Division of Extramural Research] Out-of-hospital cardiac arrest: improved survival with paramedic services. Lancet 1980 Apr 12:812-814.

Enalapril

Food and Drug Administration, Center for Drugs and Biologics. Enalapril maleate/hydro-chlorothiazide. 1987. (Summary basis of approval substitute, NDA # 19-221). [Information syntheses, Expert opinion, Epidemiological and other observational methods, Clinical trials, Bench testing]

Endoscopes

Food and Drug Administration, Center for Devices and Radiological Health. A study of the common characteristics, hazards, and performance problems of endoscopes and endoscopic accessories. 1984. (NTIS Order No. PB84-187202).

Endoscopy

Ponsky JL. Percutaneous endoscopic gastrostomy and jejunostomy. In: American Society for Gastrointestinal Endoscopy, Committee on Technology Assessment. Therapeutic gastrointestinal endoscopy: an information resource manual. 1987. [Information synthesis, Expert opinion, Group judgment, Cost analyses]

Health Council of the Netherlands. Endoscopy. Ongoing assessment.

U.S. Administrators, Professional Policy Committee. Guidelines of appropriate indications for "oscopies". Ongoing. [Group judgment]

Endoscopy and electrocoagulation

Protell RL. Ulcer hemorrhage - bicap probe treatment. In: American Society for Gastrointestinal Endoscopy, Committee on Technology Assessment. Therapeutic gastrointestinal endoscopy: an information resource manual. 1987. [Information sytheses, Expert opinion, Group judgment, Cost analyses]

Endothelial cell photography

National Center for Health Services Research and Health Care Technology Assessment, Office of Health Technology Assessment. Endothelial cell photography. 1982.

Enteral nutrition

Patrick J. [National Health Research and Development Program - Canada] Nutritional resuscitation of children with cerebral palsy: does the amount and type of dietary lipid in enteral feeds influence membrane function? 1986. (Grant No. 6606-2684-52).

Enteral nutrition pumps

ECRI Health Devices Program. Enteral feeding pumps. Health Devices 1984;14:9-30.

Enzyme-albumin polymers

Poznansky MJ. [Department Physiology, University Alberta] [Medical Research Council - Canada] Soluble enzyme-albumin polymers: new approaches to enzyme therapy. (Grant period 1976-1985).

Ephedrine

Food and Drug Administration, Center for Drugs and Biologics. Chlorpheniramine maleate pseudoephedrine sulfate. 1981. (NTIS order no.PB81-915906). [Information syntheses, Expert opinion, Epidemiological and other observational methods, Clinical trials, Bench testing]

Epikeratophakia

American Academy of Ophthalmology. Epikeratophakia procedures for the correction of severe hyperopia, myopia, and keratoconus, San Francisco, CA: American Academy of Ophthalmology, expected completion October 1987.[Information syntheses, Expert opinion]

Blue Cross and Blue Shield Association, Technology Evaluation and Coverage Program. Epikeratophakia. 1986. [Information syntheses]

California Medical Association, Medical Practice Opinion Program. Epikeratophakia in children. 1986 Dec. (Medical Practice Opinion #344) [Group judgment]

Ergonovine provocative testing

American College of Physicians, Clinical Efficacy Assessment Project. Ergonovine provocative testing. Ann Intern Med 1984;100:152-2. [Information syntheses]

Ericsson sex selection method

California Medical Association, Medical Practice Opinion Program. Ericsson sex selection method. 1983 Sep. (Medical Practice Opinion #298) [Group judgment]

Erythrocyte sedimination rate

Blue Cross and Blue Shield Association, Medical Necessity Program. Erythrocyte sedimentation rate. 1987. [Information syntheses]

Erythromycin

Food and Drug Administration, Center for Drugs and Biologics. Erythromycin base (enteric-coated pellets). 1981. (NTIS order no. PB81-915904). [Information syntheses, Expert opinion, Epidemiological and other observational methods, Clinical trials, Bench testing]

Esophageal pH monitoring

National Center for Health Services Research and Health Care Technology Assessment, Office of Health Technology Assessment. 24-hour ambulatory esophageal pH monitoring. 1985.

Esophagoscopy

California Medical Association, Medical Practice Opinion Program. Hospital admission following rigid esophagoscopy. 1986 Jul. (Medical Practice Opinion #339) [Group judgment]

Esterine

California Medical Association, Medical Practice Opinion Program. Esterine for treatment of rheumatoid arthritis. 1981 Dec. (Medical Practice Opinion #253) [Group judgment]

Estramustine

Food and Drug Administration, Center for Drugs and Biologics. Estramustine phosphate sodium. 1982. (NTIS order no.PB82-915901). [Information syntheses, Expert opinion, Epidemiological and other observational methods, Clinical trials, Bench testing]

Estrogen replacement therapy

American College of Obstetricians and Gynecologists, Committee on Technical Bulletins. Estrogen replacement therapy. 1986 Jun. (Technical bulletin no. 93). [Expert opinion]

American Medical Association, Council on Scientific Affairs. Estrogen replacement in the menopause. JAMA 1983 Jan 21;249:359. [Group judgment]

National Institutes of Health, Consensus Development Program. Estrogen use and postmenopausal women. (Consensus Development Conference Statement, Sep 13-14 1979). [Group judgment]

Estrogens

Sherwin BB [Sir Mortimer B. Davis-Jewish General Hospital, Montreal] [Medical Research Council- Canada] Long-term effects of androgen and/or estrogen on psychosexual functioning, hormone levels, and lipid metabolism in surgically menopausal women. (Grant period 1984-1985)

Ethanol

American Academy of Pediatrics, Committee on Drugs. Ethanol in liquid preparations intended for children. 1984.

Ethynodiol diacetate with ethinyl estradiol

Food and Drug Administration, Center for Drugs and Biologics. Ethynodiol diacetate with ethinyl estradiol. 1982. (NTIS order no. PB82-915901). [Information syntheses, Expert opinion, Epidemiological, and other observational methods, Clinical trials, Bench testing]

Etomidate

Food and Drug Administration, Center for Drugs and Biologics. Etomidate. 1983. (NTIS order no. PB83-91590). [Information syntheses, Expert opinion, Epidemiological and other observational methods, Clinical trials, Bench testing]

Food and Drug Administration, Center for Drugs and Biologics. Etomidate. 1982. (NTIS order no. PB82-915904). [Information syntheses, Expert opinion, Epidemiological and other observational methods, Clinical trials, Bench testing]

Evoked potentials

American Academy of Neurology, Practice Committee. Somatosensory evoked response. 1983 Nov. [Expert opinion, Group judgment]

American Academy of Neurology, Practice Committee. Visual evoked potentials. 1981 Jul. [Expert opinion, Group judgment]

ECRI Technology Assessment Program. Evoked potential (EP) response measurement. Issues Health Care Technol 1981;sec.5.E.1. [Information syntheses]

U.S. Administrators, Professional Policy Committee. Evoked potential monitoring. Ongoing. [Group judgment]

Exercise tests

Schlant RC, Blomqvist CG, Brandenburg RO, et al. [American College of Cardiology/American Heart Association Task Force on Assessment of Cardiovascular Procedures] Guidelines for exercise testing. J Am Coll Cardiol 1986;8:725-738. [Group judgment]

U.S. Administrators, Professional Policy Committee. Stress tests. [7/86] [Group judgment]

Blue Cross and Blue Shield Association, Medical Necessity Program. Cardiac exercise stress test. 1985. [Information syntheses]

American Medical Association, Council on Scientific Affairs. Indications and contraindications for exercise testing. JAMA 1981 Aug 28;246:1015. [Group judgment]

Fisher LD, Kennedy JW, Chaitman BR, et al. [National Heart, Lung, and Blood Institute] Diagnostic quantification of CASS (Coronary Artery Surgery Study) clinical and exercise test results in determining presence and extent of coronary artery disease: a multivariate approach. Circulation 1981;63:987-1000.

Exercise therapy

National Institutes of Health, Consensus Development Program. Diet and exercise in noninsulin-dependent diabetes mellitus. (Consensus Development Conference Statement, Dec 8-10 1986). [Group judgment]

U.S. Administrators, Professional Policy Committee. Exercise training for chronic obstructive lung disease. [7/86] [Group judgment]

American Medical Association, Council on Scientific Affairs. Exercise programs for the elderly. 1983. [Group judgment]

American Medical Association, Council on Scientific Affairs. Physician-supervised exercise programs in rehabilitation of patients with coronary heart disease. JAMA 1981 Apr 10;245:1463. [Group judgment]

Expert system evaluation

[National Library of Medicine] Testing of a general methodology for the evaluation of expert systems in medicine. Bethesda, MD: Lister Hill Center, National Library of Medicine. Ongoing. [Epidemiological and other observational methods]

Expert systems

Shwedyk E, Sesha S. [National Health Research and Development Program - Canada] Pattern recognition system for ambulatory electroencephalograms: design and evaluation. 1986. (Grant No. 6607-1352-51).

Smith CC. [National Center for Health Services Research and Health Care Technology Assessment, Division of Extramural Research] Microchip medicine. Ambassador 1986 Apr;19(4):20-22.

Chang EJH. [Department Computer Science, University Victoria] [Medical Research Council - Canada] Computer assisted medical reasoning. (Grant period 1984-1985).

Food and Drug Administration, Center for Devices and Radiological Health. Computerized treatment planning systems - proceedings of a symposium held at Henry Ford Hospital, Detroit, Michigan. 1984. (NTIS Order No. 84-155118).

Blum RL. [National Center for Health Services Research and Health Care Technology Assessment, Division of Extramural Research] Discovery, confirmation, and incorporation of causal relationships from a large time-oriented clinical data base: the RX Project. Comput Biomed Res 1982;15(2):164-187.

Wagner D, Knaws W, Draper E. [National Center for Health Services Research and Health Care Technology Assessment, Division of Extramural Research] In: Blum B, ed. Proceedings: Sixth Annual Symposium on Computer Applications in Medical Care, October 30-November 2, 1982, IEEE Computer Society, 727-731.

Roderer NK, King DW, McDonald DD, Bush CG. [National Library of Medicine] Evaluation of the Hepatitis Knowledge Base System. Rockville, MD: King Research, Inc., 1981. [Epidemiological and other observational methods]

National Institutes of Health, Consensus Development Program. The use of microprocessor-based "intelligent" machines in patient care. (Consensus Development Conference Statement, Oct 17-19 1979). [Group judgment]

External counterpulsation

National Center for Health Services Research and Health Care Technology Assessment, Office of Health Technology Assessment. External counterpulsation. 1984.

Extracorporeal membrane oxygenation

ECRI Technology Assessment Program. Extracorporeal membrane oxygenation (ECMO) for newborn respiratory failure. Issues Health Care Technol 1986;5.E.6. [Information syntheses]

Extracranial-intracranial arterial bypass

American Academy of Neurology, Practice Committee. Extracranial-intracranial bypass surgery for treatment or prevention of stroke. 1986 Feb. [Expert opinion, Group judgment]

Blue Cross and Blue Shield Association, Technology Evaluation and Coverage Program. Extracranial-intracranial artery bypass surgery. 1986. [Information syntheses]

EC/IC Bypass Study Group. [McMaster University, Department of Clinical Epidemiology and Biostatistics] Failure of extracranial-intracranial arterial bypass to reduce the risk of ischemic stroke. New Eng J Med 1985;313:1191-1200.

National Center for Health Services Research and Health Care Technology Assessment, Office of Health Technology Assessment. Extra-intracranial artery bypass surgery in the treatment of strokes. Ongoing.

Eyeglasses

American Dental Association, Council on Dental Materials, Instruments and Equipment. The effects of blue light on the retina and the use of protective filtering glasses. J Am Dent Assoc 1986;112:533-535.

National Center for Health Services Research and Health Care Technology Assessment, Office of Health Technology Assessment. Ultraviolet absorbing or reflecting spectacle lenses for aphakic and pseudophakic patients. 1981.

Fetal monitoring

Thompson M, Cohen A, Palmer H. [Harvard School of Public Health, Institute for Health Research] Decision making on clinical use of electronic fetal monitors. Semin Fam Med, in press. [Epidemiological methods]

Medical Technology and Practice Patterns Institute. Fetal heart monitoring. 1987.

U.S. Administrators, Professional Policy Committee. Fetal monitoring - non-stress training. [7/86] [Group judgment]

American College of Obstetricians and Gynecologists, Committee Opinion. Current role of electronic heart rate monitoring in labor. Revised 1985 Jul. [Information syntheses]

American Medical Association, Council on Scientific Affairs. Electronic fetal monitoring. JAMA 1981 Nov 20;246:2370. [Group judgment]

Thompson MS, Cohen AB. [Harvard School of Public Health, Institute of Health Research] Decision analysis: electronic fetal monitoring. In: Wortman PM, ed. Methods for evaluating health services. Beverly Hills: Sage, 1981. [Epidemiological methods]

Neutra RR, Fienberg SE, Greenland S, Friedman EA. [Harvard School of Public Health, Institute for Health Research] Effect of fetal monitoring on neonatal death rates. N Eng J Med 1978;299:324-326. [Epidemiological methods]

American College of Obstetricians and Gynecologists, Committee on Technical Bulletins. Intrapartum fetal monitoring. 1977 Jan. (Technical bulletin no. 44). [Expert opinion]

American College of Obstetricians and Gynecologists, Committee on Technical Bulletins. Fetal heart rate monitoring. 1975 Jun. (Technical bulletin no. 32). [Expert opinion]

U.S. Administrators, Professional Policy Committee. Intrapartum fetal monitoring. Ongoing. [Group judgment]

Fetal monitors

ECRI Health Devices Program. Fetal monitors. Health Devices 1982;11:123-44.

Fetal shunts

U.S. Administrators, Professional Policy Committee. Intrauterine fetal shunts. Ongoing. [Group judgment]

Fetoscopy

American College of Obstetricians and Gynecologists, Committee Opinion. Fetoscopy. Revised 1984 Jul. [Information syntheses]

Fibrinogen scanning

Hull R, Hirsch J, Sackett DL, et al. [McMaster University, Department of Clinical Epidemiology and Biostatistics] Replacement of venography in suspected venous thrombosis by impedance plethysmography and I-fibrinogen leg scanning. Ann Intern Med 1981;94:12-15.

First aid

American Academy of Pediatrics, Committee on Accident and Poison Prevention. Revised first aid for the choking child. Pediatrics 1986 Jun.

Fish oils

Office of Technology Assessment, U.S. Congress. The health effects of fish oil. Washington, D.C.: Office of Technology Assessment, February 1984.

Fluoride varnishes

Clark DC, Hanley JA, Stamm JW, Weinstein PL. [McGill University, Department of Epidemiology and Biostatistics] An empirically based system to estimate the effectiveness of caries-preventive agents: a comparison of the effectiveness estimates of APF gels and solutions and fluoride varnishes. Caries Res 1985;19:83-95.

Clark DC. [Department Dentistry, McGill University] [Medical Research Council - Canada] The preventive effect of fluoride varnishes on dental caries: three year community trial. (Grant period 1981-1985).

Fluoroscopy

Blue Cross and Blue Shield Association, Technology Evaluation and Coverage Program. Videofluoroscopic evaluation in speech pathology. 1986. [Information syntheses]

Blue Cross and Blue Shield Association, Medical Necessity Program. Upper gastrointestinal fluoroscopic study. 1984. [Information syntheses]

ECRI Technology Assessment Program. Digital radiography and fluoroscopy. Issues Health Care Technol 1983;sec.5.D.2. [Information syntheses]

Fluoroscopy units

ECRI Technology Assessment Program. Remote control fluoroscopy units. Issues Health Care Technol 1981;sec.5.F.1. [Information syntheses]

Food diaries

Dubois S. [National Health Research and Development Program - Canada] Validity of food records and dietary recalls in elderly subjects. 1986. (Grant No. 6605-2284-42).

Remmell PS, Benfari RC (for the MRFIT Group). [National Heart, Lung, and Blood Institute] Assessing dietary adherence in the Multiple Risk Factor Intervention Trial (MRFIT). II. Food record rating as an indicator of compliance. J Am Dietetic Assn, 1980;76:357-360.

Food irradiation

Health Council of the Netherlands. Food irradiation. Ongoing assessment.

Fructose

Olefsky JM, Crapo P. [American Diabetes Association] Fructose, xylitol, and sorbitol. Diabetes Care 1980;3:390-393. [Expert opinion, Group judgment]

Functional tests

Scott RN. [National Health Research and Development Program - Canada] Functional tests for upper extremity amputees. 1986. (Grant No. 6604-1048-51).

Furosemide

Food and Drug Administration, Center for Drugs and Biologics. Furosemide injection. 1981. (NTIS order no. PB81-915908). [Information syntheses, Expert opinion, Epidemiological and other observational methods, Clinical trials, Bench testing]

Food and Drug Administration, Center for Drugs and Biologics. Furosemide tablets. 1981. (NTIS order no. PB81-915911). [Information syntheses, expert opinion, Epidemiological and other observational methods, Clinical trials, Bench testing]

Gait assessment

Rang MC, Milner M. [National Health Research and Development Program - Canada] Preoperative and postoperative gait assessments as a guide in planning tendon transfers about the ankle joint in children with cerebral palsy. 1986. (Grant No. 6606-2110-51).

Winter DA. [National Health Research and Development Program - Canada] Ambulation profiles: correlation with biomechanical variables as a quantifier of gait dysfunction. 1985. (Grant No. 6606-2313-01).

Gamma cameras

United Kingdom Department of Health and Social Security, Medical Devices Evaluation Programme. Performance assessment of gamma cameras, part four. 1986 Mar. (Report no. STB/86/9) [Epidemiological and other observational methods, Bench testing]

Gas scavengers

ECRI Health Devices Program. Anesthesia unit gas scavengers. Health Devices 1983;12:267-286.

American Dental Association, Council on Dental Materials, Instruments and Equipment. Council position on nitrous oxide scavenging and monitoring devices. J Am Dent Assoc 1980;101:62.

Gastric balloon dilatation

Kozarek RA. Balloon dilation. In: American Society for Gastrointestinal Endoscopy, Committee on Technology Assessment. Therapeutic gastrointestinal endoscopy: an information resource manual. 1987. [Information synthesis, Expert opinion, Group judgment, Cost analyses]

Gastric bubble

Medical Technology and Practice Patterns Institute. Gastric bubble for treatment of morbid obesity. 1987.

American Medical Association, Diagnostic and Therapeutic Technology Assessment. Garren gastric bubble for morbid obesity. JAMA 1986 Dec 19. [Expert opinion, Information syntheses]

Blue Cross and Blue Shield Association, Technology Evaluation and Coverage Program. Gastric bubble. 1986. [Information syntheses]

California Medical Association, Medical Practice Opinion Program. Gastric bubble for treatment of obesity. 1986 Aug. (Medical Practice Opinion #343) [Group judgment]

ECRI Technology Assessment Program. Gastric bubble. Issues Health Care Technol 1986;sec.5.G.1. [Information syntheses]

U.S. Administrators, Professional Policy Committee. Gastric bubble, Garren-Edwards. [7/86] [Group judgment]

Garren L, Garren M. [Food and Drug Administration, Center for Devices and Radiological Health] Garren gastric bubble: summary of safety and efectiveness. 1985 Oct 29.(PMA no. P840025-000).

Gastric freezing

National Center for Health Services Research and Health Care Technology Assessment, Office of Health Technology Assessment. Gastric freezing for peptic ulcer disease. 1982.

Fineberg HV. [Harvard School of Public Health, Institute for Health Research] Gastric freezing: a study of diffusion of a medical innovation. In: Medical techonology and the health care system: a study of the diffusion of equipment-embodied technology. Washington, D.C.: National Academy of Sciences, 1979. [Epidemiological methods]

Gastroesophageal antireflux prosthesis

American Medical Association, Diagnostic and Therapeutic Technology Assessment. Angelchik antireflux prosthesis treatment of gastroesophageal reflux. JAMA 1986 Sep 12. [Expert opinion, Information syntheses]

Blue Cross and Blue Shield Association, Technology Evaluation and Coverage Program. Angelchik antireflux prosthesis. 1986. [Information syntheses]

National Center for Health Services Research and Health Care Technology Assessment, Office of Health Technology Assessment. Angelchik anti-reflux prosthesis. 1986.

ECRI Technology Assessment Program. Angelchik gastroesophageal antireflux prosthesis. Issues Health Care Technol 1985;sec.5.A.4. [Information syntheses]

National Center for Health Services Research and Health Care Technology Assessment, Office of Health Technology Assessment. Anti-gastroesophageal reflux implantation. 1983.

Gastro-ileal bypass

California Medical Association, Medical Practice Opinion Program. High gastric bypass for morbid obesity. 1981 Feb. (Medical Practice Opinion #246) [Group judgment]

Gastrointestinal endoscopy

Silvis SE. Endoscopic retrograde sphincterotomy (ERS). In: American Society for Gastrointestinal Endoscopy, Committee on Technology Assessment. Therapeutic gastrointestinal endoscopy: an information resource manual. 1987. [Information syntheses;Expert opinion, Group judgment, Cost analyses]

Webb WA. Esophageal and gastric foreign bodies: endoscopic removal. In: American Society for Gastrointestinal Endoscopy, Committee on Technology Assessment. Therapeutic gastrointestinal endoscopy: an information resource manual. 1987. [Information syntheses, Expert opinion, Group judgment, Cost analyses]

American Society for Gastrointestinal Endoscopy. Appropriate use of gastrointestinal endoscopy. 1986 Jun.

American Society for Gastrointestinal Endoscopy. Standards of practice for gastrointestinal endoscopy. Revised 1986 Mar.

American Society for Gastrointestinal Endoscopy. The role of endoscopy in the management of esophagitis. Revised 1986 Mar.

American Society for Gastrointestinal Endoscopy. The role of endoscopy in the management of the patient with peptic ulcer disease. Revised 1986 Mar.

American Society for Gastrointestinal Endoscopy. The role of endoscopy in the management of upper gastrointestinal hemorrhage. Revised 1986 Mar.

American Society for Gastrointestinal Endoscopy. The role of endoscopy in the patient with lower gastrointestinal bleeding. 1986 May.

American Society for Gastrointestinal Endoscopy. The role of endoscopy in the surveillance of premalignant conditions of the upper gastrointestinal tract. Revised 1986 Mar.

U.S. Administrators, Professional Policy Committee. Upper G-I endoscopy. [7/86] [Group judgment]

American College of Physicians, Clinical Efficacy Assessment Project. Esophagogastroduodenoscopy (EGD). [Information syntheses]

American Medical Association, Diagnostic and Therapeutic Technology Assessment. Endoscopic topical therapy for gastrointestinal hemorrhage. JAMA 1985 May 11. [Expert opinion, Information syntheses]

Office of Technology Assessment, U.S. Congress. The cost-effectiveness of upper gastrointestinal endoscopy. Washington, D.C.: U.S. Government Printing Office, May 1981. (Health technology case study series #8)

Showstack JA, Schroeder SA, Steinberg HR. [University of California, San Francisco, Institute for Health Policy Studies] Evaluating the costs and benefits of a diagnostic technology: the case of upper gastrointestinal endoscopy. Med Care 1981;19:498-508.

National Institutes of Health, Consensus Development Program. Endoscopy in upper GI bleeding. (Consensus Development Conference Statement, Aug 20-22 1980). [Group judgment]

Gemfibrozil

Food and Drug Administration, Center for Drugs and Biologics. Gemfibrozil. 1982. (NTIS order no. PB82—915901). [Information syntheses, Expert opinion, Epidemiological and other observational methods, Clinical trials, Bench testing]

Generators, Electric

United Kingdom Department of Health and Social Security, Medical Devices Evaluation Programme. Assessment of Philips Medical Systems Saturn 500 and Saturn 850 generators. 1985 Aug. (Report no. STB6E/85/28) [Epidemiological and other observational methods, Bench testing]

Genetic complementation test

Gravel RA. [National Health Research and Development Program - Canada] Genetic complementation analysis in clinical diagnosis. 1986. (Grant No. 6606-1932-52).

Genetic counseling

U.S. Administrators, Professional Policy Committee. Genetic counselling and screening. [7/86] [Group judgment]

American Medical Association, Council on Scientific Affairs. Genetic counseling and prevention of birth defects. JAMA 1982 Jul 9;248:221. [Group judgment]

American College of Obstetricians and Gynecologists, Committee on Technical Bulletins. Prevention of Tay-Sachs disease: carrier identification and genetic counseling. 1976 Jan. (Technical bulletin no. 34). [Expert opinion]

Genetic engineering

American Academy of Pediatrics, Committee on Bioethics. Proposed guidelines on genetic engineering. Pediatrics 1985 Jun.

Genetic screening

Steering Committee on Future Health Scenarios, Commission on Future Health Care Technology (Netherlands). Prospective assessment of future health care technology: genetic screening. 1987.

Office of Technology Assessment, U.S. Congress. Technologies for detecting heritable mutations in human beings. Washington, D.C.: U.S. Government Printing Office, September 1986.

U.S. Administrators, Professional Policy Committee. Genetic counselling and screening. [7/86] [Group judgment]

American College of Obstetricians and Gynecologists, Committee on Technical Bulletins. Prenatal detection of neural tube defects. 1982 Oct. (Technical bulletin no. 67). [Expert opinion]

National Institute of Child Health and Human Development. Antenatal diagnosis. Bethesda MD: National Institute of Child Health and Human Development, 1979. (NIH publication no. 80-1973) [Group judgment, Expert opinion]

National Institutes of Health, Consensus Development Program. Antenatal diagnosis. (Consensus Development Conference Statement, Mar 5-7 1979). [Group judgment]

Thompson M. [Harvard School of Public Health, Institute for Health Research] Prenatal diagnosis and public policy. In: Milunsky A, ed. Genetic disorders and the fetus: diagnosis, prevention and treatment. New York: Plenum Press, 1979. [Information syntheses]

Health Council of the Netherlands. Screening for neural tube defects. Ongoing.

National Institute of Child Health and Human Development. Antenatal diagnosis of hereditary disease (an update of the 1979 Conference on Antenatal Diagnosis). Planned. [Group judgment, Expert opinion]

Genetic toxicology tests

Gilman JP. [National Health Research and Development Program - Canada] Methods survey - genetic toxicology tests using cultured mammalian cells. 1986. (Grant No. 6606-3145-55).

Glaucoma screening

Eddy DM. [Duke University, Center for Health Policy Research and Education] Screening for glaucoma, reassessment. (Expected publication 1988) [Information syntheses]

Price M. [Department Ophthalmology, University British Columbia] [Medical Research Council - Canada] The development of electrodiagnostic tests to detect early chronic open angle glaucoma. (Grant period 1983-1985).

Eddy DM, Sanders L, Eddy J. [Duke University, Center for Health Policy Research and Education] The value of screening for glaucoma with tonometry. Surv Ophthalmol 1983;28:194-205. [Information syntheses]

Glucocorticoids

American Medical Association, Council on Scientific Affairs. Glucocorticoid-induced osteonecrosis. 1986. [Group judgment]

Glutathione disulfides

Food and Drug Administration, Center for Drugs and Biologics. Salts solution plus dextrose and glutathione disulfides. 1982. (NTIS order no. PB82-915901). [Information syntheses, Expert opinion, Epidemiological and other observational methods, Clinical trials, Bench testing]

Glyceryl trinitrate

ECRI Technology Assessment Program. Transdermal delivery of nitroglycerin. Issues Health Care Technol 1983;sec.5.T.2. [Information syntheses]

Food and Drug Administration, Center for Drugs and Biologics. Nitroglycerin for injection. 1981. (NTIS order no. PB81-915912). [Information syntheses, Expert opinion, Epidemiological and other observational methods, Clinical trials, Bench testing]

Gonadorelin hydrochloride

Food and Drug Administration, Center for Drugs and Biologics. Gonadorelin HCl. 1982. (NTIS order no. PB82-915904). [Information syntheses, Expert opinion, Epidemiological and other observational methods, Clinical trials, Bench testing]

Granulocyte transfusion

Strauss RG, Connett JE, Gale RP, et al. [National Heart, Lung, and Blood Institute] A controlled trial of prophylactic granulocyte transfusions during initial induction chemotherapy for acute myelogenous leukemia. N Eng J Med 1981;305:597-603.

Winston DJ, Ho WG, Gale RP. [National Heart, Lung and Blood Institute] Prophylactic granulocyte transfusions during chemotherapy of acute nonlymphocytic leukemia. Ann Intern Med 1981;94:616-622.

Guanabenz

Food and Drug Administration, Center for Drugs and Biologics. Guanabenz acetate. 1983. (NTIS order no. PB83-915903). [Information syntheses, Expert opinion, Epidemiological and other observational methods, Clinical trials, Bench testing]

Guanadrel sulfate

Food and Drug Administration, Center for Drugs and Biologics. Guanadrel sulfate. 1983. (NTIS order no. PB 83-915901). [Information syntheses, Expert opinion, Epidemiological and other observational methods, Clinical trials, Bench testing]

Hair analysis

Health Council of the Netherlands. Hair analysis. Ongoing assessment.

Halazepam

Food and Drug Administration, Center for Drugs and Biologics. Halazepam. 1981. (NTIS order no. PB81-915912). [Information syntheses, Expert opinion, Epidemiological and other observational methods, Clinical trials, Bench testing]

Health examination

American Academy of Pediatrics, Committee on School Health. School health examinations. AAP News 1986 Feb.

U.S. Administrators, Professional Policy Committee. Periodic health screening. [7/86] [Group judgment]

Strom BL, Melmon KL, Miettinen, OS. [McGill University, Department of Epidemiology and Biostatistics] Post-marketing studies of drug efficacy: a perspective. Arch Intern Med 1985;145:1791-1793.

Spitzer WO. [McGill University, Department of Epidemiology and Biostatistics] The periodic health examination: 1. Introduction. Can Med Assoc J 1984;130:1276-1278.

The Task Force on the Periodic Health Examination. W.O. Spitzer, Chairman. [McGill University, Department of Epidemiology and Biostatistics] The periodic health examination: 2. 1984 update. Can Med Assoc J 1984;130:1278-1285.

American Medical Association, Council on Scientific Affairs. Medical evaluations of healthy persons. JAMA 1983 Mar 25;249:1626-1633. [Group judgment]

Eddy DM. [Duke University, Center for Health Policy Research and Education] Guidelines for the cancer--related checkup: recommendations and rationale. CA-A Cancer J Clin 1980;30:193-240. [Information syntheses]

Health insurance

Analysis of physician pricing behavior, third-party administrative practices. In: Office of Research and Demonstrations, Health Care Financing Administration. Health care financing status report: research and demonstrations in health care financing. Jan 1986. (HCFA Pub. No. 03219).

Health care alternatives within Title XIX: evaluation of alternative reimbursement methods to providers of primary care medical services. In: Office of Research and Demonstrations, Health Care Financing Administration. Health care financing status report: research and demonstrations in health care financing. Jan 1986. (HCFA Pub. No. 03219).

Test of the out-of-pocket cost savings as an incentive for changing beneficiary choice behavior. In: Office of Research and Demonstrations, Health Care Financing Administration. Health care financing status report: research and demonstrations in health care financing. Jan 1986. (HCFA Pub. No. 03219).

Conrad D, Milgrom P, Kiyak A. [National Center for Health Services Research and Health Care Technology Assessment, Division of Extramural Research] Insurance plan effects on dental provider treatment of elderly patients. Med Care 1984;22(5):430-445.

University of Pennsylvania, Leonard Davis Institute of Health Economics. Adverse selection in multiple-option group insurance. Ongoing. (Study for National Center for Health Services Research, DHHS)

Health maintenance organizations

A demonstration of cost control and patient satisfaction resulting from the relaxation of the maximum public enrollment rule for HMO's. In: Office of Research and Demonstrations, Health Care Financing Administration. Health care financing status report: research and demonstrations in health care financing. Jan 1986. (HCFA Pub. No. 03219).

Evaluation of Medicare health maintenance organization demonstration projects. In: Office of Research and Demonstrations, Health Care Financing Administration. Health care financing status report: research and demonstrations in health care financing. Jan 1986. (HCFA Pub. No. 03219).

Evaluation of health maintenance organization (HMO) capitation demonstrations. In: Office of Research and Demonstrations, Health Care Financing Administration. Health care financing status report: research and demonstrations in health care financing. Jan 1986. (HCFA Pub. No. 03219).

Evaluation of social health maintenance organization demonstrations. In: Office of Research and Demonstrations, Health Care Financing Administration. Health care financing status report: research and demonstrations in health care financing. Jan 1986. (HCFA Pub. No. 03219).

Independent broker: coordinating open enrollment for Medicare health maintenance organizations and competitive medical plans. In: Office of Research and Demonstrations, Health Care Financing Administration. Health care financing status report: research and demonstrations in health care financing. Jan 1986. (HCFA Pub. No. 03219).

Medicare health maintenance organization additional benefits. In: Office of Research and Demonstrations, Health Care Financing Administration. Health care financing status report: research and demonstrations in health care financing. Jan 1986. (HCFA Pub. No. 03219).

Social Health Maintenance Organization Project for long-term care. In: Office of Research and Demonstrations, Health Care Financing Administration. Health care financing status report: research and demonstrations in health care financing. Jan 1986. (HCFA Pub. No. 03219).

Health promotion

Project HOPE, Center for Health Affairs. Work site health promotion program evaluation. Ongoing, expected 1987. [Information syntheses]

Jonsson B. [Linköping University, Center for Medical Technology Assessment] Economic aspects of prevention as a health technology. 1986. (Discussion series paper #3) [Swedish language only] [Information syntheses]

University of Pennsylvania, Leonard Davis Institute of Health Economics. A review of the economic benefits of selected health education and promotion activities. 1982 May. (Interim report submitted to Johnson and Johnson Live for Life Program)

Linköping University, Center for Medical Technology Assessment. Economic aspects of prevention as a health care technology. Planned.

Hearing aids

Frost BL, Mason JL. [National Health Research and Development Program - Canada] The development and evaluation of a portable vibrotactile auditory prosthetic device for the profoundly deaf. 1986. (Grant No. 6606-1959-51).

Jamieson DG. [National Health Research and Development Program - Canada] Optimizing procedures for prescribing and fitting hearing aids. 1986. (Grant No. 6609-1343-45).

Nucleus LTD. [Food and Drug Administration, Center for Devices and Radiological Health] Nucleus multichannel implantable hearing prosthesis: summary of safety and effectiveness. 1985 Dec 9. (PMA no. P840024-000).

Hearing aids—Use

McGrath P, Durieux Smith A, Goodman JT. [National Health Research and Development Program - Canada] Compliance to hearing aid use in the classroom. 1985. (Grant No. 6606-2297-51).

Heart valve implantation

Veterans Administration, Cooperative Studies Program. Prognosis and outcome following heart valve replacement (non-biological vs. tissue). Ongoing. [Clinical trials]

Heart valve prosthesis

American Edwards Division of American Supply Corporation. [Food and Drug Administration, Center for Devices and Radiological Health] Duromedics bileaflet heart valve: summary of safety and effectiveness. 1986 Sep 26. (PMA no. P850006-000).

Medical Inc. [Food and Drug Administration, Center for Devices and Radiological Health] Omniscience prosthetic cardiac valve: summary of safety and effectiveness. 1985 Sep 11. (PMA no. P830039-000).

Food and Drug Administration, Center for Devices and Radiological Health. Prosthetic heart valves: a study of in vitro performance, phase II final report part II. 1984. (NTIS order No. PB84-162387).

Food and Drug Administration, Center for Devices and Radiological Health. Prosthetic heart valves: a study of in vitro performance, phase II final report part III. 1984. (NTIS order No. PB84-162395).

Food and Drug Administration, Center for Devices and Radiological Health. Prosthetic heart valves: a study of in vitro performance, phase II final report part I. 1984. (NTIS order No. PB84-162379).

St. Jude Medical Inc. [Food and Drug Administration, Center for Devices and Radiological Health] Bileaflet--center opening cardiac valve: summary of safety and effectiveness. 1983 Mar 1. (PMA no. P810002-000).

Medtronic, Inc. [Food and Drug Administration, Center for Devices and Radiological Health] Medtronic (r) Hall prosthetic heart valve: summary of safety and effectiveness. 1982 Jan 29. (PMA no. P790018-000).

Heimlich maneuver

American Medical Association, Council on Scientific Affairs. The Heimlich maneuver - interim report (Resolution 52, I-85). 1986. [Group judgment]

American Medical Association, Council on Scientific Affairs. Choking: the Heimlich maneuver (abdominal thrust) vs. back blows. 1983. [Group judgment]

Hemodialysis

Tousignant P, Hollomby D, Guttman RD. [McGill University, Department of Epidemiology and Biostatistics] Transplantation and home hemodialysis: their cost-effectiveness in the treatment of end stage renal disease. J Chronic Dis 1985;38.

Evans RW. [National Center for Health Services Research and Health Care Technology Assessment, Division of Extramural Research] Quality of self-care (home) and facility hemodialysis. 1981. (NTIS order no. PB81-140477)

American College of Physicians, Clinical Efficacy Assessment Project. Hemodialysis for the treatment of schizophrenia. 1980. [Information syntheses]

Veterans Administration, Cooperative Studies Program. Renal failure self-care dialysis (hemo vs. peritoneal dialysis). [1980]. [Clinical trials]

Hemofiltration

Blue Cross and Blue Shield Association, Technology Evaluation and Coverage Program. Continuous arteriovenous hemofiltration. 1986. [Information syntheses]

National Center for Health Services Research and Health Care Technology Assessment, Office of Health Technology Assessment. Hemofiltration as a substitute for hemodialysis. 1986.

American Medical Association, Diagnostic and Therapeutic Technology Assessment. Continuous arteriovenous hemofiltration (CAVH) for fluid removal. JAMA 1985 Mar 1. [Expert opinion, Information syntheses]

Hemoglobin A1C measurements

American College of Physicians, Clinical Efficacy Assessment Project. Clinical usefulness of hemoglobin A1C measurements. Ann Intern Med 1984;101:710-3. [Information syntheses]

Hemoglobinopathies screening

National Institutes of Health, Consensus Development Program. Newborn screening for sickle cell disease and other hemoglobinopathies. (Consensus Development Conference Statement, Apr 6-8 1987). [Group judgment]

United Kingdom Department of Health and Social Security, Medical Devices Evaluation Programme. Evaluation of sickle cell haemoglobin (HBS) screening methods. 1985 Sep. (Report no. STB3A/85/41) [Epidemiological and other observational methods, Bench testing]

Hemophilus influenza type B vaccine

American Academy of Pediatrics, Committee on Infectious Diseases. Hemophilus type B polysaccharide vaccine. Pediatrics 1985 Aug.

Health Council of the Netherlands. Vaccination against haemophilus influenzae B. Ongoing.

Hemostatic materials

Datoscope Corporation. [Food and Drug Administration, Center for Devices and Radiological Health] Novacol (TM) textured collagen hemostatic agent: summary of safety and effectiveness. 1986 Jul 7. (PMA no. P850023-000).

Hilitrex, Inc. [Food and Drug Administration, Center for Devices and Radiological Health] Helistat (TM) absorbable collagen hemostatic sponge: summary of safety and effectiveness. 1986 Jan 2. (PMA no. P850010-000).

Johnson & Johnson. [Food and Drug Administration, Center for Devices and Radiological Health] 3-Coll (TM) collagen absorbable hemostat: summary of safety and effectiveness. 1985 Nov 15. (PMA no. 830079-000).

Avicon, Inc. [Food and Drug Administration, Center for Devices and Radiological Health] Microfibrillar collagen hemostat non-woven web: summary of safety and effectiveness. 1983 Feb 15. (PMA no. P800002-000).

Upjohn. [Food and Drug Administration, Center for Devices and Radiological Health] Gelfoam: summary of safety and effectiveness. 1983 Aug 29. (PMA no. N18286-000).

American Medical Products Corporation. [Food and Drug Administration, Center for Devices and Radiological Health] Collastat: summary of safety and effectiveness. 1982 Jan 5. (PMA no. P810006-000).

Interface Biomedical Labs., Inc. [Food and Drug Administration, Center for Devices and Radiological Health] Superstat: summary of safety and effectiveness. 1982 Jun 25. (PMA no. P810040-000).

Heparin

Hull R, Delmore T, Carter C, et al. [McMaster University, Department of Clinical Epidemiology and Biostatistics] Adjusted subcutaneous heparin versus warfarin sodium in the long-term treatment of venous thrombosis. New Eng J Med 1982;306:189-194.

Hepatitis B tests

Organon Teknika Corp. [Food and Drug Administration, Center for Devices and Radiological Health] Hepanostika (TM) HBEAG/anti HBE microelisa (TM) system: summary of safety and effectiveness. 1986 Jul 1. (PMA no. P840070-000).

Sorin Biomedica, Fiat, USA Inc. [Food and Drug Administration, Center for Devices and Radiological Health] AB-Core K hepatitis B core antigen 1251: summary of safety and effectiveness. 1986 Apr 10. (PMA no. P850044-000).

Abbott Labs. [Food and Drug Administration, Center for Devices and Radiological Health] Corzyme (TM)-M diagnostic kit: summary of safety and effectiveness. 1984 Jan 26. (PMA no. P830014-000).

Herpes simplex infection screening, Neonatal

Sacks S. [National Health Research and Development Program - Canada] Prevention of neonatal herpes simplex virus infection: a cost-effectiveness comparison of low risk versus high risk screening. 1986. (Grant No. 6610-1421-54).

Hexachlorophene

Food and Drug Administration, Center for Drugs and Biologics. Hexachlorophene. 1981. (NTIS order no. PB81-915904). [Information syntheses, Expert opinion, Epidemiological and other observational methods, Clinical trials, Bench testing]

Food and Drug Administration, Center for Drugs and Biologics. Hexachlorophene. 1981. (NTIS order no. PB81-915909). [Information syntheses, Expert opinion, Epidemiological and other observational methods, Clinical trials, Bench testing]

Hip joint replacement

Bunker JP. [National Center for Health Services Research and Health Care Technology Assessment, Division of Extramural Research] Outcomes of total hip replacement using northern California claims data: a pilot study. 1985 Aug. (NTIS order no. PB86-129574/as, inventory only)

Nevitt MD, Epstein WV, Masem M, Murray WR. [University of California, San Francisco, Institute for Health Policy Studies] Work disability before and after total hip arthroplasty: assessment of effectiveness in reducing disability. Arthritis Rheum 1984;27:410-421.

National Institutes of Health, Consensus Development Program. Total hip joint replacement. (Consensus Development Conference Statement, Mar 1-3 1982). [Group judgment]

Hip prosthesis

CBO (Centraal Begeleidingsorgaan voor de Intercollegiale Toetsing) Consensus Development Program. Total hip protheses. 1987. [Dutch language only] [Group judgment, Expert opinion]

ECRI Technology Assessment Program. Cementless hip prosthesis. Issues Health Care Technol 1984;sec.5.H.3. [Information syntheses]

Depuy (R). [Food and Drug Administration, Center for Devices and Radiological Health] Prosthesis, hip, hemi-femoral, metal: summary of safety and effectiveness. 1983 Sep 16. (PMA no. P820024-000).

Richards Medical Co. [Food and Drug Administration, Center for Devices and Radiological Health] Osteo ceramic hip: summary of safety and effectiveness. 1982 Dec 10. (PMA no. P810048-000).

Swedish Planning and Rationalization Institute of the Health Services and the Swedish Medical Research Council. The artificial hip. 1982. [Cost analyses, Epidemiological and other observational methods]

Histamine therapy

American Academy of Neurology, Practice Committee. Histamine desensitization for cluster headache. 1983 Jun. [Expert opinion, Group judgment]

American Academy of Neurology, Practice Committee. Histamine therapy for Ménière's Disease. 1981 Jul. [Expert opinion, Group judgment]

American College of Physicians, Clinical Efficacy Assessment Project. Intravenous histamine therapy. 1981. [Information syntheses]

HISTLINE

Kopp JJ. [National Library of Medicine] Research and writing in the history of health sciences, 1970-1982: a quantitative analysis of NLM's HISTLINE database. Bull Med Libr Assoc 1985;73:146-152. [Epidemiological and other observational methods]

HIV detection assays

National Institutes of Health, Consensus Development Program. Impact of routine HTLV-III antibody testing of blood and plasma donors on the health of the public. (Consensus Development Conference Statement, Jul 7-9 1986). [Group judgment]

Wainberg MA. [National Health Research and Development Program - Canada] Development of an antigen detection assay and a neutralization assay for HTLV-III. Studies on transmission and infectivity. 1986. (Grant No. 6605-2450-X).

United Kingdom Department of Health and Social Security, Medical Devices Evaluation Programme. PHLS & DHSS evaluation of five anti-HTLV3/LAV assay kits. 1985 Sep. (Report no. STB3A/85/40) [Epidemiological and other observational methods, Bench testing]

Holter monitoring

U.S. Administrators, Professional Policy Committee. Holter monitoring. [7/86] [Group judgment]

Home care

Steering Committee on Future Health Scenarios, Commission on Future Health Care Technology (Netherlands). Prospective assessment of future health care technology: home care technology. 1987.

Comparison of the cost and quality of home health and nursing home care. In: Office of Research and Demonstrations, Health Care Financing Administration. Health care financing status report: research and demonstrations in health care financing. Jan 1986. (HCFA Pub. No. 03219).

Develop the technology of aide sharing into a transferable form for use by home health agencies to reduce home health costs. In: Office of Research and Demonstrations, Health Care Financing Administration. Health care financing status report: research and demonstrations in health care financing. Jan 1986. (HCFA Pub. No.03219).

Home services for functionally disabled adults. In: Office of Research and Demonstrations, Health Care Financing Administration. Health care financing status report: research and demonstrations in health care financing. Jan 1986. (HCFA Pub. No. 03219).

Larson C. [National Health Research and Development Program - Canada] Perinatal intervention project: the effectiveness of prenatal and postpartum home visiting. 1986. (Grant No. 6605-1878-44).

Studies evaluating Medicaid home- and community--based services: a report to Congress. In: Office of Research and Demonstrations, Health Care Financing Administration. Health care financing status report: research and demonstrations in health care financing. Jan 1986. (HCFA Pub. No. 03219).

The impact of Medicaid home and community-based waiver services for the mentally retarded in Maine. In: Office of Research and Demonstrations, Health Care Financing Administration. Health care financing status report: research and demonstrations in health care financing. Jan 1986. (HCFA Pub. No. 03219).

Veterans Administration, Cooperative Studies Program. A comparison of hospital and home treatment programs for aphasic patients. [1980] [Clinical trials]

Project HOPE, Center for Health Affairs. A review of the cost-effectiveness of home health care services. Ongoing, expected 1987. [Information syntheses, Cost analyses]

Georgetown University Medical Center, Institute for Health Policy Analysis. Home health technologies. Planned.

Health Council of the Netherlands. Home care. Planned.

Hormone therapy

Trachtenberg J. [Department Surgery, University Toronto] [Medical Research Council - Canada] Hormonal control of human prostatic cancer. (Grant period 1980-1985).

Hospice

Hospice patient outcomes and quality of care. In: Office of Research and Demonstrations, Health Care Financing Administration. Health care financing status report: research and demonstrations in health care financing. Jan 1986.(HCFA Pub. No. 03219).

Implications of the National Hospice Study for hospice prospective reimbursement. In: Office of Research and Demonstrations, Health Care Financing Administration. Health care financing status report: research and demonstrations in health care financing. Jan 1986. (HCFA Pub. No. 03219).

National Hospice Study. In: Office of Research and Demonstrations, Health Care Financing Administration. Health care financing status report: research and demonstrations in health care financing. Jan 1986. (HCFA Pub. No. 03219).

Noncertified hospice cost analysis. In: Office of Research and Demonstrations, Health Care Financing Administration. Health care financing status report: research and demonstrations in health care financing. Jan 1986. (HCFA Pub. No. 03219).

Population-based study of hospice. In: Office of Research and Demonstrations, Health Care Financing Administration. Health care financing status report: research and demonstrations in health care financing. Jan 1986. (HCFA Pub. No. 03219).

The nature, process, and modes of hospice care delivery. In: Office of Research and Demonstrations, Health Care Financing Administration. Health care financing status report: research and demonstrations in health care financing. Jan 1986. (HCFA Pub. No. 03219).

Title XVIII Hospice Benefit Program evaluation (Medicare). In: Office of Research and Demonstrations, Health Care Financing Administration. Health care financing status report: research and demonstrations in health care financing. Jan 1986. (HCFA Pub. No. 03219).

U.S. Administrators, Professional Policy Committee. Hospice care/Alzheimer's. Ongoing. [Group judgment]

Hostel

Subcommittee on Special Services in Hospitals. [Health and Welfare Canada, Health Services and Promotion Branch, Institutional and Professional Services Division] Patient hostel unit guidelines. 1978. [Information syntheses, Expert opinion, group judgment]

Hubbard method

California Medical Association, Medical Practice Opinion Program. Hubbard method of detoxification. 1987 Apr. (Medical Practice Opinion #347) [Group judgment]

Human growth hormone

U.S. Administrators, Professional Policy Committee. Growth hormone - human. [7/86] [Group judgment]

American Academy of Pediatrics, Committee on Drugs. Growth hormone in treatment of children with short stature. 1983.

Health Council of the Netherlands. Synthetic growth hormone. Planned.

Human milk banking

American Academy of Pediatrics, Committee on Nutrition. Human milk banking. Pediatrics 1980 Apr.

Humidifiers

ECRI Health Devices Program. Heat and moisture exchange humidifiers. Health Devices 1983;12:155-67.

Hyaluronidase

Muller JE (ed), Braunwald E, Mock MB, et al. (assoc. eds). [National Heart, Lung, and Blood Institute] National Heart, Lung, and Blood Institute Multicenter Investigation of the Limitation of Infarct Size (MILIS). Design and methods of the clinical trial. An investigation of beta-blockade and myaluronidase for treatment of acute myocardial infarction. Am Heart Assoc Monograph 1984;100:1-134.

Hybridomas

Roder JC. [Department Microbiology and Immunology, Queens University] [Medical Research Council - Canada] The application of human hybridoma technology to cancer and autoimmune disease. (Grant period 1983-1985).

Hydralazine

Veterans Administration, Cooperative Studies Program. Prazosin vs. hydralazine in hypertension. [1980] [Clinical trials]

Hydrochlorothiazide

Food and Drug Administration, Center for Drugs and Biologics. Propranolol SR/hydrochlorothiazide. 1987. (Summary basis of approval, NDA # 19-059). [Information syntheses, Expert opinion, Epidemiological and other observational methods, Clinical trials, Bench testing]

Food and Drug Administration, Center for Drugs and Biologics. Amiloride HCl/hydrochlorothiazide. 1982. (NTIS order no. PB82-915901). [Information syntheses, Expert opinion, Epidemiological and other observational methods, Clinical trials, Bench testing]

Food and Drug Administration, Center for Drugs and Biologics. Timolol maleate & hydrochlorothiazide. 1982. (NTIS order no. PB82-915901). [Information syntheses, Expert opinion, Epidemiological and other observational methods, Clincial trials, Bench testing]

Veterans Administration, Cooperative Studies Program. Comparison of propranolol with hydrochlorothiazide for the "step 1" treatment of hypertension. [1980] [Clinical trials]

Hydrocortisone

Food and Drug Administration, Center for Drugs and Biologics. Hydrocortisone butyrate. 1983. (NTIS order no. PB83-915901). [Information syntheses, Expert opinion, Epidemiological and other observational methods, Clinical trials, Bench testing]

Food and Drug Administration, Center for Drugs and Biologics. Hydrocortisone butyrate. 1982. (NTIS order no. PB82-915902). [Information syntheses, Expert opinion, Epidemiological and other observational methods, Clinical trials, Bench testing]

Hydromorphone

Food and Drug Administration, Center for Drugs and Biologics. Hydromorphone HC1. 1987. (Summary basis of approval, NDA # 19-034). [Information syntheses, Expert opinion, Epidemiological and other observational methods, Clinical trials, Bench testing]

Hydrotherapy

National Center for Health Services Research and Health Care Technology Assessment, Office of Health Technology Assessment. Hydrotherapy (whirlpool) baths for treatment of decubitus ulcers. 1981.

Hydroxycholecalciferol level

American College of Physicians, Clinical Efficacy Assessment Project. 25 hydroxyvitamin D level. 1981. [Information syntheses]

Hyperbaric oxygen therapy

American Academy of Neurology, Practice Committee. Hyperbaric oxygen therapy for treatment of senility, multiple sclerosis, and cerebral edema. 1986 Feb. [Expert opinion, Group judgment]

National Center for Health Services Research and Health Care Technology Assessment, Office of Health Technology Assessment. Hyperbaric oxygen for treatment of chronic peripheral vascular insufficiency. 1984.

National Center for Health Services Research and Health Care Technology Assessment, Office of Health Technology Assessment. Hyperbaric oxygen in treatment of severed limbs. 1984.

National Center for Health Services Research and Health Care Technology Assessment, Office of Health Technology Assessment. Hyperbaric oxygen therapy for acute cerebral edema. 1984.

American College of Physicians, Clinical Efficacy Assessment Project. Hyperbaric oxygen therapy: acute, traumatic peripheral ischemia. 1983. [Information syntheses]

American College of Physicians, Clinical Efficacy Assessment Project. Hyperbaric oxygen therapy: chronic vascular insufficiency. 1983. [Information syntheses]

American College of Physicians, Clinical Efficacy Assessment Project. Hyperbaric oxygen therapy: decubitus ulcers. 1983. [Information syntheses]

American College of Physicians, Clinical Efficacy Assessment Project. Hyperbaric oxygen therapy: senility. [Information syntheses]

California Medical Association, Medical Practice Opinion Program. Hyperbaric oxygen therapy. 1983 Sep. (Medical Practice Opinion #243) [Group judgment]

National Center for Health Services Research and Health Care Technology Assessment, Office of Health Technology Assessment. Hyperbaric oxygen for treatment of actinomycosis. 1983.

National Center for Health Services Research and Health Care Technology Assessment, Office of Health Technology Assessment. Hyperbaric oxygen therapy for treatment of crush injury and acute traumatic peripheral ischemia. 1983.

ECRI Technology Assessment Program. Hyperbaric oxygen (HBO) therapy. Issues Health Care Technol 1982;sec.5.H.1. [Information syntheses]

National Center for Health Services Research and Health Care Technology Assessment, Office of Health Technology Assessment. Hyperbaric oxygen therapy for treatment of arthritic diseases. 1982.

National Center for Health Services Research and Health Care Technology Assessment, Office of Health Technology Assessment. Hyperbaric oxygen therapy for treatment of chronic refractory osteomyelitis. 1982.

National Center for Health Services Research and Health Care Technology Assessment, Office of Health Technology Assessment. Hyperbaric oxygen therapy for treatment of multiple sclerosis. 1982.

National Center for Health Services Research and Health Care Technology Assessment, Office of Health Technology Assessment. Hyperbaric oxygen therapy for treatment of organic brain syndrome (senility).

National Center for Health Services Research and Health Care Technology Assessment, Office of Health Technology Assessment. Hyperbaric oxygen therapy for treatment of soft tissue radionecrosis and osteoradionecrosis. 1982.

American College of Physicians, Clinical Efficacy Assessment Project. Hyperbaric oxygen therapy: actinomycosis. 1981. [Information syntheses]

American College of Physicians, Clinical Efficacy Assessment Project. Hyperbaric oxygen therapy: arthritis. 1981. [Information syntheses]

American College of Physicians, Clinical Efficacy Assessment Project. Hyperbaric oxygen therapy: osteomyelitis. 1981. [Information syntheses]

U.S. Administrators, Professional Policy Committee. Hyperbaric oxygen therapy. Ongoing. [Group judgment]

Hyperthermia systems

Clin-Therm Corporation. [Food and Drug Administration, Center for Devices and Radiological Health] Clini-Therm Mark I/IV: summary of safety and effectiveness. 1985 Sep 11. (PMA no. P840015-000).

BSD Medical Corp. [Food and Drug Administration, Center for Devices and Radiological Health] BSD 1000 hyperthermia system: summary of safety and effectiveness. 1984 Aug 27. (PMA no. P820088-002).

BSD Medical Corporation. [Food and Drug Administration, Center for Devices and Radiological Health] BSD 1000 hyperthermia system: summary of safety and effectiveness. 1984Jan 25. (PMA no. P820088-000).

Hyperthermia therapy

Blue Cross and Blue Shield Association, Technology Evaluation and Coverage Program. Hyperthermia, local. 1986. [Information syntheses]

U.S. Administrators, Professional Policy Committee. Hyperthermia. [7/86] [Group judgment]

ECRI Technology Assessment Program. Hyperthermia treatment of tumors. Issues Health Care Technol 1985;sec.5.H.2. [Information syntheses]

Podgorsak EB. [Department Radiation Oncology, McGill University] [Medical Research Council - Canada] Noninvasive thermometry and hyperthermia in cancer treatment. (Grant period 1982-1985).

American Medical Association, Diagnostic and Therapeutic Technology Assessment. Hyperthermia treatment for cancer - Update. Sep 17, 1984. [Expert opinion, Information syntheses]

National Center for Health Services Research and Health Care Technology Assessment, Office of Health Technology Assessment. Local hyperthermia for treatment of superficial and subcutaneous malignancies. 1984.

California Medical Association, Medical Practice Opinion Program. Hyperthermia treatment for cancer. 1983 Oct. (Medical Practice Opinion #296) [Group judgment]

American College of Physicians, Clinical Efficacy Assessment Project. Whole body hyperthermia for cancer patients. 1980. [Information syntheses]

Hypnosis

American Medical Association, Council on Scientific Affairs. Scientific status of refreshing recollection by the use of hypnosis. JAMA 1985 Apr 5;253:1918-1923. [Group judgment]

California Medical Association, Medical Practice Opinion Program. Anesthesia by hypnosis. 1981 Aug. (Medical Practice Opinion #250) [Group judgment]

Hypnotic drugs

American Medical Association, Council on Scientific Affairs. Hypnotic drugs and treatment of insomnia. JAMA 1981 Feb 20;245:749. [Group judgment]

Hypothyroidism screening, Neonatal

American Academy of Pediatrics, Committee on Screening Genetics. New issues in newborn screening for phenylketonuria and congenital hypothyroidism. Pediatrics 1982 Jan.

Hysterectomy

Sandberg SI, Barnes BA, Weinstein MC, Braun P. [Harvard School of Public Health, Institute for Health Research] Elective hysterectomy: benefits, risks and costs. Med Care 1985;23:1067-1085. [Information syntheses]

Braun P. [National Center for Health Services Research and Health Care Technology Assessment, Division of Extramural Research] Elective hysterectomy: benefits, risks, and costs. 1984. (NTIS order no. PB84-240126)

Office of Technology Assessment, U.S. Congress. Elective hysterectomy: costs, risks and benefits. Washington, D.C.: U.S. Government Printing Office, October 1981. (Health technology case study series #15)

Hysteroscopy

American College of Obstetricians and Gynecologists, Committee Opinion. Hysteroscopy. Revised 1986 Jan. [Information syntheses]

Ibuprofen

Food and Drug Administration, Center for Drugs and Biologics Ibuprofen. 1987. (Summary basis of approval, NDA #19-012). [Information syntheses, Expert opinion, Epidemiological and other observational methods, Clinical trials, Bench testing]

Food and Drug Administration, Center for Drugs and Biologics. Ibuprofen. 1987. (Summary basis of approval, NDA #18-989). [Information syntheses, Expert opinion, Epidemiological and other observational methods, Clinical trials, Bench testing]

Food and Drug Administration, Center for Drugs and Biologics. Ibuprofen. 1982. (NTIS order no. PB82-915902). [Information syntheses, expert opinion, Epidemiological and other observational methods, Clinical trials, Bench testing]

Food and Drug Administration, Center for Drugs and Biologics. Ibuprofen. 1981. (NTIS order no. PB81-915908). [Information syntheses, expert opinion, Epidemiological and other observational methods, Clinical trials, Bench testing]

Ileal bypass

Buchwald H, Fitch L, Varco RL. [National Heart, Lung, and Blood Institute] Ileal bypass for hyperlipidemia. World J Surg 1985:9;850-859.

Buchwald H, Fitch L, Varco RL. [National Heart, Lung, and Blood Institute] Ileal bypass for hyperlipidemia. World J Surg 1985:9;850-859.

Buchwald H, Fitch L, Varco RL. [National Heart, Lung, and Blood Institute] Partial ileal bypass; hypercholesterolemia; atherosclerosis. In: Nyhus LM, Nelson RL, (eds): Blackwell Scientific Publ Inc, Boston, MA, 1985 (in press).

Buchwald H, Fitch L, Varco RL. [National Heart, Lung, and Blood Institute] Surgical intervention in atherosclerosis: partial ileal bypass and the Program of Surgical Control of the Hyperlipidemias (POSCH). Int Encyclo Pharm Therapy, 1985 (in press).

Buchwald H, Moore RB, Rucker RD, et al. [National Heart, Lung, and Blood Institute] Clinical angiographic regression of atherosclerosis after partial ileal bypass. Artherosclerosis 1983;46:117.

Buchwald H, Moore RB, Rucker Rd, et al. [National Heart, Lung, and Blood Institute] Clinical angiographic regression of atheroscerosis after partial ileal bypass. Artherosclerosis 1983;46:117.

Buchwald H, Moore RB, Varco RL. [National Heart, Lung, and Blood Institute] Surgery in the therapy of atherosclerosis: partial ileal bypass. In: Arteriosclerosis: clinical evaluation and therapy. MTP Press Limited, International Medical Publication, 1982.

Buchwald H, Rucker RD Jr, Moore RB, et al. [National Heart, Lung, and Blood Institute] Regression of atherosclerosis by surgical cholesterol reduction. In: Noseda CI, et al. eds. Lipoproteins and coronary atherosclerosis. Elsevier Biomedical Press, 1982:417.

Moore RB, Buchwald H, Varco RL, and the Participants in the Program on the Surgical Control of the Hyperlipidemias. [National Heart, Lung, and Blood Institute] The effect of partial ileal bypass on plasma lipoproteins. Circulation 1980;62:469-476.

Ileal bypass and diet therapy

Long, JM. [National Heart, Lung, and Blood Institute] The POSCH secondary intervention trial. Proc Int Cong Prev Cardiology, Moscow, 1985.

Imaging centers

ECRI Technology Assessment Program. Freestanding imaging centers. J Health Care Technol 1985;1:257-278. [Information syntheses]

Immunoassay systems, Fluorescence

United Kingdom Department of Health and Social Security, Medical Devices Evaluation Programme. Evaluation of the Syra Advance (summary report). 1985 May. (Report no. STB3A/85/22) [Epidemiological and other observational methods, Bench testing]

United Kingdom Department of Health and Social Security, Medical Devices Evaluation Programme. Evaluation of the Syva advance automated fluorescence immuno-assay system. Final report. 1985 Dec. (Report no. STB3A/85/47) [Epidemiological and other observational methods, Bench testing]

Immunologic diagnostic tests

Urbach GI. [National Health Research and Development Program - Canada] Immunodiagnosis of human ovarian cancer. 1986. (Grant No. 6606-2908-54).

Rippey JH, Nakamura RM, eds. Diagnostic immunology: technology assessment and quality assurance. CAP Conference/1983. Skokie, IL: College of American Pathologists, 1984. [Expert opinion, Bench testing]

Immunoradiometric assay with monoclonal antibodies

Rock GA. [National Health Research and Development Program - Canada] Development of immunoradiometric assay for the measurement of factor VIII procoagulant antigen using monoclonal antibodies to procoagulant factor VIII. 1986. (Grant No. 6613-1178-52).

Immunoradiometric assays

Abbott Laboratories. [Food and Drug Administration, Center for Devices and Radiological Health] Abbott anti-delta diagnostic kit (RIA): summary of safety and effectiveness. 1986 Aug 7. (PMA no. P850062-000).

Hybritech Inc. [Food and Drug Administration, Center for Devices and Radiological Health] Tandem-R PSA immunoradiometric assay: summary of safety and effectiveness. 1986 Apr 9. (PMA no. P850048-000).

Jones BD, Chouinarad G. [National Health Research and Development Program - Canada] Clinical application of the neuroleptic radio receptor assay in the management of schizophrenia. 1986. (Grant No. 6605-1867-44).

Immunosuppressants

American Medical Association, Council on Scientific Affairs. Use of immunosuppressants in organ transplantation. 1986. [Group judgment]

Office of Technology Assessment, U.S. Congress. The use of immunosuppressive drugs in kidney transplantation. Washington, D.C.: Office of Technology Assessment, March 1984.

Immunotherapy

Office of Technology Assessment, U.S. Congress. Immuno-augmentative therapy. Washington, D.C.: U.S. Government Printing Office (to be completed in Winter 1987/1988).

American Medical Association, Council on Scientific Affairs. Use of immunosuppressants in organ transplantation. 1986. [Group judgment]

U.S. Administrators, Professional Policy Committee. Immunoaugmentative therapy. [7/86] [Group judgment]

Office of Technology Assessment, U.S. Congress. The use of immunosuppressive drugs in kidney transplantation. Washington, D.C.: Office of Technology Assessment, March 1984.

Immunotherapy—Cancer

California Medical Association, Medical Practice Opinion Program. Immunotherapy for melanoma. 1984 Feb. (Medical Practice Opinion #305) [Group judgment]

California Medical Association, Medical Practice Opinion Program. Immunotherapy for treatment of cancer. 1984 Jul. (Medical Practice Opinion #204) [Group judgment]

American College of Physicians, Clinical Efficacy Assessment Project. Immunotherapy of cancer. 1982. [Information syntheses]

Impotence diagnosis

Morales A. [Department Urology, Queens University] [Medical Research Council - Canada] The validation of nocturnal and sexual erections in the etiological diagnosis of impotence. (Grant period 1984-1985).

National Center for Health Services Research and Health Care Technology Assessment, Office of Health Technology Assessment. Diagnostic tests for impotency: devices (Snap-gauge, Rigi-scan). Ongoing.

Impotence treatment

National Center for Health Services Research and Health Care Technology Assessment, Office of Health Technology Assessment. Treatments for impotency: drug injections. Ongoing.

National Center for Health Services Research and Health Care Technology Assessment, Office of Health Technology Assessment. Treatments for impotency: other significant therapeutic modalities. Ongoing.

In vitro chemosensitivity testing

Veterans Administration, Cooperative Studies Program. Treatment of multiple myeloma directed by in vitro chemosensitivity testing. Ongoing. [Clinical trials]

In vitro fertilization

Blue Cross and Blue Shield Association, Technology Evaluation and Coverage Program. In vitro fertilization. 1986. [Information syntheses]

Caplan A. [The Hastings Center] Ethics of in vitro fertilization. Primary Care 1986 Jun.

U.S. Administrators, Professional Policy Committee. Fertilization, in vitro. [7/86] [Group judgment]

California Medical Association, Medical Practice Opinion Program. In vitro fertilization. 1985 Jun. (Medical Practice Opinion #278) [Group judgment]

American College of Obstetricians and Gynecologists, Committee Opinion. Human in vitro fertilization and embryo placement. 1984 Apr. [Information syntheses]

Health Council of the Netherlands. In vitro fertilization. Ongoing assessment.

Incentive payment

Encouraging appropriate care for the chronically ill elderly: a controlled experiment to evaluate the impacts of incentive payments on nursing home admissions, discharges, case mix, care, outcomes,and costs. In: Office of Research and Demonstrations, Health Care Financing Administration. Health care financing status report: research and demonstrations in health care financing. Jan 1986. (HCFA Pub. No. 03219).

Incentive spirometry

U.S. Administrators, Professional Policy Committee. Incentive spirometry. [7/86] [Group judgment]

Blue Cross and Blue Shield Association, Medical Necessity Program. Respiratory therapy: incentive spirometry. 1982. [Information syntheses]

Incontinent pads

ECRI Health Devices Program. Incontinent pads. Health Devices 1983;12:108-18.

Incubator therapy

Thomas KAJ. [National Center for Health Services Research and Health Care Technology Assessment, Division of Extramural Research] The influence of incubator air temperature on the respiratory responses of preterm infants. 1986 Mar. (NTIS order no. Pb86-218096/AS)

Incubators

ECRI Health Devices Program. Infant incubators. Health Devices 1982;11:191-9.

ECRI Health Devices Program. Infant transport incubators. Health Devices 1982;11:179-91.

Netherlands Organization for Applied Scientific Research, Medical Technology Unit (TNO). Intensive care convection incubators. 1981.

Indomethacin

Food and Drug Administration, Center for Drugs and Biologics. Indomethacin. 1982. (NTIS order no. PB82-915901). [Information syntheses, Expert opinion, Epidemiological and other observational methods, Clinical trials, Bench testing]

Food and Drug Administration, Center for Drugs and Biologics. Indomethacin. 1982. (NTIS order no. PB82-915902). [Information syntheses, Expert opinion, Epidemiological and other observational methods, Clinical trials, Bench testing]

Induction of labor

American College of Obstetricians and Gynecologists, Committee on Technical Bulletins. Induction of labor. 1978 May. (Technical bulletin no. 49). [Expert opinion]

Infant foods

Friel JK. [National Health Research and Development Program - Canada] Trace element supplementation of pre-term infants. 1986. (Grant No. 6602-1087-56).

American Academy of Pediatrics, Committee on Nutrition. Imitation and substitute milks. Pediatrics 1984 Jun.

American Academy of Pediatrics, Committee on Nutrition. The use of whole cow's milk in infancy. Pediatrics 1983 Aug.

American Academy of Pediatrics, Committee on Nutrition. Soy-protein formulas: recommendations for use in infant feeding. [1983]

American Medical Association, Council on Scientific Affairs. Infant formula marketing (Resolution 155, A-81). 1982. [Group judgment]

American Academy of Pediatrics, Committee on Nutrition. On the feeding of supplemental foods to infants. Pediatrics 1980 Jun.

American Medical Association, Council on Scientific Affairs. Infant nutrition (Resolution III, I-78.) 1980. [Group judgment]

American Academy of Pediatrics, Committee on Nutrition. Juice in ready-to-use bottles and nursing bottle caries. 1978.

American Academy of Pediatrics, Committee on Nutrition. Commentary on breast-feeding and infant formulas, including proposed standards for formulas. Pediatrics 1976 Feb.

Influenza vaccine

American Medical Association, Council on Scientific Affairs. Pneumococcal, influenza and hepatitis-B vaccine (Resolution 75, A-82). 1982. [Group judgment]

Office of Technology Assessment, U.S. Congress. Cost-effectiveness of influenza vaccination. Washington, D.C.: U.S. Government Printing Office, December 1981.

Health Council of the Netherlands. Vaccination against influenza. Ongoing assessment.

Information systems

[National Library of Medicine] Evaluation of medical information science in medical education. Adopted by the Executive Council of the Asociation of American Medical Colleges, Washington, DC, January 23, 1986. J Med Educ 1986;61:487-543.

Anderson JG. [National Center for Health Services Research and Health Care Technology Assessment, Division of Extramural Research] Use of an HIS by physicians and nurses. 1985 Aug. (NTIS order no. PB86-121126/AS)

American Hospital Association, Hospital Technology Series Program. A medical device recall and reporting system. 1984. (Guideline report) [Information syntheses, Expert opinion, Cost analyses]

American Hospital Association, Hospital Technology Series Program. Materials management information systems. 1983. (Guideline report) [Information syntheses, Expert opinion, Cost analyses]

American Hospital Association, Hospital Technology Series Program. Clinical laboratory information systems. 1982. (Guideline report) [Informaton syntheses, Expert opinion, Cost analyses]

Cohen, SN, et al. [National Center for Health Services Research and Health Care Technology Assessment, Division of Extramural Research] Development, implementation and evaluation of drug interactions by a pharmacy oriented reporting system. 1982 (NTIS order no. PB82-140757)

Pittman JT. [National Center for Health Services Research and Health Care Technology Assessment, Division of Extramural Research] Health information system transferability evaluation. 1981. (NTIS order no. PB81-206500)

Long JM, Brashear JR, Matts JP, et al. [National Heart, Lung, and Blood Institute] The POSCH Information Management System: experience with alternative approaches. J Med Systems 1980;4:355-366.

Office of Technology Assessment, U.S. Congress. Policy implications of medical information systems. Washington, D.C.: U.S. Government Printing Office, November 1977.

Linköping University, Center for Medical Technology Assessment. Health care information systems and cost-effectiveness: a review of methodological issues and assessment methods. Ongoing.

Infusion pumps

Swedish Planning and Rationalization Institute of the Health Services. Spri technology report 8: treatment with insulin infusion pump: cost and effects. 1987. [Cost analyses, Epidemiological and other observational methods]

Perlman K. [National Health Research and Development Program - Canada] Dietary studies with new insulin delivery systems for the treatment of diabetes mellitus. 1986. (Grant No. 6606-2451-52).

American Diabetes Association. Continuous subcutaneous insulin infusion. Diabetes 1985;34:946. [Expert opinion, Group judgment]

ECRI Health Devices Program. Infusion controllers. Health Devices 1985;14:219-256.

American College of Physicians, Clinical Efficacy Assessment Project. Heparin infusion pumps. Ann Intern Med 1984;100:305-6. [Information syntheses]

ECRI Health Devices Program. Infusion pumps. Health Devices 1983-84;13:31-62.

Netherlands Organization for Applied Scientific Research, Medical Technology Unit (TNO). Drip-rate controlled and volumetric infusion pumps. 1984.

American College of Physicians, Clinical Efficacy Assessment Project. Management of diabetes mellitus: computerized insulin infusion pumps. Ann Intern Med 1983;99::272-4. [Information syntheses]

American Hospital Association, Hospital Technology Series Program. Automated infusion devices. 1982. (Guideline report) [Information syntheses, Expert opinion, Cost analyses]

ECRI Health Devices Program. Infusion controllers. Health Devices 1982;11:75-96.

ECRI Technology Assessment Program. Insulin delivery devices. Issues Health Care Technol 1981;sec.5.I.2. [Information syntheses]

ECRI Technology Assessment Program. Insulin infusion systems (controlled). Issues Health Care Technol 1981;sec.5.I.1. [Information syntheses]

Netherlands Organization for Applied Scientific Research, Medical Technology Unit (TNO). Ambulatory insulin pumps. Ongoing. [Expert opinion, Group judgment, Bench testing]

Infusion pumps—External

National Center for Health Services Research and Health Care Technology Assessment, Office of Health Technology Assessment. External open-loop pump for the subcutaneous infusion of insulin in diabetics. 1984.

American College of Physicians, Clinical Efficacy Assessment Project. Management of diabetes mellitus: external infusion pumps. Ann Intern Med 1983;99:272-4. [Information syntheses]

National Center for Health Services Research and Health Care Technology Assessment, Office of Health Technology Assessment. External infusion pump for heparin. 1983.

National Center for Health Services Research and Health Care Technology Assessment, Office of Health Technology Assessment. Drug delivery systems: external infusion pumps for IV antibody therapy. Ongoing.

National Center for Health Services Research and Health Care Technology Assessment, Office of Health Technology Assessment. Drug delivery systems: external infusion pumps for rehydration therapy. Ongoing.

National Center for Health Services Research and Health Care Technology Assessment, Office of Health Technology Assessment. Drug delivery systems: external pump for chemotherapy for other than liver cancer. Ongoing.

National Center for Health Services Research and Health Care Technology Assessment, Office of Health Technology Assessment. Drug delivery systems: external pumps for morphine for pain of nonmalignant origin. Ongoing.

Infusion pumps—Implantable

Blue Cross and Blue Shield Association, Technology Evaluation and Coverage Program. Implantable infusion pump. 1986. [Information syntheses]

National Center for Health Services Research and Health Care Technology Assessment, Office of Health Technology Assessment. Implantable pump for chronic heparin therapy. 1984.

American Medical Association, Diagnostic and Therapeutic Technology Assessment. Implantable infusion pump for continuous drug therapy. JAMA 1983 Oct 14. [Expert opinion, Information syntheses]

National Center for Health Services Research and Health Care Technology Assessment, Office of Health Technology Assessment. Implantable chemotherapy infusion pump for the treatment of liver cancer. 1983.

ECRI Technology Assessment Program. Implantable drug infusion pumps. Issues Health Care Technol 1982;sec.5.I.4. [Information syntheses]

Intermedics Infusaid, Inc. [Food and Drug Administration, Center for Devices and Radiological Health] Infusaid implantable infusion pump model 100, 200, 4: summary of safety and effectiveness. 1982 Mar 26. (PMA no. P800036-000).

National Center for Health Services Research and Health Care Technology Assessment, Office of Health Technology Assessment. Drug delivery systems: implantable pumps for chemotherapy for other than liver cancer. Ongoing.

National Center for Health Services Research and Health Care Technology Assessment, Office of Health Technology Assessment. Drug delivery systems: implantable pumps for infusion of drugs for congestive heart failure. Ongoing.

National Center for Health Services Research and Health Care Technology Assessment, Office of Health Technology Assessment. Drug delivery systems: implantable pumps for morphine (analgesia) intractable cancer pain. Ongoing.

National Center for Health Services Research and Health Care Technology Assessment, Office of Health Technology Assessment. Drug delivery systems: implanted pumps for morphine for pain of nonmalignant origin. Ongoing.

Injury severity scales

Mackenzie EJ. [National Center for Health Services Research and Health Care Technology Assessment, Division of Extramural Research] Injury severity scales: overview and directions for future research. Am J Emerg Med 1984 Nov;2(6):537-549.

Insulin

Food and Drug Administration, Center for Drugs and Biologics. Human insulin (recombinant DNA origin) isophane suspension. 1983. (NTIS order no. PB83-915901). [Information syntheses, Expert opinion, Epidemiological and other observational methods, Clinical trials, Bench testing]

Food and Drug Administration, Center for Drugs and Biologics. Regular human insulin (recombinant DNA origin) injection. 1983. (NTIS order no. PB83-915901). [Information syntheses, Expert opinion, Epidemiological and other observational methods, Clinical trials, Bench testing]

Food and Drug Administration, Center for Drugs and Biologics. Extended purified beef insulin zinc suspension. 1981. (NTIS order no. PB81-915909). [Information syntheses, Expert opinion, Epidemiological and other observational methods, Clinical trials, Bench testing]

Food and Drug Administration, Center for Drugs and Biologics. Isophane purified beef insulin suspension. 1981. (NTIS order no. PB81-915909). [Information syntheses, Expert opinion, Epidemiological and other observational methods, Clinical trials, Bench testing]

Food and Drug Administration, Center for Drugs and Biologics. Isophane purified pork insulin suspension. 1981. (NTIS order no. PB81-915910). [Information syntheses, Expert opinion, Epidemiological and other observational methods, Clinical trials, Bench testing]

Food and Drug Administration, Center for Drugs and Biologics. Prompt purified beef insulin zinc suspension. 1981. (NTIS order no. PB81-915909). [Information syntheses, Expert opinion, Epidemiological and other observational methods, Clinical trials, Bench testing]

Food and Drug Administration, Center for Drugs and Biologics. Purified beef insulin zinc suspension. 1981. (NTIS order no. PB81-915909). [Information syntheses, Expert opinion, Epidemiological and other observational methods, Clinical trials, Bench testing]

Food and Drug Administration, Center for Drugs and Biologics. Purified pork insulin injection. 1981. (NTIS order no. PB81-915909). [Information syntheses, Expert opinion, Epidemiological and other observational methods, Clinical trials, Bench testing]

Insulin injection

California Medical Association, Medical Practice Opinion Program. Needleless insulin injection. 1982 Dec. (Medical Practice Opinion #274) [Group judgment]

Intensive care

Cohen C. [The Hastings Center] Autonomy and equity in the ICU. Hastings Cent Rep 1986.

American Academy of Pediatrics, Committee on Hospital Care. Guidelines for pediatric intensive care units. Pediatrics 1983 Sep.

Office of Technology Assessment, U.S. Congress. Intensive care units: costs, outcome, and decisionmaking. Washington, D.C.: U.S. Government Printing Office, October 1984. (Health technology case study series #28)

American Hospital Association, Hospital Technology Series Program. Evaluation methods for intensive care units. 1982. (Guideline report) [Information syntheses, Expert opinion, Cost analyses]

Knaus WA, et al. [National Center for Health Services Research and Health Care Technology Assessment, Division of Extramural Research] A comparison of intensive care in the USA and France. Lancet 1982 Sep:642-646.

Knaus WA, et al. [National Center for Health Services Research and Health Care Technology Assessment, Division of Extramural Research] Evaluating outcome from intensive care: a preliminary multihospital comparison. Crit Care Med 1982;10(8):491-496.

Scheffler RM, et al. [National Center for Health Services Research and Health Care Technology Assessment, Division of Extramural Research] Severity of illness and the relationship between intensive care and survival. Am J Public Health 1982 May;72(5):449-454

Draper EA, Wagner DP, Knaws WA. [National Center for Health Services Research and Health Care Technology Assessment, Division of Extramural Research] The use of intensive care: a comparison of a university and community hospital. Health Care Financ Rev 1981 Dec;3(2):49-64.

Subcommittee on Special Services in Hospitals. [Health and Welfare Canada, Health Services and Promotion Branch, Institutional and Professional Services Division] Intensive care unit guidelines. 1979. [Information syntheses, Expert opinion, Group judgment]

Intensive care systems, Mobile

New Jersey mobile intensive care system. In: Office of Research and Demonstrations, Health Care Financing Administration. Health care financing status report: research and demonstrations in health care financing. Jan 1986. (HCFA Pub. No. 03219).

Wagner GS. [National Center for Health Services Research and Health Care Technology Assessment, Division of Extramural Research] The effectiveness of mobile intensive care. 1985. (NTIS order no. PB85-191211/AS)

Keller MD, et al. [National Center for Health Services Research and Health Care Technology Assessment, Division of Extramural Research] The impact of mobile coronary care units. 1981. (NTIS order no. PB81-13381)

Interferons

Paty DW. [Department Medicine, University British Columbia] [Medical Research Council - Canada] A therapeutic trial of interferon in multiple sclerosis (MS). (Grant period 1983-1985).

Paty DW. [Department Medicine, University British Columbia] [Medical Research Council - Canada] Interferon therapeutic trial in MS - supplemental application. (Grant Period 1984-1985)

California Medical Association, Medical Practice Opinion Program. Interferon for the treatment of cancer. 1983 Sep. (Medical Practice Opinion #299) [Group judgment]

California Medical Association, Medical Practice Opinion Program. Interferon for the treatment of infectious diseases. 1983 Sep. (Medical Practice Opinion #300) [Group judgment]

Intermittent positive pressure breathing

U.S. Administrators, Professional Policy Committee. Intermittent positive pressure breathing. [7/86] [Group judgment]

Intermittent Positive Pressure Breathing Trial Group. [National Heart, Lung, and Blood Institute] Intermittent positive pressure breathing therapy of chronic obstructive pulmonary disease - a clinical trial. Ann Intern Med 1983;99:612-620.

Blue Cross and Blue Shield Association, Medical Necessity Program. Respiratory therapy: intermittent positive pressure breathing. 1982. [Information syntheses]

California Medical Association, Medical Practice Opinion Program. Intermittent positive pressure breathing. 1981 Aug. (Medical Practice Opinion #259) [Group judgment]

Hodgkin JE and Zorn EG. [National Heart, Lung, and Blood Institute] Intermittent positive pressure breathing (IPPB) in the outpatient management of chronic obstructive pulmonary disease (COPD): description of the NIH clinical trial. Respir Care 1981;26:1095-1104.

National Center for Health Services Research and Health Care Technology Assessment, Office of Health Technology Assessment. Intermittent positive pressure breathing (IPPB therapy). Ongoing.

Intra-aortic balloon pumps

ECRI Technology Assessment Program. Intra-aortic balloon pumps. Issues Health Care Technol 1982;sec.5.I.3. [Information syntheses]

Intracranial pressure monitoring

National Center for Health Services Research and Health Care Technology Assessment, Office of Health Technology Assessment. Intracranial pressure measurement. 1981.

Intracranial pressure monitors

Radionics, Inc. [Food and Drug Administration, Center for Devices and Radiological Health] Cosman ICP tele-sensor (R): summary of safety and effectiveness. 1984 Nov 21. (PMA no. P820012-000).

Radionics, Inc. [Food and Drug Administration, Center for Devices and Radiological Health] Cosman ICP Tele-sensor (R): summary of safety and effectiveness. 1982 Oct 1. (PMA no. P820012-000).

American Academy of Neurology, Practice Committee. Intracranial pressure monitors. 1980 Oct. [Expert opinion, Group judgment]

Intracutaneous titration

California Medical Association, Medical Practice Opinion Program. Rinkel serial intracutaneous titration-/diagnosis. 1984 Feb. (Medical Practice Opinion #295) [Group judgment]

American College of Physicians, Clinical Efficacy Assessment Project. Intracutaneous titration. 1981. [Information syntheses]

Intraocular lens implantation

Intraocular lens implants. In: Prospective Payment Assessment Commission. Technical appendixes to the report and recommendations to the Secretary, U.S. Department of Health and Human Services, April 1, 1985. Washington, DC: Government Printing Office, 1985:101-105. [Information syntheses, Cost analyses]

National Institutes of Health, Consensus Development Program. Intraocular lens implantation. (Consensus Development Conference Statement, Sep 10-11 1979). [Group judgment]

Swedish Planning and Rationalization Institute of the Health Services. Artificial lens implantation: a cost-effectiveness analysis. Ongoing. [Cost analyses, Epidemiological and other observational methods]

Intraocular lenses

Precision-Cosmet., Inc. [Food and Drug Administration, Center for Devices and Radiological Health] Kelman (TM) omnifit II model 2100: summary of safety and effectiveness. 1987 Feb 2. (PMA no. P850059-000).

Coburn Optical Industries. [Food and Drug Administration, Center for Devices and Radiological Health] Intraocular lens: summary of safety and effectiveness. 1986 Dec 16. (PMA no. P860002-000).

Coburn Optical. [Food and Drug Administration, Center for Devices and Radiological Health] J loop posterior chamber type II 0 & I0: summary of safety and effectiveness. 1986 Jul 1. (PMA no. P840039-000).

Coopervision Cilco. [Food and Drug Administration, Center for Devices and Radiological Health] Optiflex anterior chamber lenses (L1-L5): summary of safety and effectiveness. 1986 Jun 18. (PMA no. P8200035-000).

Coopervision Cilco. [Food and Drug Administration, Center for Devices and Radiological Health] SM-1, CR-1, & GR-1 IOLS: summary of safety and effectiveness. 1986 Jun 11. (PMA no. P840060-000).

Iolab Corp. [Food and Drug Administration, Center for Devices and Radiological Health] Model 91-50 IOL: summary of safety and effectiveness. 1986 Feb 14. (PMA no. P820044-000).

Optical Radiation Corporation. [Food and Drug Administration, Center for Devices and Radiological Health] Styles 31-34 posterior IOLS: summary of safety and effectiveness. 1986 Jun 18. (PMA no. P830056-000).

McGhan/3M. [Food and Drug Administration, Center for Devices and Radiological Health] Styles 30 & 31 posterior chamber IOLS: summary of safety and effectiveness. 1985 Oct 17. (PMA no. P830040-000).

Surgidev Corp. [Food and Drug Administration, Center for Devices and Radiological Health] Style 17 & 17A posterior chamber IOLS: summary of safety and effectiveness. 1985 Oct 17. (PMA no. P830033-000).

Allergan Medical Optics. [Food and Drug Administration, Center for Devices and Radiological Health] Model AC10 & AC20 I0LS: summary of safety and effectiveness. 1983 Aug 16. (PMA no. P810056-000).

Allergan Medical Optics. [Food and Drug Administration, Center for Devices and Radiological Health] Models PC10 & PC21: summary of safety and effectiveness. 1983 Jun 17. (PMA no. P820049-000).

Cilco, Inc. [Food and Drug Administration, Center for Devices and Radiological Health] Models IS & IP: summary of safety and effectiveness. 1983 Apr 26. (PMA no. P800049-000).

Cilco, Inc. [Food and Drug Administration, Center for Devices and Radiological Health] Posterior chamber intraocular lenses: summary of safety and effectiveness. 1983 Apr 1. (PMA no. P810018-001).

Coopervision Cilco. [Food and Drug Administration, Center for Devices and Radiological Health] Model AC (ACI-AC5): summary of safety and effectiveness. 1983 Apr 12. (PMA no. P810001-000).

Intermedics Intraocular Inc. [Food and Drug Administration, Center for Devices and Radiological Health] Models 011 & 011B iridocapsular IOLS: summary of safety and effectiveness. 1983 Jan 25. (PMA no. P810042-000).

Intermedics Intraocular Inc. [Food and Drug Administration, Center for Devices and Radiological Health] Models 019B, 019C, 019E, 019F, 019J, 019K: summary of safety and effectiveness. 1983 Feb 25. (PMA no. P810055-000).

Precision-Cosmet Co., Inc. [Food and Drug Administration, Center for Devices and Radiological Health] Circular open loop posterior IOLS & Kratz elliptic: summary of safety and effectiveness. 1983 Aug 9 (PMA no. P820072-000).

Coburn Optical Industries, Inc. [Food and Drug Administration, Center for Devices and Radiological Health] Binkhorst & Fedorov I iris clip IOLS: summary of safety and effectiveness. 1982 Aug 31. (PMA no. P800027-000).

Coopervision Cilco. [Food and Drug Administration, Center for Devices and Radiological Health] Posterior chamber intraocular lenses: summary of safety and effectiveness. 1982 Aug 31. (PMA no. P810018-000).

Coopervision, Inc. [Food and Drug Administration, Center for Devices and Radiological Health] Models B-13F (P-10) & B-1H (P-11): summary of safety and effectiveness. 1982 May 25. (PMA no. P810032-000).

Pharmacia, Inc. [Food and Drug Administration, Center for Devices and Radiological Health] Medallion (R): summary of safety and effectiveness. 1982 Jan 1. (PMA no. P810060-000).

Precision-Cosmet. [Food and Drug Administration, Center for Devices and Radiological Health] Tennant (TM) & Kelman (TM) type II: summary of safety and effectiveness. 1982 Apr 20. (PMA no. PB00016-000).

Intraosseous pressure measurement

California Medical Association, Medical Practice Opinion Program. Intraosseous pressure measurement. 1985 Oct. (Medical Practice Opinion #334) [Group judgment]

Intravenous fat emulsions

Food and Drug Administration, Center for Drugs and Biologics. Intravenous fat emulsion. 1982. (NTIS order no. PB82-915901). [Information syntheses, Expert opinion, Epidemiological and other observational methods, Clinical trials, Bench testing]

Food and Drug Administration, Center for Drugs and Biologics. Intravenous fat emulsion. 1981. (NTIS order no. 81-915904). [Information syntheses, Expert opinion, Epidemiological and other observational methods, Clinical trials, Bench testing]

Iodide therapy

American Academy of Pediatrics, Committee on Drugs. Adverse reactions to iodide therapy of asthma and other pulmonary diseases. Pediatrics 1976 Feb.

Iodoxamate meglumine

Food and Drug Administration, Center for Drugs and Biologics. Iodoxamate meglumine. 1981. (NTIS order no. PB81-915911). [Information syntheses, Expert opinion, Epidemiological and other observational methods, Clinical trials, Bench testing.

Iontophoresis

Blue Cross and Blue Shield Association, Technology Evaluation and Coverage Program. Iontophoresis. 1986. [Information syntheses]

Iridology

American Medical Association, Council on Scientific Affairs. Evalution of iridology. 1981. [Group judgment]

Iron-dextran complex

Food and Drug Administration, Center for Drugs and Biologics. Iron dextran Inj. USP. 1981. (NTIS order no. PB81-915906). [Information syntheses, Expert opinion, Epidemiological and other observational methods, Clinical trials, Bench testing]

Isosulfan blue

Food and Drug Administration, Center for Drugs and Biologics. Isosulfan blue. 1981. (NTIS order no. PB81-915910). [Information syntheses, Expert opinion, Epidemiological and other observational methods, Clinical trials, Bench testing]

Isotretinoin

Food and Drug Administration, Center for Drugs and Biologics. Isotretinoin. 1982. (NTIS order no. PB82-915903). [Information syntheses, Expert opinion, Epidemiological and other observational methods, Clinical trials, Bench testing]

Joint prosthesis

Sauter WF, Galway RH, Gillespie R. [National Health Research and Development Program - Canada] Development of onionized (layered) upper extremity prosthetic sockets for juvenile amputees. 1985. (Grant No. 6606-2115-55).

Office of Technology Assessment, U.S. Congress. Cost-benefit/cost-effectiveness of medical technologies: a case study of orthopedic joint implants. Washington, D.C.: U.S. Government Printing Office, September 1981. (Health technology case study series #14)

Keratomileusis

American Academy of Ophthalmology. Keratophakia and keratomileusis: safety and effectiveness. San Francisco, CA: American Academy of Ophthalmology, 1986. [Information syntheses, Expert opinion]

Keratophakia

American Academy of Ophthalmology. Keratophakia and keratomileusis: safety and effectiveness. San Francisco, CA: American Academy of Ophthalmology, 1986. [Information syntheses, Expert opinion]

Ketoconazole

Food and Drug Administration, Center for Drugs and Biologics. Ketoconazole. 1981. (NTIS order no. PB81-915909). [Information syntheses, Expert opinion, Epidemiological and other observational methods, Clinical trials, Bench testing]

Keyes technique

Office of Technology Assessment, U.S. Congress. Periodontal disease: assessing the effectiveness and costs of the Keyes technique. Washington, D.C.: U.S. Government Printing Office, May 1981. (Health technology case study series #5).

Kinetic therapy

California Medical Association, Medical Practice Opinion Program. Kinetic therapy for lumbago. 1984 Nov. (Medical Practice Opinion #312) [Group judgment]

Knee prosthesis

Christian CL. [National Center for Health Services Research and Health Care Technology Assessment, Division of Extramural Research] Total knee replacement study. 1985 Apr. (NTIS order no. PB85-236909/AS)

Depuy, Inc. [Food and Drug Administration, Center for Devices and Radiological Health] New Jersey integrated knee replacement system: summary of safety and effectiveness. 1985 May 20. (PMA no. P830055-000).

Depuy, Inc. [Food and Drug Administration, Center for Devices and Radiological Health] New Jersey integrated knee replacement system: summary of safety and effectiveness. 1985 May 20. (PMA no. P830055-002).

Kunkel test

American College of Physicians, Clinical Efficacy Assessment Project. Kunkel test (total serum gammaglobulin). 1982. [Information syntheses]

National Center for Health Services Research and Health Care Technology Assessment, Office of Health Technology Assessment. The Kunkel test for estimating total serum gamma globulin levels in patients with rheumatoid arthritis. 1981.

Labetalol

Oster G, Huse DM, Delea TE, Savage DD, Colditz GA. [Policy Analysis, Inc.] Cost effectiveness of labetalol and propranolol in the treatment of hypertension among blacks. 1987 Mar.

Lactates

Blue Cross and Blue Shield Association, Technology Evaluation and Coverage Program. Lacate infusion for panic disorder. 1986. [Information syntheses]

Laparotomy

U.S. Administrators, Professional Policy Committee. Hodgkin's disease, routine staging laparotomy. [7/86] [Group judgment]

Laser angioplasty

ECRI Technology Assessment Program. Laser angioplasty for atherosclerosis. Issues Health Care Technol 1985;sec.5.L.3. [Information syntheses]

Laser iridotomy

California Medical Association, Medical Practice Opinion Program. Assistant surgeon for laser iridotomy. 1982 Jul. (Medical Practice Opinion #272) [Group judgment]

Laser photocoagulation

Overholt BF. Ulcer hemorrhage - laser treatment. In: American Society for Gastrointestinal Endoscopy, Committee on Technology Assessment. Therapeutic gastrointestinal endoscopy: an information resource manual. 1987. [Information syntheses, Expert opinion, Group judgment, Cost analyses]

Blue Cross and Blue Shield Association, Technology Evaluation and Coverage Program. Nd:YAG laser—gastrointestinal bleeding. 1986. [Information syntheses]

American Medical Association, Diagnostic and Therapeutic Technology Assessment. Endoscopic laser photocoagulation for gastrointestinal hemorrhage. JAMA 1985 May 11. [Expert opinion, Information syntheses]

National Center for Health Services Research and Health Care Technology Assessment, Office of Health Technology Assessment. Endoscopic photocoagulation for upper gastrointestinal hemorrhage. Ongoing.

Laser radiation therapy

California Medical Association, Medical Practice Opinion Program. Laser irradiation for pain of Charcot-Marie-Tooth disease. 1985 May. (Medical Practice Opinion #321) [Group judgment]

ECRI Technology Assessment Program. Photoradiation therapy (PRT) of tumors. Issues Health Care Technol 1984;sec.5.P.6. [Information syntheses]

California Medical Association, Medical Practice Opinion Program. Laser photoradiation therapy for carcinoma. 1983 Feb. (Medical Practice Opinion #279) [Group judgment]

Laser surgery

Fleischer DE. Esophageal cancer: laser treatment. In: American Society for Gastrointestinal Endoscopy, Committee on Technology Assessment. Therapeutic gastrointestinal endoscopy: an information resource manual. 1987. [Information syntheses, Expert opinion, Group judgment, Cost analyses]

Steering Committee on Future Health Care Scenarios, Commission on Future Health Care Technology (Netherlands). Prospective assessment of future health care technology: lasers in cardiovascular surgery. 1987.

California Medical Association, Medical Practice Opinion Program. Laser therapy for plantar warts. 1985 May. (Medical Practice Opinion #320) [Group judgment]

Laser surgery—Carbon dioxide

Committee on Ophthalmic Procedures Assessment. [American Academy of Ophthalmology] Carbon dioxide laser surgery in head and neck surgery. San Francisco, CA: American Academy of Ophthalmology, 1984. [Information syntheses, Expert opinion]

National Center for Health Services Research and Health Care Technology Assessment, Office of Health Technology Assessment. Carbon dioxide lasers in head and neck surgery. 1984.

American Medical Association, Diagnostic and Therapeutic Technology Assessment. CO2 laser for the treatment of gynecologic malignancies. JAMA 1983 Aug 5. [Expert opinion, Information syntheses]

National Center for Health Services Research and Health Care Technology Assessment, Office of Health Technology Assessment. Carbon dioxide laser surgery for selected conditions. 1982.

Laser surgery—Nd:YAG

Blue Cross and Blue Shield Association, Technology Evaluation and Coverage Program. Nd:YAG laser—posterior capsulotomy. 1986. [Information syntheses]

Blue Cross and Blue Shield Association, Technology Evaluation and Coverage Program. Nd:YAG laser—tracheo-bronchial obstruction. 1986. [Information syntheses]

California Medical Association, Medical Practice Opinion Program. YAG laser for posterior lens capsules. 1985 Apr. (Medical Practice Opinion #319) [Group judgment]

Coburn Optical Industries, Inc. [Food and Drug Administration, Center for Devices and Radiological Health] Neodymium-Yag op laser OPL-3: summary of safety and effectiveness. 1984Sep 7. (PMA no. P830064-000).

National Center for Health Services Research and Health Care Technology Assessment, Office of Health Technology Assessment. Nd:YAG laser for posterior capsulotomies. 1984.

Laser trabeculoplasty

National Center for Health Services Research and Health Care Technology Assessment, Office of Health Technology Assessment. Laser trabeculoplasty (LTP) for open angle glaucoma. 1984.

American Academy of Ophthalmology. Laser trabecular surgery for open-angle glaucoma. San Francisco, CA: American Academy of Ophthalmology, 1983. [Information syntheses, Expert opinion]

Lasers

American Hospital Association, Hospital Technology Series Program. Implementing laser technology in the community hospital. 1986. (Guideline report) [Information syntheses, Expert opinion, Cost analyses]

American Medical Association, Council on Scientific Affairs. Lasers in medicine and surgery. JAMA 1986 Aug 15;256(7):900-907. [Group judgment]

Sharplan Lasers Inc. [Food and Drug Administration, Center for Devices and Radiological Health] Model 702: summary of safety and effectiveness. 1986 May 8. (PMA no. P850060-000).

U.S. Administrators, Professional Policy Committee. Laser therapy. [7/86] [Group judgment]

Lasers for Medicine, Inc. [Food and Drug Administration, Center for Devices and Radiological Health] Phototome (TM) system 2700: summary of safety and effectiveness. 1985 Sep 18. (PMA no. P850019-000).

Health Council of the Netherlands. Lasers. Ongoing assessment.

Health Council of the Netherlands. Lasers. Planned.

Lasers—Carbon dioxide

American College of Obstetricians and Gynecologists, Committee Opinion. Carbon dioxide laser. Revised 1984 Apr. [Information syntheses]

Lasers—Nd:YAG

Carl Zeiss, Inc. [Food and Drug Administration, Center for Devices and Radiological Health] Visulas Nd:Yag laser: summary of safety and effectiveness. 1986 Aug 7.(PMA no. P850083-000).

Coherent Medical Division. [Food and Drug Administration, Center for Devices and Radiological Health] Neodymium:Yag ophthalmic laser system 9900: summary of safety and effectiveness. 1986 Dec 31. (PMA no. P830054-000).

Elscint, Inc. [Food and Drug Administration, Center for Devices and Radiological Health] Gyrex, models S3500 & S5000: summary of safety and effectiveness. 1986 Sep 9. (PMA no. P840007-000).

Gish Biomedical, Inc. [Food and Drug Administration, Center for Devices and Radiological Health] Micro Yag Nd:Yag laser system: summary of safety and effectiveness. 1986 May 30. (PMA no. P850063-000).

Iolab. [Food and Drug Administration, Center for Devices and Radiological Health] Microruptor MR-2 Nd:Yag laser system: summary of safety and effectiveness. 1986 Mar 28 (PMA no. P840012-000).

Cilco. [Food and Drug Administration, Center for Devices and Radiological Health] Cilco Nd:Yag laser: summary of safety and effectiveness. 1985 Sep 11. (PMA no. P840047-000).

Coopervision Inc. [Food and Drug Administration, Center for Devices and Radiological Health] Horizon (TM) Yag laser model 2000: summary of safety and effectiveness. 1985 Aug 15. (PMA no. P850001-000).

Medical Lasers, Inc. [Food and Drug Administration, Center for Devices and Radiological Health] Meditec OPL3 Nd:Yag laser: summary of safety and effectiveness. 1985 Feb 21. (PMA no. P830025-000).

Allergan Pharmaceuticals, Inc. [Food and Drug Administration, Center for Devices and Radiological Health] ND:Yag posterior capsulotomy model 100: summary of safety and effectiveness. 1984 Nov 26. (PMA no. P830062-000).

Coherent Medical Division. [Food and Drug Administration, Center for Devices and Radiological Health] Neodymium:Yag ophthalmic laser system 9900.: summary of safety and effectiveness. 1984 Jul 30. (PMA no. P830054-000).

Trokel S. [American Academy of Ophthalmology] Academy recommendation: ophthalmic neodymium YAG lasers: safety and effectiveness. Ophthalmology 1984;91:539-42. [Information syntheses, Expert opinion]

Lead screening

Berwick DM, Komaroff AL. [Harvard School of Public Health, Institute for Health Research] Cost effectiveness of lead screening. N Eng J Med 1982;306:1392-1398. [Information syntheses]

Leisure skills training

Jongbloed L. [National Health Research and Development Program - Canada] Leisure skills training program with stroke survivors: a double blind study. 1986. (Grant No. 6610-1455-45).

Leukocyte differential counters

ECRI Technology Assessment Program. Leukocyte differential counters, automated. J Health Care Technol 1985;2:51-72. [Information syntheses]

Levodopa

Barbeau A. [Clinical Research Institute of Montreal] [Medical Research Council - Canada] Etiology and treatment of Parkinson's disease (with a study of efficacy and side effects of levodopa therapy). (Grant period 1973-1985).

Chouinard G. [Department Psychiatry, McGill University] [Medical Research Council - Canada] A clinical trial of L-dopa in the prevention of tardive dyskinesia and in the long-term treatment of parkinsonian side effects induced by neuroleptics. (Grant period 1982-1985).

Lidocaine

Food and Drug Administration, Center for Drugs and Biologics. Lidocaine HCl in 5% dextrose in plastic container (PL-146). 1981. (NTIS order no. PB81-915907). [Information syntheses, Expert opinion, Epidemiological and other observational methods, Clinical trials, Bench testing]

Food and Drug Administration, Center for Drugs and Biologics. Lidocaine hydrochloride, USP sterile powder. 1981. (NTIS order no. PB81-915905. [Information syntheses, Expert opinion, Epidemiological and other observational methods, Clinical trials, Bench testing]

Ligament prosthesis

W.L. Gore & Associates, Inc. [Food and Drug Administration, Center for Devices and Radiological Health] Gore-tex expanded PTFE prosthetic ligament: summary of safety and effectiveness. 1986 Nov 18. (PMA no. P850074-000).

Limb perfusion

Blue Cross and Blue Shield Association, Technology Evaluation and Coverage Program. Isolated limb perfusion. 1986. [Information syntheses]

Linear pumps

U.S. Administrators, Professional Policy Committee. Linear Pump, Wright. [7/86] [Group judgment]

Lipoprotein evaluation

Blue Cross and Blue Shield Association, Medical Necessity Program. Serum lipoprotein evaluation. 1985. [Information syntheses]

Lithium

Aierre YN, Waters BGH. [National Health Research and Development Program - Canada] Erythrocyte membrane enzyme and lithium in manic-depressive disorder. 1986. (Grant No. 6606-2149-52).

Chouinard G. [Department Psychiatry, McGill University] [Medical Research Council - Canada] Controlled clinical trials of lithium and tryptophan in the treatment of patients with bipolar affective disorders. (Grant period 1982-1985).

Veterans Administration, Cooperative Studies Program. Lithium treatment in alcohol dependence. [Clinical trials]

Lithotripsy

Health Services Research and Development Service. [Veterans Administration] The cost-effectiveness of lithotripsy: an information synthesis. Perry Point, MD: Special Projects Office, Health Services Research and Development, Veterans Administration, 1986.

American College of Physicians, Clinical Efficacy Assessment Project. Lithotripsy. Ann Intern Med 1985;103:626-9. [Information syntheses]

U.S. Administrators, Professional Policy Committee. Lithotripsy - reconsideration re expanded indications. Ongoing. [Group judgment]

Lithotripsy—Extracorporeal shock wave

Medical Technology and Practice Patterns Institute. Extracorporeal shockwave lithotripsy (inpatient). 1987.

Medical Technology and Practice Patterns Institute. Extracorporeal shockwave lithotripsy (outpatient). 1987.

Carlsson P, Tiselius HG. [Linköping University, Center for Medical Technology Assessment] Evaluation of extracorporeal shock-wave lithotripsy treatment for upper urinary tract calculi—the first year experiences. 1986. (Discussion series paper #10) [Swedish language only] [Cost analyses, Clinical trials, Epidemiological methods]

Extracorporeal shockwave lithotripsy. In: Prospective Payment Assessment Commission. Technical appendixes to the report and recommendations to the Secretary, U.S. Department of Health and Human Services, April 1, 1986 Washington, DC: Government Printing Office, 1986:112-114. [Information syntheses, Cost analyses]

Health Services Research and Development Service. [Veterans Administration] Technology assessment of extracorporeal shock wave lithotripsy (ESWL). Perry Point, MD: Special Projects Office, Health Services Research and Development, Veterans Administration, 1986.

Office of Technology Assessment, U.S. Congress. Extracorporeal shock-wave lithotripsy. Washington, D.C.: U.S. Government Printing Office, May 1986. (Health technology case study series #36)

U.S. Administrators, Professional Policy Committee. E.S.W.L. [7/86] [Group judgment]

American Medical Association, Diagnostic and Therapeutic Technology Assessment. Non-invasive extracorporeal lithotripsy for disruption of kidney stones—Update. Feb 15, 1985. [Expert opinion, Information syntheses]

California Medical Association, Medical Practice Opinion Program. Extracorporeal shock-wave lithotripsy. 1985 Sep. (Medical Practice Opinion #32) [Group judgment]

National Center for Health Services Research and Health Care Technology Assessment, Office of Health Technology Assessment. Extracorporeal shock wave lithotripsy (ESWL) procedures for the treatment of kidney stones. 1985.

ECRI Technology Assessment Program. Extracorporeal shock-wave lithotripsy (ESWL). Issues Health Care Technol 1984;sec.5.L.2. [Information syntheses]

Lithotripsy—Percutaneous

Medical Technology and Practice Patterns Institute. Percutaneous lithotripsy. 1987.

National Center for Health Services Research and Health Care Technology Assessment, Office of Health Technology Assessment. Percutaneous ultrasound procedures for the treatment of kidney stones. 1985.

ECRI Technology Assessment Program. Percutaneous lithotripsy of kidney stones. Issues Health Care Technol 1983;sec.5.L.1. [Information syntheses]

Lithotripsy—Transurethral

National Center for Health Services Research and Health Care Technology Assessment, Office of Health Technology Assessment. Transurethral ureteroscopic lithotripsy procedures for the treatment of kidney stones. 1985.

National Center for Health Services Research and Health Care Technology Assessment, Office of Health Technology Assessment. Treatment of kidney stones—transurethral ureteroscopic lithotripsy. Ongoing.

Lithotripters, Extracorporeal shock wave

American Hospital Association, Hospital Technology Series Program. Lithotripters. 1985. (Guideline report) [Information syntheses, Expert opinion, Cost analyses]

Dornier System GMBH. [Food and Drug Administration, Center for Devices and Radiological Health] Dornier lithotripter, model HM3: summary of safety and effectiveness. 1985 Jan 16. (PMA no. P840008-000).

Health Council of the Netherlands. Lithotryptor. Ongoing assessment.

Lixiscope

National Center for Health Services Research and Health Care Technology Assessment, Office of Health Technology Assessment. Portable hand-held x-ray instrument (lixiscope). 1985.

United Kingdom Department of Health and Social Security, Medical Devices Evaluation Programme. Assessment of Lixiscop hand held imager with radioactive source. 1985 Sep. (Report no. STB6E/85/33) [Epidemiological and other observational methods, Bench testing]

Long term care

A longitudinal study of case-mix outcomes and resource use in nursing homes. In: Office of Research and Demonstrations, Health Care Financing Administration. Health care financing status report: research and demonstrations in health care financing. Jan 1986. (HCFA Pub. No. 03219).

An evaluation of "Life-Continuum of Care" residential centers in the United States. In: Office of Research and Demonstrations, Health Care Financing Administration. Health care financing status report: research and demonstrations in health care financing. Jan 1986. (HCFA Pub. No. 03219).

Can geriatric nurse practitioners improve nursing home care? In: Office of Research and Demonstrations, Health Care Financing Administration. Health care financing status report: research and demonstrations in health care financing. Jan 1986. (HCFA Pub No. 03219).

Chamberg LW, Mohide AE, Tugwell P, Bayne R, Pill ML, Nightingale H. [National Health Research and Development Program - Canada] Randomized trial of resident care quality assurance by criteria mapping in nursing homes. 1986. (Grant No. 6606-2450-44).

Comparison by state of SNF/ICF types: beds, staffing, utilization, and ownership. In: Office of Research and Demonstrations, Health Care Financing Administration. Health care financing status report: research and demonstrations in health care financing. Jan 1986. (HCFA Pub. No. 03219).

Comparison of the cost and quality of home health and nursing home care. In: Office of Research and Demonstrations, Health Care Financing Administration. Health care financing status report: research and demonstrations in health care financing. Jan 1986. (HCFA Pub. No. 03219).

Evaluation of coordinated community-oriented, long--term care demonstration. In: Office of Research and Demonstrations, Health Care Financing Administration. Health care financing status report: research and demonstrations in health care financing. Jan 1986. (HCFA Pub. No. 03219).

Long-term care of aged individuals with hip fractures: public versus private costs. In: Office of Research and Demonstrations, Health Care Financing Administration. Health care financing status report: research and demonstrations in health care financing. Jan 1986. (HCFA Pub. No. 03219).

Long-term care residential services for developmentally disabled people. In: Office of Research and Demonstrations, Health Care Financing Administration. Health care financing status report: research and demonstrations health care financing. Jan 1986. (HCFA Pub. No. 03219).

National and cross-national study of long-term care populations. In: Office of Research and Demonstrations, Health Care Financing Administration. Health care financing status report: research and demonstrations in health care financing. Jan 1986. (HCFA Pub. No. 03219).

Planning study: phase I of a major study of national long-term care policies. In: Office of Research and Demonstrations, Health Care Financing Administration. Health care financing status report: research and demonstrations in health care financing. Jan 1986. (HCFA Pub. No. 03219).

Quality of life among life-care facility and community residents: A comparison. In: Office of Research and Demonstrations, Health Care Financing Administration. Health care financing status report: research and demonstrations in health care financing. Jan 1986. (HCFA Pub. No. 03219).

State Medicaid nursing home policies, utilization, and expenditures. In: Office of Research and Demonstrations, Health Care Financing Administration. Health care financing status report: research and demonstrations in health care financing. Jan 1986. (HCFA Pub. No. 03219).

Study of long-term care quality and reimbursement in teaching and nonteaching nursing homes. In: Office of Research and Demonstrations, Health Care Financing Administration. Health care financing status report: research and demonstrations in health care financing. Jan 1986. (HCFA Pub. No. 03219).

Subcommittee on Special Services in Hospitals. [Health and Welfare Canada, Health Services and Promotion Branch, Institutional and Professional Services Division] Adult long-term institutional care. 1984. [Information syntheses, Expert opinion, Group judgment]

Veterans Administration, Cooperative Studies Program. Community vs. VA nursing home care vs. hospitalization in psychiatric patients. [1980] [Clinical trials]

Lymphangiography

U.S. Administrators, Professional Policy Committee. Hodgkin's disease, routine lymphangiography. [7/86] [Group judgment]

Magnesium chloride

Food and Drug Administration, Center for Drugs and Biologics. CaCl2, MgCl, Kcl, & NaCl. 1982. (NTIS order no. PB82-915902). [Information syntheses, Expert opinion, Epidemiological and other observational methods, Clinical trials, Bench testing]

Magnesium sulfate

Food and Drug Administration, Center for Drugs and Biologics. NaCl, KCl, MgSO4, NaPO4, & KPO4. 1982. (NTIS order no. PB82-915901). [Information syntheses, Expert opinion, Epidemiological and other observational methods, Clinical trials, Bench testing]

Magnetic resonance imaging

Medical Technology and Practice Patterns Institute. Magnetic resonance imaging (inpatient). 1987.

Medical Technology and Practice Patterns Institute. Magnetic resonance imaging (outpatient). 1987.

National Institutes of Health, Consensus Development Program. Magnetic resonance imaging. (Consensus Development Conference Statement, Oct 26-28, 1987). [Group judgment]

Health Services Research and Development Service. [Veterans Administration] Nuclear magnetic resonance imaging: information synthesis on clinical applications and cost considerations. Perry Point, MD: Special Projects Office, Health Services Research and Development, Veterans Administration, April 1986.

University of Pennsylvania, Leonard Davis Institute of Health Economics. Magnetic resonance imaging. 1986 Dec. (Pilot study for University of Pennsylvania)

Magnetic resonance imaging. In: Prospective Payment Assessment Commission. Technical appendixes to the report and recommendations to the Secretary, U.S. Department of Health and Human Services, April 1, 1986. Washington, DC: Government Printing Office, 1986:107-111.

Nicholson RL. [National Health Research and Development Program - Canada] Nuclear magnetic resonance imaging: clinical evaluation and future impact on health care. 1986. (Grant No. 6606-2240-03).

Prato FS. [National Health Research and Development Program - Canada] Effects on human and rat learning and behavior of radio frequency waves and magnetic fields associated with NMR imaging. 1986. (Grant No. 6606-2300-03).

Swedish Planning and Rationalization Institute of the Health Services. Spri technology report 7: MRT - magnetic resonance tomography: experience in Sweden. 1986. [Cost analyses, Epidemiological and other observational methods]

U.S. Administrators, Professional Policy Committee. Nuclear magnetic resonance imaging. [7/86] [Group judgment]

Allen PS. [Department Medicine, University Alberta] [Medical Research Council - Canada] In-vivo medical applications of nuclear magnetic resonance. (Grant period 1984-1985).

American Hospital Association, Hospital Technology Series Program. NMR - issues for 1985 and beyond. 1985. (Guideline report) [Information syntheses, Expert opinion, Cost analyses]

Bronskill MJ. [Princess Margaret Hospital, Toronto] [Medical Research Council - Canada] Physical studies of NMR imaging. (Grant period 1983-1985).

California Medical Association, Medical Practice Opinion Program. Magnetic resonance imaging. 1985 Sep. (Medical Practice Opinion #277) [Group judgment]

ECRI Technology Assessment Program. Magnetic resonance imaging (MRI). J Health Care Technol 1985;2:23-50. [Information syntheses]

National Center for Health Services Research and Health Care Technology Assessment, Office of Health Technology Assessment. Magnetic resonance imaging (MRI). 1985.

Stason WB, Localio AR. [Harvard School of Public Health, Institute for Health Research] Magnetic resonance imaging: clinical efficacy, costs and policy considerations. Blue Cross and Blue Shield Association, 1985. [Information syntheses]

American Academy of Neurology, Practice Committee. Nuclear magnetic resonance. 1984 Feb. [Expert opinion, Group judgment]

Office of Technology Assessment, U.S. Congress. Nuclear magnetic resonance imaging technology: a clinical, industrial, and policy analysis. Washington, D.C.: U.S. Government Printing Office, September 1984. (Health technology case study series #27)

American Hospital Association, Hospital Technology Series Program. Nuclear magnetic resonance (NMR). 1983. (Guideline report) [Information syntheses, Expert opinion, Cost analyses]

Health Council of the Netherlands. NMR/MRI. Ongoing.

National Center for Health Services Research and Health Care Technology Assessment, Office of Health Technology Assessment. Coverage of gating devices and the use of surface radio frequency coils in conjunction with magnetic resonance imaging (MRI) procedures. Ongoing.

University of Pennsylvania, Leonard Davis Institute of Health Economics. Adoption and diffusion of magnetic resonance imaging under DRGs. Ongoing. (Study for the National Center for Health Services Research, DHHS)

University of Pennsylvania, Leonard Davis Institute of Health Economics. Evaluation of magnetic resonance imaging. Planned. (Submitted to Riverside Methodist Hospital, Columbus, OH).

Magnetic resonance imaging—Brain and spine

American College of Physicians, Clinical Efficacy Assessment Project. Magnetic resonance imaging of the brain and spine, 1987. [Information syntheses]

Magnetic resonance imaging—Lung injury

Inch WR. [Department Radiation Oncology, University Western Ontario] [Medical Research Council - Canada] Nuclear magnetic resonance to monitor lung injury. (Grant period 1983-1985).

Magnetic resonance imaging—Multiple sclerosis

Paty DW. [Department Medicine, University British Columbia] [Medical Research Council - Canada] NMR imaging in MS, I: The nature of the lesion. (Grant period 1984-1985).

Paty DW. [Department Medicine, University British Columbia] [Medical Research Council - Canada] NMR imaging in MS, II, diagnosis of the disease and quantitation. (Grant period 1984-1985).

Magnetic resonance imaging—Neoplasms

Sharp AR. [National Health Research and Development Program - Canada] Resolution enhanced pulsed NMR investigation of normal, preneoplastic and neoplastic systems. 1986. (Grant No. 6604-1042-03).

Magnetic resonance imaging systems

Phillips Medical Systems, Inc. [Food and Drug Administration, Center for Devices and Radiological Health] Gyroscan (TM): summary of safety and effectiveness. 1986 Sep 16. (PMA no. P840063-000).

Thompson CGR Medical Corp. [Food and Drug Administration, Center for Devices and Radiological Health] Magniscan 5000 MRI System: summary of safety and effectiveness. 1986 Oct 6. (PMA no. 850043-000).

General Electric, Co. [Food and Drug Administration, Center for Devices and Radiological Health] GE signa magnetic resonance diagnostic imaging system: summary of safety and effectiveness. 1985 Jun 5. (PMA no. P830074-000)

Siemans Medical Systems, Inc. [Food and Drug Administration, Center for Devices and Radiological Health] Magnetom: summary of safety and effectiveness. 1985 Jan 2. (PMA no. P830081-000).

Diasonics, Inc. [Food and Drug Administration, Center for Devices and Radiological Health] Diasonics NMR imaging system: summary of safety and effectiveness. 1984 Apr 25. (PMA no. P830053-000).

Fonar Corp. [Food and Drug Administration, Center for Devices and Radiological Health] Fonar NMR whole body scanner beta 3000: summary of safety and effectiveness. 1984 Nov 13. (PMA no. P830076).

Picker International. [Food and Drug Administration, Center for Devices and Radiological Health] Nuclear magnetic resonance scanner models NMR 1000: summary of safety and effectiveness. 1984 Jun 8. (PMA no. P830052-000).

Technicare Corporation. [Food and Drug Administration, Center for Devices and Radiological Health] Teslacon (TM) NMR imaging system: summary of safety and effectiveness. 1984 Apr 25. (PMA no. P830051-000).

Magnetic resonance spectroscopy

Health Council of the Netherlands. Magnetic resonance spectroscopy. 1986. [English summary only].

Magnetoencephalography

Health Systems Research and Development Division. [Veterans Administration] Technology assessment of magnetoencephalography (MEG). Perry Point, MD: Special Projects Office, Health Systems Research and Development Division, Veterans Administration, in preparation, expected August 1987.

Malathion

Food and Drug Administration, Center for Drugs and Biologics. Malathion. 1982. (NTIS order no. PB82-915904). [Information syntheses, Expert opinion, Epidemiological and other observational methods, Clinical trials, Bench testing]

Mammographic devices

American College of Radiology, Task Force on Breast Cancer. Policy statement on oscillating grids for mammography equipment. Expected 1987. [Group judgment]

United Kingdom Department of Health and Social Security, Medical Devices Evaluation Programme. Assessment of Elscint Mam LS3 mammographic unit. 1986 Jan. (Report no. STB6E/86/3) [Epidemiological and other observational methods, Bench testing]

United Kingdom Department of Health and Social Security, Medical Devices Evaluation Programme. Assessment of Wolverson X-ray (Acoma) MXR 102 mammography unit. 1986 Jan. (Report no. STB6E/86/1) [Epidemiological and other observational methods, Bench testing]

United Kingdom Department of Health and Social Security, Medical Devices Evaluation Programme. Assessment of medical X-ray supplies (Soredex) Mammex DC mammographic unit. 1986 Jan. (Report no. STB6E/86/2) [Epidemiological and other observational methods, Bench testing]

Mammography

Eddy DM, Hasselblad V, McGivney W, Hendee W. [Duke University, Center for Health Policy Research and Education] The value of mammography screening for women age 40-49. (Submitted for publication) [Information syntheses]

Eddy DM. [Duke University, Center for Health Policy Research and Education] Screening by mammography for women over age 65, reassessment. (Expected publication 1988) [Information syntheses]

Office of Technology Assessment, U.S. Congress. Mammography screening for the Medicare population. Washington, D.C.: Office of Technology Assessment (to be completed in Summer 1987).

American College of Radiology, Task Force on Breast Cancer. Resolution no. 1: supplementary mammography statement. 1986 Sep. [Group judgment]

American College of Radiology, Task Force on Breast Cancer. Resolution no. 2: mammography performance guidelines. 1986 Sep. [Group judgment]

American Medical Association, Diagnostic and Therapeutic Technology Assessment. Mammographic screening for breast cancer. Oct 19, 1986. [Expert opinion, Information syntheses]

Eddy DM. [Duke University, Center for Health Policy Research and Education] The effectiveness, cost, & cost-effectiveness of breast cancer screening with annual mammography & breast physical exam. for women over 65. Report prepared for Committee on Ways & Means, Subcommittee on Health, U.S. House of Representatives. 1986 Jan 7. [Information syntheses]

CBO (Centraal Begeleidingsorgaan voor de Intercollegiale Toetsing) Consensus Development Program. Mammography policy. 1983. [Dutch language only] [Group judgment, Expert opinion]

American College of Radiology, Task Force on Breast Cancer. Policy statement: guidelines for mammography. 1982 Sep 22. [Group judgment]

American College of Obstetricians and Gynecologists, Committee Opinion. ACOG statement on mammography. 1979 Sep. [Information syntheses]

Swedish Planning and Rationalization Institute of the Health Services. Mammography screening for breast cancer: a randomized controlled cost-effectiveness analysis. Ongoing. [Cost analyses, Epidemiological and other observational methods]

Maple syrup urine disease screening

Hasselblad V. [Duke University, Center for Health Policy Research and Education] Analysis of the prevention of mental retardation by screening for maple syrup urine disease. (Expected publication 1988) [Information syntheses]

Mass spectroscopy

ECRI Technology Assessment Program. Clinical use of mass spectrometers. Issues Health Care Technol 1986;sec.5.M.2. [Information syntheses]

Mastectomy

U.S. Administrators, Professional Policy Committee. Subcutaneous (subareolar) mastectomy (bilateral). [7/86] [Group judgment]

Zemore R, Shepel LF. [National Health Research and Development Program - Canada] Coping with breast cancer and mastectomy. 1986. (Grant No. 6608-1170-42).

Maternal serum alpha fetoprotein monitoring

Burton BK, Dillard RG, Clark EN. [National Center for Health Services Research and Health Care Technology Assessment, Division of Extramural Research] MSAFP screening: the effect of participation on anxiety and attitudes toward pregnancy in women with normal results. Am J Obset Gynecol 1985;152:540-543.

Gutzwiller F, Grob PJ, Boppart I, Marguerat PH, eds. [University of Lausanne, Institute of Social and Preventive Medicine] Swiss alpha-foetoprotein screening working group: results of the collaborative study of early detection of neural tube defects. 1985. [Epidemiological and other observational methods]

ECRI Technology Assessment Program. Prenatal alpha-fetoprotein (AFP) testing. Issues Health Care Technol 1984;sec.5.A.2. [Information syntheses]

American Medical Association, Council on Scientific Affairs. Maternal serum a-fetoprotein monitoring. JAMA 1982 Mar 12;247:1478. [Group judgment]

Measles-mumps-rubella vaccine

Stewart M. [National Health Research and Development Program - Canada] Illness after measles-mumps-rubella (MMR) vaccination - a study using the health diary method. 1986. (Grant No. 6606-3028-43).

Medical record systems

Woogh CM. [National Health Research and Development Program - Canada] Kingston psychiatric record linkage system. 1986. (Grant No. 6606-2880-43).

Long JM. [National Heart, Lung, and Blood Institute] Discovery and confirmation of causal relationships in a large medical record database: a POSCH experiment. Society for Clinical Trials, Annual Conference, 1985.

Whiting-O'Keefe QE, et al. [National Center for Health Services Research and Health Care Technology Assessment, Division of Extramural Research] A computerized summary medical record system can provide more information than the standard medical record. JAMA 1985 Sep 6;254(9):1185-1192.

Barnett GO. [National Center for Health Services Research and Health Care Technology Assessment, Division of Extramural Research] The application of computer-based medical record systems in ambulatory practice. N Engl J Med 1984 Jun;310(25):1643-1650.

Simborg DW. [National Center for Health Services Research and Health Care Technology Assessment, Division of Extramural Research] Evaluation of a summary medical record system. 1984 (NTIS order no. PB84-100247)

Widerhold G. [National Center for Health Services Research and Health Care Technology Assessment, Division of Extramural Research] Automated ambulatory medical records systems in the U.S. 1984. (NTIS order no. PB84-118884)

[National Center for Health Services Research and Health Care Technology Assessment, Division of Extramural Research] The effect of immediate access to a computerized medical record on physician test ordering: a controlled clinical trial in the emergency room. Am J Public Health 1982 Jul;72(7):698-702.

MEDLARS

Office of Technology Assessment, U.S. Congress. MEDLARS and health information policy. Washington, D.C.: U.S. Government Printing Office, September 1982.

MEDLINE

[National Library of Medicine] Health professionals use of MEDLINE. Bethesda, MD: National Library of Medicine, 1987. [Epidemiological and other observational methods]

MEDLINE—Optical disk

[National Library of Medicine] Field test and evaluation of MEDLINE on optical disk. Bethesda, MD: National Library of Medicine. Ongoing. [Epidemiological and other observational methods]

Medroxyprogesterone

American Academy of Pediatrics, Committee on Drugs. Medroxyprogesterone acetate (Depo-Provera). Pediatrics 1980 Mar.

Melodic intonation therapy

American Academy of Neurology, Practice Committee. Melodic intonation therapy for aphasia. [Expert opinion, Group judgment]

National Center for Health Services Research and Health Care Technology Assessment, Office of Health Technology Assessment. Melodic intonation therapy. 1982.

Methaqualone

American Medical Association, Council on Scientific Affairs. Methaqualone, abuse limits its usefulness. JAMA 1983 Dec 9;250:3052. [Group judgment]

Methotrexate

American College of Physicians, Clinical Efficacy Assessment Project. Methotrexate for rheumatoid arthritis, 1987. [Information syntheses]

U.S. Administrators, Professional Policy Committee. Arthritis, low-dose methotrexate therapy. [7/86] [Group judgment]

Methoxsalen

Food and Drug Administration, Center for Drugs and Biologics. Methoxsalen. 1982. (NTIS order no. PB82-915903). [Information syntheses, Expert opinion, Epidemiological and other observational methods, Clinical trials, Bench testing]

Methyldopa

Food and Drug Administration, Center for Drugs and Biologics. Methyldopa. 1981. (NTIS order no. PB81-91591). [Information syntheses, Expert opinion, Epidemiological and other observational methods, Clinical trials, Bench testing]

Methylethylketone

California Medical Association, Medical Practice Opinion Program. Methylethylketone damage of the immune system. 1982 Nov. (Medical Practice Opinion #261) [Group judgment]

Methylphenidate

Simeon JG. [National Health Research and Development Program - Canada] Biological and behavioural factors associated with methylphenidate therapy of attention deficit and conduct disorders in children. 1986. (Grant No. 6606-2407-52).

Metoclopramide

Food and Drug Administration, Center for Drugs and Biologics. Metoclopramide HC1. 1982. (NTIS order no. PB82-915903). [Information syntheses, Expert opinion, Epidemiological and other observational methods, Clinical trials, Bench testing]

Metolazone

Food and Drug Administration, Center for Drugs and Biologics. Metolazone. 1981. (NTIS order no. PB81-915905). [Information syntheses, Expert opinion, Epidemiological and other observational methods, Clinical trials, Bench testing]

Metoprolol

Levin, LA. [Linköping University, Center for Medical Technology Assessment] Economic consequences of postinfarction prophylaxis with beta-blockers: a cost effect study of metoprolol treatment. 1982. (Discussion series paper #2) [Swedish language only] [Cost analyses, Epidemiological methods]

Metronidazole

California Medical Association, Medical Practice Opinion Program. Treatment of rheumatoid arthritis with flagyl. 1985 Oct. (Medical Practice Opinion #330) [Group judgment]

Food and Drug Administration, Center for Drugs and Biologics. Metronidazole injection, 0.5%. 1982. (NTIS order no. PB82-915904). [Information syntheses, Expert opinion, Epidemiological and other observational methods, Clinical trials, Bench testing]

Mezlocillin

Food and Drug Administration, Center for Drugs and Biologics. Mezlocillin sodium. 1981. (NTIS order no. PB81-915912). [Information syntheses, Expert opinion, Epidemiological and other observational methods, Clinical trials, Bench testing]

Miconazole

Food and Drug Administration, Center for Drugs and Biologics. Miconazole nitrate. 1982. (NTIS order no. PB82-915902). [Information syntheses, Expert opinion, Epidemiological and other observational methods, Clinical trials, Bench testing]

Food and Drug Administration, Center for Drugs and Biologics. Miconazole nitrate. 1982. (NTIS order no. PB82-915904). [Information syntheses, Expert opinion, Epidemiological and other observational methods, Clinical trials, Bench testing]

Microbiological testing systems

Analytab Products, Inc. [Food and Drug Administration, Center for Devices and Radiological Health] Uniscept (TM): summary of safety and effectiveness. 1984 Apr 25. (PMA no. P830028-000).

Boehringer Mannheim Diagnostics Inc. [Food and Drug Administration, Center for Devices and Radiological Health] Micur-mic systems: summary of safety and effectiveness. 1983 Jul 19. (PMA no. P820073-000).

Warner Lambert. [Food and Drug Administration, Center for Devices and Radiological Health] Autobac MTS plus test system: summary of safety and effectiveness. 1982 Mar 26. (PMA no. P810024-0000).

Microbiology equipment

United Kingdom Department of Health and Social Security, Medical Devices Evaluation Programme. Evaluation of Don Whitley Mark II anaerobic cabinet-/work station. 1986 Mar. (Report no. STB/86/11) [Epidemiological and other observational methods, Bench testing]

United Kingdom Department of Health and Social Security, Medical Devices Evaluation Programme. An evaluation of the Hamilton Microlab 2100. 1985 Apr. (Report no. STB3A/85/18) [Epidemiological and other observational methods, Bench testing]

United Kingdom Department of Health and Social Security, Medical Devices Evaluation Programme. Evaluation of the Autobac IDX. 1985 Dec. (Report no. STB3A/85/46) [Epidemiological and other observational methods, Bench testing]

United Kingdom Department of Health and Social Security, Medical Devices Evaluation Programme. Evaluation of the Matascan. 1985 May. (Report no. STB3A/85/23) [Epidemiological and other observational methods, Bench testing]

Micronucleus test

Stich HF. [National Health Research and Development Program - Canada] Application of the micronucleus test to exfoliated human urinary cells for quantitating exposures to lifestyle factors and industrial carcinogens. 1986. (Grant No. 6610-1329-52).

Microsurgery

American Medical Association, Diagnostic and Therapeutic Technology Assessment. Microsurgical reconstruction for brachial plexus injury. Jul 16, 1986. [Expert opinion, Information syntheses]

California Medical Association, Medical Practice Opinion Program. Microsurgery in the treatment of infertility. 1985 Aug. (Medical Practice Opinion #308) [Group judgment]

Daniel RK. [Department Plastic Surgery, McGill University] [Medical Research Council - Canada] Surgical reconstruction utilizing microsurgical tissue transplants. (Grant period 1984-1985).

American College of Obstetricians and Gynecologists, Committee Opinion. Microsurgery. 1984 Apr. [Information syntheses]

California Medical Association, Medical Practice Opinion Program. Microsurgical lumbar discectomy. 1980 Feb. (Medical Practice Opinion #238) [Group judgment]

Migration inhibition test

Warrington RJ. [National Health Research and Development Program - Canada] Assessment of the migration inhibition test in the diagnosis of hypersensitivity to food additives and salicylates in chronic urticaria. 1986. (Grant No. 6607-12878-08).

Minerals

American Academy of Pediatrics, Committee on Nutrition. Vitamins and mineral supplement needs. 1980.

Minnesota Q-Qs codes

Karnegis JN, Matts JP, Tuna N, et al and the POSCH Group. [National Heart, Lung, and Blood Institute] Quantitative assessment of left ventricular function after myocardial infarction using the Minnesota Q-Qs codes for resting electrocardiograms. Cathet Cardiovasc Diagn 1985;11:393-400.

Karnegis JN, Matts JP, Tuna N and the POSCH Group. [National Heart, Lung, and Blood Institute] Development and evolution of electrocardiographic Minnesota Q-Qs codes in patients with acute myocardial infarction. Am Heart J 1985;110:452-459.

Mobility aids

Lotto WN, Milner M. [National Health Research and Development Program - Canada] Evaluations and development of powered mobility aids for two-to-five year olds with neuromusculoskeletaal disorders. 1985. (Grant No. 6606-2114-51).

Moire topography

Tredwell SJ, Saunders CG. [National Health Research and Development Program - Canada] A clinical study of shadow moire contourography as a useful assessment of the effects of orthotic treatment of curvature of the spine. 1986. (Grant No. 6610-1366-51).

Scott RN. [National Health Research and Development Program - Canada] Evaluation of moire topography in sclerosis monitoring. 1985. (Grant No. 6604-1055-51).

Scott RN. [National Health Research and Development Program - Canada] Moire topography in scoliosis monitoring. 1985. (Contract No. 6604-1049-51).

Monoclonal antibodies

Steering Committee on Future Health Scenarios, Commission on Future Health Care Technology (Netherlands). Prospective assessment of future health care technology: monoclonal antibodies and diagnostic kits. 1987.

Health Council of the Netherlands. Monoclonal antibodies. 1986.

Health Council of the Netherlands. Monoclonal antibodies. 1986. [English summary only].

Walker MC. [National Health Research and Development Program - Canada] The development of human monoclonal antibodies against HLA antigens. 1986. (Grant No. 6605-2035-52).

Health Council of the Netherlands. Monoclonal antibodies, advice on regulatory issues. Ongoing.

Mouth protectors

American Dental Association, Council on Dental Materials, Instruments and Equipment. Mouth protectors and sports team dentists. J Am Dent Assoc 1984;109:84-87.

Moxalactam

Food and Drug Administration, Center for Drugs and Biologics. Moxalactam disodium. 1982. (NTIS order no. PB82-915901). [Information syntheses, Expert opinion, Epidemiological and other observational methods, clinical trials, Bench testing]

Mycoplasma complement fixation test

National Center for Health Services Research and Health Care Technology Assessment, Office of Health Technology Assessment. The use of the mycoplasma complement fixation test in the diagnosis of rheumatoid arthritis. 1981.

Myoelectric prostheses

Scott RN, Dunfield VA. [National Health Research and Development Program - Canada] Design and evaluation of myoelectric controls. 1986. (Grant No. 6604-1029-51).

Scott RN. [National Health Research and Development Program - Canada] Infants and myoelectric prostheses. 1986. (Grant No. 6604-1056-51).

Shwedyk E, Quanbury AO, Marinic J. [National Health Research and Development Program - Canada] Sequential myoelectric processor evaluation. 1986. (Grant No. 6607-1332-51).

Nadolol

Food and Drug Administration, Center for Drugs and Biologics. Nadolol-bendroflumethiazide. 1983. (NTIS order no. PB 83-915903). [Information syntheses, Expert opinion, Epidemiological and other observational methods, Clinical trials, Bench testing]

Veterans Administration, Cooperative Studies Program. Evaluation of nadolol in treatment of hypertension. [1980]. [Clinical trials]

Nafcillin

Veterans Administration, Cooperative Studies Program. Nafcillin therapy of staphylococcal bacteremia. [1980]. [Clinical trials]

Naloxone

Chernick V. [Department Pediatrics, University Manitoba] [Medical Research Council - Canada] Clinical trial of naloxone in birth asphyxia. (Grant period 1983-1985).

Food and Drug Administration, Center for Drugs and Biologics. Pentazocine HCl and naloxone HCl. 1983. (NTIS order no. PB83-915901). [Information syntheses, Expert opinion, Epidemiological and other observational methods, Clinical trials, Bench testing]

American Academy of Pediatrics, Committee on Drugs. Naloxone use in newborns. Pediatrics 1980 Mar.

Nebulizers

Food and Drug Administration, Center for Drugs and Biologics. Bronalide inhaler system. 1987. (Summary basis of approval, NDA #18-340). [Information syntheses, Expert opinion, Epidemiological and other observational methods, Clinical trials, Bench testing]

Needle aspiration cytology

American College of Obstetricians and Gynecologists, Committee Opinion. Needle aspiration cytology in the evaluation of breast lesions. 1984 Jun. [Information syntheses]

Negative pressure respirators

National Center for Health Services Research and Health Care Technology Assessment, Office of Health Technology Assessment. Negative pressure respirators. 1983.

American Academy of Neurology, Practice Committee. Negative pressure respirators for home use in chronic neuromuscular disease. 1982 Oct. [Expert opinion, Group judgment]

Neonatal intensive care

Budetti P, McManus P. [University of California, San Francisco, Institute for Health Policy Studies] Assessing the effectiveness of neonatal intensive care. Med Care 1982;20:1027-1039.

Health Council of the Netherlands. Neonatal intensive care. 1982.

Kaufman SL, Shepard DS. [Harvard School of Public Health, Institute for Health Research] Costs of neonatal intensive care by day of stay. Inquiry 1982;19:167-178.

Office of Technology Assessment, U.S. Congress. The costs and effectiveness of neonatal intensive care. Washington, D.C.: U.S. Government Printing Office, August 1981. (Health technology case study series #10)

Subcommittee on Special Services in Hospitals. [Health and Welfare Canada, Health Services and Promotion Branch, Institutional and Professional Services Division] Perinatal intensive care unit guidelines. 1979. [Information syntheses, Expert opinion, Group judgment]

Neonatal monitors

Corometrics Medical Systems, Inc. [Food and Drug Administration, Center for Devices and Radiological Health] Model 515 neonatal monitor: summary of safety and effectiveness. 1986 Jan 31. (PMA no. P840037-000).

Nephrolithotomy

American Medical Association, Diagnostic and Therapeutic Technology Assessment. Endoscopic transurethral nephrolithotomy for disruption of kidney stones. JAMA 1984 Dec 21. [Expert opinion, Information syntheses]

American Medical Association, Diagnostic and Therapeutic Technology Assessment. Percutaneous nephrolithotomy for kidney stone removal. JAMA 1984 Dec 2. [Expert opinion, Information syntheses]

Nephrostomy

ECRI Technology Assessment Program. Percutaneous nephrostomy. Issues Health Care Technol 1984;sec.5.N.1. [Information syntheses]

Neurotoxins

American Academy of Neurology, Practice Committee. Amyotrophic lateral sclerosis - injected modified neurotoxin for treatment. 1983 Feb. [Expert opinion, Group judgment]

American Academy of Neurology, Practice Committee. Modified neurotoxin in the treatment of ALS. 1983 Jun. [Expert opinion, Group judgment]

Neutralization therapy—Food allergies

National Center for Health Services Research and Health Care Technology Assessment, Office of Health Technology Assessment. Intracutaneous (intradermal) and subcutaneous provocative and neutralization testing and neutralization therapy for food allergies. 1981.

National Center for Health Services Research and Health Care Technology Assessment, Office of Health Technology Assessment. Sublingual provocative testing and neutralization therapy for food allergies. 1981

Niclosamide

Food and Drug Administration, Center for Drugs and Biologics. Niclosamide. 1982. (NTIS order no. PB82-915903). [Information syntheses, Expert opinion, Epidemiological and other observational methods, Clinical trials, Bench testing]

Nicotine gum

Oster G, Huse DM, Delea TE, Colditz GA. [Policy Analysis, Inc.] Cost-effectiveness of nicotine gum as an adjunct to physician's advice against cigarette smoking. JAMA 1986;256:1315-1318.

American Medical Association, Council on Scientific Affairs. Nicotine chewing gum for cessation of smoking. 1984. [Group judgment]

Nifedipine

Food and Drug Administration, Center for Drugs and Biologics. Nifedipine. 1982. (NTIS order no. PB82-915901). [Information syntheses, Expert opinion, Epidemiological and other observational methods, Clinical trials, Bench testing]

Nissen fundoplication

California Medical Association, Medical Practice Opinion Program. Nissen's fundoplication - gastric reservoir reduction for morbid obesity. 1983 May. (Medical Practice Opinion #290) [Group judgment]

Nitroprusside

Food and Drug Administration, Center for Drugs and Biologics. Sodium nitroprusside. 1981. (NTIS order no. PB81-915912) [Information syntheses, Expert opinion, Epidemiological and other observational methods, Clinical trials, Bench testing]

Noncardiac pain diagnosis

American Gastroenterological Association, Patient Care Committee. Diagnostic procedures in noncardiac chest pain. Ongoing.

Nonionizing radiation measurement devices

Food and Drug Administration, Center for Devices and Radiological Health. Instrumentation for nonionizing radiation measurement. 1984. (NTIS Order No. 84-180603).

Norethindrone with ethinyl estradiol

Food and Drug Administration, Center for Drugs and Biologics. Norethindrone & ethinyl estradiol. 1982. (NTIS order no. PB82-915902). [Information syntheses, Expert opinion, Epidemiological and other observational methods, Clinical trials, Bench testing]

Normaline kit

Apothecary Products, Inc. [Food and Drug Administration, Center for Devices and Radiological Health] The normaline kit: summary of safety and effectiveness. 1983 Jun 17. (PMA no. P800055-002).

Apothecary Products, Inc. [Food and Drug Administration, Center for Devices and Radiological Health] The normaline kit: summary of safety and effectiveness. 1982 Jan 12. (PMA no. P800055-000).

Nutritional counseling

Chandra RK. [National Health Research and Development Program - Canada] Influence of nutritional counselling and support on immunocompetence, nutritional status and illness in the elderly. 1986. (Grant No. 6601-1063-56).

Apothecary Products, Inc. [Food and Drug Administration, Center for Devices and Radiological Health] The normaline kit: summary of safety and effectiveness. 1983 Jun 17. (PMA no. P800055-002).

Apothecary Products, Inc. [Food and Drug Administration, Center for Devices and Radiological Health] The normaline kit: summary of safety and effectiveness. 1982 Jan 12. (PMA no. P800055-000).

Oral contraceptives

American College of Obstetricians and Gynecologists, Committee on Technical Bulletins. Oral contraception 1976 Jul. (Technical bulletin no. 41). [Expert opinion]

National Institute of Child Health and Human Development. Safety and efficacy of oral contraceptives. Planned. [Group judgment, Expert opinion]

Oral rehydration therapy

American Academy of Pediatrics, Committee on Nutrition. Use of oral fluid therapy and posttreatment feeding following enteritis in children in a developed country. Pediatrics 1985 Feb.

Organ preservation

Bitter-Suermann H. [Department Surgery, Dalhousie University] [Medical Research Council - Canada] Liver preservation. (Grant Period 1984-1985).

Guttman FM. [Montreal Children's Hospital] [Medical Research Council - Canada] Long term organ preservation. (Grant period 1979-1985).

Organ procurement

Caplan A. [The Hastings Center] Should fetuses or infants be used as organ donors? Bioethics (forthcoming)

Developing incentive systems to increase the supply of cadaveric kidneys for transplants. In: Office of Research and Demonstrations, Health Care Financing Administration. Health care financing status report: research and demonstrations in health care financing. Jan 1986. (HCFA Pub. No. 03219).

Organ Donor Education Project. In: Office of Research and Demonstrations, Health Care Financing Administration. Health care financing status report: research and demonstrations in health care financing. Jan 1986. (HCFA Pub. No. 03219).

Prottas JM, Batten HL. [Brandeis University, Health Policy Center, Organ Procurement Project] Attitudes and incentives in organ procurement: report to the Health Care Financing Administration. 1986 Apr. [Epidemiological and other observational methods]

Prottas JM. [Brandeis University, Health Policy Center, Organ Procurement Project] Organ procurement in Europe and the United States. Millbank Mem Fund Q 1985;63(1):94-126. [Epidemiological and other observational methods]

Prottas JM. [Brandeis University, Health Policy Center, Organ Procurement Project] The structure and effectiveness of the U.S. procurement system. Inquiry 1985;22(4)365-376. [Epidemiological and other observational methods]

The Hastings Center. Ethical, legal and policy issues pertaining to solid organ procurement: a report of the Project on Organ Transplantation. 1985 Oct.

Prottas JM. [Brandeis University, Health Policy Center, Organ Procurement Project] Encouraging altruisms: public attitudes and the marketing of organ donation. Milbank Mem Fund Q 1983;61:278-306. [Epidemiological and other observational methods]

Prottas JM. [Brandeis University, Health Policy Center, Organ Procurment Project] Obtaining replacements: the organizational framework of organ procurement. J Health Polit Policy Law 1983;8(2):235-250. [Epidemiological and other observational methods]

American Medical Association, Council on Scientific Affairs. Organ donor recruitment. JAMA 1981 Nov 13;246:2157. [Group judgment]

Orphan devices

Georgetown University Medical Center, Institute for Health Policy Analysis. Orphan devices in health care. (Planned).

Orthodontic appliances

Mclachlan KR. [Department Dentistry, University Manitoba] [Medical Research Council - Canada] The effectiveness of loops and auxiliary appliances in continuous arch orthodontic therapy.

American Dental Association, Council on Dental Materials, Instruments and Equipment. Status report on beta titanium orthodontic wire. J Am Dent Assoc 1982;105:684-685.

Orthotic devices

Foort J. [National Health Research and Development Program - Canada] Tabular orthoses for stabilizing body joints. 1986. (Grant No. 6610-1290-51).

Osteoporosis screening

Critchfield GC, Eddy DM. [Duke University, Center for Health Policy Research and Education] Screening for osteoporosis. (Expected publication 1988) [Information syntheses]

U.S. Administrators, Professional Policy Committee. Screening tests for osteoporosis. Ongoing. [Group judgment]

Oximeters

ECRI Technology Assessment Program. Pulse oximeters. Issues Health Care Technol 1986;sec.5.O.1. [Information syntheses]

Oximetry

Medical Technology and Practice Patterns Institute. Pulse oximetry. 1987.

Oxprenolol

Veterans Administration, Cooperative Studies Program. Oxprenolol vs. propranolol in hypertension. [1980]. [Clinical trials]

Oxybutynin chloride with metoclopramide

Jewett M. [National Health Research and Development Program - Canada] Evaluation of oxybutynin chloride and metoclopramide in the treatment of detrusor instability in the elderly. 1986. (Grant No. 6606-2677-53).

Oxygen-air proportioners

ECRI Health Devices Program. Oxygen-air proportioners. Health Devices 1985;14:263-76.

Oxygen analyzers

ECRI Health Devices Program. Oxygen analyzers. Health Devices 1983;12:183-97.

Oxygen therapy

Blue Cross and Blue Shield Association, Medical Necessity Program. Oxygen therapy. 1982. [Information syntheses]

Nocturnal Oxygen Therapy Trial Group. [National Heart, Lung, and Blood Institute] Continuous or nocturnal oxygen therapy in hypoxemic chronic obstructive lung disease: a clinical trial. Ann Intern Med 1980;93:391-398.

Oxygen therapy—Inhalation

Heaton RK, Grant I, McSweeny J, et al. [National Heart, Lung, and Blood Institute] Psychologic effects of continuous and nocturnal oxygen therapy in hypoxemic chronic obstructive pulmonary disease. Arch Intern Med 1983;143:1941-1947.

Nocturnal Oxygen Therapy Trial Group. [National Heart, Lung, and Blood Institute] Continuous or nocturnal oxygen therapy in hypoxemic chronic obstructive lung disease: a clinical trial. Ann Intern Med 1980;93:391-398.

Nocturnal Oxygen Therapy Trial Study Group. [National Heart, Lung, and Blood Institute] Is 12-hour oxygen as effective as 24-hour oxygen in advanced chronic obstructive pulmonary disease with hypoxemia? (The Nocturnal Oxygen Therapy Trial - NOTT). Chest 1980;78:419-420.

Oxygen therapy—Topical

National Center for Health Services Research and Health Care Technology Assessment, Office of Health Technology Assessment. Topical oxygen therapy in the treatment of decubitus ulcers and persistent skin lesions. 1983.

Pain assessment

McGrath PA. [National Health Research and Development Program - Canada] Paediatric pain and behavioural medicine: pain assessment and the role of an endogenous opiate system in pain relief by psychological intervention. 1986. (Grant No. 6606-2244-04).

Pain rehabilitation

U.S. Administrators, Professional Policy Committee. Pain rehabilitation programs. [7/86] [Group judgment]

Pain therapy

Health Council of the Netherlands. Pain treatment. 1986. [English summary only].

National Institutes of Health, Consensus Development Program. Integrated approach to the management of pain. (Consensus Development Conference Statement, May 19-21 1986). [Group judgment]

ECRI Technology Assessment Program. Patient-controlled analgesia. Issues Health Care Technol 1985;sec.5.P.8. [Information syntheses]

American Academy of Neurology, Practice Committee. Functional integration in the alleviation of chronic muscular pain and spasticity. 1984 Feb. [Expert opinion, Group judgment]

National Institutes of Health, Consensus Development Program. Pain, discomfort, and humanitarian care. (Consensus Development Conference Statement, Feb 16 1979). [Group judgment]

Health Council of the Netherlands. Pain treatment and clinics. Ongoing.

U.S. Administrators, Professional Policy Committee. Pain clinics. Ongoing. [Group judgment]

Palatopharyngoplasty

California Medical Association, Medical Practice Opinion Program. Palatopharyngoplasty for the treatment of snoring. 1983 Dec. (Medical Practice Opinion #301) [Group judgment]

Pap smear

National Institutes of Health, Consensus Development Program. Cervical cancer screening: the pap smear. (Consensus Development Conference Statement, Jul 23-25 1980). [Group judgment]

Papaverine

National Center for Health Services Research and Health Care Technology Assessment, Office of Health Technology Assessment. Diagnostic tests for impotency: papaverine injections. Ongoing.

National Center for Health Services Research and Health Care Technology Assessment, Office of Health Technology Assessment. Treatments for impotency: papaverine. Ongoing.

Parenteral nutrition

Veterans Administration, Cooperative Studies Program. A randomized clinical trial of total parenteral nutrition in malnourished surgical patients. Pending. [Clinical trials]

American College of Physicians, Clinical Efficacy Assessment Project. Parenteral nutrition, 1987. [Information syntheses]

Medical Technology and Practice Patterns Institute. Total parenteral nutrition (inpatient). 1987.

Medical Technology and Practice Patterns Institute. Total parenteral nutrition (outpatient). 1987.

Sitzmann JV, Pitt HA. [American Gastroenterological Association, Patient Care Committee] Guidelines for total parenteral nutrition. Gastroenterology 1987 (in press).

Callahan D. [The Hastings Center] Public policy and the cessation of nutrition. In: Lynn J, ed. By no extraordinary means: the choice to forgo life-sustaining food and water. University of Indiana Press, 1986.

American Academy of Pediatrics, Committee on Nutrition. Commentary on parenteral nutrition. Pediatrics 1983 Apr.

Veterans Administration, Cooperative Studies Program. Randomized clinical trial of total parenteral nutrition in malnourished surgical patients. Ongoing. [Clinical trials]

Partial thromboplastin time

Blue Cross and Blue Shield Association, Medical Necessity Program. Activated partial thromboplastin time and prothrombin time. 1987. [Information syntheses]

Patch tests

American Dental Association, Council on Dental Materials, Instruments and Equipment, Council on Dental Therapeutics. Patch tests for sensitivity to mercury or nickel. J Am Dent Assoc 1984;108:381.

PEEP valves

ECRI Health Devices Program. Positive end expiratory pressure (PEEP) valves. Health Devices 1985;14:379-99.

Peer group counseling

Buchanan WW, Kragg G, Tugwell R. [National Health Research and Development Program - Canada] A trial to assess the efficacy of peer group rehabilitative counselling in patients with rheumatoid arthritis. 1986. (Grant No. 6606-1941-43).

Penile artery bypass

National Center for Health Services Research and Health Care Technology Assessment, Office of Health Technology Assessment. Treatments for impotency: penile artery bypass. Ongoing.

Penile prosthesis

Penile prostheses. In: Prospective Payment Assessment Commission. Technical appendixes to the report and recommendations to the Secretary, U.S. Department of Health and Human Services, April 1, 1986. Washington, DC: Government Printing Office, 1986:104-106. [Information syntheses, Cost analyses]

ECRI Technology Assessment Program. Penile prostheses. Issues Health Care Technol 1983;sec.5.P.5. [Information syntheses]

National Center for Health Services Research and Health Care Technology Assessment, Office of Health Technology Assessment. Treatments for impotency: Erect-aid system. Ongoing.

U.S. Administrators, Professional Policy Committee. Penile implants. Ongoing. [Group judgment]

Pentazocine

Food and Drug Administration, Center for Drugs and Biologics. Pentazocine HCl and naloxone HCl. 1983. (NTIS order no. PB83-915901). [Information syntheses, Expert opinion, Epidemiological and other observational methods, Clinical trials, Bench testing]

Food and Drug Administration, Center for Drugs and Biologics. Pentazocine hydrochloride and acetaminophen. 1982. (NTIS order no. PB82-915904). [Information syntheses, Expert opinion, epidemiological and other observational methods, Clinical trials, Bench testing]

Pentetate indium disodium

Food and Drug Administration, Center for Drugs and Biologics. Pentetate indium disodium In 111. 1982. (NTIS order no. PB82-915902). [Information syntheses, Expert opinion, Epidemiological and other observational methods, Clinical trials, Bench testing]

Percutaneous balloon valvuloplasty

ECRI Technology Assessment Program. Percutaneous balloon valvuloplasty. Issues Health Care Technol 1986;sec.5.P.9. [Information syntheses]

Percutaneous transluminal angioplasty

Adar R, Critchfield GC, Eddy DM. [Duke University, Center for Health Policy and Education] A confidence profile analysis of the results of percutaneous transluminal angioplasty in the treatment of ischemic femoropopliteal artery disease. (Expected publication 1988) [Information syntheses]

American Academy of Neurology, Practice Committee. Percutaneous transluminal angioplasty (PTA). 1985 Feb. [Expert opinion, Group judgment]

American Medical Association, Council on Scientific Affairs. Percutaneous transluminal angioplasty. JAMA 1984 Feb 10;251:764-768. [Group judgment]

National Center for Health Services Research and Health Care Technology Assessment, Office of Health Technology Assessment. Percutaneous transluminal angioplasty for obstructive lesions of arteriovenous dialysis fistulas. 1984.

National Center for Health Services Research and Health Care Technology Assessment, Office of Health Technology Assessment. Percutaneous transluminal angioplasty for obstructive lesions of the aortic arch vessels. 1984.

American College of Physicians, Clinical Efficacy Assessment Project. Percutaneous transluminal angioplasty: carotid, vertebral, and subclavian arteries. Ann Intern Med 1983;99:864-9. [Information syntheses]

American College of Physicians, Clinical Efficacy Assessment Project. Percutaneous transluminal angioplasty: iliac, femoral, and popliteal arteries. Ann Intern Med 1983;99:864-9. [Information syntheses]

American College of Physicians, Clinical Efficacy Assessment Project. Percutaneous transluminal angioplasty: renal arteries. Ann Intern Med 1983;99:864-9. [Information syntheses]

ECRI Technology Assessment Program. Percutaneous transluminal angioplasty (PTA) of peripheral arteries. Issues Health Care Technol 1983;sec.5.P.4. [Information syntheses]

National Center for Health Services Research and Health Care Technology Assessment, Office of Health Technology Assessment. Percutaneous transluminal angioplasty in treatment of stenotic lesions of the renal arteries. 1982.

National Center for Health Services Research and Health Care Technology Assessment, Office of Health Technology Assessment. Percutaneous transluminal angioplasty in treatment of the lower extremities. 1981.

Veterans Administration, Cooperative Studies Program. Percutaneous transiuminal angioplasty in the lower extremity. Ongoing. [Clinical trials]

Percutaneous transluminal coronary angioplasty

American College of Physicians, Clinical Efficacy Assessment Project. A comparative assessment of coronary artery bypass surgery and percutaneous transluminal coronary angioplasty, expected completion 1988. [Information systheses]

Medical Technology and Practice Patterns Institute. Percutaneous transluminal coronary angioplasty. 1987.

American Edwards Laboratories. [Food and Drug Administration, Center for Devices and Radiological Health] Amer. Ed. Labs. PTCA: summary of safety and effectiveness. 1986 Jul 9. (PMA no. P850021-000).

ECRI Technology Assessment Program. Percutaneous transluminal coronary angioplasty (PTCA). Issues Health Care Technol 1986;sec.5.P.2. [Information syntheses]

California Medical Association, Medical Practice Opinion Program. Reconsideration of percutaneous and transluminal coronary angioplasty. 1985 Feb. [Group judgment]

National Center for Health Services Research and Health Care Technology Assessment, Office of Health Technology Assessment. Patient selection criteria for percutaneous coronary angioplasty of a stenotic lesion in a single coronary artery. 1985.

Percutaneous transluminal coronary angioplasty. In: Prospective Payment Assessment Commission. Technical appendixes to the report and recommendations to the Secretary, U.S. Department of Health and Human Services, April 1, 1985. Washington, DC: Government Printing Office, 1985:105-111. [Information syntheses, Cost analyses]

American College of Physicians, Clinical Efficacy Assessment Project. Percutaneous transluminal angioplasty: coronary arteries. Ann Intern Med 1983;99:864-9. [Information syntheses]

Holmes DR, Vliestra RE, Fisher LD, et al. [National Heart, Lung, and Blood Institute] Follow-up of patients from the Coronary Artery Surgery Study (CASS) potentially suitable for percutaneous transluminal coronary angioplasty. Am Heart J 1983;106:981-988.

National Center for Health Services Research and Health Care Technology Assessment, Office of Health Technology Assessment. Percutaneous transluminal angioplasty for treatment of stenotic lesions of a single coronary artery. 1982.

Gosselin AJ, Fisher L, Judkins MP, et al. [National Heart, Lung, and Blood Institute] An estimate of the number of possible candidates from the CASS registry. Proceedings of the workshop on percutaneous transluminal coronary angioplasty June 15-16, 1979, March 1980:89-100. (U.S. Department of Health, Education and Welfare, NIH Publication No. 80-2030).

American College of Cardiology/American Heart Association Task Force on Assessment of Cardiovascular Procedures. Guidelines for percutaneous transluminal coronary angioplasty (PTCA). Ongoing. [Group judgment]

Johns Hopkins Program for Medical Technology and Practice Assessment. Analysis of the comparative cost-effectiveness of alternative strategies for managing acute heart attacks, including use of thrombolytic drugs, such as tissue plasminogen activator and steptokinase, and emergency coronary angioplasty. Ongoing.

National Center for Health Services Research and Health Care Technology Assessment, Office of Health Technology Assessment. Percutaneous transluminal coronary angioplasty when multi-vessel disease is involved (reassessment). Ongoing.

Veterans Administration, Cooperative Studies Program. Percutaneous transluminal coronary angioplasty (PTCA). Ongoing. [Clinical trials]

Perimetry

Keltner JL. [American Academy of Ophthalmology] Academy recommendation: automated perimetry. Ophthalmology 1984;91:51-56. [Information syntheses, Expert opinion]

National Center for Health Services Research and Health Care Technology Assessment, Office of Health Technology Assessment. Computer enhanced perimetry. 1983.

Periodontal ligament injection

American Dental Association, Council on Dental Materials, Instruments and Equipment. Status report: the periodontal ligament injection. J Am Dent Assoc 1983;106:222-224.

Peritoneal dialysis

Veterans Administration, Cooperative Studies Program. Renal failure self-care dialysis (hemo vs. peritoneal dialysis). [1980]. [Clinical trials]

Peritoneal dialysis cyclers

ECRI Health Devices Program. Peritoneal dialysis cyclers. Health Devices 1986;15:31-61.

Peritoneal dialysis solutions

Food and Drug Administration, Center for Drugs and Biologics. Peritoneal dialysis solutions in plastic containers. 1982. (NTIS order no. PB82-915901). [Information syntheses, Expert opinion, Epidemiological and other observational methods, Clinical trials, Bench testing]

Permanent eyeliner

California Medical Association, Medical Practice Opinion Program. Permanent eyeliner. 1985 Nov. (Medical Practice Opinion #332) [Group judgment]

Pertussis vaccine

American Academy of Pediatrics, Committee on Infectious Diseases. Pertussis vaccine. Pediatrics 1984 Aug.

Koplan JP, Schoenbaum SC, Weinstein MC, Fraser DW. [Harvard School of Public Health, Institute for Health Research] Pertussis vaccine - an analysis of benefits, risks and costs. N Eng J Med 1979;301:906-911. [Information syntheses]

Phenobarbital

Veterans Administration, Cooperative Studies Program. Evaluation of anti-epileptic drugs (phenobarb vs. phenytoin vs. primidone vs. carbamazepine). [1980] [Clinical trials]

Phenylketonuria screening

American Academy of Pediatrics, Committee on Screening Genetics. Maternal phenylketonuria. Pediatrics 1985 Aug.

American Academy of Pediatrics, Committee on Screening Genetics. New issues in newborn screening for phenylketonuria and congenital hypothyroidism. Pediatrics 1982 Jan.

Phenylpropanolamine

American Medical Association, Council on Scientific Affairs. OTC diet preparations containing phenylpropanolamine (Resolution 100, I-85). 1986. [Group judgment]

Food and Drug Administration, Center for Drugs and Biologics. Phenylpropanolamine hydrochloride chlorpheniramine maleate. 1981. (NTIS order no. PB81-915910). [Information syntheses, expert opinion, Epidemiological and other observational methods, Clinical trials, Bench testing]

Phenytoin

Veterans Administration, Cooperative Studies Program. Evaluation of anti-epileptic drugs (phenobarb vs. phenytoin vs. primidone vs. carbamazepine). [1980] [Clinical trials]

Phlebography

Hull R, Hirsch J, Sackett DL, et al. [McMaster University, Department of Clinical Epidemiology and Biostatistics] Replacement of venography in suspected venous thrombosis by impedance plethysmography and I-fibrinogen leg scanning. Ann Intern Med 1981;94:12-15.

Hull R, Hirsh J, Sackett DL, et al. [McMaster University, Department of Clinical Epidemiology and Biostatistics] Clinical validity of a negative venogram in patients with clinically suspected venous thrombosis. Circulation 1981;64:622.

Phonocardiography

American College of Physicians, Clinical Efficacy Assessment Project. Phonocardiography. 1982. [Information syntheses]

Photokymography

National Center for Health Services Research and Health Care Technology Assessment, Office of Health Technology Assessment. Photokymography. 1983.

Phototherapy

Blue Cross and Blue Shield Association, Technology Evaluation and Coverage Program. Home phototherapy for neonatal jaundice. 1986. [Information syntheses]

American Academy of Pediatrics, Committee on Fetus and Newborn. Home phototherapy. Pediatrics 1985 Jul.

Physical therapy

Kragg GR, Stokes B. [National Health Research and Development Program - Canada] The effects of comprehensive home physiotherapy and supervision on patients with ankylosing spondylitis - A randomized controlled trial. 1986. (Grant No. 6606-2385-43).

Levison H. [National Health Research and Development Program - Canada] The effects of home care chest physiotherapy on the pulmonary function of patients with cystic fibrosis - a three year study to evaluate the effects of postural drainage with mechanical percussion. 1986. (Grant No. 6606-2355-44).

U.S. Administrators, Professional Policy Committee. Physical therapy. [7/86] [Group judgment]

Piper MC. [National Health Research and Development Program - Canada] Effect of early physical therapy on the neuromotor status of the high risk infant. 1985. (Grant No. 6605-1754-51).

Physical therapy with home exercise

Wall JC. [National Health Research and Development Program - Canada] An evaluation of out-patient physiotherapy and a home exercise program in the restoration and improvement of locomotor function in residual hemiplegia. 1986. (Grant No. 6603-1161-01).

Physician education

Laxdal OE. [National Health Research and Development Program - Canada] A study of the effectiveness of continuing medical education in improving physician performance. 1986. (Grant No. 6608-1144-07).

Schroeder SA, Myers LP, McPhee SJ, et al. [University of California, San Francisco, Institute for Health Policy Studies] The failure of physician education as a cost containment strategy: report of a prospective controlled trial at a university hospital. JAMA 1984;252:225-230.

Avorn JL, Soumerai SB. [National Center for Health Services Research and Health Care Technology Assessment, Division of Extramural Research] Improving drug-therapy decisions through educational outreach: a randomized controlled trial of academically based "detailing." N Engl J Med 1983 Jun; 308(24):1457-1463.

Physiologic monitoring systems

ECRI Health Devices Program. Physiologic monitoring systems. Health Devices 1985;14:143-182.

ECRI Health Devices Program. Physiologic monitoring systems. Health Devices 1982;11:211-47.

Picture archiving and communication systems

ECRI Technology Assessment Program. Image transmission and data compression. J Health Care Technol 1986;3:83-93. [Information syntheses]

American Hospital Association, Hospital Technology Series Program. Picture archiving and communication systems. 1985. (Guideline report) [Information syntheses, Expert opinion, Cost analyses]

ECRI Technology Assessment Program. Digital imaging storage and retrieval. J Health Care Technol 1984;1:13-38. [Information syntheses]

American College of Radiology, Task Force on Breast Cancer. Statement of the preservation of mammograms. 1983. [Group judgment]

Pindolol

Food and Drug Administration, Center for Drugs and Biologics. Pindolol, 1982. (NTIS order no. PB82-915904). [Information syntheses, Expert opinion, Epidemiological and other observational methods, Clinical trials, Bench testing]

Piperacillin

Food and Drug Administration, Center for Drugs and Biologics. Sterile piperacillin sodium. 1982. (NTIS order no. PB82-915901). [Information syntheses, Expert opinion, Epidemiological and other observational methods, Clinical trials, Bench testing]

Piroxicam

Food and Drug Administration, Center for Drugs and Biologics, Piroxicam. 1982. (NTIS order no. PB82-915903). [Information syntheses, Expert opinion, Epidemiological and other observational methods, Clinical trials, Bench testing]

Plasma exchange

Rock GA. [National Health Research and Development Program - Canada] A clinical research project to study the role of plasma exchange and plasma infusion in the treatment of thrombotic thrombocytopenic purpura. 1986. (Grant No. 6613-1158-46).

Rock GA. [National Health Research and Development Program - Canada] The role of plasma exchange in the management of immune thrombocytopenia. 1986. (Grant No. 6613-1164-52).

Rock GA. [National Health Research and Development Program - Canada] A clinical research project to study the role of plasma exchange in the treatment of Rh disease. 1985. (Grant No. 6613-1156-52).

National Center for Health Services Research and Health Care Technology Assessment, Office of Health Technology Assessment. Plasmapheresis and plasma exchange for thrombotic thrombocytopenic purpura. 1982.

Plasma exchange devices

Sarn, Inc. [Food and Drug Administration, Center for Devices and Radiological Health] Therapore (TM) system: summary of safety and effectiveness. 1986 Dec 24. (PMA no. 850092-000).

Parker Hannifin Corporation. [Food and Drug Administration, Center for Devices and Radiological Health] Cryomax (TM): summary of safety and effectiveness. 1983 Feb 18. (PMA no. P820002-000).

Cobe Laboratories, Inc. [Food and Drug Administration, Center for Devices and Radiological Health] Cobe century (R) TPE system: summary of safety and effectiveness. 1982 Mar 9. (PMA no. P810023-000).

Plasma filters

Gambro, Inc. [Food and Drug Administration, Center for Devices and Radiological Health] Gambro fiber plasmafilter: summary of safety and effectiveness. 1986 Jul 7. (PMA no. P83006-000).

Plasma, Frozen

National Institutes of Health, Consensus Development Program. Fresh frozen plasma: indications and risks. (Consensus Development Conference Statement, Sep 24-26 1984). [Group judgment]

Plasma infusion

Rock GA. [National Health Research and Development Program - Canada] A clinical research project to study the role of plasma exchange and plasma infusion in the treatment of thrombotic thrombocytopenic purpura. 1986. (Grant No. 6613-1158-46).

Plasma perfusion

National Center for Health Services Research and Health Care Technology Assessment, Office of Health Technology Assessment. Plasma perfusion of charcoal filters for treatment of pruritis of cholestatic liver disease. 1983.

Plasma separation systems

Organon Teknika Corp. [Food and Drug Administration, Center for Devices and Radiological Health] Curesis plasma separator: summary of safety and effectiveness. 1984 Nov 9. (PMA no. P830010-000).

Asahi Chemical Industry America, Inc. [Food and Drug Administration, Center for Devices and Radiological Health] Plasmaflo AP-O5H Asahi plasma separator: summary of safety and effectiveness. 1983 Aug 12. (PMA no. P820033-000).

Travenol Laboratories. [Food and Drug Administration, Center for Devices and Radiological Health] Plasma separation system: summary of safety and effectiveness. 1983 Nov 3. (PMA no. P820032-000).

Plasmapheresis

Cole EH, Cattran DC. [National Health Research and Development Program - Canada] A controlled trial of plasmapheresis in idiopathic rapidly progressive glomerulonephritis. 1986. (Grant No. 6606-2372-52).

National Institutes of Health, Consensus Development Program. The utility of therapeutic plasmapheresis for neurological disorders. (Consensus Development Conference Statement, Jun 2-4 1986). [Group judgment]

American Medical Association, Council on Scientific Affairs. Current status of therapeutic plasmapheresis and related techniques. JAMA 1985 Feb 8;253:819-825. [Group judgment]

American College of Obstetricians and Gynecologists, Committee on Technical Bulletins. Blood component therapy. 1984 Jul. (Technical bulletin no. 78). [Expert opinion]

American Academy of Neurology, Practice Committee. Plasmapheresis in treatment of multiple sclerosis. 1983 Feb. [Expert opinion, Group judgment]

American Academy of Neurology, Practice Committee. Plasmapheresis in treatment of myasthenia gravis. 1983 Feb. [Expert opinion, Group judgment]

California Medical Association, Medical Practice Opinion Program. Plasmapheresis for rheumatoid arthritis. 1982 Aug. (Medical Practice Opinion #263) [Group judgment]

California Medical Association, Medical Practice Opinion Program. Plasmapheresis for six conditions. 1982 Sep. (Medical Practice Opinion #249) [Group judgment]

California Medical Association, Medical Practice Opinion Program. Plasmapheresis treatment of multiple sclerosis. 1981 Dec. (Medical Practice Opinion #212) [Group judgment]

ECRI Technology Assessment Program. Therapeutic plasmapheresis. Issues Health Care Technol 1981;sec.5.P.1. [Information syntheses]

Plasticizers

Rock GA. [National Health Research and Development Program - Canada] An evaluation of the effects of various plasticizers and/or leachables contained in plastic medical devices on blood components, blood donors, and patients. 1986. (Grant No. 6613-1239-52).

Rock GA. [National Health Research and Development Program - Canada] Toxicological evaluation of plasticizers and their metabolites leaching from plastic medical devices into human plasma. 1986. (Grant No. 6613-1177-52).

Platelet transfusion

National Institutes of Health, Consensus Development Program. Platelet transfusion therapy. (Consensus Development Conference Statement, Oct 6-8 1986). [Group judgment]

CBO (Centraal Begeleidingsorgaan voor de Intercollegiale Toetsing) Consensus Development Program. Thrombocytes transfusion policy. 1984. [Dutch language only] [Group judgment, Expert opinion]

Plethysmography

ECRI Technology Assessment Program. Plethysmography for diagnosing deep vein thrombosis. Issues Health Care Technol 1984;sec.5.P.7. [Information syntheses]

National Center for Health Services Research and Health Care Technology Assessment, Office of Health Technology Assessment. Photoplethysmography. 1982.

Hull R, Hirsch J, Sackett DL, et al. [McMaster University, Department of Clinical Epidemiology and Biostatistics] Replacement of venography in suspected venous thrombosis by impedance plethysmography and I-fibrinogen leg scanning. Ann Intern Med 1981;94:12-15.

National Center for Health Services Research and Health Care Technology Assessment, Office of Health Technology Assessment. Diagnostic tests for impotency: plethysmography. Ongoing.

Pneumococcal vaccine

American College of Physicians, Clinical Efficacy Assessment Project. Pneumococcal vaccine. Ann Intern Med 1986;104:118-120

American Academy of Pediatrics, Committee on Infectious Diseases. Recommendations for using pneumococcal vaccine in children. Pediatrics 1985 Jun.

American Academy of Pediatrics, Committee on Infectious Diseases. Recommendations for using pneumococcal vaccine in children. Pediatrics 1985 Jun.

Office of Technology Assessment, U.S. Congress. Update of Federal activities regarding the use of pneumococcal vaccine. Washington, D.C.: U.S. Government Printing Office, May 1984.

American Medical Association, Council on Scientific Affairs. Pneumococcal, influenza and hepatitis-B vaccine (Resolution 75, A-82). 1982. [Group judgment]

Veterans Administration, Cooperative Studies Program. Pneumococcal capsular vaccine immunity in high risk patients. [1980]. [Clinical trials]

Polydextrose

American Diabetes Association. Position statment on polydextrose. 1986. [Expert opinion, Group judgment]

Polypectomy

Wayne JD. Colonoscopic polypectomy. In: American Society for Gastrointestinal Endoscopy, Committee on Technology Assessment. Therapeutic gastrointestinal endoscopy: an information resource manual. 1987. [Information syntheses, Expert opinion, Group judgment, Cost analyses]

Polyurethane tubing

Food and Drug Administration, Center for Devices and Radiological Health. Surface cracking of polyurethane tubing resulting from subcutaneous implantation in dogs. 1985. (NTIS Order No. PB85-171619/AS).

Positron emission tomography

American Hospital Association, Hospital Technology Series Program. Positron emission tomography. 1987. (Guideline report) [Information syntheses, Expert opinion, Cost analyses]

Health Council of the Netherlands. Positron emission tomography. 1986. [English summary only].

Health Council of the Netherlands. PET-scan. Ongoing assessment.

Postmarketing surveillance

Strom BL, Melmon KL, Miettinen OS. [McGill University, Department of Epidemiology and Biostatistics] Post marketing studies of drug efficacy: why? Am J Med 1985;78:475-480.

Office of Technology Assessment, U.S. Congress. Postmarketing surveillance of prescription drugs. Washington, D.C.: U.S. Government Printing Office, November 1982.

Health Council of the Netherlands. Post marketing surveillance of drugs. Planned.

Postural drainage

Levison H. [National Health Research and Development Program - Canada] The effects of home care chest physiotherapy on the pulmonary function of patients with cystic fibrosis - a three year study to evaluate the effects of postural drainage with mechanical percussion. 1986. (Grant No. 6606-2355-44).

Blue Cross and Blue Shield Association, Medical Necessity Program. Respiratory therapy: postural drainage. 1982. [Information syntheses]

Posture control devices

Foort J. [National Health Research and Development Program - Canada] A modular exoskeletal system for supporting heavy disabled people in the sitting position. 1986. (Grant No. 6610-1291-51).

Tredwell SJ. [National Health Research and Development Program - Canada] Pelvic stabilizer for postural control. 1986. (Grant No. 6610-1422-51).

Potassium chloride

Food and Drug Administration, Center for Drugs and Biologics. Potassium chloride. 1987. (Summary basis of approval substitute, NDA # 19-123). [Information syntheses, Expert opinion, Epidemiological and other observational methods, Clinical trials, Bench testing]

Food and Drug Administration, Center for Drugs and Biologics. Potassium chloride. 1987. (Summary basis of approval, NDA # 19-439). [Information syntheses, Expert opinion, Epidemiological and other observational methods, Clinical trials, Bench testing]

Food and Drug Administration, Center for Drugs and Biologics. Potassium chloride. 1987. (Summary basis of approval, NDA# 19-123). [Information syntheses, Expert opinion, Epidemiological and other observational methods, Clinical trials, Bench testing]

Food and Drug Administration, Center for Drugs and Biologics. CaCl2, MgCl, Kcl, & NaCl. 1982. (NTIS order no. PB82-915902). [Information syntheses, Expert opinion, Epidemiological and other observational methods, Clinical trials, Bench testing]

Food and Drug Administration, Center for Drugs and Biologics. NaCl, KCl, MgSO4, NaPO4, & KPO4. 1982. (NTIS order no. PB82-915901). [Information syntheses, Expert opinion, Epidemiological and other observational methods, Clinical trials, Bench testing]

Food and Drug Administration, Center for Drugs and Biologics. Potassium chloride 1981. (NTIS order no. PB81-915901). [Information syntheses, Expert opinion, Epidemiological and other observational methods, Clinical trials, Bench testing]

Potassium citrate

Food and Drug Administration, Center for Drugs and Biologics. Potassium citrate. 1987. (Summary basis of approval, NDA #19-071). [Information syntheses, Expert opinion, Epidemiological and other observational methods, Clinical trials, Bench testing]

Potassium phosphate

Food and Drug Administration, Center for Drugs and Biologics. NaCl, KCl, MgSO4, NaPO4, & KPO4. 1982. (NTIS order no. PB82-915901). [Information syntheses, Expert opinion, Epidemiological and other observational methods, Clinical trials, Bench testing]

Praziquantel

Food and Drug Administration, Center for Drugs and Biologics. Praziquantel, 1983. (NTIS order No. PB83-915901). [Information syntheses, Expert opinion, Epidemiological and other observational methods, Clinical trials, Bench testing]

Prazosin

Veterans Administration, Cooperative Studies Program. Prazosin vs. hydralazine in hypertension. [1980] [Clinical trials]

Prenatal care

Prenatal care and its relationship to Medicaid costs. In: Office of Research and Demonstrations, Health Care Financing Administration. Health care financing status report: research and demonstrations in health care financing. Jan 1986. (HCFA Pub. No. 03219).

National Institute of Child Health and Human Development, Division of Maternal and Child Health. Content of prenatal care. Ongoing. [Group judgment, Expert opinion]

Prenatal education

Robitaille Y, Kramaer MS. [McGill University, Department of Epidemiology and Biostatistics] Does participation in prenatal courses lead to heavier babies? Am J Public Health 1985;75:1186-1189.

Pressure transducers

ECRI Health Devices Program. Disposable pressure transducers. Health Devices 1984;13:268-90.

Primadone

Veterans Administration, Cooperative Studies Program. Evaluation of anti-epileptic drugs (phenobarb vs. phenytoin vs. primidone vs. carbamazepine). [1980] [Clinical trials]

Progestin receptor assays

New England Nuclear. [Food and Drug Administration, Center for Devices and Radiological Health] Rianen (TM) (3H) progestin receptor assay kit: summary of safety and effectiveness. 1983 Oct 12. (PMA no. P820052-000).

Prolotherapy

American Academy of Neurology, Practice Committee. Prolotherapy. 1981 Jul. [Expert opinion, Group judgment]

Propranolol

Food and Drug Administration, Center for Drugs and Biologics. Propranolol HCl liquid. 1987. (Summary basis of approval substitute, NDA# 19-536). [Information syntheses, Expert opinion, Epidemiological and other observational methods, Clinical trials, Bench testing]

Food and Drug Administration, Center for Drugs and Biologics. Propranolol SR/hydrochlorothiazide. 1987. (Summary basis of approval, NDA # 19-059). [Information syntheses, Expert opinion, Epidemiological and other observational methods, Clinical trials, Bench testing]

Food and Drug Administration, Center for Drugs and Biologics. Propranolol hydrochloride. 1987. (Summary basis of approval, NDA #18-553). [Information syntheses, Expert opinion, Epidemiological and other observational methods, Clinical trials, Bench testing]

Oster G, Huse DM, Delea TE, Savage DD, Colditz GA. [Policy Analysis, Inc.] Cost effectiveness of labetalol and propranolol in the treatment of hypertension among blacks. 1987 Mar.

Friedman LM, Byington RP, Capone RJ, et al. for the Beta-Blocker Heart Attack Trial Research Group. [National Heart, Lung, and Blood Institute] Effect of propranolol in patients with myocardial infarction and ventricular arrhythmia. J Am Coll Cardiol 1986;7:1-8.

Morganroth J, Lichstein E, Byington R. [National Heart, Lung, and Blood Institute] Beta-Blocker Heart Attack Trial: impact of propranolol therapy on ventricular arrhythmias. Prev Med 1985;14:346-357.

Furberg CD, Hawkins CM, Lichstein E for the Beta-Blocker Heart Attack Study Group. [National Heart, Lung, and Blood Institute] Effect of propranolol in postinfarction patients with mechanical or electrical complications. Circulation 1984;69:761-765.

Roberts R, Croft C, Gold HK, et al and the MILIS Study Group. [National Heart, Lung, and Blood Institute] Effect of propranolol on myocardial-infarct size in a randomized blinded multicenter trial. N Eng J Med 1984;311:218-225.

Beta-Blocker Heart Attack Trial Research Group. [National Heart, Lung, and Blood Institute] A randomized trial of propranolol in patients with acute myocardial infarction. II. Morbidity results. JAMA 1983;250:2814-2819.

Goldstein, S. [National Heart, Lung, and Blood Institute] Propranolol therapy in patients with acute myocardial infarction: the Beta-Blocker Heart Attack Trial. Circulation 1983;67(Suppl 1):53-57.

Lichstein E, Morganroth J, Harrest R, et al. [National Heart, Lung, and Blood Institute] Effect of propranolol on ventricular arrhythmia: the Beta-Blocker Heart Attack Trial Experience. Circulation 1983;67(Suppl I):5-10.

Beta-Blocker Heart Attack Trial Research Group. [National Heart, Lung, and Blood Institute] A randomized trial of propranolol in patients with acute myocardial infarction. I. Mortality results. JAMA 1982;247:1707-1713.

Veterans Administration, Cooperative Studies Program. Comparison of propranolol with hydrochlorothiazide for the "step 1" treatment of hypertension. [1980] [Clinical trials]

Veterans Administration, Cooperative Studies Program. Oxprenolol vs. propranolol in hypertension. [1980]. [Clinical trials]

Prospective payment systems

Annual reports to Congress on the impact of the Medicare Hospital prospective payment system. In: Office of Research and Demonstrations, Health Care Financing Administration. Health care financing status report: research and demonstrations in health care financing. Jan 1986. (HCFA Pub. No. 03219).

Evaluability assessment of the Medicare prospective payment system on long-term care. In: Office of Research and Demonstrations, Health Care Financing Administration. Health care financing status report: research and demonstrations in health care financing. Jan 1986. (HCFA Pub. No. 03219).

Home health agency prospective payment demonstration. In: Office of Research and Demonstrations, Health Care Financing Administration. Health care financing status report: research and demonstrations in health care financing. Jan 1986. (HCFA Pub. No. 03219).

Impact of DRG-based prospective payment system on quality of care for hospitalized Medicare patients. In: Office of Research and Demonstrations, Health Care Financing Administration. Health care financing status report: research and demonstrations in health care financing. Jan 1986. (HCFA Pub. No. 03219).

Impact of Medicare's prospective payment system and private sector initiatives: the Blue Cross and Blue Shield Organization's experiences. In: Office of Research and Demonstrations, Health Care Financing Administration. Health care financing status report: research and demonstrations in health care financing. Jan 1986. (HCFA Pub. No. 03219).

Impact of the prospective payment system on the quality of inpatient care. In: Office of Research and Demonstrations, Health Care Financing Administration. Health care financing status report: research and demonstrations in health care financing. Jan 1986. (HCFA Pub. No. 03219).

Incentive prospective payment system for hospitals through fiscal intermediaries (Massachusetts). In: Office of Research and Demonstrations, Health Care Financing Administration. Health care financing status report: research and demonstrations in health care financing. Jan 1986. (HCFA Pub. No. 03219).

Longitudinal study of the impact of prospective reimbursement under Medicaid on nursing home care in Maine. In: Office of Research and Demonstrations, Health Care Financing Administration. Health care financing status report: research and demonstrations in health care financing. Jan 1986. (HCFA Pub. No. 03219).

New York State case-mix, prospective reimbursement system for long-term care. In: Office of Research and Demonstrations, Health Care Financing Administration. Health care financing status report: research and demonstrations in health care financing. Jan 1986. (HCFA Pub. No. 03219).

Office of Technology Assessment, U.S. Congress. OTA's second report on the Prospective Payment Assessment Commission (special report). Washington, D.C.: Office of Technology Assessment, March 1986.

Payment options for nonphysician anesthetists under the prospective payment system. In: Office of Research and Demonstrations, Health Care Financing Administration. Health care financing status report: research and demonstrations in health care financing. Jan 1986. (HCFA Pub. No. 03219).

Project HOPE, Center for Health Affairs. PPS payments for expensive devices: issues and evidence. (for Prospective Payment Assessment Commission). 1986 Aug. [Cost analyses]

Prospective Payment Assessment Commission. Medicare prospective payment and the American health care system: report to the Congress. February 1986. Washington, D.C.: Government Printing Office, 1986. [Information syntheses, Cost analyses]

Prospective Payment Assessment Commission. Report and recommendataions to the Secretary, U.S. Department of Health and Human Services, April 1, 1986. Washington, DC: Government Printing Office, 1986. [Information syntheses, Cost analyses]

Prospective Payment Assessment Commission. Technical appendixes to the report and recommendations to the Secretary, U.S. Department of Health and Human Services, April 1, 1986. Washington, DC: Government Printing Office, 1986. [Information syntheses, Cost analyses]

Prospective payment beneficiary impact study. In: Office of Research and Demonstrations, Health Care Financing Administration. Health care financing status report: research and demonstrations in health care financing. Jan 1986. (HCFA Pub. No. 03219).

Prospective payment in rehabilitation hospitals and programs. In: Office of Research and Demonstrations, Health Care Financing Administration. Health care financing status report: research and demonstrations in health care financing. Jan 1986. (HCFA Pub. No. 03219).

Prospective payment of physicians. In: Office of Research and Demonstrations, Health Care Financing Administration. Health care financing status report: research and demonstrations in health care financing. Jan 1986. (HCFA Pub. No. 03219).

Prospective payment system and post-hospital care: use, cost, and market changes. In: Office of Research and Demonstrations, Health Care Financing Administration. Health care financing status report: research and demonstrations in health care financing. Jan 1986. (HCFA Pub. No. 03219).

Prospective payment system for acute and chronic care hospitals in Maryland. In: Office of Research and Demonstrations, Health Care Financing Administration. Health care financing status report: research and demonstrations in health care financing. Jan 1986. (HCFA Pub. No. 03219).

Prospective reimbursement system based on patient case mix for New Jersey hospitals. In: Office of Research and Demonstrations, Health Care Financing Administration. Health care financing status report: research and demonstrations in health care financing. Jan 1986. (HCFA Pub. No. 03219).

Selected analyses of the prospective payment system's impact on hospital's behavior In: Office of Research and Demonstrations, Health Care Financing Administration. Health care financing status report: research and demonstrations in health care financing. Jan 1986. (HCFA Pub. No. 03219).

Office of Technology Assessment, U.S. Congress. Medicare's prospective payment system: strategies for evaluating cost, quality, and medical technology. Washington, D.C.: U.S. Government Printing Office, October 1985.

Office of Technology Assessment, U.S. Congress. OTA's first report on the Prospective Payment Assessment Commission (special report). Washington, D.C.: Office of Technology Assessment, March 1985.

Prospective Payment Assessment Commission. Report and recommendations to the Secretary, U.S. Department of Health and Human Services, April 1, 1985. Washington, DC: Government Printing Office, 1985. [Information syntheses, Cost analyses]

Prospective Payment Assessment Commission. Technical appendixes to the report and recommendations to the Secretary, U.S. Department of Health and Human Services, April 1, 1985. Washington, DC: Government Printing Office, 1985. [Information syntheses, Cost analyses]

American Hospital Association, Hospital Technology Series Program. Equipment acquisition under prospective payment. 1984. (Guideline report) [Information syntheses, Expert opinion, Cost analyses]

Project HOPE, Center for Health Affairs. The effect of PPS on the diffusion and use of medical technologies. (for Prospective Payment Assessment Commission). Ongoing, expected 1987. [Information syntheses]

Prostatic acid phosphatase kits

United Kingdom Department of Health and Social Security, Medical Devices Evaluation Programme. Comparative evaluation of prostatic acid phosphatase kits. 1985 May. (Report no. STB3A/85/21) [Epidemiological and other observational methods, Bench testing]

Prostheses

Foort J. [National Health Research and Development Program - Canada] Amputee fitting—standard shape processing. 1986. (Grant No. 6610-1289-51).

Saunders CG, Morrison JB, Foort J. [National Health Research and Development Program - Canada] Amputee fitting standard shape processing (sealing) Part II. 1986. (Grant No. 6610-1369-51).

Protein-calorie therapy with anabolic steroids

Veterans Administration, Cooperative Studies Program. Protein-calorie therapy in combination with anabolic steroids in alcoholic hepatitis. Ongoing. [Clinical trials]

Prothrombin time

Blue Cross and Blue Shield Association, Medical Necessity Program. Activated partial thromboplastin time and prothrombin time. 1987. [Information syntheses]

Prothrombin-complex concentrate

Lusher JM, Shapiro SS, Palascak JE, et al. [National Heart, Lung, and Blood Institute] Efficiency of prothrombin-complex concentrates in hemophiliacs with antibodies to Factor VIII. N Eng J Med 1980;303:421.

Psychoactive drugs

American Academy of Pediatrics, Committee on Drugs. Psychotropic drugs in pregnancy and lactation. Pediatrics 1982 Feb.

Psychosurgery

Health Council of the Netherlands. Psychosurgery. Ongoing.

Psychotherapy

Piper WE. [National Health Research and Development Program - Canada] A controlled study of patient suitability and outcome in short term, individual psychotherapy. 1986. (Grant No. 6609-1367-46).

Office of Technology Assessment, U.S. Congress. The efficacy and cost effectiveness of psychotherapy. Washington, D.C.: U.S. Government Printing Office, Oct 1980. (Health technology case study series #18)

Pulmonary function tests

American College of Physicians, Clinical Efficacy Assessment Project. Preoperative pulmonary function tests, expected completion 1988. [Information syntheses]

Blue Cross and Blue Shield Association, Medical Necessity Program. Diagnostic studies for respiratory patients: pulmonary function tests. 1982. [Information syntheses]

Subcommittee on Special Services in Hospitals. [Health and Welfare Canada, Health Services and Promotion Branch, Institutional and Professional Services Division] Pulmonary function laboratories guidelines. 1982. [Information syntheses, Expert opinion, Group judgment]

Punctal occlusion

American Academy of Ophthalmology. Punctal occlusion for the dry eye. San Francisco, CA: American Academy of Ophthalmology, 1987. [Information syntheses, Expert opinion]

PUVA therapy

Stern RS and members of the 16-center PUVA Follow-up Study. [Harvard School of Public Health, Institute for Health Research] Long-term utilization of PUVA therapy for psoriasis - evidence for efficacy and cost savings. J Am Acad Dermatol, in press. [Clinical trials]

Blue Cross and Blue Shield Association, Technology Evaluation and Coverage Program. Psoralens and ultraviolet A (PUVA). 1986. [Information syntheses]

American Academy of Pediatrics, Committee on Drugs. PUVA: a caution. Pediatrics 1978 Aug.

Pyelography

American College of Physicians, Clinical Efficacy Assessment Project. Intravenous pyelography, expected completion 1988. [Information syntheses]

Pyrimethamine

Food and Drug Administration, Center for Drugs and Biologics. Sulfadoxine and pyrimethamine. 1982. (NTIS order no. PB82-915901). [Information syntheses, Expert opinion, Epidemiological and other observational methods, Clinical trials, Bench testing]

Quality assurance programs

Howanitz PJ, ed. Quality assurance in physician office, bedside, and home testing. Skokie, IL: College of American Pathologists. (expected 1987) [Expert opinion, Bench testing]

Evaluation of three-state demonstration in nursing home quality assurance. In: Office of Research and Demonstrations, Health Care Financing Administration. Health care financing status report: research and demonstrations in health care financing. Jan 1986. (HCFA Pub. No. 03219).

Improving New York State's Nursing Home Quality Assurance Program. In: Office of Research and Demonstrations, Health Care Financing Administration. Health care financing status report: research and demonstrations in health care financing. Jan 1986. (HCFA Pub. No. 03219).

Scherer K, Farrell P. [National Health Research and Development Program - Canada] A project for measuring the quality of nursing care in Manitoba. 1986. (Grant No. 6607-1238-46).

Food and Drug Administration, Center for Devices and Radiological Health. Recommendations for quality assurance programs in nuclear medicine facilities. (GPO Stock No. 017-015-00225-0, NTIS Order No. 85-145720/AS).

Penner DW. [National Health Research and Development Program - Canada] Quality control (quality evaluation) for diagnostic surgical pathology and cytopathology. 1985. (Grant No. 6607-1279-55).

Food and Drug Administration, Center for Devices and Radiological Health. A basic quality assurance program for small diagnostic radiology facilities. 1984. (NTIS Order No. PB84-119098).

Poddercord M, Taylor RN. [National Center for Health Services Research and Health Care Technology Assessment, Division of Extramural Research] Evaluation of laboratory quality assurance activities. 1984. (NTIS order no. PB84-205913)

Food and Drug Administration, Center for Devices and Radiological Health. Quality assurance in nuclear medicine - proceedings of an international symposium and workshop, held in Washington, D.C., April 27-29. 1981. 1982. (GPO Stock No. 017-015-00221-7, NTIS Order No. PB84-199306).

McDonald CJ. [National Center for Health Services Research and Health Care Technology Assessment, Division of Extramural Research] A controlled trial of a quality assurance mechanism. 1982. (NTIS order no. PB82-265539)

Radial keratotomy

American Academy of Ophthalmology. Radial keratotomy for myopia. San Francisco, CA: American Academy of Ophthalmology, expected completion October, 1987. [Information syntheses, Expert opinion]

California Medical Association, Medical Practice Opinion Program. Radial keratotomy for myopia. 1985 Apr. (Medical Practice Opinion #244) [Group judgment]

American Medical Association, Diagnostic and Therapeutic Technology Assessment. Radial keratotomy for the treatment of myopia. JAMA 1983 Jul 15. [Expert opinon, Information syntheses]

ECRI Technology Assessment Program. Radial keratotomy. Issues Health Care Technol 1982;sec.5.R.1. [Information syntheses]

Radiant warmers

ECRI Health Devices Program. Infant radiant warmers. Health Devices 1984;13:119-45.

Radiation measurement

Food and Drug Administration, Center for Devices and Radiological Health. Computer program for absorbed dose to the breast in mammography. 1986. (GPO Stock No. 017-015-00228-4, NTIS Order No. PB86-114774/AS).

Food and Drug Administration, Center for Devices and Radiological Health. Evaluation of radiation exposure from diagnostic radiology examinations - technique/exposure guides for the craniocaudal projection in mammography. 1986. (NTIS Order No. PB86-126075/AS).

Food and Drug Administration, Center for Devices and Radiological Health. Evaluation of radiation exposure from diagnostic radiology examinations: general recommendations. 1986. (NTIS Order No. PB86-125903/AS).

Food and Drug Administration, Center for Devices and Radiological Health. Recommendations for evaluation of radiation exposure from diagnostic radiology examinations. 1986. (NTIS Order No. PB86-125846/AS).

Stuchly SS. [National Health Research and Development Program - Canada] Radiowave and microwave dosimetry in human models. 1986. (Grant No. 6606-2455-52).

Food and Drug Administration, Center for Devices and Radiological Health. Evaluation of radiation exposure from diagnostic radiology examinations (technique/exposure guides for the dental bitewing projection). 1985. (FDA Pub No. 85-8245).

Radiation protection

Food and Drug Administration, Center for Devices and Radiological Health. Embryo, fetus, infant . . . recommendations to minimize diagnostic nuclear medicine exposure. 1986. (FDA Pub. No. FDA86-8254).

Food and Drug Administration, Center for Devices and Radiological Health. Patient exposure reduction during scoliosis radiography. 1985. (GPO Stock No. 017-015-00227-6).

Food and Drug Administration, Center for Devices and Radiological Health. Reducing patient exposure during scoliosis radiography. 1985. (FDA Pub No. FDA 85-8252).

Radiation therapy

American Hospital Association, Hospital Technology Series Program. Radiation therapy planning. 1987. (Guideline report) [Information syntheses, Expert opinion, Cost analyses

California Medical Association, Medical Practice Opinion Program. Stereotactic heavy-ion irradiation for arteriovenous malformations. 1985 Sep. (Medical Practice Opinion #316) [Group judgment]

U.S. Administrators, Professional Policy Committee. Radiation therapy for lung carcinoma. Ongoing. [Group judgment]

Radioallergosorbent test

California Medical Association, Medical Practice Opinion Program. Radioallergosorbent test (RAST) 1984 Dec. (Medical Practice Opinion #255) [Group judgment]

American College of Physicians, Clinical Efficacy Assessment Project. Radio allergosorbent technique (RAST). 1981. [Information syntheses]

California Medical Association, Medical Practice Opinion Program. Paper radioallergosorbent test (PRAST). 1981 Aug. (Medical Practice Opinion #256) [Group judgment]

Radiographic contrast dyes

ECRI Technology Assessment Program. Low-osmolality radiographic contrast agents. Issues Health Care Technol 1986;sec.5.L.4. [Information syntheses]

American Academy of Pediatrics, Committee on Radiology. Water-soluble contrast material. Pediatrics 1978 Jul.

Johns Hopkins Program for Medical Technology and Practice Assessment. A synthesis of the published literature regarding the comparative toxicity of high osmolar and low osmolar radiographic contrast dyes. Ongoing.

Johns Hopkins Program for Medical Technology and Practice Assessment. An analysis of economic and policy issues related to the introduction of low osmolar radiographic contrast dyes. Ongoing.

Johns Hopkins Program for Medical Technology and Practice Assessment. A clinical trial at determining the comparative nephrotoxicity and comparative cost-effectiveness of low osmolar versus high osmolar radiographic contrast dyes. Planned.

Radiographic darkrooms

American Dental Association, Council on Dental Materials, Instruments and Equipment. Recommendations for radiographic darkrooms and darkroom practices. J Am Dent Assoc 1982;104:636-637.

Radiographic equipment

United Kingdom Department of Health and Social Security, Medical Devices Evaluation Programme. Assessment of Siemens Optilux 57 intensifier associated with the Sircam 100mm camera and Polyphos 300E generator. 1986 Jan. (Report no. STB6E/86/4) [Epidemiological and other observational methods, Bench testing]

United Kingdom Department of Health and Social Security, Medical Devices Evaluation Programme. An evaluation of eight non-invasive electronic KV measuring instruments which are commercially available in the UK. 1985 Jun. (Report no. STB6E/85/19) [Epidemiological and other observational methods, Bench testing]

United Kingdom Department of Health and Social Security, Medical Devices Evaluation Programme. Assessment of Picker Clinix C servo chest unit. 1985 Jun. (Report no. STB6E/85/14) [Epidemiological and other observational methods, Bench testing]

United Kingdom Department of Health and Social Security, Medical Devices Evaluation Programme. Assessment of Siemens basic radiological system (BRS) to WHO modified specification. 1985 Sep. (Report no. STB6E/85/34) [Epidemiological and other observational methods, Bench testing]

United Kingdom Department of Health and Social Security, Medical Devices Evaluation Programme. Assessment of Sine Mobil 3N and 3H mobile imaging intensifiers. 1985 Sep. (Report no. STB6E/85/30) [Epidemiological and other observational methods, Bench testing]

United Kingdom Department of Health and Social Security, Medical Devices Evaluation Programme. Assessment of Todd Research BRS to WHO modified specification. 1985 Sep. (Report no. STB6A/85/36) [Epidemiological and other observational methods, Bench testing]

United Kingdom Department of Health and Social Security, Medical Devices Evaluation Programme. Assessment of Wolverson Mylo X radiographic unit, Royal Preston Hospital, North Manchester. 1985 Apr. (Report no. STB6E/85/8) [Epidemiological and other observational methods, Bench testing]

United Kingdom Department of Health and Social Security, Medical Devices Evaluation Programme. Assessment of a Siemens Polydoros 80 X-ray generator. 1985 Aug. (Report no. STB6E/85/27) [Epidemiological and other observational methods, Bench testing]

United Kingdom Department of Health and Social Security, Medical Devices Evaluation Programme. Introduction to imaging cameras with assessment of Matric HPC 1010/4. 1985 Nov. (Report no. STB6E/85/42) [Epidemiological and other observational methods, Bench testing]

Radiographic film

United Kingdom Department of Health and Social Security, Medical Devices Evaluation Programme. Physical evaluation of the imaging performance of the Agfa Gevaert range of screen film systems. 1985 Aug. (Report no. STB6E/85/26) [Epidemiological and other observational methods, Bench testing]

Radiographic film processors

United Kingdom Department of Health and Social Security, Medical Devices Evaluation Programme. Assessment of Kodak M8 radiographic film processor. 1985 Jun. (Report no. STB6E/85/24) [Epidemiological and other observational methods, Bench testing]

ECRI Health Devices Program. X-ray film processors. Health Devices 1982;11:99-115.

Radiography

Blue Cross and Blue Shield Association, Medical Necessity Program. Routine preoperative and general hospital admission chest x-rays. 1987. [Information syntheses]

Schwarz RD. [National Health Research and Development Program - Canada] An assessment of the need for radiological evaluation of all girls with recurrent urinary infection. 1986. (Grant No. 6603-1201-42).

U.S. Administrators, Professional Policy Committee. Multiple views - diagnostic radiology. [7/86] [Group judgment]

Food and Drug Administration, Center for Devices and Radiological Health. Assessment and modification of clinical utility in diagnostic radiology: the oral cholecystogram and the upper gastrointestinal examinations. 1985. (NTIS Order No. PB-85-246916/AS).

Food and Drug Administration, Center for Devices and Radiological Health. Extremity radiography following trauma: an overview. 1985. (GPO Stock No. 017-015-00224-1, NTIS Order No. PB85-115053).

Podgorsak FB. [Department Radiation Oncology, McGill University] [Medical Research Council - Canada] Radiographic imaging by solid state electrostatic techniques. (Grant period 1981-1985).

Blue Cross and Blue Shield Association, Medical Necessity Program. Chest x-ray examinations. 1984. [Information syntheses]

Blue Cross and Blue Shield Association, Medical Necessity Program. Radionuclide bone scan and x-ray of bones in the evaluation of bone metastases. 1984. [Information syntheses]

Blue Cross and Blue Shield Association, Medical Necessity Program. Ultrasound and x-ray pelvimetry in maternity care. 1984. [Information syntheses]

Brand DA. [National Center for Health Services Research and Health Care Technology Assessment, Division of Extramural Research] An x-ray screening protocol for extremity injuries. 1984. (NTIS order no. PB84-111384)

American Academy of Pediatrics, Committee on Hospital Care. Preoperative chest radiographs. Pediatrics 1983 May.

Liang M, Komaroff A. [Harvard School of Public Health, Institute for Health Research] Roentgenograms in primary care patients with acute low back pain. Arch Intern Med 1982;142:1108-1112. [Epidemiological methods]

Office of Technology Assessment, U.S. Congress. Assessment of four common X-ray procedures. Washington, D.C.: U.S. Government Printing Office, April 1982. (Health technology case study series #19)

American Academy of Pediatrics, Committee on Radiology. Comparison radiographs of extremities in childhood: recommended usage. Pediatrics 1980 Mar.

American Academy of Pediatrics, Committee on Radiology. Radiation of pregnant women. Pediatrics 1978 Jan.

Neuhauser D. [Harvard School of Public Health, Institute for Health Research] Cost effective clinical decision making: are routine pediatric preoperative chest X-rays worth it? Ann Radiol (Paris) 1978;21:80-83. [Information syntheses]

U.S. Administrators, Professional Policy Committee. Protocol for use of multiple EKG's and chest X-rays in CCUs and ICUs. Ongoing. [Group judgment]

Radionuclide angiography

Pryor DB, et al. [National Center for Health Services Research and Health Care Technology Assessment, Division of Extramural Research] Prognostic indicators from radionuclide angiography in medically treated patients with coronary artery disease. Am J Cardiol 1984 Jan;53:18-22.

Gibbons RJ, et al. [National Center for Health Services Research and Health Care Technology Assessment, Division of Extramural Research] The use of radionuclide angiography in the diagnosis of coronary artery disease; a logistic regression analysis. Circulation 1983 Oct;68(4):740-746.

Radionuclide imaging

O'Rourke RA, Chatterjee K, Dodge HT, et al. [American College of Cardiology/American Heart Association Task Force on Assessment of Cardiovascular Procedures] Guidelines for clinical use of cardiac radionuclide imaging. J Am Coll Cardiology 1986 Dec;8:1471-83. [Group judgment]

U.S. Administrators, Professional Policy Committee. Radionuclide scans (post-operative). [7/86] [Group judgment]

U.S. Administrators, Professional Policy Committee. Radionuclide scans (pre-operative). [7/86] [Group judgment]

Blue Cross and Blue Shield Association, Medical Necessity Program. Outmoded radionuclide imaging procedures. 1984. [Information syntheses]

Blue Cross and Blue Shield Association, Medical Necessity Program. Radionuclide bone scan and x-ray of bones in the evaluation of bone metastases. 1984. [Information syntheses]

Blue Cross and Blue Shield Association, Medical Necessity Program. Radionuclide brain scan in the evaluation of adult intracranial disease. 1984. [Information syntheses]

Office of Technology Assessment, U.S. Congress. Cardiac radionuclide imaging and cost-effectiveness. Washington, D.C.: U.S. Government Printing Office, May 1982. (Health technology case study series #13)

Stason WB, Fortess E. [Harvard School of Public Health, Institute for Health Research] Case study #13: Cardiac radionuclide imaging and cost effectiveness. In: Implications of cost-effectiveness analysis of medical technology. Office of Technology Assessment, U.S. Congress, 1982. [Information syntheses]

Radionuclide laboratories

Health Council of the Netherlands. Classification of and standards for radionuclide laboratories. 1985. (English summary only).

Subcommittee on Institutional Program Guidelines. [Health and Welfare Canada, Health Services and Promotion Branch, Institutional and Professional Services Division] Nuclear medicine units in hospitals. 1985. [Information syntheses, Expert opinion, Group judgment]

Radiopaque plastics

American Dental Association, Council on Dental Materials, Instruments and Equipment. The desirability of using radiopaque plastics in dentistry: a status report. J Am Dent Assoc 1981;102:347-349.

Radiopharmaceuticals

American Medical Association, Council on Scientific Affairs. Safe use of radioactive materials in medical practice (Resolution 66, A-85). 1986. [Group judgment]

Szarek W. [Department Chemistry, Queens University] Radiopharmaceutical development for positron imaging. (Grant period 1981-1985).

Ranitidine

Food and Drug Administration, Center for Drugs and Biologics. Ranitidine HCl. 1987. (Summary basis of approval NDA # 18-703). [Information syntheses, Expert opinion, Epidemiological and other observational methods, Clinical trials, Bench testing]

Food and Drug Administration, Center for Drugs and Biologics. Ranitidine HCl. 1987. (Summary basis of approval substitute, NDA # 19-593). [Information syntheses, Expert opinion, Epidemiological and other observational methods, Clinical trials, Bench testing]

Rectal mucosal replacement

California Medical Association, Medical Practice Opinion Program. Rectal mucosal replacement. 1983 Nov. (Medical Practice Opinion #288) [Group judgment]

Registries

Loeser J, Zvagulis I, Hercz L, Pless IB. [McGill University, Department of Epidemiology and Biostatistics] The organization and evaluation of a computer-assisted centralized immunization registry. Am J Public Health 1983;73(11):1298-1301.

Rehabilitation

Edgar LJ. [National Health Research and Development Program - Canada] Implementation and evaluation of a rehabilitative approach as a part of normal nursing care of cancer patients. 1986. (Grant No. 6605-2223-46).

Subcommittee on Institutional Program Guidelines. [Health and Welfare Canada, Health Services and Promotion Branch, Institutional and Professional Services Division] Rehabilitation medicine program guidelines. 1986. [Information syntheses, Expert opinion, Group judgment]

Gauthier L, Gauthier S. [National Health Research and Development Program - Canada] Group rehabilitation as an adjunct to medical therapy in idiopathic Parkinson's disease. 1985. (Grant No. 6605-1946-05).

Rehabilitation programs—Spinal cord injury

Subcommittee on Institutional Program Guidelines. [Health and Welfare Canada, Health Services and Promotion Branch, Institutional and Professional Services Division] Spinal cord injury program guidelines. 1986. [Information syntheses, Expert opinion, Group judgment]

Rehabilitation programs—Stroke

Subcommittee on Institutional Program Guidelines. [Health and Welfare Canada, Health Services and Promotion Branch, Institutional and Professional Services Division] Stroke program guidelines. 1986. [Information syntheses, Expert opinion, Group judgment]

Rehfuss test

National Center for Health Services Research and Health Care Technology Assessment, Office of Health Technology Assessment. Rehfuss test for gastric acidity. 1982.

Relative value scales

A national study of resource-based relative value scales for Physician Services. In: Office of Research and Demonstrations, Health Care Financing Administration. Health care financing status report: research and demonstrations in health care financing. Jan 1986. (HCFA Pub. No. 03219).

Relaxation therapy

Milner M, Levison H. [National Health Research and Development Program - Canada] Evaluation of relaxed breathing and its augmentation with biofeedback upon bronchospasm induced by methacholine in paediatric patients with chronic asthma. 1986. (Grant No. 6606-2113-53).

U.S. Administrators, Professional Policy Committee. Relaxation therapy for hypertension. Ongoing. [Group judgment]

Reminder systems

Rooser W. [National Health Research and Development Program - Canada] Evaluation of a patient, nurse and physician reminder system for screening procedures in family practice. 1986. (Grant No. 6606-2374-43).

Tierney WM, Hui SC, McDonald CJ. [National Center for Health Services Research and Health Care Technology Assessment, Division of Extramural Research] Delayed feedback of physician performance versus immediate reminders to perform preventive care. Med Care 1986 Aug;24(8):659-666.

Grover S, Gagnon G, Flegel K, Hoey JR. [McGill University, Department of Epidemiology and Biostatistics] Improving appointment-keeping by patients new to a hospital medical clinic with telelphone or mailed reminders. Can Med Assoc J 1983;129:1101-1103.

Reserpine

Curb JD, Hardy RJ, Labarthe DR, et al. [National Heart, Lung, and Blood Institute] Reserpine and breast cancer in the Hypertension Detection and Follow-up Program. Hypertension 1982;4(2):307-311.

Reserpine with chlorthalidone

Veterans Administration, Cooperative Studies Program. Efficacy of low doses of reserpine plus chlorthalidone in comparison with standard dosage of reserpine plus chlorthalidone in hypertension. [1980] [Clinical trials]

Respirators

Subcommittee on Special Services in Hospitals. [Health and Welfare Canada, Health Services and Promotion Branch, Institutional and Professional Services Division] Respiratory technology service unit guidelines. 1978. [Information syntheses, Expert opinion, Group judgment]

Respiratory therapy

Home respiratory therapy services. In: Office of Research and Demonstrations, Health Care Financing Administration. Health care financing status report: research and demonstrations in health care financing. Jan 1986. (HCFA Pub. No. 03219).

Man GCW. [Department Medicine, University Alberta] [Medical Research Council - Canada] The effect of high frequency oscillatory ventillation. (Grant period 1983-1985).

Office of Technology Assessment, U.S. Congress. Assessing selected respiratory therapy modalities: trends and relative costs in the Washington, D.C. area. Washington, D.C.: U.S. Government Printing Office, July 1981. (Health technology case study series #12)

Resuscitation

Zimmerman JE, et al. [National Center for Health Services Research and Health Care Technology Assessment, Division of Extramural Research] The use and implications of do not resuscitate orders in intensive care units. JAMA 1986 Jan 17;255(3):351-356.

Resuscitation—Mouth-to-mouth

California Medical Association, Medical Practice Opinion Program. Transmission of disease via mouth to mouth resuscitation. 1985 June. (Medical Practice Opinion #323) [Group judgment]

Resuscitators

Food and Drug Administration, Center for Devices and Radiological Health. Safety and performance of resuscitators. 1984. (NTIS Order No. PB84-195635).

Reuse of disposables

Georgetown University Medical Center, Institute for Health Policy Analysis. Reuse of disposable medical devices: legal liability and public policy issues. (In press) [Information syntheses, Expert opinion, Group judgment, Cost analyses]

Chu F, Novak N, Radany MH, Perry S. [Georgetown University Medical Center, Institute for Health Policy Analysis] Reuse and reprocessing of disposable medical devices. J Health Care Technol 1986;3:5-12. [Information syntheses, Expert opinion, Group judgment, Cost analyses]

[Georgetown University Medical Center, Institute for Health Policy Analysis] Changing attitudes toward reusing medical devices. Health Span-Report of Health Bus Law 1986;3:14-8. [Information syntheses, Expert opinion, Group judgment, Cost analyses]

National Center for Health Services Research and Health Care Technology Assessment, Office of Health Technology Assessment. Hemodialyzer reuse. 1986.

Perry S. [Georgetown University Medical Center, Institute for Health Policy Analysis] Reuse of medical devices intended for single use only. Health Care Instrum 1985;1:4-8. [Information syntheses, Expert opinion, Group judgment, Cost analyses]

Perry S. [Georgetown University Medical Center, Institute for Health Policy Analysis] Reusing disposable medical devices raises ethical, legal and cost questions. Bus Health 1985;2:53-4. [Information syntheses, Expert opinion, Group judgment, Cost analyses]

Subcommittee on Special Services in Hospitals. [Health and Welfare Canada, Health Services and Promotion Branch, Institutional and Professional Services Division] The reuse of disposables: an information report. 1985. [Information syntheses, Expert opinion, Group judgment]

Georgetown University Medical Center, Institute for Health Policy Analysis. Conference proceedings: International Conference on the Reuse of Disposable Medical Devices in the 1980s. Washington, DC: Institute for Health Policy Analysis, 1984. [Information syntheses, Expert opinion, Group judgment, Cost analyses]

Rheumatology tests

U.S. Administrators, Professional Policy Committee. Arthritis - diagnostic procedures. [7/86] [Group judgment]

Rhinoplasty

California Medical Association, Medical Practice Opinion Program. Assistant surgeon for septorhinoplasty. 1984 Jan. (Medical Practice Opinion #307) [Group judgment]

Ringer's irrigation

Food and Drug Administration, Center for Drugs and Biologics. Ringer's irrigation, USP in flex containers. 1981. (NTIS order no. PB81-915906). [Information syntheses, Expert opinion, Epidemiological and other observational methods, Clinical trials, Bench testing]

Rubella tests

Food and Drug Administration, Center for Devices and Radiological Health. Problem definition study: rubella antibody testing. 1986. (NTIS Order No. PB86-131935).

Rubidium

Chouinard G. [Louis-H. La Fontaine Hospital, Montreal] [Medical Research Council - Canada] A controlled clinical trial of rubidium in chronic schizophrenia. (Grant period 1983-1985).

Saccharin

American Medical Association, Council on Scientific Affairs. Saccharin: review of safety issues. JAMA 1985 Nov 8;254(18):2622-2624. [Group judgment]

Office of Technology Assessment, U.S. Congress. Cancer testing technology and saccharin. Washington, D.C.: U.S. Government Printing Office, October 1977.

Saralasin

Food and Drug Administration, Center for Drugs and Biologics. Saralasin acetate. 1981. (NTIS order no. PB81-915908). [Information syntheses, Expert opinion, Epidemiological and other observational methods, Clinical trials, Bench testing]

Satellite communication

American Hospital Association, Hospital Technology Series Program. Purchasing a satellite receiving earth terminal. 1986. (Guideline report) [Information syntheses, Expert opinion, Cost analyses]

[National Library of Medicine] Performance evaluation of a satellite-linked experimental network. IEEE Trans Aerosp Electron Syst 1980;16:771-82. [Epidemiological and other observational methods]

[National Library of Medicine] Biomedical communications experiments using the communications technology satellite: technical evaluation. Bethesda, MD: Lister Hill Center, National Library of Medicine, 1979. (NTIS order no. PB-80-111-016/GBB). [Epidemiological and other observational methods]

Scales, Patient

ECRI Health Devices Program. Patient bed scales. Health Devices 1984;13:75-91.

Schizophrenia screening

Schwartzman AE, Serbin LA, Ledingham JE. [National Health Research and Development Program - Canada] Identification of children at risk for adult schizophrenia for preventive and early treatment programs: a longitudinal study. 1986. (Grant No. 6605-1865-44).

Scintiphotography—Heart

Croft CH, Rude RE, Lewis SE, et al. [National Heart, Lung, and Blood Institute] Comparison of left ventricular function and infarct size in patients with and without positive technetium-99m pyrophosphate myocardial scintigrams after myocardial infarction: analysis of 357 patients. Am J Cardiol 1984;53:421-428.

Scintiphotography—Joint

National Center for Health Services Research and Health Care Technology Assessment, Office of Health Technology Assessment. The role of joint scans using technetium-99m pertechnetate in diagnosing and assessing therapeutic gain in arthritis. 1981.

Sclerotherapy

Sivak MV. Sclerotherapy of esophageal varices. In: American Society for Gastrointestinal Endoscopy, Committee on Technology Assessment. Therapeutic gastrointestinal endoscopy: an information resource manual. 1987. [Information syntheses, Expert opinion, Group judgment, Cost analyses]

American Collegee of Physicians, Clinical Efficacy Assessment Project. Endoscopic injection sclerotherapy. Ann Intern Med 1984;100:608-10. [Information syntheses]

California Medical Association, Medical Practice Opinion Program. Use of sclerosant injections for neck, back and lower extremity pain. 1984. (Medical Practice Opinion #313) [Group judgment]

U.S. Administrators, Professional Policy Committee. Sclerosing therapy for esophageal varices. Ongoing. [Group judgment]

Veterans Administration, Cooperative Studies Program. Cooperative clinical trial of sclerotherapy for esophageal varices in alcoholic liver disease. Ongoing. [Clinical trials]

Scoliosometry

Fernie GR. [National Health Research and Development Program - Canada] Use of trunk shape measurements to quantify scoliotic deformity. 1986. (Grant No. 6606-2995-51).

Second opinions

Evaluation of the impact of second opinions for elective surgery. In: Office of Research and Demonstrations, Health Care Financing Administration. Health care financing status report: research and demonstrations in health care financing. Jan 1986. (HCFA Pub. No. 03219).

Secretin

Food and Drug Administration, Center for Drugs and Biologics. Secretin. 1981. (NTIS order no. PB81-915908). [Information syntheses, Expert opinion, Epidemiological and other observational methods, Clinical trials, Bench testing]

Selenium sulfide

Food and Drug Administration, Center for Drugs and Biologics. Selenium sulfide. 1983. (NTIS order no. PB83-915902). [Information syntheses, Expert opinion, Epidemiological and other observational methods, Clinical trials, Bench testing]

Sensory integrative therapy

Humphries TW. [National Health Research and Development Program - Canada] The effects of sensory integrative therapy on selected aspects of functioning in learning disabled children. 1986. (Grant No. 6606-2441-43).

Seromucoid assay

National Center for Health Services Research and Health Care Technology Assessment, Office of Health Technology Assessment. Serum seromucoid assay. 1982.

Sex hormones

California Medical Association, Medical Practice Opinion Program. Treatment of rheumatoid arthritis with sex hormones. 1985 Oct. (Medical Practice Opinion #331) [Group judgment]

Shape sensor

Fernie GR. [National Health Research and Development Program - Canada] High speed dimensional shape sensor for clinical application. 1986. (Grant No. 6606-2404-51).

Shoe insoles

Newell E. [National Health Research and Development Program - Canada] Development of a clinical evaluation scheme to test the efficacy of shoe insole materials used in the treatment of metatarsalgia associated with rheumatoid arthritis. 1985. (Grant No. 6606-2144-51).

Sigmoidoscopy

American Society for Gastrointestinal Endoscopy. Flexible sigmoidoscopy. Revised 1986 Mar.

Silver sulfadiazine

Food and Drug Administration, Center for Drugs and Biologics. Silver sulfadiazine. 1982. (NTIS order no. PB82-915902). [Information syntheses, Expert opinion, Epidemiological and other observational methods, Clinical trials, Bench testing]

Singer-Blom valve operation

California Medical Association, Medical Practice Opinion Program. Singer-Blom valve operation. 1981 Jul. (Medical Practice Opinion #262) [Group judgment]

Sisomicin

Food and Drug Administration, Center for Drugs and Biologics. Sisomicin sulfate. 1981. (NTIS order no. PB81-915901). [Information syntheses, Expert opinion, Epidemiological and other observational methods, Clinical trials, Bench testing]

Smoke detectors

American Medical Association, Council on Scientific Affairs. Preventing death and disability from fires by the new rapid response automatic sprinklers and smoke detectors (Resolution 2, A-85). 1986. [Group judgment]

Socket prosthesis

Durance JP. [National Health Research and Development Program - Canada] Modular sockets in the prosthetic fitting of below-knee amputees (evaluation). 1986 (Grant No. 6606-2315-01).

Fernie GR. [National Health Research and Development Program - Canada] An evaluation of computer-aided design of trans-tibial prosthetic sockets. 1986. (Grant No. 6606-3024-51).

Sodium cellulose phosphate

Food and Drug Administration, Center for Drugs and Biologics. Sodium cellulose phosphate. 1987. (Summary basis of approval, NDA #18-757). [Information syntheses, Expert opinion, Epidemiological and other observational methods, Clinical trials, Bench testing]

Sodium chloride

Akorn, Inc. [Food and Drug Administration, Center for Devices and Radiological Health] Sodium chloride tablets, USP: summary of safety and effectiveness. 1986 Mar 14. (PMA no. 850037-000).

Ocumed Inc. [Food and Drug Administration, Center for Devices and Radiological Health] Sodium chloride tablets 250 mg: summary of safety and effectiveness. 1986 Mar 12. (PMA no. P850016-000).

Food and Drug Administration, Center for Drugs and Biologics. CaCl2, MgCl, Kcl, & NaCl. 1982. (NTIS order no. PB82-915902). [Information syntheses, Expert opinion, Epidemiological and other observational methods, Clinical trials, Bench testing]

Food and Drug Administration, Center for Drugs and Biologics. 0.45% sodium chloride injection, USP. 1981. (NTIS order no. PB81-915909). [Information syntheses, Expert opinion, Epidemiological and other observational methods, Clinical trials, Bench testing]

Food and Drug Administration, Center for Drugs and Biologics. 0.9% sodium chloride injection, USP. 1981. (NTIS order no. PB81-915909). [Information syntheses, Expert opinion, Epidemiological and other observational methods, Clinical trials, Bench testing]

Sodium phosphate

Food and Drug Administration, Center for Drugs and Biologics. NaCl, KCl, MgSO4, NaPO4, & KPO4. 1982. (NTIS order no. PB82-915901). [Information syntheses, Expert opinion, Epidemiological and other observational methods, Clinical trials, Bench testing]

Sodium restriction

Langford HG, Schlundt D, Levine K. [National Heart, Lung, and Blood Institute] Sodium restriction in hypertension. Compr Ther 1984;10:6-11.

Wassertheil-Smoller S, Langford HG, Blaaufox MD, et al. [National Heart, Lung, and Blood Institute] Diuretics and salt-restriction in blood pressure control. In: Winick M ed. Nutrition and drugs. New York: John Wiley and Sons Inc, 1983:175-189.

Somatic cell mutation tests

Tomkins DJ. [National Health Research and Development Program - Canada] Validation of in vivo somatic cell mutation tests in human populations. 1986. (Grant No. 6606-2688-52).

Tomkins DJ. [National Health Research and Development Program - Canada] In vivo tests for somatic cell mutation in man. 1985. (Grant No. 6606-2074-52).

Sorbitol

Olefsky JM, Crapo P. [American Diabetes Association] Fructose, xylitol, and sorbitol. Diabetes Care 1980;3:390-393. [Expert opinion, Group judgment]

SPECT imaging

ECRI Technology Assessment Program. SPECT imaging. J Health Care Technol 1986;3:33-62. [Information syntheses]

Sperm penetration assay

Blue Cross and Blue Shield Association, Technology Evaluation and Coverage Program. Sperm penetration assay. 1986. [Information syntheses]

American Medical Association, Diagnostic and Therapeutic Technology Assessment. Sperm penetration assay in identifying male infertility. JAMA 1985 Oct 11. [Expert opinion, Information syntheses]

Sphincterotomy

Silvis SE. Endoscopic retrograde sphincterotomy (ERS). In: American Society for Gastrointestinal Endoscopy, Committee on Technology Assessment. Therapeutic gastrointestinal endoscopy: an information resource manual. 1987. [Information syntheses;Expert opinion, Group judgment, Cost analyses]

American College of Physicians, Clinical Efficacy Assessment Project. Efficacy of endoscopic retrograde cholangiopancreatography (ERCP) and endoscopic retrograde sphincterotomy (ERS). 1984. [Information syntheses]

Spinal puncture

American College of Physicians, Clinical Efficacy Assessment Project. The diagnostic spinal tap. Ann Intern Med 1986;104:880-5,840-8. [Information syntheses]

Sporicidin

American Dental Association, Council on Dental Therapeutics. Council accepts dilution claims for Sporicidin. J Am Dent Assoc 1980;100:918.

Sprinklers

American Medical Association, Council on Scientific Affairs. Preventing death and disability from fires by the new rapid response automatic sprinklers and smoke detectors (Resolution 2, A-85). 1986. [Group judgment]

Standardized Medreview Instrument

An independent evaluation of the reliability of the Standardized Medreview Instrument. In: Office of Research and Demonstrations, Health Care Financing Administration. Health care financing status report: research and demonstrations in health care financing. Jan 1986. (HCFA Pub. No. 03219)

Appropriateness of hospitalization: a comparative analysis of reliability and validity of the Appropriateness Evaluation Protocol and the Standardized Medreview Instrument. In: Office of Research and Demonstrations, Health Care Financing Administration. Health care financing status report: research and demonstrations in health care financing. Jan 1986. (HCFA Pub. No. 03219).

Stapedectomy

California Medical Association, Medical Practice Opinion Program. Stapedectomy for otosclerosis. 1983 Sep. (Medical Practice Opinion #302) [Group judgment]

Stereotaxic depth electrode implantation

National Center for Health Services Research and Health Care Technology Assessment, Office of Health Technology Assessment. Stereotaxic depth electrode implantation prior to surgical treament of focal epilepsy. 1981.

Stereotaxic neurosurgery, Computed tomography-assisted

ECRI Technology Assessment Program. CT-assisted stereotactic neurosurgery. Issues Health Care Technol 1985;sec.5.S.3. [Information syntheses]

Sterile water for injection

Food and Drug Administration, Center for Drugs and Biologics. Sterile water for injection, USP. 1981. (NTIS order no . PB81-915909. [Information syntheses, Expert opinion, Epidemiological and other observational methods, Clinical trials, Bench testing]

Sterilization equipment

American Hospital Association, Hospital Technology Series Program. Ethylene oxide sterilization. 1982. (Guideline report) [Information synthesis, expert opinion, Cost analyses]

Sterilizers

American Dental Association, Council on Dental Therapeutics. Acceptance of OMNI-II disinfectant for instruments and equipment. J Am Dent Assoc 1985;110.

ECRI Health Devices Program. Ethylene oxide sterilizers. Health Devices 1982;11:287-301.

Steroids

American College of Obstetricians and Gynecologists, Committee Opinion. Teratogenicity of steroids. Pending. [Information syntheses]

Veterans Administration, Cooperative Studies Program. Alcoholic hepatitis (steroid therapy). [1980] [Clinical trials]

Stool guaiac

Neuhauser D, Lewicki A. [Harvard School of Public Health, Institute for Health Research] What do we gain from the sixth stool guaiac? N Eng J Med 1975;293:226-228. [Epidemiological methods]

Streptokinase

U.S. Administrators, Professional Policy Committee. Streptokinase. [7/86] [Group judgment]

ECRI Technology Assessment Program. Streptokinase thrombolysis of coronary arteries. Issues Health Care Technol 1985;sec.5.T.1. [Information syntheses]

Hillis LD, Borer J, Braunwald E, et al. [National Heart, Lung, and Blood Institute] High dose intravenous streptokinase for acute myocardial infarction: preliminary results of a multicenter trial. J Am Coll Cardiol 1985;6:957-962.

National Center for Health Services Research and Health Care Technology Assessment, Office of Health Technology Assessment. Streptokinase infusion for acute myocardial infarction. 1984.

California Medical Association, Medical Practice Opinion Program. Intravenous streptokinase after myocardial infarction. 1983 June. (Medical Practice Opinion #287) [Group judgment]

John Hopkins Program for Medical Technology and Practice Assessment. Analysis of the comparative cost-effectiveness of alternative strategies for managing acute heart attacks, including use of thrombolytic drugs, such as tissue plasminogen activator and steptokinase, and emergency coronary angioplasty. Ongoing.

Streptozocin

Food and Drug Administration, Center for Drugs and Biologics. Streptozocin. 1982. (NTIS order no. PB82-915903).

Sucralfate

Food and Drug Administration, Center for Drugs and Biologics. Sucralfate. 1982. (NTIS order no. PB82-915901). [Information syntheses, Expert opinion, Epidemiological and other observational methods, Clinical trials, Bench testing]

Suction equipment

ECRI Health Devices Program. Suction canisters (aspirator collection bottles). Health Devices 1985;14:411-34.

ECRI Health Devices Program. Suction regulators. Health Devices 1985;14:191-209.

ECRI Health Devices Program. Suction canisters (aspirator collection bottles). Health Devices 1983;12:127-49.

Suction lipectomy

California Medical Association, Medical Practice Opinion Program. Suction lipectomy. 1985 Dec. (Medical Practice Opinion #286) [Group judgment]

Sulfadoxine

Food and Drug Administration, Center for Drugs and Biologics. Sulfadoxine and pyrimethamine. 1982. (NTIS order no. PB82-915901). [Information syntheses, Expert opinion, Epidemiological and other observational methods, Clinical trials, Bench testing]

Sulfamethoxazole

Food and Drug Administration, Center for Drugs and Biologics. Sulfamethoxazole and trimethoprim. 1981. (NTIS order no. PB81-915909). [Information syntheses, Expert opinion, Epidemiological and other observational methods, Clinical trials, Bench testing]

Veterans Administration, Cooperative Studies Program. Prospective evaluation of the efficacy & tolerance of oral trimethoprim sulfamethoxazole prophylaxis in granulocytopenic patients with acute non-lymphocytic leukemia. Ongoing. [Clinical trials]

Sulfinpyrazone

Gent M, Barnett HJM, Sackett DL, Taylor DW. [McMaster University, Department of Clinical Epidemiology and Biostatistics] A randomized trial of aspirin and sulfinpyrazone in patients with threatened stroke: results and methodologic issues. Circulation 1980;62(Suppl V):V-97.

Suloctidil

Gent M, Blakely JA, Hachinski V, et al. [McMaster University. Department of Clinical Epidemiology and Biostatistics] A secondary prevention, randomized trial of suloctidil in patients with a recent history of thromboembolic stroke. Stroke 1985;16(3).

Sunlamps

Food and Drug Administration, Center for Devices and Radiological Health. Quality control guide for sunlamp products. 1985. (NTIS Order No. PB85-124808).

Supportive care

Mitchell A. [National Health Research and Development Program - Canada] Pilot study: a randomized controlled trial of supportive care for patients with ulcerative colitis. 1986. (Grant No. 6606-2769-43).

National Institutes of Health, Consensus Development Program. Supportive therapy in burn care. (Consensus Development Conference Statement, Nov 10-11 1978). [Group judgment]

Surgery

Duncan PG. [National Health Research and Development Program - Canada] The influence of anesthesia and surgery on the outcome of pregnancy - pilot analysis. 1986. (Grant No. 6607-1289-53).

Johnston CC. [National Health Research and Development Program - Canada] Comparison of preparation for surgery in children undergoing major and minor surgery. 1986. (Grant No. 6605-1955-04).

Post-surgical mortality among the aged for common operations. In: Office of Research and Demonstrations, Health Care Financing Administration. Health care financing status report: research and demonstrations in health care financing. Jan 1986. (HCFA Pub. No. 03219).

Rehospitalization after surgery among Medicare enrollees. In: Office of Research and Demonstrations, Health Care Financing Administration. Health care financing status report: research and demonstrations in health care financing. Jan 1986. (HCFA Pub. No. 03219).

Roos LL, Ross NP. [National Health Research and Development Program - Canada] A collaborative analysis of common surgical procedures. 1986. (Grant No. 6607-1197-44).

Sloan FA, Perrin JM, Valvona J. [National Center for Health Services Research and Health Care Technology Assessment, Division of Extramural Research] Inhospital mortality of surgical patients: is there an empiric basis for standard setting? Surgery 1986 Apr;99(4):446-453.

The relation of surgical volume and other factors to mortality after surgery. In: Office of Research and Demonstrations, Health Care Financing Administration. Health care financing status report: research and demonstrations in health care financing. Jan 1986. (HCFA Pub. No. 03219).

Sloan FA. [National Center for Health Services Research and Health Care Technology Assessment, Division of Extramural Research] Diffusion of surgical technology. 1985 Jul. (NTIS order no. PB86-124559/AS)

Ruthow IM. [National Center for Health Services Research and Health Care Technology Assessment, Division of Extramural Research] Surgical decision making and operative rates. 1983. (NTIS order no. PB83-141929)

Barnes BA, Barnes AB. [Harvard School of Public Health, Institute for Health Research] Evaluation of surgical therapy by cost-benefit analysis. Surgery 1977;82:21-33. [Information syntheses]

Bunker J, Barnes B, Mosteller F, eds. Costs, risks, and benefits of surgery. New York: Oxford University Press, 1977. [Information syntheses]

Health Council of the Netherlands. Pediatric surgery. Ongoing assessment.

Surgery—Ambulatory

University of Pennsylvania, Leonard Davis Institute of Health Economics. Designing and evaluating incentives for ambulatory surgery: a nationwide study. 1986 Dec. (Study for Robert Wood Johnson Foundation)

Subcommittee on Special Services in Hospitals. [Health and Welfare Canada, Health Services and Promotion Branch, Institutional and Professional Services Division] Day surgery unit guidelines. 1982. [Information syntheses, Expert opinion, Group judgment]

Johns Hopkins Program for Medical Technology and Practice Assessment. An analysis of the comparative costs of inpatient versus outpatient surgery for several types of surgery. Planned.

Surgery—Arthritis

U.S. Administrators, Professional Policy Committee. Arthritis - surgical intervention. [7/86] [Group judgment]

Surgery—Breast

Office of Technology Assessment, U.S. Congress. Surgery for breast cancer. Washington, D.C.: U.S. Government Printing Office, October 1981. (Health technology case study series #17)

Surgery—Esophageal reflux

Veterans Administration, Cooperative Studies Program. A prospective randomized trial of medical and surgical therapies for gastroesophageal reflux disease. Ongoing. [Clinical trials]

Surgery—Eye

U.S. Administrators, Professional Policy Committee. Eye surgery. [7/86] [Group judgment]

Surgery—Fetal

Bermel J. [The Hastings Center] Mothers vs. their babies in fetal therapy. Dialog Pediat Urol 1986 Jan.

American Medical Association, Council on Scientific Affairs. In-utero fetal surgery: (Resolution 73 (I-81). JAMA 1983 Sep 16;250:1443-1444. [Group judgment]

Health Council of the Netherlands. Fetal surgery. Ongoing assessment.

Surgery—Heart

Health Council of the Netherlands. Cardiac surgery. 1984.

Health Council of the Netherlands. Coronary heart surgery. 1976.

Surgery—Impotence

National Center for Health Services Research and Health Care Technology Assessment, Office of Health Technology Assessment. Treatments for impotence: surgical treatments. Ongoing.

Surgery—Morbid obesity

U.S. Administrators, Professional Policy Committee. Morbid obesity. [7/86] [Group judgment]

American Medical Association, Diagnostic and Therapeutic Technology Assessment. Gastric restrictive surgery for morbid obesity. JAMA 1984 Jun 8. [Expert opinion, Information syntheses]

ECRI Technology Assessment Program. Surgery for morbid obesity. Issues Health Care Technol 1984;sec.5.S.2. [Information syntheses]

Eddy DM, Eddy JF, Sanders LE. [Duke University, Center for Health Policy Research and Education] Surgical treatment of obesity. Evidence of effectiveness and risks. Report prepared for the North Carolina Blue Cross and Blue Shield Asociation. 1983. [Information syntheses]

National Institutes of Health, Consensus Development Program. Surgical treatment of morbid obesity. (Consensus Development Conference Statement, Dec 4-5 1978). [Group judgment]

Surgery—Prostate

Veterans Administration, Cooperative Studies Program. A randomized study of prostatic surgery for moderately symptomatic benign prostatic hyperplasia in elderly men. Ongoing. [Clinical trials]

Surgery—Scoliosis

U.S. Administrators, Professional Policy Committee. Kyphoscoliosis surgery. [7/86] [Group judgment]

Viviani GR. [Department Surgery, McMaster University] [Medical Research Council - Canada] Biomechanical studies of surgical systems to correct spinal deformities. (Grant period 1982-1985).

Surgical aids—Ophthalmic

Cilco, Inc. [Food and Drug Administration, Center for Devices and Radiological Health] Sodium chrondroitin sulfate: summary of safety and effectiveness. 1986 Nov 5. (PMA no. P820079-000).

Cilco. [Food and Drug Administration, Center for Devices and Radiological Health] Viscoat (TM): summary of safety and effectiveness. 1986 Jun 6. (PMA no.P840064-000).

Pharmacia Diagnostics. [Food and Drug Administration, Center for Devices and Radiological Health] Healon: summary of safety and effectiveness. 1983 Feb 8. (PMA no. P810031-000).

Precision-Cosmet, Co. [Food and Drug Administration, Center for Devices and Radiological Health] AMVISC (R): summary of safety and effectiveness. 1983 Nov 28. (PMA no. P810025-000).

Surgical case carts

ECRI Health Devices Program. Surgical case carts. Health Devices 1982;11:311-24.

ECRI Health Devices Program. Surgical case carts. Health Devices 1982;12:33-9.

Surgical drapes

ECRI Health Devices Program. Surgical drapes. Health Devices 1986;15:111-40.

Surgical gloves

ECRI Health Devices Program. Surgical gloves, latex. Health Devices 1983;12:83-98.

Surgical shunt

Veterans Administration, Cooperative Studies Program. Surgical shunt vs. medical treatment in alcoholic cirrhosis ascites. Pending. [Clinical trials]

Surgical stapling

California Medical Association, Medical Practice Opinion Program. Arthroscopic stapling of an unstable shoulder. 1985 Sep. (Medical Practice Opinion #335) [Group judgment]

Sutures

Ethicon, Inc. [Food and Drug Administration, Center for Devices and Radiological Health] PDS suture (dyed): summary of safety and effectiveness. 1986 Jul 22. (PMA no. N18331-016).

W.L. Gore & Assoc., Inc. [Food and Drug Administration, Center for Devices and Radiological Health] Gore-Tex (R) expanded PTFE suture: summary of safety and effectiveness.1986 Feb 28. (PMA no. P820083-000).

Davis & Geck. [Food and Drug Administration, Center for Devices and Radiological Health] Novafil (TM): summary of safety and effectiveness. 1985 Nov 18. (PMA no. P840041-000).

Howmedica, Inc. [Food and Drug Administration, Center for Devices and Radiological Health] Deklene (TM): summary of safety and effectiveness. 1982 Jun 4. (PMA no. P810028-000).

Syphilis tests

Blue Cross and Blue Shield Association, Medical Necessity Program. Syphilis tests. 1987. [Information syntheses]

Syringe pumps

Netherlands Organization for Applied Scientific Research, Medical Technology Unit (TNO). Syringe pumps for non-ambulatory use. 1986.

Systeme International units

American Medical Association, Council on Scientific Affairs. SI units for clinical laboratory data. JAMA 1985 May 3;253:2553-2554. [Group judgment]

American Medical Association, Council on Scientific Affairs. Progress in adoption of SI units. 1980. [Group judgment]

Tamoxifen

Gavin NI, Hasselblad V, Eddy DM. [Duke University, Center for Health Policy Research and Education] The role of adjuvant tamoxifen treatment of postmenopausal women with stage II breast cancer. (Expected publication 1988) [Information syntheses]

Team care

Wood-Dauphinee SS, et al. [McGill University, Department of Epidemiology and Biostatistics] A randomized trial of team care following stroke. Stroke 1984;15:864-872.

Technetium Tc 99m kits

Food and Drug Administration, Center for Drugs and Biologics. Technetium Tc 99m albumin colloid kit. 1983. (NTIS order no. PB83-915902). [Information syntheses, Expert opinion, Epidemiological and other observational methods, Clinical trials, Bench testing]

Food and Drug Administration, Center for Drugs and Biologics. Technetium Tc 99M succimer kit. 1982. (NTIS order no. PB82-915903). [Information syntheses, Expert opinion, epidemiological and other observational methods, Clinical trials, Bench testing]

Food and Drug Administration, Center for Drugs and Biologics. Technetium Tc 99m disofenin kit. 1982. (NTIS order no. PB82-915902). [Information syntheses, Expert opinion, Epidemiological and other observational methods, Clinical trials, Bench testing]

Food and Drug Administration, Center for Drugs and Biologics. Technetium 99m oxidronate kit. 1981. (NTIS order no. PB81-915905). [Information syntheses, Expert opinion, Epidemiological and other observational methods, Clinical trials, Bench testing]

Food and Drug Administration, Center for Drugs and Biologics. Technetium Tc 99m medronate kit. 1981. (NTIS order no. PB81-915905). [Information syntheses, Expert opinion, Epidemiological and other observational methods, Clinical trials, Bench testing]

Telemetry

University of Pennsylvania, Leonard Davis Institute of Health Economics. The effect of telemetry on advanced life support care. 1984 Apr. (Final Report to the National Center for Health Services Research, DHHS)

Temazepam

Food and Drug Administration, Center for Drugs and Biologics. Temazepam. 1981. (NTIS order no. PB81-915905). [Information syntheses, Expert opinion, Epidemiological and other observational methods, Clinical trials, Bench testing]

Temporomandibular joint procedure

California Medical Association, Medical Practice Opinion Program. Temporomandibular joint procedure. 1984 Feb. (Medical Practice Opinion #270) [Group judgment]

Thallium imaging

American College of Physicians, Clinical Efficacy Assessment Project. Exercise thallium scanning, expected completion 1988. [Information syntheses]

U.S. Administrators, Professional Policy Committee. Thallium and/or equilibrium-gated myocardial imaging. [7/86] [Group judgment]

Theophylline

Fox ZR, Dupont C, Kramer MS, Stewart JH. [McGill University, Department of Epidemiology and Biostatistics] A double-blind crossover comparison between Phyllocontin and Theo-Dur in asthmatic children. In: Turner-Warwick M, Levy J, eds. New perspectives in theophylline therapy. London: Royal Society of Medicine, 1984:29-37.

Food and Drug Administration, Center for Drugs and Biologics. Theophylline in 5% dextrose injection in plastic container. 1982. (NTIS order no. PB82-915904). [Information syntheses, Expert opinion, Epidemiological and other observational methods, Clinical trials, Bench testing]

Therapeutic drug monitoring

ECRI Technology Assessment Program. Therapeutic drug monitoring (TDM). J Health Care Technol 1984;1:39-61. [Information syntheses]

Therapeutic embolization

ECRI Technology Assessment Program. Transcatheter therapeutic embolization. Issues Health Care Technol 1984;sec.5.E.3. [Information syntheses]

Thermography

California Medical Association, Medical Practice Opinion Program. Thermography for spinal problems. 1982 Jul. (Medical Practice Opinion #269) [Group judgment]

American Medical Association, Diagnostic and Therapeutic Technology Assessment. Thermography (electronic and liquid crystal) for diagnosing low-back pain. Ongoing. [Expert opinion, Information syntheses]

National Center for Health Services Research and Health Care Technology Assessment, Office of Health Technology Assessment. Thermography for indications for other than breast lesions. Ongoing.

Thermography—Breast

ECRI Technology Assessment Program. Thermography for breast cancer prescreening. Issues Health Care Technol 1985;sec.5.T.5. [Information syntheses]

American College of Radiology, Task Force on Breast Cancer. Policy statement on thermography for the detection of breast cancer. 1983 Sep 28. [Group judgment]

National Center for Health Services Research and Health Care Technology Assessment, Office of Health Technology Assessment. Thermography for breast cancer detection. 1983.

Thermometers

Food and Drug Administration, Center for Devices and Radiological Health. Problem definition study in liquid crystal forehead temperature strips. 1984. (NTIS Order No. PB84-187483).

ECRI Health Devices Program. Electronic intermittent thermometers. Health Devices 1982;12:3-20.

Thoracentesis

American College of Physicians, Clinical Efficacy Assessment Project. Congestive heart failure and thoracentesis, 1986. [Information syntheses]

American College of Physicians, Clinical Efficacy Assessment Project. Diagnostic thoracentesis and pleural biopsy. Ann Intern Med 1985;103:799-802. [Information syntheses]

Throat cultures

Blue Cross and Blue Shield Association, Medical Necessity Program. Throat cultures and rapid test for diagnosing group A streptococcal pharyngitis. 1987. [Information syntheses]

Thrombolytic therapy

American College of Physicians, Clinical Efficacy Assessment Project. Thrombolysis for evolving myocardial infarction. Ann Intern Med 1985;103:463-9. [Information syntheses]

TIMI Study Group. [National Heart, Lung, and Blood Institute] Special report. The Thrombolysis in Myocardial Infarction (TIMI) Trial. Phase I findings. N Engl J Med 1985;312:932-936.

California Medical Association, Medical Practice Opinion Program. Thrombolytic therapy for pulmonary embolism. 1983 Feb. (Medical Practice Opinion #281) [Group judgment]

National Institutes of Health, Consensus Development Program. Thrombolytic therapy in thrombosis. (Consensus Development Conference Statement, Apr 10-12 1980). [Group judgment]

Thymoxamine

American Academy of Ophthalmology. Thymoxamine: the need for orphan drug status. San Francisco, CA: American Academy of Ophthalmology, 1986. [Information syntheses, Expert opinion]

Thyroxine assays

United Kingdom Department of Health and Social Security, Medical Devices Evaluation Programme. Comparative evaluation of free thyroxine assay kits. 1985 Nov. (Report no. STB3A/85/44) [Epidemiological and other observational methods, Bench testing]

Tibial osteotomy

Milner M. [National Health Research and Development Program - Canada] The effects of proximal tibial osteotomy and tibial tubercle elevation on knee and ankle joint loading. 1986. (Grant No. 6606-2740-51).

Tibial tubercle elevation

Milner M. [National Health Research and Development Program - Canada] The effects of proximal tibial osteotomy and tibial tubercle elevation on knee and ankle joint loading. 1986. (Grant No. 6606-2740-51).

Timolol

Food and Drug Administration, Center for Drugs and Biologics. Timolol maleate & hydrochlorothiazide. 1982. (NTIS order no. PB82-915901). [Information syntheses, Expert opinion, Epidemiological and other observational methods, Clinical trials, Bench testing]

Tinnitus maskers

National Center for Health Services Research and Health Care Technology Assessment, Office of Health Technology Assessment. Tinnitus maskers. 1981.

Tioconazole

Food and Drug Administration, Center for Drugs and Biologics. Tioconazole. 1983. (NTIS order no. PB83-915902). [Information syntheses, Expert opinion, Epidemiological and other observational methods, Clinical trials, Bench testing]

Tissue banks

Bergeron C. [Department Pathology, University Toronto] [Medical Research Council - Canada] Canadian brain tissue bank. (Grant period 1983-1985).

Tissue plasminogen activators

Eddy DM. [Duke University, Center for Health Policy Research and Education] The use of confidence profiles to assess tissue-type plasminogen activator. In: Califf RM, Wanger GS, eds. Acute coronary care. Boston: Martinus Nijhoff Publishing, 1987. [Information syntheses]

ECRI Technology Assessment Program. Plasminogen activator thrombolysis of coronary arteries. Issues Health Care Technol 1984;sec.5.T.4. [Information syntheses]

Williams DO, Passamani ER, et al. [National Heart, Lung, and Blood Institute] Intravenous recombinant tissue-type plasminogen activator in patients with acute myocardial infarction: a report from the NHLBI Thrombolysis in Myocardial Infarction Trial. Circulation 1986;73:338-346.

Johns Hopkins Program for Medical Technology and Practice Assessment. Analysis of the comparative cost-effectiveness of alternative strategies for managing acute heart attacks, including use of thrombolytic drugs, such as tissue plasminogen activator and steptokinase, and emergency coronary angioplasty. Ongoing.

Tissue preservation technics

Rock GA. [National Health Research and Development Program - Canada] Storage of platelets for 5 days - optimization of conditions by factorial analysis. 1986. (Grant No. 6613-1208-52).

Tobramycin

Food and Drug Administration, Center for Drugs and Biologics. Tobramycin. 1982. (NTIS order no. 82-915901). [Information syntheses, Expert opinion, Epidemiological and other observational methods, Clinical trials, Bench testing]

Tocodynamometry

Office of Technology Assessment, U.S. Congress. Effectiveness and costs of ambulatory tocodynamometry. Washington, D.C.: U.S. Government Printing Office, to be completed in Spring 1987.

Blue Cross and Blue Shield Association, Technology Evaluation and Coverage Program. Ambulatory uterine monitoring. 1986. [Information syntheses]

California Medical Association, Medical Practice Opinion Program. Ambulatory monitoring of uterine activity. 1986 Jul. (Medical Practice Opinion #342) [Group judgment]

Tomography, Standard

American College of Physicians, Clinical Efficacy Assessment Project. A comparative assessment of standard and computed tomography in the evaluation of neoplasms of the chest. 1986. [Information syntheses]

Tonometry

Eddy DM, Sanders L, Eddy J. [Duke University, Center for Health Policy Research and Education] The value of screening for glaucoma with tonometry. Surv Ophthalmol 1983;28:194-205. [Information syntheses]

Tonsillectomy

California Medical Association, Medical Practice Opinion Program. Indications for tonsillectomy. 1985 Dec. (Medical Practice Opinion #326) [Group judgment]

National Institutes of Health, Consensus Development Program. Indications for tonsillectomy and adenoidectomy: phase I. (Consensus Development Conference Statement, Jul 20 1978). [Group judgment]

Tooth extraction

National Institutes of Health, Consensus Development Program. Removal of third molars. (Consensus Development Conference Statement, Nov 28-30 1979). [Group judgment]

Toothpaste

American Dental Association, Council on Dental Therapeutics. Acceptance of Promise with Fluoride and Sensodyne-F toothpastes for sensitive teeth. J Am Dent Assoc 1986;113:673-5.

American Dental Association, Council on Dental Therapeutics. Acceptance of Sensodyne toothpaste for sensitive teeth. J Am Dent Assoc 1985;110.

Clark DC, Hanley JA, Geoghegan S, Vinet D. [McGill University, Department of Epidemiology and Biostatistics] The effectiveness of a desensitizing toothpaste in treating dentinal hypersensitivity. J Periodontol Res 1985;20:212-219.

American Dental Association, Council on Dental Therapeutics. Evaluation of Denquel Sensitive Teeth toothpaste. J Am Dent Assoc 1982;105.

American Dental Association, Council on Dental Therapeutics. Council accepts Aim with sodium monofluorophosphate. J Am Dent Assoc 1980;101:822.

Topographic brain mapping

American Hospital Association, Hospital Technology Series Program. Topographic brain mapping. 1987. (Guideline report) [Information syntheses, Expert opinion, Cost analyses]

California Medical Association, Medical Practice Opinion Program. Topographic brain mapping. 1987 Mar. (Medical Practice Opinion #345) [Group judgment]

American Academy of Neurology, Practice Committee. Topographic mapping. 1985. Feb. [Expert opinion, Group judgment]

Tourniquets

ECRI Health Devices Program. Pneumatic tourniquets. Health Devices 1984;13:299-316.

TOXLINE

[National Library of Medicine] Evaluation of the scope and coverage of NLM's TOXLINE. Bethesda, MD: National Library of Medicine. Ongoing. [Epidemiological and other observational methods]

Transcutaneous electrical nerve stimulation

National Center for Health Services Research and Health Care Technology Assessment, Office of Health Technology Assessment. Transcutaneous electrical nerve stimulation for acute pain treatment for ambulatory patients. 1984.

American Academy of Neurology, Practice Committee. Trancutaneous electrical nerve stimulation for treatment of acute pain for ambulatory patients. 1983 Nov. [Expert opinion, Group judgment]

California Medical Association, Medical Practice Opinion Program. Transcutaneous electrical nerve stimulation. 1982 Jul. (Medical Practice Opinion #82) [Group judgment]

National Center for Health Services Research and Health Care Technology Assessment, Office of Health Technology Assessment. Transcutaneous electrical nerve stimulation for acute postoperative incision pain. 1981.

Transfer factor therapy

American Academy of Neurology, Practice Committee. Transfer factor treatment in multiple sclerosis. 1980 Apr. [Expert opinion, Group judgment]

Transillumination—Breast

Brown RE, Schipper, H. [National Health Research and Development Program - Canada] Electronic diaphanography (E/DPG) as an adjunct to the early diagnosis of breast cancer. 1986. (Grant No. 6607-1304-07).

American Medical Association, Diagnostic and Therapeutic Technology Assessment. Diaphanography (transillumination of the the breast) for cancer screening. JAMA 1984 Apr 18. [Expert opinion, Information syntheses]

National Center for Health Services Research and Health Care Technology Assessment, Office of Health Technology Assessment. Transillumination light scanning for the diagnosis of breast cancer. 1984.

National Center for Health Services Research and Health Care Technology Assessment, Office of Health Technology Assessment. Transillumination light scanning for use in detection of diseases of the breast. Ongoing.

Transplantation

Health Council of the Netherlands. Transplantation issues. 1987.

Caplan A. [The Hastings Center] The morality and immorality of reuse. Renal Life. 1986 Oct.

U.S. Administrators, Professional Policy Committee. Organ transplantation. [7/86] [Group judgment]

American Medical Association, Council on Scientific Affairs. Xenografts: Review of the literature and current status. JAMA 1985 Dec 20;254(23):3353. [Group judgment; Information syntheses]

Health Council of the Netherlands. Transplantation: ethical and legal; kidney; heart; liver; pancreas; bone marrow. Ongoing assessment.

Transplantation—Bone marrow

Medical Technology and Practice Patterns Institute. Bone marrow transplantation. 1987.

U.S. Administrators, Professional Policy Committee. Bone marrow transplantation. [7/86] [Group judgment]

ECRI Technology Assessment Program. Bone marrow transplantation. Issues Health Care Technol 1985;sec.5.B.5. [Information syntheses]

American Medical Association, Diagnostic and Therapeutic Technology Assessment. Bone marrow transplantation in childhood leukemia. JAMA 1984 Apr 27. [Expert opinion, Information syntheses]

Office of Technology Assessment, U.S. Congress. The cost-effectiveness of bone marrow transplant therapy and its policy implications. Washington, D.C.: U.S. Government Printing Office, May 1981. (Health technology case study series #6)

Health Council of the Netherlands. Bone marrow transplantation. Ongoing.

U.S. Administrators, Professional Policy Committee. Bone marrow transplant - reconsideration. Ongoing. [Group judgment]

Transplantation—Bone marrow, Allogenic

Blue Cross and Blue Shield Association, Technology Evaluation and Coverage Program. Bone marrow transplantation, allogeneic. 1986. [Information syntheses]

Health Council of the Netherlands. Allogenic bone marrow transplantation. 1985. (English summary only).

National Center for Health Services Research and Health Care Technology Assessment, Office of Health Technology Assessment. Allogenic bone marrow transplantation for indications other than aplastic anemia and leukemia. 1985.

Transplantation—Bone marrow, Autologous

American Medical Association, Diagnostic and Therapeutic Technology Assessment. Autologous bone marrow transplantation. JAMA 1986 Jul 4. [Expert opinion, Information syntheses]

Blue Cross and Blue Shield Association, Technology Evaluation and Coverage Program. Bone marrow transplantation, autologous. 1986. [Information syntheses]

National Center for Health Services Research and Health Care Technology Assessment, Office of Health Technology Assessment. Autologous bone marrow transplantation (ABMT). 1985.

National Center for Health Services Research and Health Care Technology Assessment, Office of Health Technology Assessment. Reassessment of autologous bone marrow transplantation (ABMT). Ongoing.

Transplantation—Cornea

U.S. Administrators, Professional Policy Committee. Epikeratophakia grafts. [7/86] [Group judgment]

Transplantation—Heart

Medical Technology and Practice Patterns Institute. Heart transplantation. 1987.

Project HOPE, Center for Health Affairs. Paying for heart transplantation under Medicare. (for Prospective Payment Assessment Commission). 1986 Feb. [Information syntheses, Cost analyses]

Study of Medicare-funded heart transplants. In: Office of Research and Demonstrations, Health Care Financing Administration. Health care financing status report: research and demonstrations in health care financing. Jan 1986. (HCFA Pub. No. 03219).

Battelle Human Affairs Research Centers. National Heart Transplantation Study, Final Report to the Health Care Financing Administration. 1984.

California Medical Association, Medical Practice Opinion Program. Heart transplants. 1981 Dec. (Medical Practice Opinion #252) [Group judgment]

Transplantation—Heart-lung

California Medical Association, Medical Practice Opinion Program. Heart-lung transplantation. 1984 Sep. (Medical Practice Opinion #309) [Group judgment]

Transplantation—Kidney

Comparative analysis of the costs and outcomes of kidney transplants. In: Office of Research and Demonstrations, Health Care Financing Administration. Health care financing status report: research and demonstrations in health care financing. Jan 1986. (HCFA Pub. No. 03219).

Health Council of the Netherlands. Dialysis and kidney transplantation. 1986. [English summary only].

National Kidney Dialysis and Kidney Transplantation Study. In: Office of Research and Demonstrations, Health Care Financing Administration. Health care financing status report: research and demonstrations in health care financing. Jan 1986. (HCFA Pub. No. 03219).

Relative effectiveness and cost of transplantation and dialysis in end-stage renal disease. In: Office of Research and Demonstrations, Health Care Financing Administration. Health care financing status report: research and demonstrations in health care financing. Jan 1986. (HCFA Pub. No. 03219).

Hutchinson TA, Michaud L, Thomas DC. [McGill University, Department of Epidemiology and Biostatistics] Comparison of survival with dialysis and renal transplantation - the effect of the method of statistical analysis on results. J Am Soc Artif Intern Organs 1985;75:732-736.

Parfrey PS, Hutchinson TA, Harvey C, Guttman RD. [McGill University, Department of Epidemiology and Biostatistics] Transplantation versus dialysis in diabetic patients with renal failure. Am J Kidney Dis 1985;5:112-116.

Parfrey PS, et al. [McGill University, Department of Epidemiology and Biostatistics] The impact of renal transplantation on the course of hepatitis B liver disease. Transplantation 1985;39:610-615.

Tousignant P, Hollomby D, Guttman RD. [McGill University, Department of Epidemiology and Biostatistics] Transplantation and home hemodialysis: their cost-effectiveness in the treatment of end stage renal disease. J Chronic Dis 1985;38.

Battelle Human Affairs Research Centers. National Kidney Dialysis and Kidney Transplantation Study, Final Report submitted to the Health Care Financing Administration. 1984.

Hutchinson TA, Thomas DC, Lemieux JC, Harvey CF. [McGill University, Department of Epidemiology and Biostatistics] A prognostically controlled comparison of dialysis and renal transplantation. Kidney Int 1984;26:44-51.

Transplantation—Liver

Medical Technology and Practice Patterns Institute. Liver transplantation. 1987.

American Medical Association, Council on Scientific Affairs. Statement on liver transplantation. 1986. [Group judgment]

California Medical Association, Medical Practice Opinion Program. Liver transplantation. 1983 Sep. (Medical Practice Opinion #297) [Group judgment]

National Center for Health Services Research and Health Care Technology Assessment, Office of Health Technology Assessment. Liver transplantation. 1983.

National Institutes of Health, Consensus Development Program. Liver transplantation. (Consensus Development Conference Statement, Jun 20-23 1983). [Group judgment]

Health Council of the Netherlands. Liver transplantation. Ongoing.

National Center for Health Services Research and Health Care Technology Assessment, Office of Health Technology Assessment. Adult liver transplantation. Ongoing.

Transplantation—Nail bed

U.S. Administrators, Professional Policy Committee. Nail bed transplants. [7/86] [Group judgment]

Transplantation—Pancreas

National Center for Health Services Research and Health Care Technology Assessment, Office of Health Technology Assessment. Transplantation of the pancreas. 1984.

American College of Physicians, Clinical Efficacy Assessment Project. Management of diabetes mellitus: pancreatic transplants. Ann Intern Med 1983;99:272-4. [Information syntheses]

Transsexual surgery

National Center for Health Services Research and Health Care Technology Assessment, Office of Health Technology Assessment. Transsexual surgery. 1981.

Health Council of the Netherlands. Transsexualism. 1977.

Trazodone

Food and Drug Administration, Center for Drugs and Biologics. Trazodone HCI. 1982. (NTIS order no. PB82-915901). [Information syntheses, Expert opinion, Epidemiological and other observational methods, Clinical trials, Bench testing]

Triamterene

Food and Drug Administration, Center for Drugs and Biologics. Triamterene and hydrochlorothiazide. 1987. (Summary basis of approval, NDA # 19-129). [Information syntheses, Expert opinion, Epidemiological and other observational methods, Clinical trials, Bench testing]

Triazolam

Food and Drug Administration, Center for Drugs and Biologics. Triazolam. 1983. (NTIS order no. PB83-915901). [Information syntheses, Expert opinion, Epidemiological and other observational methods, Clinical trials, Bench testing]

Trimethoprim

Food and Drug Administration, Center for Drugs and Biologics. Trimethoprim tablets. 1982. (NTIS order no. PB82-915904). [Information syntheses, Expert opinion, Epidemiological and other observational methods, Clinical trials, Bench testing]

Food and Drug Administration, Center for Drugs and Biologics. Sulfamethoxazole and trimethoprim. 1981. (NTIS order no. PB81-915909). [Information syntheses, Expert opinion, Epidemiological and other observational methods, Clinical trials, Bench testing]

Food and Drug Administration, Center for Drugs and Biologics. Trimethoprim/sulfamethoxazole. 1981. (NTIS order no. 81-915908). [Information syntheses, Expert opinion, Epidemiological and other observational methods, Clinical trials, Bench testing]

Veterans Administration, Cooperative Studies Program. Prospective evaluation of the efficacy & tolerance of oral trimethoprim sulfamethoxazole prophylaxis in granulocytopenic patients with acute non-lymphocytic leukemia. Ongoing. [Clinical trials]

Tryptophan

Chouinard G. [Department Psychiatry, McGill University] [Medical Research Council - Canada] Controlled clinical trials of lithium and tryptophan in the treatment of patients with bipolar affective disorders. (Grant period 1982-1985).

Tubal ligation

California Medical Association, Medical Practice Opinion Program. Assistant surgeon at elective abdominal tubal ligation. 1985 Nov. (Medical Practice Opinion #333) [Group judgment]

Tuberculosis screening

California Medical Association, Medical Practice Opinion Program. Tuberculosis surveillance program for hospital employees. 1984 Oct. (Medical Practice Opinion #304) [Group judgment]

Tumor markers

ECRI Technology Assessment Program. Tumor markers. J Health Care Technol 1985;2:105-28. [Information syntheses]

Tumor stem cell assay

California Medical Association, Medical Practice Opinion Program. Human tumor stem cell assay. 1982 Jul. (Medical Practice Opinion #273) [Group judgment]

American College of Physicians, Clinical Efficacy Assessment Project. Human tumor cell drug sensitivity assay in the treatment of solid tumors. 1981. [Information syntheses]

National Center for Health Services Research and Health Care Technology Assessment, Office of Health Technology Assessment. The use of human tumor stem cell drug sensitivity assays for predicting anticancer drug effects. 1981.

Type A score

Shekelle RB, Gale M, Norusis M for the Aspirin Myocardial Infarction Study Research Group. [National Heart, Lung, and Blood Institute] Type A score (Jenkins activity survey) and the risk of recurrent coronary heart disease in the Aspirin Myocardial Infarction Study. Am J Cardiol 1985;56:221-225.

Ultrasonography—Arteries

American College of Physicians, Clinical Efficacy Assessment Project. Ultrasonic arteriography, B mode. 1981. [Information syntheses]

American College of Physicians, Clinical Efficacy Assessment Project. Ultrasonic arteriography, B-scan and Doppler ultrasound. 1981. [Information syntheses]

National Center for Health Services Research and Health Care Technology Assessment, Office of Health Technology Assessment. B-mode scan in peripheral arterial disease. 1981.

American Academy of Neurology, Practice Committee. Ultrasonic arteriography. 1980 May. [Expert opinion, Group judgment]

Ultrasonography—Breast

American College of Radiology, Task Force on Breast Cancer. Policy statement on sonography for the detection and diagnosis of breast disease. 1984. [Group judgment]

Ultrasonography—Follicular growth

American College of Obstetricians and Gynecologists, Committee Opinion. Ultrasonography in the monitoring of follicular growth. Pending. [Information syntheses]

Ultrasonography—Head

Pape KE. [Hospital for Sick Children, Toronto] [Medical Research Council - Canada] A prospective study of the evolution and outcome of cystic brain damage in the preterm infant utilizing diagnostic ultrasound brain scans. (Grant period 1980-1985).

Blue Cross and Blue Shield Association, Medical Necessity Program. Head CT scan and ultrasound in the pediatric patient. 1984. [Information syntheses]

Ultrasonography—Pancreas

Fineberg HV. [Harvard School of Public Health, Institute for Health Research] Assessing the diagnostic contribution of imaging tests: computed tomography and ultrasound of the pancreas. In: Alperovitch A, de Dombal FT, Gremy F, eds. Evaluation of efficacy of medical action. New York: Elsevier-North Holland, 1979. [Epidemiological methods]

Ultrasonography—Pregnancy

National Institute of Child Health and Human Development. Diagnostic ultrasound imaging in pregnancy. Bethesda, MD: National Institute of Child Health and Human Development, 1984. (NIH publication no. 84-667) [Group judgment, Expert opinion]

National Institutes of Health, Consensus Development Program. Diagnostic ultrasound imaging in pregnancy. (Consensus Development Conference Statement, Feb 6-8 1984). [Group judgment]

Ultrasonography—Prostate

ECRI Technology Assessment Program. Transrectal ultrasound of the prostate. Issues Health Care Technol 1983;sec.5.T.3. [Information syntheses]

Ultrasonography—Sinuses

California Medical Association, Medical Practice Opinion Program. Echocine for diagnosis of sinusitis. 1985 Jun. (Medical Practice Opinion #318) [Group judgment]

Ultrasound

Health Council of the Netherlands. Ultrasound. 1987.

American Academy of Neurology, Practice Committee. Neurosonology. 1980 Mar. [Expert opinion, Group judgment]

Health Council of the Netherlands. Ultrasound. Ongoing.

Netherlands Organization for Applied Scientific Research, Medical Technology Unit (TNO). Ultrasound physiotherapy equipment. Ongoing. [Expert opinion, Group judgment, Bench testing]

Ultrasound—Cardiac output

National Center for Health Services Research and Health Care Technology Assessment, Office of Health Technology Assessment. Noninvasive method of monitoring cardiac output by doppler ultrasound. 1984.

Ultrasound—Intraoperative

American Medical Association, Diagnostic and Therapeutic Technology Assessment. Diagnostic intraoperative ultrasound. JAMA 1985 Jul 12. [Expert opinion, Information syntheses]

Ultrasound—Obstetrics and gynecology

American College of Obstetricians and Gynecologists, Committee on Technical Bulletins. Diagnostic ultrasound in obstetrics and gynecology. 1981 Oct. (Technical bulletin no. 63). [Expert opinion]

Ultrasound—Obstetrics and gynecology—Pelvimetry

Blue Cross and Blue Shield Association, Medical Necessity Program. Ultrasound and x-ray pelvimetry in maternity care. 1984. [Information syntheses]

Ultrasound equipment—Diagnostic

Subcommittee on Special Services in Hospitals. [Health and Welfare Canada, Health Services and Promotion Branch, Institutional and Professional Services Division] Diagnostic ultrasound facilities in hospital guidelines. 1985. [Information syntheses, Expert opinion, Group judgment]

Ultrasound equipment—Therapeutic

Food and Drug Administration, Center for Devices and Radiological Health. A practitioner's guide to the ultrasonic therapy equipment standard. 1986. (NTIS order no. PB86-113933/AS).

Ultraviolet therapy

National Center for Health Services Research and Health Care Technology Assessment, Office of Health Technology Assessment. Ultraviolet light for treatment of decubitus ulcers. 1981.

Unbundling

U.S. Administrators, Professional Policy Committee. Unbundling. [7/86] [Group judgment]

Johns Hopkins Program for Medical Technology and Practice Assessment. An analysis of the potential cost implications of Medicare of unbundling of services (particularly diagnostic services provided by hospitals). Planned.

Ureteroscopy

National Center for Health Services Research and Health Care Technology Assessment. Office of Health Technology Assessment. Transurethral ureteroscopic lithotripsy procedures for the treatment of kidney stones. 1985.

Urinalysis

Blue Cross and Blue Shield Association, Medical Necessity Program. Urinalysis, urine culture, and other tests in the diagnosis of women with acute dysuria. 1987. [Information syntheses]

ECRI Technology Assessment Program. Urinalysis, automated. J Health Care Technol 1986;2:201-10. [Information syntheses]

Urinary sphincter, Artificial

ECRI Technology Assessment Program. Artificial urinary sphincters. Issues Health Care Technol 1986;sec.5.U.1. [Information syntheses]

Urine autoinjection

National Center for Health Services Research and Health Care Technology Assessment, Office of Health Technology Assessment. Urine autoinjection (autogenous urine immunization). 1981.

American College of Physicians, Clinical Efficacy Assessment Project. Urine autoinjection. 1980. [Information syntheses]

Urography

U.S. Administrators, Professional Policy Committee. Urography (excretory). [7/86] [Group judgment]

American Academy of Pediatrics, Committee on Radiology. Excretory urography for evaluation of enuresis. Pediatrics 1980 Mar.

Urologic disease screening

American Academy of Pediatrics, Committee on Screening Genetics. Screening school children for urologic disease. Pediatrics 1977 Aug.

Vaccination policy

Office of Technology Assessment, U.S. Congress. Compensation for vaccine-related injuries. Washington, D.C.: U.S. Government Printing Office, November, 1980.

Office of Technology Assessment, U.S. Congress. A review of selected federal vaccine and immunization policies. Washington, D.C.: U.S. Government Printing Office, September 1979.

Health Council of the Netherlands. National vaccination program. Ongoing.

Vaccines

Steering Committee on Future Health Scenarios, Commission on Future Health Care Technology (Netherlands). Prospective assessment of future health care technology: biotechnology and new vaccines. 1987.

California Medical Association, Medical Practice Opinion Program. Viral and bacterial vaccines for arthritis. 1982 Jun. (Medical Practice Opinion #268) [Group judgment]

Health Council of the Netherlands. Admission of new sera and vaccines. Ongoing.

Valproate

American Academy of Pediatrics, Committee on Drugs. Valproate teratogenicity. Pediatrics 1983 Jun.

American Academy of Pediatrics, Committee on Drugs. Valproic acid: benefits and risks. Pediatrics 1982 Aug.

Veterans Administration, Cooperative Studies Program. Efficacy and toxicity of carbamazepine vs. valproic acid for partial seizures. Ongoing. [Clinical trials]

Vascular access ports

ECRI Technology Assessment Program. Implantable vascular access ports. Issues Health Care Technology 1985;sec.5.V.2. [Information syntheses]

Genetics Lab. [Food and Drug Administration, Center for Devices and Radiological Health] Bioflow (TM): summary of safety and effectiveness. 1982 Jul 20. (PMA no. P800064-000).

Vasodilators

Veterans Administration, Cooperative Studies Program. Vasodilators used in chronic heart failure (CSP 153). [1980]. [Clinical trials]

Veterans Administration, Cooperative Studies Program. Vasodilators used in chronic heart failure (CSP 19). [1980]. [Clinical trials]

Veterans Administration, Cooperative Studies Program. Vasodilators used in chronic heart failure-II. [Clinical trials]

Ventilation-perfusion lung scans

Hull RD, Hirsch J, Carter CJ, et al. [McMaster University, Department of Clinical Epidemiology and Biostatistics] Diagnostic value of ventilation-perfusion lung scanning in patients with suspected pulmonary embolism. Chest 1985;88:819.

Ventilators

ECRI Health Devices Program. Neonatal ventilators. Health Devices 1986;15:219-46.

American Hospital Association, Hospital Technology Series Program. Adult volume ventilators. 1984. (Guideline report) [Information syntheses, Expert opinion, Cost analyses]

Food and Drug Administration, Center for Devices and Radiological Health. Safety and performance of ventilators. 1984.(NTIS Order No. PB84-188721).

ECRI Health Devices Program. Volume ventilators. Health Devices 1982;11:264-83.

ECRI Technology Assessment Program. High-frequency ventilators. Issues Health Care Technol 1981;sec.5.V.1. [Information syntheses]

Ventricular assist devices

Medical Technology and Practice Patterns Institute. Left ventricular assist device. 1987.

Ventricular mapping, Intraoperative

National Center for Health Services Research and Health Care Technology Assessment, Office of Health Technology Assessment. Intraoperative ventricular mapping. 1984.

Verapamil

Food and Drug Administration, Center for Drugs and Biologics. Verapamil HCl. 1987. (Summary basis of approval substitute, NDA # 19-152). [Information syntheses, Expert opinion, Epidemiological and other observational methods, Clinical trials, Bench testing]

Food and Drug Administration, Center for Drugs and Biologics. Verapamil. 1987. (Summary basis of approval substitute, NDA # 18-817/S-003). [Information syntheses, Expert opinion, Epidemiological and other observational methods, Clinical trials, Bench testing]

Food and Drug Administration, Center for Drugs and Biologics. Verapamil HCI. 1982. (NTIS order no. PB82-915902). [Information syntheses, Expert opinion, Epidemiological and other observational methods, Clinical trials, Bench testing]

Food and Drug Administration, Center for Drugs and Biologics. Verapamil. 1981. (NTIS order no. PB81-915911). [Information syntheses, expert opinion, Epidemiological and other observational methods, Clinical trials, Bench testing]

Vertebral artery surgery

California Medical Association, Medical Practice Opinion Program. Vertebral artery surgery. 1986 Sep. (Medical Practice Opinion #341) [Group judgment]

Vidarabine

Food and Drug Administration, Center for Drugs and Biologics. Vidarabine. 1983. (NTIS order no. PB83-915903). [Information syntheses, Expert opinion, Epidemiological and other observational methods, Clinical trials, Bench testing]

Viral hepatitis vaccine

Jonsson B. [Linköping University, Center for Medical Technology Assessment] Cost benefit analysis of hepatitis-B vaccination. 1986. (Discussion series paper #12) [Information syntheses]

American College of Physicians, Clinical Efficacy Assessment Project. Hepatitis B vaccine. Ann Intern Med 1984;100:149-50. [Information syntheses]

American Medical Association, Council on Scientific Affairs. Pneumococcal, influenza and hepatitis-B vaccine (Resolution 75, A-82). 1982. [Group judgment]

Szmuness W, Stevens CE, Harley EJ, et al. [National Heart, Lung, and Blood Institute] Hepatitis B vaccine: demonstration of efficacy in a controlled clinical trial in high-risk population in the United States. N Eng J Med 1980;303:833-841.

Vision aids

Overburg O, Jackson WB, West ML. [National Health Research and Development Program - Canada] Determinates of successful use of low vision aids: an interdisciplinary study to correlate ophthalmological and psychological variables. 1986. (Grant No. 6605-1799-43).

Vision screening

American Academy of Pediatrics, Committee on Practice and Ambulatory Medicine. Screening for vision problems. Pediatrics (To be published).

American Academy of Pediatrics, Committee on Practice and Ambulatory Medicine. Vision screening and eye examination in children. Pediatrics 1986 Jun.

Vitamin A

Willett WC, Polk BF, Underwood BA, et al. [National Heart, Lung, and Blood Institute] Relation of serum vitamins A and E and carotenoids to the risk of cancer. N Engl J Med 1984;310:410-434.

Vitamin B1

American Medical Association, Council on Scientific Affairs. Addition of thiamine to alcoholic beverages (Resolution 140, A-81). 1982. [Group judgment]

Vitamin B12 assay

Cooper BA. [National Health Research and Development Program - Canada] Evaluation and development of assays for B12 and folate. 1985. (Grant No. 6605-1784-52).

Vitamin E

Robertson JMD. [National Health Research and Development Program - Canada] Does supplementary vitamin E prevent cataracts? 1986. (Grant No. 6606-2445-43).

American Academy of Pediatrics, Committee on Fetus and Newborn. Vitamin E and the prevention of retinopathy of prematurity. Pediatrics 1985 Aug.

Willett WC, Polk BF, Underwood BA, et al. [National Heart, Lung, and Blood Institute] Relation of serum vitamins A and E and carotenoids to the risk of cancer. N Engl J Med 1984;310:410-434.

Trevithick JR,. [Department Biochemistry, University Western Ontario] [Medical Research Council - Canada] Microwave and heat-induced cataracts: prevention by vitamin E and chronic studies of low level pulsed irradiation. (Grant period 1983-1985).

Vitamins

American Medical Association, Council on Scientific Affairs. Vitamin preparations as dietary supplements and as therapeutic agents. 1985. [Group judgment]

American Academy of Pediatrics, Committee on Nutrition. Vitamins and mineral supplement needs. 1980.

Warfarin

Hull R, Delmore T, Carter C, et al. [McMaster University, Department of Clinical Epidemiology and Biostatistics] Adjusted subcutaneous heparin versus warfarin sodium in the long-term treatment of venous thrombosis. New Eng J Med 1982;306:189-194.

Veterans Administration, Cooperative Studies Program. Anticoagulants in RX of CA (warfarin). [1980] [Clinical trials]

Wheelchair tray systems

Parnes PH. [National Health Research and Development Program - Canada] Towards development of a modular universal wheelchair tray system for communication control and ADL. 1986. (Grant No. 6605-3006-51).

Wheelchairs

Richardson MF. [National Health Research and Development Program - Canada] Construction and testing of a motorized variable-height wheelchair. 1986. (Grant No. 6606-2123-55).

Office of Technology Assessment, U.S. Congress. The market for wheelchairs: innovations and public policy. Washington, D.C.: U.S. Government Printing Office, November 1984. (Health technology case study series #30)

Shepard DS, Karon SL. [Harvard School of Public Health, Institute for Health Research] The market for wheelchairs: innovations and federal policy. Washington, D.C.: U.S. Congress, Office of Technology Assessment, 1984. Health Technology Case Study 30, OTA-HCS-30) [Information syntheses]

Xenon

Food and Drug Administration, Center for Drugs and Biologics. Xenon Xe 127 gas. 1983 (NTIS order no. PB83-915901). [Information syntheses, Expert opinion, Epidemiological and other observational methods, Clinical trials, Bench testing]

Xylitol

Olefsky JM, Crapo P. [American Diabetes Association] Fructose, xylitol, and sorbitol. Diabetes Care 1980;3:390-393. [Expert opinion, Group judgment]

Yohimbine

Morales A. [Department Urology, Queens University] [Medical Research Council - Canada] A controlled clinical trial of yohimbine in the treatment of impotence. (Grant period 1981-1985).

Zomepirac sodium

Food and Drug Administration, Center for Drugs and Biologics. Zomepirac sodium. 1981. (NTIS order no. PB81-915901). [Information syntheses, Expert opinion, Epidemiological and other observational methods, Clinical trials, Bench testing]

Part 3
Information and Data Resources

Part 3: Information and Data Resources

This part has three sections: a categorical chart of information and data resources beginning on page 501, the 73 resource descriptions beginning on page 504, and a subject index to the resource descriptions beginning on page 551.

The categorical chart indicates which of three broad types of descriptors, i.e. file type, format, and access, characterizes each resource. The descriptions of each of the 73 information and data resources are arranged alphabetically by name of resource; each is described in terms of source, subject, content, compilation, and access. The subject index is for identifying information and data resources relevant to particular topics.

Categories of Information and Data Resources

	File type: directories/compendiums	bibliographic information/abstracts	reports/texts/references	data sets	news/bulletins	Format: hard copy/print/microfiche	online computer	machine-readable/disk/magnetic tape	Access: public	limited
Abstracts of Health Care Machine-Readable Data Files	•					•			•	
ADAMHA Publications and Data	•			•		•		•	•	
AMA/NET	•	•	•		•		•		•	
Baseline Reports				•		•	•		•	
BIOETHICSLINE		•				•	•		•	
Birth Defects and Developmental Disabilities Reports				•		•				•
BMEDSS		•			•		•		•	
Boston Collaborative Drug Surveillance Program				•		•		•		•
BRS/SEARCH		•	•		•		•		•	
CANCERLIT		•					•		•	
CASSIS			•				•		•	
CCC Bibliography on Regional Variations in Health Care	•	•				•			•	
Center for Health Promotion and Education				•				•	•	
CLINPROT			•				•		•	
COLLEAGUE		•	•				•		•	
COMPASS, DURbase				•		•			•	
Compendium of HHS Evaluations and Relevant Other Studies	•					•			•	
CPHA Files				•		•		•	•	
CRISP	•					•	•			•
Current Assessments New Technology Abstracts		•				•			•	

continued

Categories of Information and Data Resources

	File type					**Format**			**Access**	
	directories/compendiums	bibliographic information/abstracts	reports/texts/references	data sets	news/bulletins	hard copy/print/microfiche	online computer	machine-readable/disk/magnetic tape	public	limited
Device Experience Network			●			●	●		●	●
DIALOG	●	●	●		●		●		●	
Directory of Health Services and Research Organizations	●					●			●	
DIRLINE	●						●		●	
Drug Product Problem Reporting Program			●			●			●	
Duke Comprehensive Cancer Center Database				●		●		●		●
Environmental Hazards and Health Effects Reports			●	●		●			●	●
Environmental Health Laboratory Sciences Reports			●	●		●			●	●
FDA Bulletin Board			●		●	●	●		●	
F-D-C Reports	●				●	●			●	
Futures Program			●		●	●			●	
HEALTH		●				●	●		●	
Health Devices Alerts			●		●	●	●		●	
Health Devices Sourcebook	●					●			●	
Health Information Resources in the Federal Government	●					●			●	
HEALTHLAWYER		●	●				●		●	
HECLINET		●					●		●	
HIAA Medical Appropriateness Compilation			●			●			●	
High Blood Pressure Information Center	●	●	●			●	●		●	
IMPAC				●		●		●	●	●
IMS Audits				●		●	●		●	
International Market Research Studies			●			●			●	●
INTERNIST-1/ QUICK MEDICAL REFERENCE			●					●		●
Market Research Reports	●		●			●			●	
Market/Technology Reports	●		●			●			●	
Medical Device and Laboratory Product Problem Reporting Program			●			●	●		●	●
Medical Device Register	●					●	●	●	●	

Categories of Information and Data Resources

	File type					**Format**			**Access**	
	directories/compendiums	bibliographic information/abstracts	reports/texts/references	data sets	news/bulletins	hard copy/print/microfiche	online computer	machine-readable/disk/magnetic tape	public	limited
Medical Device Reporting			●			●	●		●	●
MEDIS		●	●				●		●	
MEDLINE		●				●	●		●	
MEDLINK		●			●		●		●	
Multi-Client Reports			●			●			●	
NAHDO Resource Manual	●					●			●	
NCHS Publications and Data				●		●		●	●	
National Cholesterol Educ Prog/ NHLBI Smoking Educ Prog Info Ctr	●		●			●			●	
National Reference File			●	●		●			●	●
NTIS Publications and Data	●	●	●	●		●	●	●	●	
NEXIS		●	●		●		●		●	
NHLBI Publications			●			●			●	
Oxford Database of Perinatal Trials		●				●		●	●	
PDQ		●	●				●		●	
Pharmaprojects	●				●	●	●		●	
POPLINE		●					●		●	
Product Development Directory Product SOS	●		●		●	●			●	
Randomized Controlled Clinical Trials Report Collection		●	●			●				●
Report on Cost-Effective Products and Technologies			●			●			●	
Scrip	●		●		●	●	●		●	
SEER				●		●		●	●	
SPRILINE		●				●	●		●	
Technical Data Center	●	●	●			●	●		●	
U.S. Industrial Outlook			●	●		●			●	
WHO/LINFO Database on Health Technology Assessment	●	●				●			●	
WHO Publications			●		●	●			●	

Abstracts of Health Care Machine-Readable Data Files

Source: Hospital Data Center, Department of Special Studies, American Hospital Association (AHA), 840 North Lake Shore Drive, Chicago, IL 60611, 312-280-6520

Subject: Machine-readable databases related to health care that are national in scope and are available to users outside the source organizations, with or without restrictions on use or conditions of release.

Content: The 1986 version contains 137 abstracts of non-bibliographic machine-readable files. Each abstract includes the file citation, brief narrative description, descriptors based on NLM controlled vocabulary MeSH, geographic coverage, time coverage, technical notes, information about related files, availability, and contact person. The abstracts are arranged alphabetically by title and are indexed by source and by MeSH. The 1986 version is an expansion and updating of shorter descriptions of 257 databases contained in the 1984 version. The forthcoming version will be an expansion and update of the two earlier documents.

Compilation: All versions were compiled by the AHA from survey forms sent to source organizations. Databases listed include data pertaining to periods later than January 1, 1970.

Access: The 1986 volume *Abstracts of Health Care Machine-Readable Data Files* (157 pages) is available from the AHA Hospital Data Center; price to be set by AHA. Its predecessor, the 1984 *Inventory of U.S. Health Care Data Bases 1976-1983*, was originally published by HRSA, and is available from NTIS (order HRP0906300LP) for $18.95 plus $3 handling. An updated version, *Inventory of Machine-Readable Healthcare Data Bases* will be available in 1988; price to be set by AHA.

Alcohol, Drug Abuse, and Mental Health Administration Publications and Data

Source: Alcohol, Drug Abuse, and Mental Health Administration (ADAMHA), Parklawn Building, Room 13C-05, 5600 Fishers Lane, Rockville, MD 20857, 301-443-3820

Subject: Alcohol, drug abuse, and mental health (ADM) disorders.

Content: Publications and data cover statistical, epidemiological and services research information pertaining to substance abuse and mental health disorders and their public health implications. Includes ADM client/patient data, research findings on ADM disorders, facility service and resources information, and financial data. Also available: directory of organizations involved in ADM research, treatment, and related issues.

Compilation: Most ADAMHA activities initiated in 1972. Information gathered from clients in treatment; facilities providing alcohol, drug abuse, and mental health treatment and prevention services in U.S., Puerto Rico, and six territories. Publications issued periodically.

Access: Alcohol, Drug Abuse, and Mental Health Administration (ADAMHA) publications are available free of charge by contacting individual institutes within ADAMHA, i.e., National Institute on Drug Abuse (NIDA) 301-443-4577, National Institute on Mental Health (NIMH) 301-443-4515, National Institute on Alcohol Abuse and Alcoholism (NIAAA) 301-443-2954. Studies independently conducted for use by NIAAA, NIDA, NIMH; IBM-compatible data tapes available from sponsoring Institute, price to be determined. Sample formats of particular data collections or surveys are available from sponsoring Institutes.

AMA/NET

Source: SoftSearch, Inc., 1560 Broadway, Suite 900, Denver, CO 80202, 303-832-7111, 800-426-2873. Sponsored by the American Medical Association (AMA).

Subject: Medicine and health care delivery; designed for health care professionals.

Content: AMA/NET provides the following databases. AP MEDICAL NEWS SERVICE is a compendium of health care-related articles selected from Associated Press news wires and U.S. newspapers. EMPIRES CURRENT AWARENESS provides access to specialty specific citations; contains references to articles from over 300 international medical and scientific journals covering some 65 medical specialties and subspecialties. DISEASE INFORMATION is a reference summary of more than 3,500 distinct diseases, disorders, and conditions; provides synopsis of classic signs and symptoms, as well as laboratory and radiologic findings of the entities. MEDICAL PROCEDURE CODING & NOMENCLATURE, based on AMA publication *Physicians' Current Procedural Terminology* includes descriptive terms and billing codes for more than 6,000 medical procedures and services performed by physicians. SOCIO/ECONOMIC BIBLIOGRAPHIC INFORMATION contains over 5,500 citations to documents pertaining to health care delivery and economic issues in medicine.

Also available are electronic communications services, including electronic mail and bulletin boards; public information services providing direct access to such government organizations as the Centers for Disease Control, the Surgeon General's Office, and the National Library of Medicine/National Institutes of Health; AMA; literature ordering service providing reprints of articles referenced in either the SOCIO/ECONOMIC BIBLIOGRAPHIC INFORMATION or EMPIRES databases; interactive, computer-based continuing medical education courses developed at the Massachusetts General Hospital Laboratory of Computer Science.

Compilation: Databases compiled from journal articles, legislative reports, books, wire services, and newspapers. AP MEDICAL NEWS SERVICE updated daily; EMPIRES updated weekly.

Access: Online databases and other services available at any time; accessible via modem from remote terminal. Subscription required. One-time subscription fee ($30 for AMA members, $50 for non-members) includes one user name and introductory materials. Registration fee for each additional user $15. Basic service charge $14/hour peak time; $10/hour off-peak. Information service charge varies with service used.

Baseline Reports

Source: Massachusetts Health Data Consortium, Inc., 400-1 Totten Pond Road, Waltham, MA 02154, 617-890-6040

Subject: Diagnosis, treatment, costs, and outcomes of all patients discharged from acute care hospitals in Massachusetts.

Content: Database covers information on hospital utilization, hospital charges, patient socio-demographic characteristics, clinical status including principle diagnoses and procedures, and discharge status. The following types of reports and data sets are available. Patient origin report sets identify hospital service areas and community dependency for pediatrics, medical/surgical, obstetrics/gynecology, and psychiatry. Market position reports analyze market penetration by town, age, and payer. Market position trend analyses chart market share changes over time by hospital for 24 clinical specialties. Statewide summary charge data reports rank top 100 diagnosis-related groups (DRGs) by payers, hospital bed size, patient discharge status, sex, and age. Hospital-specific charge data reports highlight charges and length of stay by DRGs. Case mix profiles display a case mix adjustment factor and length-of-stay performance measures. Per diem charge profiles provide case mix adjusted per diem charges for Blue Cross and commercially insured patients. Payer mix trend analyses display changes in payer mix for 24 clinical specialties. Community use rate reports contain population-based discharge and use rates. DRG outlier and mortality reports include hospital-specific length of stay, deaths, and outliers by DRG. Data express service provides custom reports in response to special requests for data or analyses.

Compilation: Information gathered from data tapes supplied by 109 acute care hospitals and two Veterans Administration hospitals in Massachusetts and surrounding communities. Coverage from 1978 to present; updated annually.

Access: Free catalog of publications available upon request. Report prices range from $75 to $1,850. Database available online; accessible via modem from remote terminal.

BIOETHICSLINE

Source: Bioethics Information Retrieval Project, Kennedy Institute of Ethics, Georgetown University, Washington, DC 20057, 202-687-3885

Subject: Multidisciplinary coverage of the ethical, legal, and public policy aspects of medicine, health care, and biomedical and behavioral research.

Content: Database includes bibliographic citations to documents relating to euthanasia, organ donation and transplantation, allocation of health care resources, patients' rights, codes of professional ethics, in vitro fertilization and other reproductive technologies, genetic intervention, abortion, behavior control and mental health therapies, and human experimentation. About 20 percent of citations include abstracts. Approximately 80 percent of database keywords are mapped to terms in NLM controlled vocabulary MeSH, making it possible to search BIOETHICSLINE using MeSH. See MEDLINE description for listing of NLM MEDLARS databases.

Compilation: Compiled from journal articles, monographs, newspaper articles, court decisions, bills, laws, audiovisual materials, and unpublished documents. Coverage from 1973 to present. Updated bimonthly with approximately 2,000 citations added annually.

Access: Available online at any time through NLM MEDLARS computer system to more than 6,000 online centers in hospitals, medical schools, universities, government agencies, commercial firms, and other organizations throughout U.S., as well as MEDLARS centers located in 13 other countries. Also accessible via modem from remote terminal through TELENET, TYMNET, direct dial. To contact MEDLARS Management Division call 800-638-8480 or 301-496-6193 in Maryland. Call source for search strategies and further information about *Bibliography of Bioethics* and related services. Connect cost averages $22/hour peak time, $15/hour off-peak.

Individual searches available free of charge from the affiliated National Reference Center for Bioethics Literature 800-633-3849; citations are printed offline and arrive in about one week. Printed bibliographies on selected topics are available bimonthly ($10/topic, $60/complete package). BIOETHICSLINE citations appear in print form in the annual *Bibliography of Bioethics* ($25).

Birth Defects and Developmental Disabilities Reports

Source: Division of Birth Defects and Developmental Disabilities (BDDD), Center for Environmental Health, Centers for Disease Control, 1600 Clifton Road, Atlanta, GA 30333, 404-454-4706

Subject: Adverse reproductive outcomes, congenital malformations, genetic diseases, and other diseases or conditions that originate before birth or that develop during childhood.

Content: BDDD surveillance activities include the following programs. Metropolitan Atlanta Congenital Defects Program (MACDP) monitors occurrence of congenital malformations (e.g., structural, chromosomal, or biochemical abnormalities) in Atlanta-area hospitals and maintains a case registry for epidemiologic and genetic studies. Birth Defects Monitoring Program (BDMP) monitors U.S. incidence of birth defects; functions primarily as an early warning system for correlating incidence patterns with temporal and geographic distribution of drugs, chemicals, other possible human teratogens. Developmental Disabilities Surveillance Program collects and analyzes data on developmental disabilities in 10 year-olds in Atlanta area. Data include statistical information for trend analysis and selected regional comparisons.

Compilation: MACDP initiated in 1967; BDMP initiated in 1975; Developmental Disabilities Surveillance initiated in 1985. BDMP data gathered from hospital discharge data on newborns. MACDP drawn from Atlanta-area hospital records. Disabilities Surveillance Program drawn from educational and health care providers records. MACDP updated monthly; BDMP updated quarterly. Surveillance reports published intermittently.

Access: Copies of *Congenital Malformations Surveillance* reports available upon request. All data maintained in computer files is for access by CDC staff; no public use data tapes available. Staff may prepare documents or data sets in response to justified individual requests made directly to BDDD for specific data or information.

BMEDSS (Biomedical Engineering Decision Support Services)

Source: Medical Engineering Department, Akron City Hospital, 525 East Market Street, Akron, OH 44309-2090, 216-375-3501

Subject: Pharmaceuticals, medical devices and equipment. Designed primarily for biomedical engineers, device/equipment manufacturers, purchasing agents, materiel managers, biomedical research and teaching professionals.

Content: BMEDSS databases include FDA ENFORCEMENT REPORTS on medical devices and lab reagents, FDA RECALL REPORTS on pharmaceuticals, FDA TALK PAPERS, FDA MEDICAL DEVICE BULLETIN, FDA DEN (Device Experience Network) and MDR (Medical Device Reporting) as formatted and coded by ECRI, abstracts from *Journal of Clinical Engineering* from 1976 to present, abstracts of AAMI (Association for the Advancement of Medical Instrumentation) publications including *National Standards and Recommended Practices, Technology Assessment Reports, Updates and Information Reports*, and *Medical Instrumentation*; ECRI databases including HDA (Health Devices Alerts), abstracts and indexes of ECRI publications. Other services include User Report Forum that allows device experiences to be entered onto FDA DEN; Inventory Comparison Program permits in-house medical device inventories to be compared to current FDA recall file and ECRI's HDA and DEN files, and automatically flags recalled equipment; electronic mail and bulletin board.

Compilation: Information gathered from FDA sources, ECRI publications and databases, professional journals, and other relevant publications. Databases updated monthly. BMEDSS initiated in 1984.

Access: Databases available online through COMPUSERVE 800-848-8990; accessible via modem from remote terminal. Charges are $50 subscription fee plus approximately $35/month and $35/connect hour, adjusted for usage. Special group rates available. Connect cost varies with service used. Reprints of abstracts are available; contact BMEDSS for further information.

Boston Collaborative Drug Surveillance Program

Source: Boston University Medical Center, 400 Totten Pond Road, Waltham, MA 02154, 617-890-1300. Supported by the FDA and the pharmaceutical industry.

Subject: Postmarketing drug surveillance.

Content: Program monitors clinical effects of drugs routinely prescribed to hospitalized and ambulatory-care patients. Database includes information on frequency and importance of adverse drug reactions, adverse reaction rates, adverse reaction causation, assessment of adverse drug interactions, unsuspected drug side effects, drug efficacy, and evaluation of the role of certain patient characteristics in influencing clinical drug effects. Information is also available regarding drug utilization and prevailing practices in drug therapy such as magnitude of drug use, frequencies of various indications, utilization of specific drugs, and variability of utilization patterns by hospital and geographic area.

Compilation: Program implemented in 1966. Studies use data from two primary sources: drug use experience of 50,000 people hospitalized in one of eight hospitals in the U.S., Canada, and Israel; and members of Group Health Cooperative of Puget Sound (GHC) in Seattle, Washington. Hospital data include records of all drug exposures and all adverse events at the selected hospitals. Automated data files received from GHC on annual basis include all prescriptions and refills filled by GHC members at one GHC pharmacy, hospitalizations of GHC members, and routine information on GHC members.

Access: Boston Collaborative Drug Surveillance Program (BCDSP) computer tapes are not in the public domain. Contact BCDSP regarding access to data resources in collaboration with BCDSP. Over 200 articles describing past BCDSP studies have been published in various medical and professional journals. Reprints are available upon request. Listing of publications is available in: Cohen, M.R. A Compilation of Abstracts and Index Published by the Boston Collaborative Drug Surveillance Program 1966-1985. *Hospital Pharmacy* 21:497-559, 1986.

BRS/SEARCH

Source: BRS Information Technologies, 1200 Route 7, Latham, NY 12110, 800-345-4277

Subject: Health, medicine, pharmacology, biosciences, science and technology, education, business and finance, social sciences, politics, humanities.

Content: BRS/SEARCH Service includes over 90 multidisciplinary databases. Among those relevant to medical technology are MEDLINE, HEALTH, PDQ, HEALTHLAWYER, DRUG INFORMATION FULL TEXT (full-text information on current and investigational drugs, including research, treatment, and pharmacological practice), INTERNATIONAL PHARMACEUTICAL ABSTRACTS (indexes and abstracts from international pharmaceutical and health-related journals, covering drug development, use, and professional pharmaceutical practice), DIOGENES (FDA Medical Device Reporting, other regulatory information), EMBASE (from Excerpta Medica; references and summaries of international medical literature covering biomedicine, health, and health care management), IRCS MEDICAL SCIENCE DATABASE (full-text articles on biomedical research). Many databases provide bibliographic citations, many include abstracts; others provide complete document texts; most are indexed by title, subject, author, publication date. Monthly *BRS Bulletin* provides information on new databases, developments, and features.

Compilation: Databases are compiled from journal articles, books, periodicals, dissertations, monographs, government reports, corporate reports, newspaper articles. Most references are updated monthly; newspaper files are updated daily.

Access: Databases available online; accessible via modem from remote terminal through TELENET, TYMNET, OCLC GATEWAY, IN-WATS, direct dial. Outside U.S. and Canada, accessed through BRSNET. Online or offline document printing. Subscription required. Two basic subscription plans offered: (1) basic plan allows access to BRS on an as-needed basis; annual password fee ($75); connect cost ($25/hour plus database royalties), telecommunications, and document charges; (2) advance purchase plan provides volume discounts; a variety of subscription levels available. User manual ($45), database guides ($5 each), database summaries, and catalog available to subscribers. Training seminars offered in BRS/SEARCH features and search procedures.

CANCERLIT

Source: International Cancer Information Center, Office of International Affairs, National Cancer Institute (NCI), Building 82 Room 103, Bethesda, MD 20892, 301-496-7403

Subject: Major cancer topics.

Content: Database includes more than 600,000 citations and abstracts of published cancer literature and other sources. All records from non-MEDLINE sources contain abstracts; more than 60 percent of MEDLINE-derived records include abstracts. Records added since January 1980 have been indexed using NLM controlled vocabulary MeSH. All records are retrievable by free-text searching. See MEDLINE description for listing of NLM MEDLARS databases.

Compilation: Compiled from articles appearing in approximately 2,000 biomedical journals, government reports, meeting abstracts, papers presented at conferences, books, monographs, theses and dissertations. Most journal literature is derived from MEDLINE. Approximately 200 additional foreign journals and published literature references are also screened. 5,000 new references are added monthly.

Access: Available online at any time through NLM MEDLARS computer system to more than 6,000 online centers in hospitals, medical schools, universities, government agencies, commercial firms, and other organizations throughout U.S., as well as MEDLARS centers located in 13 other countries. Also accessible via modem from remote terminal through TELENET, TYMNET, direct dial. To contact MEDLARS Management Division call 800-638-8480 or 301-496-6193 in Maryland. Connect cost averages $22/hour peak time, $15/hour off-peak. Also available through BRS 800-345-4277, COLLEAGUE (BRS/Saunders) 800-468-0908, and DIALOG 800-334-2564.

CASSIS (Classification and Search Support Information System)

Source: Patent Depository Library Program Office, Patent and Trademark Office, U.S. Department of Commerce, Washington, DC 20231, 703-557-9686

Subject: Patent information of the U.S. Patent and Trademark Office.

Content: Encompasses information on the 4.9 million U.S. patents. Generally used to search classes and subclasses of patents in order to identify patent numbers that may be used to locate patent documents in microfilm holdings of Patent Depository Libraries. CASSIS searches or displays classifications of patents, patents in classifications, structured classification titles, keywords in classification titles, keywords in patent abstracts, and terms in the patent classification index.

Within the patent classification system, the following are examples of classes of patents that pertain to medical technologies: surgery (classes 128 and 604); drugs, bio-affecting, and body treating compositions (424,514); dentistry (433); prosthesis, i.e., artificial body members, parts thereof, or aids and accessories therefore (623); genetic engineering technology (935); multicellular living organisms and unmodified parts thereof (800); chemistry: molecular biology and microbiology (435); chemistry: analytical and immunological testing (436); eye examination, vision testing, and correcting (351). Each class has many subclasses.

Compilation: Operational since the late 1970s. Updated continuously; information about a new patent appears in the system approximately two months after it is issued. Although all patent numbers and classification information remain on the system, patent abstracts are rotated off after one to three years.

Access: Available online at no charge through any of the 60 Patent Depository Libraries located in 38 states in the U.S. No direct access from other remote terminals.

CCC (Copenhagen Collaborating Center) Bibliography on Regional Variations in Health Care

Source: Copenhagen Collaborating Center for the Study of Regional Variations in Health Care, Institute of Social Medicine, University of Copenhagen, Panum Institute, Blegdamsvej 3, 2200 Copenhagen N., Denmark, (45-1) 35-79-00 Ext. 3011. CCC is a World Health Organization (WHO) Collaborating Center established by four Danish research institutes.

Subject: Regional variation in the provision, utilization, and outcomes of health care.

Content: Studies covered in bibliography focus on small area variations, employ epidemiological methods, and include interpretation and discussion of variations. 1986 bibliography contains 153 entries, abstracts/extracts, author and subject index. Quarterly *International Newsletter on Regional Variations in Health Care* reports regional variations in medical practice, practice outcomes, clinical decision-making processes. Other articles include meeting announcements, summaries of proceedings, international activities in technology assessment, e.g., WHO Global Programme for Appropriate Health Care Technology. Also available is a directory of persons and institutions interested in regional variations in health care. Other CCC activities include research, organization of international meetings, and international research training.

Compilation: Bibliography compiled through unpublished literature reviews and information from researchers in the field. Data for other organizational and information activities are acquired through questionnaires sent to individuals and research institutes. CCC activities initiated in 1985. First bibliography was published in 1986; to be updated periodically. Directory is updated continuously.

Access: Online text retrieval and literature searches available from Danish Hospital Institute. Printed copy of bibliography and copies of newsletter available upon request. Contact CCC about receiving newsletter on regular basis.

Center for Health Promotion and Education

Source: Centers for Disease Control (CDC), 1600 Clifton Road, Atlanta, GA 30333, 404-321-2263

Subject: Nutritional status of select U.S. populations, behavioral risk factors, women's reproductive health.

Content: Reports and data tapes from Center for Health Promotion and Education's (CHPE) national surveillance activities cover nutritional status of high-risk pediatric populations and low-income, high-risk pregnant women, adolescent pregnancy, infant mortality, abortion, and behavioral risk factors such as smoking, hypertension, obesity, and alcohol use. Areas of applied research include female reproductive cancer and endogenous hormones, and the safety and efficacy of tubal ligation/female sterilization procedures. Data include statistical and demographic information which permit trend analysis and select regional comparisons.

Compilation: CHPE established in 1981. Information gathered primarily from state health departments, clinics, and select health and nutrition programs, e.g., Supplemental Food Program for Women, Infants, and Children (WIC), Early and Periodic Screening, Diagnosis, and Treatment (EPSDT) program. Information on behavioral risk factors gathered through telephone surveys by states. Reports usually issued annually.

Access: Reports available upon request, free of charge. Contact CHPE) for further information regarding access and availability of public use data tapes.

CLINPROT

Source: International Cancer Information Center, Office of International Affairs, National Cancer Institute (NCI), Building 82 Room 103, Bethesda, MD 20892, 301-496-7403

Subject: Clinical investigations of new anti-cancer agents and treatment modalities.

Content: Database contains comprehensive information on approximately 6,000 experimental cancer therapy protocols from the U.S. and other countries; approximately 1,500 are active protocols and over 4,000 are completed studies. Protocol summaries provide descriptions of clinical trials, including protocol objectives, study outline, patient entry criteria, treatment regimen, special study parameters, and status of the protocol. Active protocols indexed according to type and stage of cancer treated, phase of clinical investigation, specific agents or combination of agents, treatment modalities. Records retrieved by free-text searching or by using the 300 clinical protocol terms used for indexing. See MEDLINE description for listing of NLM MEDLARS databases.

Compilation: Coverage from 1960 to present. Currency and accuracy of information are maintained through monthly updates.

Access: Available online at any time through NLM MEDLARS computer system to more than 6,000 online centers in hospitals, medical schools, universities, government agencies, commercial firms, and other organizations throughout U.S., as well as MEDLARS centers located in 13 other countries. Also accessible via modem from remote terminal through TELENET, TYMNET, direct dial. To contact MEDLARS Management Division call 800-638-8480 or 301-496-6193 in Maryland. Connect cost averages $22/hour peak time, $15/hour off-peak.

COLLEAGUE

Source: BRS/Saunders, 1290 Avenue of the Americas, New York, NY 10104, 800-468-0908

Subject: Health care, medicine, pharmaceuticals; designed for health care professionals.

Content: Medical Search Service offers bibliographic sources including MEDLINE, HEALTH, EMBASE (from Exerpta Medica), BIOSIS PREVIEWS, INTERNATIONAL PHARMACEUTICAL ABSTRACTS, COMPREHENSIVE CORE MEDICAL LIBRARY, and PDQ. Medical and Psychological Previews Service permits access to citations from over 200 journals indexed by title and author prior to their inclusion in MEDLINE; also includes editorials, letters, and clinical notes. Complete Text Library incorporates full text of more than 20 medical books and textbooks in critical care medicine, and more than 50 medical and health-related journals. General Searching Service allows access to 70 other nonmedical databases offered by BRS. Electronic mail and bulletin boards are available through COLLEAGUE Mail service.

Compilation: Databases compiled from journal articles, periodicals, textbooks, monographs, medical manuals. Most references updated monthly; Medical and Psychological Previews updated weekly.

Access: Databases available online; accessible via modem from remote terminal through TELENET, TYMNET, direct dial. Online or offline document printing are available. Connect cost $32 to $79/hour peak time, $20 to $69/hour off-peak. Connect time volume discounts available. Subscription required. One-time registration fee ($95/individual, $175/group), includes password, user manual, and support services. Tutorial diskettes explaining COLLEAGUE and search strategies available upon request.

COMPASS (Computerized On-Line Medicaid Pharmaceutical Analysis and Surveillance System), DURbase (Drug Utilization Review base)

Source: Health Information Designs, Inc. (HID), 1616 North Fort Meyer Drive, Suite 1420, Arlington, VA 22209, 703-528-2032

Subject: Postmarketing drug surveillance.

Content: COMPASS database is composed of patient-specific billing data, including age, sex, state, inpatient and outpatient diagnoses recorded by ICD-9-CM codes, and outpatient drugs dispensed. Drug data are retrievable by strength, generic name, therapeutic class, or manufacturer. Database is supplemented by data on mortality, maternal-child linkages, and nursing home status. Reports available on individual patient diagnosis and prescription profiles, rankings of drugs and diagnoses, demographic characteristics, drug use patterns, average daily doses for specific drugs, comparisons of clinical outcomes between patients receiving specific drugs and control groups, and temporal relationships between specific drugs and subsequent diagnoses.

DURbase is a computerized drug utilization review system for identifying patients at high risk for drug-induced illness. Reports include chronological listings of all pharmaceuticals for patients identified as being at risk for drug-induced illness, summaries of individual patient prescription patterns, and other services.

Compilation: COMPASS and DURbase are drawn from HID database consisting primarily of billing data covering hospital, dental, and pharmaceutical services provided to 9 million patients, including 7 million Medicaid patients from 11 states and 2 million patients from HMOs, major employers, and other private sector sources. Medicaid data come from state Medicaid Management Information Systems. More than 20 million encounter records are added to the database monthly, including 7 million prescription drug claims. System includes data collected since 1980.

Access: COMPASS is used primarily by the FDA and pharmaceutical companies for postmarketing surveillance. DURbase is used primarily by government and private sector providers and payers for drug utilization monitoring and related quality review activities for their patient groups. Most HDI products are in the form of reports generated from COMPASS and DURbase data and analysis. Report prices depend upon the amount of data, level of analysis, and computer time required; charges for COMPASS products may range from $2,000 to $250,000. Online access to COMPASS is available only to the FDA. DURbase charges generally are based upon the size of the patient group studied and a per patient record charge. Patient group sizes range from 10,000 to 1.5 million people for certain Medicaid data sets. Charge per patient record ranges from $0.60 to $1.25 depending upon the extent to which HDI is asked to undertake clinical review of the data.

Compendium of HHS Evaluations and Relevant Other Studies

Source: HHS Evaluation Documentation Center (EDC), Office of the Assistant Secretary for Planning and Evaluation, U.S. Department of Health and Human Services (HHS), Room 438F Humphrey Building, 200 Independence Avenue, SW, Washington, DC 20201, 202-245-6445

Subject: Examples from 300-term subject index are ambulatory and outpatient health care, biomedical research, drugs therapeutic and devices, economic analysis, health care delivery systems, health insurance and financing, information systems, medical practice, medical technology, quality assurance, and utilization review.

Content: Project descriptions of in-process and completed evaluations from the Office of the Secretary of HHS, HCFA, PHS (e.g., ADAMHA, CDC, FDA, HRSA, NIH, OASH), Social Security Administration, and other agencies. *Compendium* is organized by HHS operating divisions and agencies; it includes project descriptions (1,800 in 1985 edition), a subject index, agency sponsor index, and program name index. Project descriptions include agency sponsor, project title, report title, performer, agency contact, programs evaluated, abstract, access descriptors, and other information. The 1985 edition is 926 pages long; the 1987 edition is approximately 1,100 pages long.

Compilation: Compiled from one-page descriptions of all ongoing and completed HHS evaluation studies carried out since the early 1970s. EDC first published project descriptions of HHS evaluation activities in 1976. System was computerized in 1979. Database was expanded in later years to include more agencies.

Access: Copies of *Compendium*, a bound volume, may be obtained from NTIS 703-487-4650. 1985 (fifth) edition (order PB86112281) price is $66.95 plus $3 handling. Sixth edition due summer 1987. For electronic access to the EDC database, users must register with EDC and have an account with the Parklawn Computer Center. EDC makes available *Users Guide to the Evaluation Documentation Center* and *Sponsors Guide to the Evaluation Documentation Center*. The quarterly *Memorandum* provides information on EDC acquisitions as they occur.

CPHA (Commission on Professional and Hospital Activities) Files

Source: CPHA, 1968 Green Road, PO Box 1809, Ann Arbor, MI 48106. 800-521-6210, 800-828-6762 in Michigan

Subject: Computerized patient discharge data.

Content: *National Inpatient Profile* is a diagnosis and procedure utilization data set drawn from the CPHA *National Patient Sample File*. Two-volume annual set is sequenced by ICD-9-CM diagnoses and procedures. The summary profile section provides overview of projected number of principal and secondary diagnoses or procedures treated in U.S. hospitals. The detail profile displays demographic, clinical, and facility characteristics of these diagnoses and procedures. For each ICD-9-CM code, data are provided on patient demographics, patient clinical information, number and percent of patients having the code as a principal procedure, number and percent of occurrences of the code as a secondary procedure, and hospital facility information.

Other standard CPHA data sets include *Cost Containment Series: Length of Stay and Medicare Ancillary Charge Norms*, *Quality of Care Series: Case Fatalities by DRG*, and *National Outpatient Profile*. *National Patient Sample File* is also used to generate other data files and customized data sets on, e.g., newborns, inpatient charges, and trends in occurrences of diseases and procedures.

Compilation: CPHA files are compiled from patient discharge data from more than 1,400 hospitals, covering 10 million patients and 25 percent of North America's acute care hospitalizations. *National Patient Sample File* is based on 2 million patient sample drawn every year. CPHA archive maintains a total of 300 million patient records. For some files, CPHA merges its patient data with institutional data from the American Hospital Association and other sources.

Access: CPHA files are available as hard copy reports, on floppy disk, or magnetic tape. Charge for *National Inpatient Profile* is $5,000 to commercial and $750 to non-commercial buyers. Charge for *National Outpatient Profile* is $3,000 to commercial and $500 to non-commercial buyers. Charge for *Length of Stay* information sets (one each on diagnoses and procedures) is $85 for books and $4,500 for tapes. Prices for customized statistical reports vary; typical charge may be $500, or less if client is a regular subscriber to CPHA information services.

CRISP (Computer Retrieval of Information on Scientific Projects)

Source: Statistics and Analysis Branch, Division of Research Grants (DRG), National Institutes of Health, Bethesda, MD 20892, 301-496-7543

Subject: Scientific information on extramural research projects supported through grants and contracts programs of NIH, ADAMHA, and other PHS agencies, as well as intramural research projects conducted by NIH and ADAMHA.

Content: In general, information from CRISP can take the form of topical scientific information or institution-based scientific profiles. The five files of CRISP computer information system use disk storage for random and sequential access. CRISP is capable of subdividing program projects, center, and other multifaceted projects into smaller research components. File 1 is a master dictionary of scientific subject headings corresponding to those appearing in MHRST (Medical and Health Related Sciences Thesaurus used for describing research projects). File 2 stores the indexed subject heading numbers with their associated project numbers. File 4 serves to combine the data elements contained in the Files 1 and 2. File 3 is a project identification master file, consisting of information transferred from IMPAC (a related system dealing with administrative aspects of NIH extramural programs; see description), including project and subproject numbers and titles, investigators names and addresses, initial review group designations, institution codes, and amounts awarded. File 5 contains the investigator-prepared narrative for each project. The two-volume Research Awards Index, compiled from CRISP, contains project and contract information listed by subject, project or contract number, and principal investigator.

Compilation: Projects are indexed based on applications or progress reports for extramural research, and on annual reports or project narratives for intramural research. CRISP is updated twice weekly; intramural projects are reported and entered into CRISP annually. The project identification master file (File 3) is updated through weekly links with IMPAC. MHRST is updated semiannually. The Research Awards Index is published annually.

Access: Direct access to CRISP files is available to all NIH staff with registered accounts by contacting DRG. Online access to selected data from the latest fiscal year files is available to outside individuals or organizations through subscription from NTIS 703-487-4808.

Current Assessments, New Technology Abstracts

Source: New York State Center for Assessing Health Services, Health Services Center 4L 215, State University of New York at Stony Brook, Stony Brook, NY 11794, 516-444-2101

Subject: *Current Assessments* covers public health, clinical and health services research; *New Technology Abstracts* covers innovations in health care technology and biomedical research.

Content: *Current Assessments* provides annotated summaries of journal articles that report findings from public health, clinical, and health services research; and address the impact of technology on health policy. Summaries include reference citation, research findings, description of data source, study population, research methodology, study limitations, and implications of research for health care industry and subsequent policy decisions.

New Technology Abstracts lists citations to journal articles and reports that cover new technologies in health care and biomedical research, or innovative applications of existing technologies. Also includes listings of FDA notices and notices from U.S. Patent Office. Center also conducts studies of the impact of changes in health services for health policy. Studies conducted during 1987 address innovations in intensive home health care, regulation of risk in ambulatory surgery, organization of organ replacement services by states, and cost of inpatient treatment for patients with AIDS in four hospitals in metropolitan New York.

Compilation: Journal articles were selected through monthly computer search of *Index Medicus*, *Index to Dental Literature*, *International Nursing Index*, *Hospital Literature Index*, and staff review of recent publications. Center also conducted monthly search of U.S. government technical and research reports listed in NTIS Bibliographic Data Base, FDA notices listed in *Federal Register*, and patents for medical devices reported in the *Official Gazette of the U.S. Patent and Trademark Office*. Publications were first issued in 1985. *Current Assessments* and *New Technology Abstracts* published every few months.

Access: In 1987, the New York State Department of Health ended its cosponsorship of the Center, hence, publication of *Current Assessments* and *New Technology Abstracts* has been suspended. Back publications, reports, and copies of articles listed in *New Technology Abstracts* are available upon request.

Device Experience Network (DEN)

Source: Division of Product Surveillance, Office of Compliance, Center for Devices and Radiological Health, HFZ-343, Food and Drug Administration, 8757 Georgia Avenue, Silver Spring, MD 20910, 301-427-8100

Subject: Postmarketing surveillance of FDA-approved medical devices and in vitro diagnostic and laboratory products.

Content: Computerized database contains voluntary reports from health care providers and provider organizations concerning device-related hazards, defects, and deficiencies; these include performance failures, improper labeling, incomplete, inadequate, or erroneous instructions, unsatisfactory packaging, or defective components. DEN identifies industry-wide problems and significant trends, e.g., product recalls and regulatory actions related to a particular product.

Compilation: DEN consists primarily of information from the Medical Device and Laboratory Product Problem Reporting Program (PRP) administered by the United States Pharmacopeial Convention and the Medical Device Reporting (MDR) program of the FDA. Information is gathered from health care professionals, hospitals, state and local government, public health officials, FDA field offices, contracting groups, consumer organizations, and consumers. Established in 1973. Updated continuously.

Access: DEN reports accessible through BMEDSS 216-375-3501, National Technical Information Service 703-487-4630, Medical Device Register's *Product SOS* 203-348-6319, and ECRI 215-825-6000. Confidential trade, commercial, financial, personnel, medical, and patient information are deleted from publicly available reports. DEN reports in microfiche and additional information about specific reports available from FDA, Freedom of Information Office, Room 12A16, HFI-31, 5600 Fishers Lane,

Rockville, MD 20857, 301-443-6310. Monthly publication *Device Experience Network Reports*, which includes PRP but not MDR information, is available from FOI Services 301-881-0410 for $190. To report a device problem call U.S. Pharmacopeial Convention 800-638-6725 or contact FDA.

DIALOG

Source: DIALOG Information Services, Inc., 3460 Hillview Avenue, Palo Alto, CA 94304, 800-334-2564, 415-858-3785

Subject: Databases cover biosciences, health care, medicine, science and technology, business and finance, law, government, social sciences, current affairs/news, humanities, education.

Content: Includes over 250 multidisciplinary databases. Those relevant to medical technology include BIOSIS PREVIEWS, CANCERLIT, CLINICAL ABSTRACTS (abstracts from journals covering clinical medicine, clinical practice, and research), DRUG INFORMATION FULL TEXT (full-text information on current and investigational drugs, including research, treatment, and pharmacological practice), EMBASE (from Excerpta Medica, with references and summaries of international medical literature, covering biomedicine, health, and health care management), HEALTH, and MEDLINE. Many databases offer bibliographic citations, summaries of articles and reports, detailed financial data on companies, directory listings of companies and associations, or full-text articles and newswires; most indexed by title, subject, author, publication date. Monthly newsletter provides information on DIALOG system and databases. Electronic mail and bulletin boards available through DIALMAIL service.

Compilation: Databases are compiled from journal articles, books, periodicals, patent indexes, business/company directories, newspaper articles, government documents, dissertations and theses, wire services, corporate reports. Most references are updated monthly; newspaper files are updated daily.

Access: Databases are available online; accessible via modem from remote terminal through DIALNET, TYMNET, TELENET, MEADNET, IN-WATS, INFONET, DUNSNET, direct dial. Online or offline document printing available. Subscription required. Standard service plan requires no initiation fee or monthly charge; first password free for new users. Optional starter package ($150) includes training seminar and user guide. Connect cost includes all database royalties; varies with database searched. Several other service plan/advance purchase options available, e.g., connect cost discounts of up to $15/hour.

Directory of Health Services Research Organizations

Subject: Health services and policy research centers.

Content: Describes more than 100 university-based health services and policy research centers, Veterans Administration health services research and demonstration field programs, and AHSR institutional members. Notes each organization's budget, primary area of emphasis and expertise, staffing, training capabilities, organizational location, address, telephone number, and name of director. Highlights major research projects, funding source, and principle investigator. Indexed by subject, funding source, and principle investigators.

Compilation: Information collected through mail survey and follow-up telephone interviews. Current edition of directory available early 1988.

Access: Directory available upon request. Cost for AHSR members $10; non-members $15.

DIRLINE (Directory of Information Resources Online)

Source: MEDLARS Management Section, National Library of Medicine (NLM), Building 38, Room 4N421, 8600 Rockville Pike, Bethesda, MD 20894, 800-638-8480, 301-496-6193 in Maryland

Subject: Public and private sector health and biomedical organizations.

Content: Database contains information on over 14,000 resource centers, with specialized information in a variety of disciplines. Also includes over 1,500 records for organizations providing information in various areas of health and disease. Contains two subfiles on specialty topics: poison control and substance abuse. Information provided for each organization includes its full name, address, contact person, and telephone number, as well as a summary of its services, activities, publications and interests. Can be searched by organization name using text words or subject-related keywords. See MEDLINE description for listing of NLM MEDLARS databases.

Compilation: Information gathered from Library of Congress National Referral Center database and the ODPHP National Health Information Center database (a product of the Office of Disease Prevention and Health Promotion, U.S. Department of Health and Human Services). Specialty subfiles derived from Poison Control Centers and Drug Abuse Communications Network. All records updated at least once every two years. File updated quarterly.

Access: Available online at any time through NLM MEDLARS computer system to more than 6,000 online centers in hospitals, medical schools, universities, government agencies, commercial firms, and other organizations throughout U.S., as well as MEDLARS centers located in 13 other countries. Also accessible via modem from remote terminal through TELENET, TYMNET, direct dial. Connect cost averages $22/hour peak time, $15/hour off-peak.

Drug Product Problem Reporting Program (DPPR)

Source: Practitioner Reporting System, United States Pharmacopeial Convention, Inc. (USP), 12601 Twinbrook Parkway, Rockville, MD 20852, 301-881-0666. DPPR supported by FDA.

Subject: Postmarketing surveillance of FDA-approved prescription, over-the-counter, and radiopharmaceutical drug products.

Content: Database contains voluntary reports from health care practitioners on problems experienced when pharmaceutical products are received, used, or dispensed; these include unsatisfactory packaging, erroneous or deficient labeling, inadequate package insert information, poor pharmaceutical quality, questionable bioavailability, stability, and therapeutic effectiveness. Reports retrievable by date report submitted, product name, manufacturer and/or type of problem. DPPR identifies trend by specific product, across product lines by drug entity, and by manufacturer.

Compilation: Information gathered via toll-free telephone line or prepared reporting forms from health care professionals including physicians, nurses, pharmacists, biomedical engineers, medical laboratory personnel, risk managers, purchasing and quality assurance personnel, and consumers. Reports are entered as unverified information into FDA databases; FDA is responsible for follow up, i.e., determining manufacturer's evaluation of problem and establishing final assessment of problem. Program initiated in 1971. Updated continuously.

Access: For copies of DPPR reports and product experience data, contact FDA, Freedom of Information Office, 5600 Fishers Lane, Room 12A16, HFI-31, Rockville, MD 20857, 301-443-6310. To report a drug product problem call 800-638-6725 or contact USP for reporting form.

Duke Comprehensive Cancer Center Database

Source: Duke Comprehensive Cancer Center (DCCC), Duke University Medical Center, Box 3153, Durham, NC 27710, 919-684-2057

Subject: Cancer cases diagnosed or treated at DCCC; designed for clinical and research oncologists.

Content: Database includes epidemiological, histological, and patient demographic information such as patient medical history and history of prior cancers, state of birth, state of residency, zip code, type and stage of cancer/tumor, and treatment regimen. In addition to this comprehensive tumor registry, special registries are often established to investigate specific research questions, to examine sequelae of particular cancers, or to facilitate statistical analyses. *Annual Data Management Unit Report* provides statistical summaries of registry data, e.g., cancer-specific frequencies, county-specific frequencies, tumor-specific trends, survival rates, as well as an in-depth analysis of one or more types of cancer. Research findings also reported in medical journals and at medical conferences.

Compilation: Tumor registry initiated in 1970. All living cancer patients in registry are routinely monitored; individual follow-up every 13 months. Information gathered from daily oncology clinic visits, as well as surveys designed for specific research purposes. Registry data obtained primarily from medical charts; special registries may also obtain data from laboratory and pathology reports.

Access: DCCC computer tapes are not in public domain due to patient confidentiality constraints. Contact DCCC Director regarding access to data resources; written requests indicating purpose of data acquisition and specific data required are preferred. Database search costs, if any, vary according to information requested. Searches available include frequencies and survival graphs.

Environmental Hazards and Health Effects Reports

Source: Division of Environmental Hazards and Health Effects (DEHHE), Center for Environmental Health, Centers for Disease Control, 1600 Clifton Road, Atlanta, GA 30333, 404-454-4772

Subject: Health hazards resulting from environmental contaminants, e.g., toxic chemicals and radiation.

Content: DEHHE databases cover disasters, environmental hazards, toxic chemicals, and other miscellaneous events. National data are collected on deaths, populations exposed to environmental toxicants, persons injured by man-made or natural disasters (e.g., nuclear or chemical disasters, hurricanes, earthquakes, tornados, etc.), variety of public health hazards, and resultant health outcomes. Reports and other publications are based on these databases.

Compilation: Division activities initiated in 1984. Information gathered from individual studies, surveillance systems, laboratory data of subjects in special studies, and National Medical Examiner/Coroner Survey. Reports and other publications issued on an ad hoc basis. Databases updated as necessary.

Access: Reports of studies are usually available from the requesting agency within or outside CDC for which studies are done, rather than from DEHHE. Reports from DEHHE often appear in CDC *Morbidity and Mortality Weekly Report* and scientific journals; reprints available upon request by writing to source. Justified requests for use of databases must usually be made in writing to individual investigator, study collaborators, or CDC Freedom of Information Office.

Environmental Health Laboratory Sciences Reports

Source: Division of Environmental Health Laboratory Sciences (EHLS), Center for Environmental Health, Centers for Disease Control, Chamblee 17/1103, 1600 Clifton Road, Atlanta, GA 30333, 404-452-4152

Subject: Application of laboratory technology for the diagnosis, treatment, and prevention of chronic diseases and toxic chemical exposures.

Content: EHLS activities include international surveillance of lipid and apolipoprotein measurements for determination of risk to coronary heart disease; international surveillance of toxic chemical exposure incidents (on request); and laboratory support for the National Health and Nutrition Examination Survey (HANES). Data collected on levels of dioxin and related compounds in population; cholesterol and apolipoprotein levels; exposure to and levels of polychlorinated biphenyls; cytology of cervical cancer; levels of lead, cadmium, and arsenic in the population; nutritional markers; exposure to pesticides; phenylketonuria and hypothyroidism; and biomarkers. Reports and other publications are based on these databases; also covered are descriptions of the development, validation, and evaluation of analytical methods used in surveillance activities, e.g., methods for monitoring human exposure to toxicants; responses to acute and chronic occurrences, e.g., exposures; and general epidemiological information.

Compilation: Division activities initiated in 1970. Information gathered from research and clinical laboratories; public health community studies; and national, stratified, probability sample of U.S. households (HANES data). Reports and other publications issued upon study/survey completion.

Access: Reports of studies are usually available from the requesting agency within or outside CDC for which studies are done, rather than from EHLS. Reprints of journal articles written by EHLS staff and other publications available upon request by writing to source. Justified requests for use of databases must usually be made in writing to individual investigator, study collaborators, or CDC Freedom of Information Office.

FDA Bulletin Board

Source: Food and Drug Administration, Press Office, 5600 Fishers Lane, Parklawn Building, Room 1505, HFI-20, Rockville, MD 20857, 301-443-3285

Subject: FDA communications and meetings.

Content: NEWS file contains FDA news releases covering public health and product safety issues, and some product recalls. ENFORCE file contains the weekly *FDA Enforcement Report*, a list of FDA-regulated products under recall; also includes seizure items, prosecution actions, injunction actions, and health fraud notices. CONSUMER file provides table of contents and selected articles from FDA's monthly magazine *FDA Consumer*; also covers topical updates, regulatory matters, and reports on actions by FDA investigators. APPROVALS file contains complete text of the monthly *Drug and Device Products Approvals List*; includes human drug approvals, medical device approvals, biological licenses issued, and veterinary drug approvals. DATE-REG file provides summaries of all FDA announcements made in the *Federal Register* arranged by publication date; includes short summary of article, name of contact person, and time and place of public meetings. SUBJ-REG provides summaries of all FDA *Federal Register* announcements arranged by subject. BULLETIN contains the current *Drug Bulletin*, a newsletter useful for physicians and other health professionals. CDRH file includes the *Centers for Devices and Radiological Health Bulletins* that are issued monthly and contain information on recent CDRH developments and meetings. MEETINGS file covers upcoming FDA meetings announced in the *Federal Register*; describes time and place of meetings, topics to be discussed, and contact person. CONGRESS file contains full text of prepared statements delivered by FDA officials at congressional oversight hearings. SPEECH file provides full text of prepared speeches delivered by FDA Commissioner and Deputy Commissioner at various meetings. Keyword searching available; document can be scanned or read in its entirety.

Compilation: Most items are added to bulletin board as soon as they are issued and are held for one month.

Access: Available through DAILCOM 202-488-0550. Charges are $25/hour peak time and $22.30/hour off-peak, plus $0.05/kilocharacter; $25 monthly minimum. Contact Press Office for information on obtaining bulletin board documents in print form.

F-D-C Reports

Source: F-D-C Reports, Inc., Suite One, 5550 Friendship Boulevard, Chevy Chase, MD 20815, 301-657-9830

Subject: Pharmaceutical product development information.

Content: *NDA Pipeline* is a 600-page annual reference volume covering drug developments during the previous calendar year. Contents include listing by company and generic name of new drug approvals (NDAs) and biological product licenses; original NDAs listed according to FDA classification system for NDAs and investigational new drug applications (INDs); index of products reviewed by FDA advisory committees; descriptions of 1,200 drug and biological products under development; articles from *Prescription and OTC Pharmaceuticals*; FDA drug advisory committee members and meetings; list of orphan products; and index and contact information for companies mentioned in volume.

Additional F-D-C Reports include the following weekly newsletters. *Prescription and OTC Pharmaceuticals* covers regulatory activities, industry developments, new product introductions, and financial changes. *Medical Devices, Diagnostics & Instrumentation Reports* covers similar topics for the medical devices, diagnostics, and instrumentation industries. *Health Policy & Biomedical Research* covers Medicare and Medicaid, public health, health professions education and supply, federal health policy, developments concerning NIH and ADAMHA, university and industrial biomedical research, and FDA regulatory activity affecting these. *Technology Reimbursement Reports* covers health care reimbursement and the medical technology industry. *Weekly Pharmacy Reports* covers news on introduction and pricing of new pharmaceuticals, regulatory activity, lawsuits, and related developments of interest to pharmacists. *Quality Control Reports*, published monthly, addresses quality assurance and quality control procedures in prescription, over-the-counter pharmaceutical, cosmetics, and medical device industries.

Compilation: F-D-C Reports are compiled from FDA public documents, meetings, and press releases; other federal agencies such as Federal Trade Commission and Justice Department; congressional publications, hearings and other sources; health product company reports and announcements, industry and professional society conferences, news services, and investment sources.

Access: F-D-C Reports may be ordered from source. Annual *NDA Pipeline* costs $175. Cost of *Weekly Pharmacy Reports* is $25/year; other weekly newsletters range from $260 to $470/year. Cost of *Quality Control Reports* is $85/year. Discounts for multiple copies.

Futures Program

Source: Center for Health Management Research, 1423 South Grand Avenue, Los Angeles, CA 90015, 213-742-6335. Member of American Healthcare Systems.

Subject: Market trends in health care industry; intended primarily for health care management personnel.

Content: Futures Program includes series of publications covering the social, technological, environmental, economic, and political events and trends affecting health care.

Forecast is an annual report on market trends and projections; recent subjects include cost-containment, intrauterine devices, laser surgery, lithotripter, long-term care, product liability, transplants. *Forecast* slides and scripts or videotapes also available. *Health Scan* assesses the impact of emerging technology and business innovations on the health care industry in terms of strategic implications for management; topics include AIDS, Alzheimer's disease, fiber optics, HMOs, marketing, technological change. *Market Scan* informs health care managers of new product and service opportunities; recent topics include bioethics, cardiac imaging, cardiac monitoring, cryosurgery, echocardiography, gamma camera, gene therapy, home care, diagnostic imaging, interferon, interleukin-2, mammography, non-invasive technology, PPOs, perinatal services, prostheses, recombinant DNA, tomography, ultrasound. *Mini Trends* covers market trends and intelligence information derived from sources not generally scanned by health care managers; recent issues include AZT, artificial kidney, bioengineering, cataracts, dialysis, genetic engineering, steroids. *Book Digest* provides synopses of management literature and other select publications pertinent to health care.

Compilation: Information gathered from trade journals, periodicals, books, and other relevant literature. Active since 1980.

Access: Annual subscription fee of $2,500 includes five copies of each publication mailed bimonthly. Additional subscriptions may be purchased on sliding-fee basis.

HEALTH (Health Planning and Administration)

Source: American Hospital Association (AHA) Resource Center, 840 North Lake Shore Drive, Chicago, IL 60611, 312-280-6263

Subject: Non-clinical aspects of health care delivery, including administration and planning of health care facilities, services and manpower; health insurance; health policy; financial management; law and regulation; personnel administration; quality assurance; licensure and accreditation; and patient education and health promotion.

Content: Database includes approximately 330,000 bibliographic citations, 90 percent of which are to English language publications. Indexed using NLM's controlled vocabulary MeSH (Medical Subject Headings). *Hospital Literature Index* produced from HEALTH file. See MEDLINE description for listing of NLM MEDLARS databases.

Compilation: Citations derived from MEDLINE, AHA, and National Health Planning Information Center (1975-1981). Source documents include journal articles, technical reports, government documents, theses, monographs, and monographic chapters. Approximately 3,000 citations added monthly.

Access: Available online at any time through NLM MEDLARS computer system to more than 6,000 online centers in hospitals, medical schools, universities, government agencies, commercial firms, and other organizations throughout U.S., as well as MEDLARS centers located in 13 other countries. Also accessible via modem from remote terminal through TELENET, TYMNET, direct dial. To contact MEDLARS Management Division call 800-638-8480 or 301-496-6193 in Maryland. Call source for information about *Hospital Literature Index* and related information. Connect cost averages $22/hour peak time, $15/hour off-peak. Also available through BRS 800-345-4277, COLLEAGUE (BRS/Saunders) 800-468-0908, and DIALOG 800-334-2564.

Health Devices Alerts

Source: ECRI, 5200 Butler Pike, Plymouth Meeting, PA 19462, 215-825-6000

Subject: Problems, hazards, and recalls involving medical devices or equipment.

Content: The publication reflects recalls, hazards, and problems with medical devices where these have been verified by ECRI. A typical issue of *Health Devices Alerts Abstracts* consists of 80 to 100 abstracts, organized by device type. Also included are presentations of the problem and of the action needed, as well as a list of hospital departments that might be affected.

Compilation: Information is compiled from review of more than 500 English-language medical, engineering, legal, and government publications. *Health Devices Alerts* was initiated in 1976.

Access: *Health Devices Alerts* is published in two forms: *Health Devices Alerts Abstracts* is published twice monthly; *Health Devices Alerts Action Items* is published weekly. Subscriptions are $235/year. The database is currently on ECRI computer systems; searches are available. The database is to be available online through BMEDSS in 1988.

Health Devices Sourcebook

Source: ECRI, 5200 Butler Pike, Plymouth Meeting, PA 19462, 215-825-6000

Subject: Medical device nomenclature and manufacturers.

Content: Cross-referenced list of more than 5,000 categories of medical devices and related products, based on ECRI numerical coding system. Each product is listed along with its U.S. and Canadian manufacturers, importers, and distributors, with contact information; a trade name section is included. Directory has references to brand-name product ratings and comparisons, and database searches made available by ECRI.

Compilation: Any firm that is the manufacturer, exclusive distributor, or importer of a medical device that is sold to hospitals, either directly or through distributors or dealers qualifies for inclusion in the directory.

Access: *Health Devices Sourcebook* published annually; 1987 edition price $140.

Health Information Resources in the Federal Government

Source: ODPHP National Health Information Center (ONHIC), Office of Disease Prevention and Health Promotion, U.S. Department of Health and Human Services, PO Box 1133, Washington, DC 20013-1133, 800-336-4797, 202-429-9091

Subject: Selected federal agencies and federally sponsored organizations with information in various areas of health and disease.

Content: Information provided for each organization/resource in the directory includes contact information, summary of services, activities, databases, publication topics and access information. Entries arranged alphabetically by principal keyword.

Compilation: Entries selected based on resource's ability to provide health information to health professionals and general public, and resource's existence as an office within, or a project of, the federal government.

Access: 1987 directory is available from source for $2 handling fee. ONHIC database of referral organizations available online through NLM MEDLARS computer system as a component of DIRLINE. Directory provides DIRLINE record accession number for each organization to facilitate online searching.

HEALTHLAWYER

Source: American Hospital Association (AHA), Office of Legal Communications, 840 North Lake Shore Drive, Chicago, IL 60611, 312-280-6679

Subject: Legal and regulatory issues of health care.

Content: Search capability by subject headings from thesaurus, keywords. Contains case digests, including those from *Hospital Law* and *Health Law Digest*; abstracts of articles selected from over 100 journals, including *American Journal of Law and Medicine*, *Law Medicine and Health Care*, and *Hospitals*; full text of selected articles from newsletters such as *Health Law Vigil*, *Hospital Ethics*, and *Medical Staff News*, abstracts of educational conference materials.

Compilation: Compiled from government reports/documents, papers presented at conferences, wire services, corporate reports, and periodicals. Database established in January 1984, updated monthly; 6,000 new records added per year.

Access: Available online from BRS 800-345-4277. Connect costs $16 to $35/hour, plus $33 to $40 royalty. Printing costs $0.37/record online, $0.40/record offline; plus $3 to $9 telecommunication fee. Accessed through TELENET, direct dial. Subscription required. Thesaurus/search aid available to subscribers for $10.

HECLINET (Health Care Literature Information Network)

Source: Deutsches Institute für Medizinische Dokumentation und Information (DIMDI), Welbhausstrasse 27, Postfach 42 05 80, D-50000 Cologne 41, Federal Republic of Germany, (49-221) 47-24-1

Subject: Hospital administration, design and construction, maintenance, financing, hygiene, and economics; and non-clinical aspects of health services, including policy, economics, education, insurance, organization, planning, law, jurisdiction, and regional planning.

Content: HECLINET indexes articles from approximately 400 journals on hospital affairs and public health services; 200 journals on architecture, city planning and engineering; 20 journals on operations research; and 700 journals on economics; as well as 400 books, monographs, conference proceedings, and company publications annually. Approximately 50 percent of the articles indexed are in German; approximately 30 percent are in English. 60 percent of the literature indexed in HECLINET appears in the printed version of the database, *Informationsdienst Krankenhauswesen/ Health Care Information Service*. HECLINET's Thesaurus Krankhauswesen uses 1,100 indexing terms, available in German and English. Under new indexing system, all records will be indexed in both languages.

DIMDI also provides access to U.S. National Library of Medicine databases MEDLINE, CANCERLIT, CLINPROT, HEALTH, and TOXLINE, as well as databases from other sources such as BIOSIS PREVIEWS, EMBASE (Excerpta Medica), IRCS (Elsevier International Research Communications System), MEDITEC (Medizinische Technik), and SCISEARCH (Science Citation Index).

Compilation: HECLINET has been compiled cooperatively since 1969 by the hospital institutes of the Federal Republic of Germany, Denmark, Sweden, Austria, and Switzerland. The system has a total of approximately 70,000 document records; 4,500 new records are added to HECLINET each year. The system is updated bimonthly.

Access: Accessible via modem from remote terminal from DIMDI. Connection to DIMDI is possible via COMPUSERVE, DATAPAK, ITT-UDTS, TELENET, TYMNET, WUI-DBS, RCA-LSDS, TRT and UNINET. User number codes and English language user handbook available from DIMDI. Charges for HECLINET from DIMDI include $25/year for user number code, $15/connect hour for royalties, $0.2/ printed citation, and other charges for systems time, think time, number of characters, and downloading. Some charges are reduced for non-profit users; rebates apply after 60 hours of connect time. About 65 percent of HECLINET users as German.

HIAA (Health Insurance Association of America) Medical Appropriateness Compilation

Source: Health Insurance Association of America, 1025 Connecticut Avenue, NW, Washington, DC 20036-3998, 202-223-7837

Subject: Appropriateness of diagnostic and therapeutic medical procedures.

Content: Each procedure transmittal in the *Compilation* includes name of procedure, definition of procedure, name of assessment program—usually the Council of Medical Specialty Societies (CMSS), date submitted by HIAA to CMSS, date of opinion provided by CMSS to HIAA, source of opinion (e.g., CMSS and one or more specialty societies), and opinion (most are from one sentence to one paragraph in length). In addition, the *Compilation* has sections on how to participate, assessment organizations, technology news, procedure listings, sources of definitions, and a topical index of procedures.

Compilation: Medical appropriateness opinions in the *Compilation* have been generated through an arrangement initiated in 1977 between HIAA and the CMSS. HIAA has accepted requests for opinions from its member companies and forwarded these to CMSS (specifically, its Program for Clinical Procedure Review), which distributed them to one or more of its 24 respective specialty societies, as appropriate. When the specialty societies rendered opinions to CMSS, these have been forwarded to HIAA for distribution. A few opinions have been used from other assessment sources. Since 1985, these opinions, referred to as procedure transmittals, have been organized in the loose-leaf *Compilation*, which is updated approximately annually. Since 1978, CMSS has returned opinions on 115 of approximately 200 HIAA requests. The CMSS is reviewing and considering revisions to its clinical procedures review process and related technology assessment activities.

Access: The *Compilation* is available from HIAA for $25.

High Blood Pressure Information Center

Source: Office of Prevention, Education, and Control, National Heart, Lung, and Blood Institute (NHLBI), 120/80 National Institutes of Health, Bethesda, MD 20892, 301-496-1809

Subject: High blood pressure and prevention of hypertension-related death and disability.

Content: Bibliographic database provides citations to over 6,000 journal articles pertaining to hypertension, cardiovascular disease risk factors, and related topics. Information resources cover consumer and professional health education interventions for control and detection of high blood pressure (HBP), materials and guides on planning, implementing, and evaluating HBP control programs, guidelines for detection, diagnosis, and treatment of HBP, recommendations on the roles of health care providers in HBP control, catalogs of audiovisual and printed educational materials, and ongoing community and state activities in HBP control. Center maintains information on research, funding, and principal investigators in hypertension and assists in referrals to appropriate sources of research information. Other services: preparation of customized information packets containing journal reprints, resource materials on current topics of interest and relevant publications, literature searches, and technical assistance for program planning or workshop development. Publishes quarterly newsletter featuring ongoing projects and activities.

Compilation: Information gathered from medical and professional journals, National Health and Nutrition Examination Survey, Health Interview Survey, National Center for Health Statistics reports, NHLBI demonstration and education projects, NHLBI research grants, state and local health departments, voluntary health agencies, pharmaceutical company publications, and member organizations on National High Blood Pressure Education Program Coordinating Council. Database updated monthly. Active since 1972.

Access: Publications list available upon request. All services and materials are free of charge; however, materials available in limited quantities. Database is available online through BRS 800-345-4277, and is also part of the Combined Health Information Database (CHID). Database indexed by keywords; thesaurus available to users.

IMPAC (Information for Management Planning Analysis and Coordination)

Source: Statistics and Analysis Branch, Division of Research Grants (DRG), National Institutes of Health, Bethesda, MD 20892, 301-496-7543

Subject: Administrative information on reviews and awards for extramural research programs of NIH, ADAMHA, and other PHS programs.

Content: The IMPAC Pending and Open Master Files include master records of basic data on NIH extramural programs. The Institutional Profile File is used to retrieve institution-specific information. The Project Address File is used to retrieve address and related information for Notices of Grant Award. The Trainee Appointment File contains information on NIH, ADAMHA, and CDC training grant programs. The Committee Management Information System includes information on NIH public advisory committees. The National Research Service Award (NRSA) Payback File contains information on fellows and trainees who have incurred a payback obligation under a National Research Service Award.

Compilation: Much of IMPAC data is compiled from the approximately 50,000 competing and noncompeting applications for PHS extramural support processed through the system annually; data are updated continuously during the review and award process and with feedback from recipients of IMPAC output. Each week, administrative data from IMPAC are transferred to CRISP (a related system dealing with scientific aspects of extramural and intramural research supported by PHS; see CRISP description).

Access: IMPAC is designed primarily for access by DHHS staff. DRG offers a variety of IMPAC services to DHHS users, including an extensive query software system. Specified data sets on magnetic tape are provided to most PHS awarding agencies. A variety of reports on active grants and training awards are provided in hard copy, magnetic tapes, and microfiche. DRG provides publications generated from IMPAC on trends in extramural research, characteristics of NIH public advisory committees and peer review of grant applications, and related information.

IMS Audits

Source: IMS America Ltd., 660 West Germantown Pike, PO Box 905, Plymouth Meeting, PA 19462-0905, 215-834-5000

Subject: Sales and market research on health care products.

Content: Data provided on prescription, distribution, promotion, and sale of pharmaceuticals; purchase of hospital supplies; patterns of diagnosis and treatment of disease. Among the audits provided by IMS are the following. *U.S. Pharmaceutical Market—Hospitals* reports hospital purchases of pharmaceuticals and diagnostics, including a monthly report of new drugs on clinical trial. *Hospital Supply Index* reports on hospital purchases of medical/surgical supplies. *New Product Digest* covers new products and their progress in the market. *LabList* audits census information on laboratory instrumentation and equipment in clinical laboratories. *GrouPractice Market: Instrumentation and Testing* audits census data on instrumentation in physician group practices. *Clinical Laboratory Audit*, based on survey data from the College of American Pathologists, covers test volume and brand share for clinical laboratory tests. *National Disease and Therapeutic Index* covers data on patterns and treatment of disease encountered in medical practice. Other audits cover circulation and cost of pharmaceutical advertising, sales of pharmaceuticals and diagnostic reagents, and prescribing activities of individual physicians. Data from these audits may be customized in a variety of formats.

IMSPACT is an online system for access to the complete IMS pharmaceutical database, including data on drugstore, hospital, physician, and promotional activities in the U.S.

Compilation: IMS collects census or sample data from 27,000 anonymous sources in U.S. and Canada, including drugstores, hospitals, physicians, and laboratories.

Access: Data are accessible on a contractual basis through remote online terminals, printed matter, and microfilm. Charges vary depending upon choice of audit and the amount of data required. For instance, charges for *LabList* may range from approximately $2,600 for smaller portions of the audit, to approximately $93,000 for the entire audit. The charge for the 12-14 volume annual *LabFile* from the *LabList* is approximately $25,000. Charges for *Clinical Laboratory Audit* may range from $1,000 for certain portions to $36,000 for the entire audit. IMSPACT is accessible online for subscribers to printed IMS audits. The charge for online access to the complete set of files in IMSPACT is approximately $94,000, plus computer charges. When approved by IMS, certain data sets may be accessible at reduced or no charges to university or other researchers for non-commercial purposes.

International Market Research Studies

Source: Division of Market Analysis, Office of Commercial Information Management, Room 2012, U.S. Department of Commerce, 14th Street and Constitution Avenue, NW, Washington, DC 20230, 202-377-4203

Subject: Export market information for many U.S. industries, including medical equipment and supplies and health care service industries.

Content: *International Market Research Studies* analyze market size, trends, competition, distribution channels, competition, distribution channels, business practices, barriers, and other market factors for an industry in a selected country. Studies on medical equipment and/or health care services were conducted for approximately 30 countries during the period 1982-1987.

Compilation: Majority of reports conducted using Commerce specifications under contracts issued by U.S. embassies to consultants in respective countries. *Special Situation Reports* generally conducted by U.S. and Foreign Commercial Service and/or embassies.

Access: Print copies formerly available from U.S. Department of Commerce. During 1987, information for all studies was loaded on new U.S. Department of Commerce computer system CIMS (Commercial Information Management System). Tailored reports of varying lengths may be printed for set-up fee (e.g., $15) and per-page fee (e.g., $2). Computer files not directly accessible to public. Some back reports are available from local district and regional Commerce offices for approximately $100. More than 80 new reports reviewed during 1987 to be placed directly onto CIMS. Related reports include *Export Statistics Profiles, Export Overviews*, and *Special Situation Reports. Country Market Surveys* and *Annual Worldwide Industry Reviews* no longer produced, though back issues may be available in district offices.

INTERNIST-1/QUICK MEDICAL REFERENCE (QMR)

Source: Section of Medical Informatics, Department of Medicine, 190 Lothrop Street #165A, University of Pittsburgh School of Medicine, Pittsburgh, PA 15261, 412-648-3190

Subject: Diseases in internal medicine; designed as diagnostic consultant system for health care professionals.

Content: Information organized in disease profiles, a list containing an average of 85 findings per disease. Findings include demographic data, predisposing factors, patient symptoms, signs, and laboratory abnormalities. Knowledge base describes 573 diagnoses, recognizes 4,100 patient findings, and includes more than 4,000 links detailing causal, temporal, and probable interrelationships among disorders. Approximately 250,000 medical facts and other items of information are included in the knowledge base. QMR augments INTERNIST-1 capabilities, allows direct access to information in knowledge base, provides users with multiple ways of reviewing and manipulating diagnostic information, and assists users with generating hypotheses in complex patient cases.

Compilation: INTERNIST-1 developed in 1973; successor program QMR developed in 1985. Data about a disease or clinical syndrome and its diagnosis derived primarily from two sources: review of medical literature, including general and subspecialty textbooks, monographs, and approximately 50-100 relevant primary journal articles; and debriefing medical experts, i.e., gathering information about their factual and heuristic knowledge of a given disease. Knowledge base updated weekly. Several publications appear annually describing progress in further refining program capabilities and related research activities.

Access: Computer programs run on IBM-PC-AT compatible microcomputers. Knowledge base is copyrighted and proprietary to the University of Pittsburgh; contact directly for further information. Several articles describing knowledge base and related research activities have appeared in medical and professional journals; reprints available upon request.

Market Research Reports

Source: Theta Corporation, Theta Building, Middlefield, CT 06455, 203-349-1054

Subject: Market analysis/research on health care, biotechnology, pharmaceuticals, analytical instruments; intended primarily for medical device manufacturers.

Content: Reports cover specific markets, including description and analysis of technology, review of other technologies in field, evaluation of competitors, current market assessment, market trends and projections. Reports generally include executive summary, technology, market factors, market size, market shares, and company profiles. Recent topics include electrophoresis, spectroscopy, DNA synthesizers, monoclonal antibodies, endoscopy, diagnostic imaging equipment, fetal monitoring, cardiac monitoring, medical ultrasound, arthroscopy surgical systems, lithotripsy, cryosurgery equipment, kidney dialysis supplies and equipment, contraceptive devices, and dental equipment. Monthly newsletter *Changing Medical Markets* covers business/finance, medical products, premarket approvals, recalls and patents, new technology, sales and acquisitions, management changes, publications/journals, the courts, and meetings. *1986 Med Tech Directory* profiles 800 publicly owned health care companies. *MPA Healthcare Distributor Guide* describes product distributor selection.

Compilation: Information gathered from industry personnel, trade journals, government publications, annual reports, trade shows, conferences. Active since 1968.

Access: Free catalog, report table of contents, and sample newsletter available upon request. Report prices range from $300 to $900. Newsletter subscriptions $195/year or $325/two years. *1986 Med Tech Directory* price $150. *MPA Healthcare Distributor Guide* price $495.

Market/Technology Reports

Source: Biomedical Business International, 17722 Irvine Boulevard, Tustin, CA 92680, 714-838-8350

Subject: Market research on health care products and services.

Content: Three major types of reports are *Market/Technology Reports* (ranging from 40 to 500 pages in length) covering current markets, technologies, competition and environmental factors, and market forecasts; *Strategic Marketing Studies* (50-230 pages) covering marketing and sales approaches; and *Conference Proceedings* (86-183 pages). Major subject areas for reports are anesthesiology, biomaterials, cardiovascular products, catheters, clinical testing, critical care/monitoring, dentistry, disposables, drugs and drug delivery, extracorporeal therapy, HMOs/alternate site services, fertility control, hematology, home health/self care, imaging, information management, IV fluids/nutrition, neurology, ob/gyn/perinatology, oncology, ophthalmology, orthopedics/trauma, respiratory therapy, and surgery. Newsletters include: *Biomedical Business International* (20 issues/year) covers market segments, companies and business issues, new technologies; *Worldwide Medical Markets* (44/year) covers international product sales opportunities; *Healthcare Marketing* (12/year); *Medical Product Development* (12/year). Directories on genetic engineering and biotech firms, biotech firms medical products of Japan, West Germany Directory of Medical Devices, and U.K. Health Service Buyers Guide. *Healthcare Technology Transfer and Product Opportunities* directory covers descriptions and contact information for technologies available for purchase, license, or distribution. Other reports cover international regulations for health care products, and market research reports for specific countries. Arranges approximately 20 conferences annually, usually in conjunction with professional society meetings.

Compilation: Information gathered from interviews of health care providers and industry personnel, trade journals, government publications, annual and quarterly company reports, conferences, press contacts, literature searches.

Access: Free catalog, sample newsletters, tables of contents for *Market Technology Reports, Strategic Marketing Studies, Conference Proceedings*, and directories available upon request. Market/Technology Reports prices range from $450 to $2,900, newsletters $275-$695, conference report proceedings $100-$700, product and firm directories $80-$195, *Healthcare Technology Transfer and Product Opportunities* directory $775 plus monthly updates. Customized information services also available.

Medical Device and Laboratory Product Problem Reporting Program (PRP)

Source: Practitioner Reporting System, United States Pharmacopeial Convention, Inc., 12601 Twinbrook Parkway, Rockville, MD 20852, 301-881-0666. PRP supported by FDA Center for Devices and Radiological Health.

Subject: Postmarketing surveillance of FDA-approved medical and radiological health devices and laboratory products.

Content: Computerized database contains voluntary reports from health care practitioners on problems experienced with medical or lab products such as improper labeling, design problems, defective components, performance failures, poor packaging, incomplete or confusing instructions, and erroneous information. Products covered include intravenous pumps, catheters, in vitro diagnostic reagents and kits, cardiac and respiratory monitors, ultrasound and X-ray equipment. Reports retrievable by date report submitted, product name, manufacturer and/or type of problem. PRP identifies industry-wide problems or trends and highlights specific product problems.

Compilation: Information gathered via toll-free telephone line or reporting forms from health care professionals including physicians, nurses, pharmacists, biomedical engineers, medical laboratory personnel, risk managers, purchasing and quality assurance personnel, and consumers. PRP reports are used to compile the Device Experience Network (DEN) files for FDA. Reports are submitted as unverified information to FDA, which is responsible for follow up, i.e., determining manufacturer's evaluation of problem and establishing final assessment of problem. Program initiated in 1973. Updated continuously.

Access: PRP reports are included in DEN reports accessible through BMEDSS 216-375-3501, National Technical Information Service 703-487-4630, Medical Device Register's *Product SOS* 203-348-6319, and ECRI 215-825-6000. Confidential trade, commercial, financial, personnel, medical, and patient information are deleted from publicly available reports. DEN reports in microfiche and additional information about specific reports available from FDA, Freedom of Information Office, Room 12A16, HFI-31, 5600 Fishers Lane, Rockville, MD 20857, 301-443-6310. Monthly publication *Device Experience Network Reports*, which includes PRP but not Medical Device Reporting information, is available from FOI Services, Inc., 301-881-0410 for $190. To report a device problem call U.S. Pharmacopeial Convention 800-638-6725 or contact USP for reporting form.

Medical Device Register

Source: Medical Device Register, Inc., 655 Washington Boulevard, Stamford, CT 06901, 800-222-3045, 203-348-6319

Subject: Medical devices, equipment, and supplies; includes manufacturers and distributors.

Content: *Volume 1* covers over 8,000 manufacturers and 13,000 distributors in U.S. and Canada, with data on company size, ownership, key executives, financial status, distribution method, and product line. Products are organized into 6,000 FDA categories;

includes definitions and product descriptions, as well as comparison of prices and specifications for competing products. *Volume 1* contains keyword index, device information, and trade name index. *Volume 2* covers over 3,000 manufacturers and 3,300 distributors located outside the U.S. and Canada. Both volumes are divided into four sections: directory of products, supplier profiles, supplier geographical index, and directory of local dealers. Bimonthly newsletter *Supplier Hotlist* profiles new companies and their products added to MDR database during previous two-month period. *Catalog Library Service* consists of catalogs on microfiche of 2,000 medical product manufacturers. *Distributor Profiles* contains company descriptions and contact information. *Public Company Profiles* highlights the 500 publicly owned companies covered in *Medical Device Register*.

Compilation: Information is gathered primarily from product manufacturers and distributors, as well as news releases, reports from various other sources, including FDA. Database is updated daily; approximately 3,000 manufacturers and distributors added annually. Publications are issued annually. Active since 1981.

Access: Charge for *Medical Device Register Volume 1* (1987) is $150; charge for *Medical Device Register Volume 2* (1987) is $120. Charge for computer tapes is $400 for set up plus $400/1,000 companies, or $6,800 for all companies; floppy disks also available. Medical Device Register information is to be available online through DIALOG in 1988. *Supplier Hotlist* subscription $125/year. Brochure and price list available upon request.

Medical Device Reporting (MDR)

Source: Division of Product Surveillance, Office of Compliance, Center for Devices and Radiological Health, HFZ-343, Food and Drug Administration, 8757 Georgia Avenue, Silver Spring, MD 20910, 301-427-8100

Subject: Postmarketing surveillance of medical devices and in vitro diagnostic products.

Content: Medical Device Reporting regulation (1984) requires that manufacturers and importers of medical and diagnostic products report to FDA any information that suggests one of their devices may have caused or contributed to a death or serious injury, or has malfunctioned and, if such malfunction recurs, is likely to cause or contribute to death or serious injury. MDR database contains reports from manufacturers and importers pertaining to device performance failures and/or malfunctions that have resulted in injury, death, or any hazard to safety.

Compilation: Information reported to FDA is gathered from physicians nurses, patients, consumers,and hospitals; medical and scientific literature; and from independent research, testing, evaluation, servicing, or maintenance of devices by the manufacturer. Program established in 1984. Updated continuously.

Access: MDR reports are included in DEN reports accessible through BMEDSS 216-375-3501, National Technical Information Service 703-487-4630, Medical Device Register's *Product SOS* 203-348-6319, and ECRI 215-825-6000; and are available from the BRS/SEARCH database DIOGENES. Confidential trade, commercial, financial, personnel, medical, and patient information are deleted from publicly available reports.

DEN reports in microfiche and additional information about specific reports available from FDA, Freedom of Information Office, Room 12A16, HFI-31, 5600 Fishers Lane, Rockville, MD 20857, 301-443-6310.

MEDIS

Source: Mead Data Central, PO Box 933, Dayton, OH 45401, 800-227-4908, 513-865-6800

Subject: Medicine, drugs, health care, pediatrics, psychology.

Content: MEDIS service is divided into the following files: GENMED, PHARM, CANCER, MEDLINE, and ADMIN. Provides full text of more than 60 clinical journals, newsletters, and textbooks covering a broad range of medical topics. Covers publications of American Medical Association, American Society of Hospital Pharmacists, American Health Consultants, and F-D-C Reports. Also includes PDQ and MEDLINE. Full-text searching capability by subject. Electronic clipping service ECLIPSE automatically repeats stored MEDIS searches.

Compilation: Compiled from journal articles, monographs, books, and newsletters. Updates vary with publication.

Access: Database available online from remote terminal. Connect cost is $30/hour including telecommunication cost. Search charge is $3 to $13/search during peak time; 30 percent discount for off-peak. Accessed through MEADNET, TELENET, direct dial. Subscription required, fee for physicians $50/month, includes access to NEXIS. Different price structure available for hospitals and medical groups.

MEDLINE

Source: MEDLARS Management Section, National Library of Medicine (NLM), Building 38, Room 4N421, 8600 Rockville Pike, Bethesda, MD 20894, 800-638-8480, 301-496-6193 in Maryland

Subject: Medicine, biomedicine, health care.

Content: Database includes bibliographic citations to over 5 million articles from approximately 3,200 biomedical journals published in the U.S. and abroad. Contains all citations published in *Index Medicus*, as well as citations found in *International Nursing Index* and *Index to Dental Literature*. Citations include English abstracts, if published with article. Indexed using NLM controlled vocabulary MeSH. Published literature searches on selected topics available from NLM, including, e.g., percutaneous ultrasonic lithotripsy, adjuvant chemotherapy for breast cancer, therapeutic plasmapheresis in neurological disorders, surgical treatment of morbid obesity, peer review organizations, HMOs, and indigent care. Also available are brochure and fact sheets covering online services, specialized information sources, and extramural programs; and online services training courses.

Other databases provided by MEDLARS that are described in this section include BIOETHICSLINE, CANCERLIT, CLINPROT, DIRLINE (Directory of Information Resources Online), HEALTH (Health Planning and Administration), PDQ (Physician

Data Query), and POPLINE (Population Information Online). Additional databases provided by MEDLARS are AVLINE (Audiovisuals Online), CATLINE (book Catalog Online), CHEMLINE (Chemical Dictionary Online), HISTLINE (History of Medicine Online), MeSH VOCABULARY FILE, NAME AUTHORITY FILE, RTECS (Registry of Toxic Effects of Chemical Substances), SERLINE (Serials Online), and TOXLINE (Toxicology Information Online).

Compilation: Compiled primarily from journal articles and selected chapters and articles from monographs. Coverage from 1966 to present. Updated monthly with approximately 25,000 citations.

Access: Available online at any time through NLM MEDLARS computer system to more than 6,000 online centers in hospitals, medical schools, universities, government agencies, commercial firms, and other organizations throughout U.S., as well as MEDLARS centers located in 13 other countries. Also accessible via modem from remote terminal through TELENET, TYMNET, direct dial. Connect cost averages $22/hour peak time, $15/hour off-peak. Also available through BRS 800-345-4277, COLLEAGUE (BRS/Saunders) 800-468-0908, DIALOG 800-334-2564, MEDIS (Mead Data Central) 800-227-4908, and PAPERCHASE (Beth Israel Hospital) 617-735-2253 in Massachusetts, 800-722-2075 elsewhere. *NLM Publications* available upon request; provides current ordering information, titles, and prices for NLM publications. *Online Services Reference Manual, 1986* ($46) and *Basics of Searching MEDLINE: A Guide for the Health Professional* ($12) available from NTIS 703-487-4650.

GRATEFUL MED is a software package on two floppy disks for facilitating online searching and search downloading of MEDLINE, CATLINE, CHEMLINE, DIRLINE, HEALTH, TOXLINE, and other MEDLARS databases. Contact MEDLARS Management for additional information. GRATEFUL MED can be ordered for $29.95 plus $3 for shipping from NTIS 703-487-4650.

MEDLINK (Massachusetts Medical Information Link)

Source: PO Box 9080, Waltham, MA 02254-9080, 800-342-1338, 617-890-0385 in Massachusetts. Directed by the Publishing Operation of the Massachusetts Medical Society.

Subject: Electronic mail and interlibrary loan networking service.

Content: Information services such as document delivery, literature searching, topic bibliographies, newsletters. Information sources available on the network include newswires and EASYNET, a service linking many databases including MEDLINE and HEALTH. Network also offers general use electronic mail, bulletin boards, online directory of subscribers, access to American Library Association's ALANET electronic information service. Provides network services for groups seeking to establish their own subnetworks. Training classes available for searching MEDLINE, BRS/COLLEAGUE, and PAPERCHASE.

Compilation: Network links approximately 80 Massachusetts health science libraries and five out-of-state resource libraries, including the National Library of Medicine and its regional medical library at the New York Academy of Sciences. Began operations in 1985.

Access: Accessible via modem from remote terminal. One-time registration fee ($50) includes three user IDs, set-up, and introductory materials. Registration fee for each additional user $5. Annual service fee $100/year; statistics fee $85/year. Connect time $18/hour peak time; $14/hour off-peak. Surcharges for newswires, bulletin board, gateway to other databases, text storage, and training classes.

Multi-Client Reports

Source: International Resource Development, Inc., 6 Prowitt Street, Norwalk, CT 06855, 203-866-7800

Subject: Market analysis/research reports on biotechnology, medical devices and systems, telecommunications, consumer electronics, financial services, personal computers, robotics, electro-optics.

Content: Reports cover international high-technology industries and markets, including the development of selected industries and companies, critical trends and technologies, and 10-year growth projections. Reports normally include: executive summary, background description of the field, market segments, market analysis, market assessment, market forecasts, and company profiles. Recent report topics include biotechnology equipment and supplies, prostheses for sensory and internal organs, European medical imaging equipment markets, impact of biotechnology on specialty chemicals and pharmaceutical markets, high-tech drug delivery systems, laser market opportunities, emerging membrane separation technologies. Publishes several newsletters on software distribution technologies, electronic mail and micro systems, telecommunications equipment and services, and electronic home information.

Compilation: Information derived from interviews with industry personnel, industry data, current publications, reports, and other relevant literature. Approximately 50 studies conducted annually, five to ten of which are in the biotechnology and life sciences field. Active since 1971.

Access: Free catalog of publications available upon request. Report prices range from $900 to $2,500. Newsletter subscriptions $260 to $375/year.

NAHDO Resource Manual

Source: National Association of Health Data Organizations (NAHDO), 316 Pennsylvania Avenue, SE, Suite 202, Washington, DC 20003, 202-546-5881

Subject: Compendium of information regarding statewide health data organizations. Intended audience includes state governments, health services researchers, health insurers, consulting firms.

Content: Contents arranged by state. Included are copies of legislation and regulations authorizing data collection, analysis and dissemination; data dictionaries for financial and discharge databases; documentation of sources of data used, e.g., providers or third parties; description of data system software and hardware; descriptions of coding systems; standard report formats; procedures for requesting data and reports; plan or procedure for report dissemination; and budget and staffing information.

Compilation: State health data organizations submit information and data annually to NAHDO for compilation of manual.

Access: First edition available early 1988; price to be determined.

National Center for Health Statistics Publications and Data

Source: Scientific Information Branch, Division of Data Services, National Center for Health Statistics (NCHS), 3700 East-West Highway, Hyattsville, MD 20782, 301-436-8500

Subject: Vital and health statistics for the U.S.

Content: Public use data tapes include: Vital Statistics (natality, mortality, marriage, divorce, other vital events); National Health and Nutrition Examination Survey (disease prevalence, normative ranges for physiological and body measurements, and nutritional status); National Health Interview Survey (extent of illness and disability in the population); National Survey of Family Growth (contraception, reproduction, family formation and dissolution); National Hospital Discharge Survey, National Ambulatory Medical Care Survey, National Nursing Home Survey (supply and utilization of health resources/services); National Master Facility Inventory (inpatient health facilities); National Inventory of Family Planning Services (facilities providing medical and nonmedical family planning services); National Medical Utilization and Expenditure Survey (costs of illness and health care expenditures).

Data from surveys and studies are presented in a variety of publications, including the *Vital and Health Statistics* series, *Advance Data from Vital and Health Statistics*, *Vital Statistics of the U.S.*, *Monthly Vital Statistics Report*, *Statistical Notes for Health Planners*, and selected articles published in medical and scientific journals. Public use data tapes and unpublished tabulations are also available. NCHS provides technical assistance through conferences, seminars, workshops, and individual consultations to foster and improve health statistics analysis and use.

Compilation: Data obtained from several statistical data collection systems: national vital registration system, surveys based on samples of birth and death records, continuing nationwide interview survey of households, series of national surveys in which physical examinations are conducted on samples of populations, periodic surveys of institutions and their patients, continuous national sampling of short-stay hospital records, and surveys of various categories of health manpower. Reports cover monthly, annual, and periodic data collection activities. Active since 1960.

Access: Catalog of NCHS publications available upon request. Catalog provides list of free reports, order form, prices, and instructions for purchasing reports from U.S. Government Printing Office 202-783-3238; publications indexed by major health topics. Catalog providing availability and price information on NCHS public use data tapes available upon request. Public use data tapes sold through NTIS 703-487-4650. *Data Tape Update* provides current information on data tapes and prices.

National Cholesterol Education Program (NCEP)/NHLBI Smoking Education Program (NSEP) Information Center

Source: Office of Prevention, Education, and Control, National Heart, Lung, and Blood Institute (NHLBI), Building 31, Room 4A-21, National Institutes of Health, Bethesda, MD 20892, 301-230-1340

Subject: Health effects of cholesterol and smoking; prevention of coronary heart disease and chronic obstructive pulmonary disease.

Content: Publications cover arteriosclerosis, heart disease, management strategies for detection and treatment of persons with high blood cholesterol levels, consensus statements concerning high blood cholesterol, counseling techniques and consumer education sheets, cardiovascular disease risk factors, materials for work-site heart disease risk reduction programs, physician continuing medical education materials related to cholesterol and smoking, primary care physician's role in promoting smoking cessation, and suggestions for public, professional, and patient education. NCEP publications list is organized alphabetically by title and annotated; NSEP resource list is annotated and divided into professional and patient education resources. Center is developing a database on smoking and cholesterol programmatic materials, including curriculum guides and other educational materials, descriptions or evaluations of specific programs, directories and bibliographies, relevant laws and legislation.

Compilation: Information gathered from NHLBI-sponsored research and working groups, expert panels, results of biomedical, epidemiological and health behavior studies. Active since 1985.

Access: Current NCEP publications list and NSEP resource list available upon request. Single copies of publications available free of charge. NCEP/NSEP Information Center database not yet publicly available; however, planning is underway to make it available through BRS 800-345-4277, as part of the Combined Health Information Database (CHID).

National Reference File

Source: Health Data Institute (HDI) (subsidiary of Caremark, Inc.), 20 Maguire Road, Lexington, MA 02173, 617-863-2000

Subject: Compilation of national normative statistics on health care utilization and cost trends and patterns of care.

Content: Database contains information provided by client organizations' employee health insurance claims data. Clients include major corporations, unions, commercial insurance companies, and Blue Cross and Blue Shield plans, as well as state and federal health care providers. The file provides data by population subgroup, region of the country, industry, diagnosis or provider or other information relevant to the location of care (inpatient, outpatient, office), length of stay, appropriateness of care, average cost per service, and utilization rates.

Compilation: All clients of HDI Claims Data Analysis Division are asked to add their claims data to the national database. HDI edits and merges all relevant data into the National Reference File.

Access: HDI clients who provide data into National Reference File (NRF) can get comparative statistics included with other HDI analytic reports. Clients who have no data to provide are charged a fee based on data requested. HDI plans to publish normative descriptive statistics and trends in a subscription series format in late 1987.

National Technical Information Service Publications and Data

Source: National Technical Information Service, U.S. Department of Commerce, 5285 Port Royal Road, Springfield, VA 22161, 703-487-4650

Subject: Among the subject categories of the NTIS information classification system are biomedical technology and human factors engineering; computers, control, and information theory; government inventions for licensing; health planning and health services research; library and information sciences; and medicine and biology.

Content: NTIS BIBLIOGRAPHIC DATABASE has bibliographic summaries of NTIS reports. *1986 Published Search Catalog* provides bibliographic citations of NTIS reports in such areas as diagnostic agents, health care costs, health information systems, health insurance, HMOs, mechanical organs, medical computer applications, medical equipment, and medical imaging. Among weekly NTIS abstract newsletters covering new entries to NTIS collection are *Biomedical Technology & Human Factors Engineering*, *Health Planning & Health Services Research*, *Government Inventions for Licensing*, and *Medicine & Biology*. FEDRIP (Federal Research in Progress) database provides bibliography of ongoing federally funded research projects, including NIH, VA, other sources.

NTIS provides data files from such agencies as NCHS (health and vital statistics), NCHSR (hospital care, home care, national medical expenditures, HMOs, services to the elderly), and FDA (summary reports of newly approved medical products, national drug code directory). Monthly *Tech Notes* provides fact sheets on new applied technology and R&D results in medicine and biology and other fields; these are compiled by subject in *Federal Technology Catalogs*. Other products are *Directory of Federal Laboratory & Technology Resources* and *Government Reports Annual Index*.

Compilation: NTIS holdings are compiled from scientific, technical, engineering, and business studies sponsored by the U.S. government and international sources. Among the federal sources are CDC, DOD, EPA, FDA, NASA, NCHS, NCHSR, NIH, NLM, USDA, and VA. NTIS BIBLIOGRAPHIC DATABASE includes 1.2 million records, increased by 70,000/year. Collection contains 350,000 technical reports from other countries.

Access: NTIS information is available in technical reports, software, data files, databases, abstract newsletters, published searches, and other formats. *Guide to NTIS* brochure provides overview to resources and access information. Charges for printed reports generally cover the cost of duplication plus $3 handling fee. Annual subscription charges range from $79 to $205 for weekly abstract newsletters, $127 for monthly *Tech Notes*. NTIS BIBLIOGRAPHIC DATABASE is available through DIALOG 800-227-1960, SDC Search Services 800-421-7229, and Bibliographic Retrieval Services

800-833-4707. Database search help is available at no charge from NTIS 703-487-4640; call 703-487-4929 for international access information. NTIS sales desk 703-487-4650; for rush orders call 800-336-4700, 703-487-4700 in Virginia.

NEXIS

Source: Mead Data Central, PO Box 933, Dayton, OH 45401, 800-227-4908, 513-865-6800

Subject: General reference, business and industry, marketing, finance, science, technology.

Content: NEXIS service includes the following library files: NEXIS, ASAP II, ENCYLOPAEDIA BRITANNICA, GOVERNMENT DOCUMENTS, INFORMATION BANK, and U.S. PATENT AND TRADEMARK OFFICE. Files cover more than 160 newspapers, magazines, wire services, newsletters, trade and professional journals in full text. Files organized by publication type and subject. Full-text searching capability by subject.

Compilation: Compiled from journal articles, government reports/documents, published proceedings, theses and dissertations, news releases, broadcasts, security analysts' reports. Updates vary with publication; daily for newspapers.

Access: Database available online via modem from remote terminal. Connect cost: $30/hour including telecommunication cost, plus $7 peak time search charge for individual files; 30 percent discount for off-peak. Accessed through MEADNET, TELENET, direct dial. Document delivery through NEXIS mail service, offline or online printers. Subscription fee is $50/month. Contact producer for one-time installation charge and monthly charges. Free user manual and database documentation available to subscribers.

National Heart, Lung, and Blood Institute Publications

Source: Communications and Public Information Branch, National Heart, Lung, and Blood Institute (NHLBI), Building 31, Room 4A-21, National Institutes of Health, Bethesda, MD 20892, 301-496-5343

Subject: Causes, detection, treatment, and prevention of heart, lung, and blood disease and management of blood resources.

Content: Publications cover summaries of NHLBI-sponsored working groups; state-of-the-art assessments; recommendations for future research; annual Institute Director's reports; NHLBI Advisory Council reports; and health education, community intervention, and medical intervention strategies for control of high blood pressure, high blood cholesterol, and smoking cessation. Publications organized by NHLBI programmatic area and subject.

Compilation: Publications prepared by NHLBI Office of Prevention, Education, and Control (OPEC). Information gathered from studies supported by NHLBI, working groups or conferences sponsored by NHLBI, programmatic materials developed by NHLBI or by NHLBI-supported researchers, and OPEC's three cardiovascular disease/chronic obstructive pulmonary disease risk factor reduction programs: National High Blood Pressure Education Program, National Cholesterol Education Program, and NHLBI Smoking Education Program. Publications list updated annually. NHLBI activities initiated in 1948; Office of Prevention, Education, and Control created in 1972.

Access: Current listing of publications available upon request. Many publications are free, however, supplies are limited.

Oxford Database of Perinatal Trials

Source: National Perinatal Epidemiology Unit, Radcliffe Infirmary, Oxford OX2 6HE, England, (44-865) 81-68-76. Research sponsored by Department of Health and Social Services and Oxford University Press.

Subject: Perinatal medicine

Content: Database provides bibliographic citations to, evaluation of, and analyses based on more than 3,000 reports of randomized controlled trials in perinatal medicine conducted in approximately 57 countries. Includes data derived from meta-analyses of subject-specific subgroups of trials, as well as information on unpublished, ongoing, and planned trials. Reports are classified according to stage of perinatal period covered in trial, entry characteristics and total number of participants, intervention, outcome, methods of treatment allocation, number of treatment groups; also indexed by author, title, journal, year of publication, country, title keyword, and subject. Records may be accessed using any of above categories alone or in combination.

Compilation: Database has been compiled since 1978 from articles in obstetric, pediatric, and other medical journals, MEDLINE searches, lists of citations used in reviews and other reports of research, conference reports and abstracts, correspondence, and informal meetings. Coverage from 1940 to present; updated daily.

Access: Database on computer disk, including user manual and tutorial package, available in 1988; charge is approximately $750. For further information, contact Anne Yates, Oxford Electronic Publishing, Oxford University Press, Walton Street, Oxford OX2 6DP, England. Listing of reports published between 1940 and 1984 is available in: *National Perinatal Epidemiology Unit: A Classified Bibliography of Controlled Trial in Perinatal Medicine, 1940-1984*, Oxford University Press, 1985.

PDQ (Physician Data Query)

Source: International Cancer Information Center, Office óf International Affairs, National Cancer Institute (NCI), Building 82 Room 103, Bethesda, MD 20892, 301-496-7403

Subject: Advances in cancer treatment and clinical trials; designed for use by physicians.

Content: Databank provides detailed summaries of all major tumor types, including prognosis, staging, cellular classification, and state-of-the-art treatment options. Contains comprehensive information on more than 1,000 active cancer-treatment protocols approved by NCI. Protocol summaries include study objectives, patient entry criteria, and treatment regimen, as well as names, addresses, and telephone numbers of the principle investigators. Each protocol indexed according to disease, stage-specific eligibility criteria, and details of treatment. Physician directory contains information on more than 12,000 physicians who treat cancer patients. Organization directory has contact information for approximately 2,000 organizations associated with cancer treatment. See MEDLINE description for listing of NLM MEDLARS databases.

Compilation: An editorial board of 70 cancer specialists solicits opinions from experts in oncology concerning treatment options to list; statements of treatment are formulated and subsequently reviewed by consultants with expertise in cancer management. Editorial board maintains currency and accuracy of information on available cancer therapies, treatment research, physician, and organization directories through monthly updates.

Access: Available online at any time through NLM MEDLARS computer system to more than 6,000 online centers in hospitals, medical schools, universities, government agencies, commercial firms, and other organizations throughout U.S., as well as MEDLARS centers located in 13 other countries. Also accessible via modem from remote terminal through TELENET, TYMNET, direct dial. To contact MEDLARS Management Division call 800-638-8480 or 301-496-6193 in Maryland. Connect cost averages $22/hour peak time, $15/hour off-peak. Also available through BRS 800-345-4277, COLLEAGUE (BRS/Saunders) 800-468-0908, and MEDIS (Mead Data Central) 800-227-4908. Will be available in Europe on TELMED, a Swiss medical information system.

Pharmaprojects

Source: U.S. office: PharmaBooks, Ltd., 1775 Broadway, Suite 511, New York, NY, 10019. 212-262-8230. Head office: Pharmaprojects, 18/20 Hill Rise, Richmond, Surrey, TW10 6UA, United Kingdom, (44-1) 94-83-26-2

Subject: Pharmaceutical product development information.

Content: *Manufacturers Volume* lists more than 4,000 products under development by more than 800 companies. Each product entry includes generic names, research codes, trade names, financial and other information about originating companies and licencees, standardized activity descriptors, stage of development, related text and literature references. *Therapeutic Categories Volume* lists product developments in particular therapeutic fields arranged by an anatomically-based classification system. Monthly updates identifying recent developments parallel both annual volumes. Cumulative indexes available on products, manufacturers, product activity, and licensing opportunities. PHARMAPROJECTS ONLINE includes manufacturers and therapeutic categories information corresponding to printed version (PHAR file); additional online files contain information on products whose development has been discontinued (PHAD), and products that have been placed in major markets (PHAL).

Compilation: Compiled from medical and scientific publications, brokers' reports, company annual reports, conference papers, and direct contacts with companies. Printed version updated monthly. Online version updated monthly (PHAR) and quarterly (PHAD and PHAL).

Access: Annual subscription for printed versions is $2,525 from U.S. office; subscriptions elsewhere available from Head office. PHARMAPROJECTS ONLINE available in U.S. on Data-Star via modem from remote terminal through TELENET, TYMNET, RS-NET; available on other networks in other countries. Online access cost approximately $110/hour plus $0.55/record for printed version subscribers and $30/record for nonsubscribers; discounts available. Call 800-221-7754 for further information about access and use of Data-Star.

POPLINE (Population Information Online)

Source: MEDLARS Management Section, National Library of Medicine (NLM), Building 38, Room 4N421, 8600 Rockville Pike, Bethesda, MD 20894, 800-638-8480, 301-496-6193 in Maryland.

Subject: Population issues and family planning.

Content: Database includes bibliographic citations and abstracts to documents relevant to human fertility, contraceptive methods, community-based services, program evaluation, demography, censuses, vital statistics, and related health, law and policy issues. See MEDLINE description for listing of NLM MEDLARS databases.

Compilation: Compiled from journal articles, monographs, technical reports, and unpublished works. Coverage 1970 to present; selected citations date back to 1886. Updated monthly with approximately 10,000 citations added annually. POPLINE produced in cooperation with the Johns Hopkins University Population Information Program, Columbia University Center for Population and Family Health, Princeton University Population Index Library/Information Program, and the University of North Carolina at Chapel Hill Carolina Population Center; supported by U.S. Agency for International Development and National Institute of Child Health and Human Development.

Access: Available online at any time through NLM MEDLARS computer system to more than 6,000 online centers in hospitals, medical schools, universities, government agencies, commercial firms, and other organizations throughout U.S., as well as MEDLARS centers located in 13 other countries. Also accessible via modem from remote terminal through TELENET, TYMNET, direct dial. Connect cost averages $22/hour peak time, $15/hour off-peak.

Product Development Directory, Product SOS

Source: Medical Device Register, Inc., 655 Washington Boulevard, Stamford, CT 06901, 800-222-3045, 203-348-6319 in Connecticut

Subject: Non-drug medical products and product safety problems.

Content: *Product Development Directory* indexes 40,000 510(k) filings on medical products approved by the FDA since 1976, organized by product category. Product approvals arranged historically within product category by FDA approval date; manufacturer and name of product approved are listed. *Product SOS* (Situation Occurrence Service) presents information on medical product problem reports. 1986 edition includes more than 3,000 user reports from DEN (Device Experience Network of FDA) for 1985 and

22,000 reports from MDR (Medical Device Reporting regulations of FDA) from beginning of MDR in December 1984 through first quarter of 1987. Included with 1986 edition are bimonthly alerts on new problems as they are reported.

Compilation: Information is gathered primarily from FDA sources, which delete certain confidential trade, commercial, financial, personnel, medical, and patient information. *Product Development Directory* was first issued in January 1987. *Product SOS* updated regularly.

Access: *Product Development Directory* price $87; *Product SOS* (1986 edition) price $360. Detailed documents, FDA 510(k) filings on each product may be obtained from Medical Device Register or FDA.

Randomized Controlled Clinical Trials Report Collection

Source: Thomas C. Chalmers, M.D., Harvard School of Public Health, 677 Huntington Avenue, Kresge 4th Floor, Boston, MA 02115, 617-732-1090

Subject: Randomized controlled clinical trials (RCTs) and meta-analyses of RCTs.

Content: Database contains approximately 8,000 articles describing RCTs, quality assessments and meta-analyses in various fields, and methodological books and articles. Contents partially indexed.

Compilation: Collection activities initiated in 1973. Information gathered through published and unpublished literature searches. Five to ten papers or abstracts based on the collection published yearly.

Access: Collection partially supported by NLM. Database currently not machine-readable. Contact source for further information about access to collection.

Report on Cost-Effective Products and Technologies

Source: Friedman, Eisenstein, Raemer, and Schwartz (FER&S), Certified Public Accountants/Business and Personal Consultants, 401 North Michigan Avenue, Chicago, IL 60611, 312-644-6000

Subject: Cost-effectiveness of medical devices, pharmaceuticals, medical services, and other health care products. Designed for hospital administrators, medical directors, and other health care facility and industry managers.

Content: Each report provides synopses of cost-effectiveness analyses of up to five medical products. Each synopsis describes the product, how it is used, and applicable diagnosis-related group (DRG) where appropriate. Study results and analysis are presented. Features of analysis discussed are product orientation (beneficiary of product's cost-effectiveness), study objectives, study methodology, production relationships (impact of product application on other labor, supply, equipment, and overhead resources), cost identification, differential benefit identification (product's cost-effectiveness versus alternative product-type or technique), and factors affecting study's scope and validity. Independent organization conducting or reviewing study and contact person at medical product company are identified.

Compilation: Medical product and pharmaceutical companies submit cost-effectiveness analyses of their products to FER&S. Studies to be included in report are reviewed to determine whether they are methodologically valid, were conducted or reviewed by an independent third party, and involve an FDA-approved product. First report issued in October 1986; subsequent reports published quarterly.

Access: Reports routinely distributed to selected hospital administrators nationwide. Copies of reports available upon request.

Scrip

Source: U.S. Office: Scrip World Pharmaceutical News, 1775 Broadway, Suite 511, New York, NY, 10019, 212-262-8230. Head office: Scrip 18/20 Hill Rise, Richmond, Surrey, TW10 6UA, United Kingdom, (44-1) 94-83-26-2

Subject: Pharmaceutical industry news, including international industry, regulatory environment, development of new products, and company affairs.

Content: 20-28 page newsletter on pharmaceutical products, finance, world news and markets, company news, advertising. Among other Scrip reports are *Scrip Yearbook*; *Scrip's Pharmaceutical Company League Tables*; *New Product Reviews*; monographs on such subjects as biotechnology companies, product liability, European drug registration, Japanese companies; and monographs on product types such as cardiovascular, chemotherapy, thrombolytics, and asthma. Scrip provides copies of selected FDA Summary Bases of Approval reports, and recent FDA guidelines for new drug applications.

The Scrip database PHIND (Pharmaceutical and Healthcare Industries News Database) is available online. It includes the text from Scrip and other publications in two files; PHID is updated daily, and PHIN contains Scrip archival material up to three weeks prior to the current date.

Compilation: Scrip is published twice a week; 100 issues/year. PHIND is updated daily. Compiled from medical and scientific publications, brokers' reports, company annual reports, conference papers, and direct contacts with companies.

Access: Annual Scrip subscription $523; $282 for additional copies sent in same envelope. PHIND is available in U.S. on Data-Star via modem from personal computer through TELENET, TYMNET, RS-NET; available on other networks in other countries. PHIND online access costs approximately $110/hour, $1.55/current article, $0.35/back article. Call 800-221-7754 for further information about access and use of Data-Star.

SEER (Surveillance, Epidemiology, and End Results Program)

Source: Surveillance and Operations Research Branch, Blair Building, Room 532, National Cancer Institute (NCI), National Institutes of Health, Bethesda, MD 20892-4200, 301-427-8829

Subject: Cancer surveillance and epidemiology.

Content: Database provides statistical data on cancer incidence, mortality, and survival in about 10 percent of the U.S. population; based on several defined geographic areas: Connecticut, Iowa, Detroit, Atlanta and four rural counties in Georgia, Utah, Hawaii, New Mexico and Arizona Native Americans, San Francisco, Seattle, New Jersey, and Puerto Rico. Serves as basis for cancer research, cancer prevention and control research program evaluation. Data include cancer site, year of diagnosis, diagnostic procedures, histology, staging, treatment regimen and date initiated, follow up, i.e., date and cause of death or vital status, patient demographics. SEER issues *Annual Cancer Statistics Review* and reprints of monographs and numerous journal articles that detail research findings and examine other relevant topics.

Compilation: Program activities initiated in 1973; 1 million records are on file. Information gathered from hospital/medical records and pathology reports of cancer cases.

Access: Published SEER reports are available from source upon request; some are also available from U.S. Government Printing Office 202-783-3238. Requests for public use data tapes and for special data runs must be justified in writing. Online access to database is available to NIH users only.

SPRILINE

Source: Library and Research Report Bank, Swedish Planning and Rationalization Institute for the Health Services (SPRI), Box 27310, S-102 54, Stockholm, Sweden, (46-8) 63-05-60

Subject: Health services administration and planning, health economics, health personnel, health statistics, hospital construction, hospital equipment, hospital supplies, medical ethics, medical technology, nursing, social services.

Content: Interactive online bibliographic database and library system includes references to literature, reports, organizations, and individuals; Swedish health services data; information on surveys and pilot projects. SPRILINE database includes 13,000 records of books, journal articles, and unpublished research reports on Swedish health care from Research Report Bank. About 15 percent of the records are from English language sources. All records for journal articles and research reports contain an abstract; searches can be made using free-text technique or controlled terms from thesaurus, which covers 1,200 Swedish indexing terms. Author, title, abstract, keywords, corporative author, publication year, serial title, and language fields may be searched. Printed products include indexes of books and journals, unpublished research reports, annual catalog of research report bank holdings, bibliography of primary care. Subject-coded references of recently acquired books and journal articles are mailed 10 times/year to public health agencies and medical libraries in Sweden and abroad, including the American Hospital Association and the National Library of Medicine. Information about new acquisitions is published in news bulletin *Spri Informerar*.

Compilation: More than 3,000 records are added each year, including 1,300 books, 1,000 journal articles, and 700 research reports. System is linked to other libraries in Sweden, and participates in the HECLINET (Health Care Literature Information Network) European documentation service. SPRILINE has been available for online searching since 1984.

Access: User ID and password are available from source. SPRILINE is available online via modem from remote terminals all hours except 2am-4am Wednesdays and Fridays. Telephone inquiries accepted 9am-3pm weekdays. Document delivery service supplies copies of journal articles and lends books and reports; document requests can be made online via electronic mailbox, mail, and telephone. Except for a nominal fee for multiple photocopies, SPRILINE has no access charges.

Technical Data Center

Source: Occupational Safety and Health Administration (OSHA), U.S. Department of Labor, 200 Constitution Avenue, NW, Room N2439, Washington, DC 20210, 202-523-9700

Subject: Occupational safety and health, including biochemistry, analytical chemistry, biology, physiology, industrial toxicology, sampling and analysis, ergonomics, engineering, health physics, radiology, industrial medicine and health, environmental health, industrial hygiene, sanitation, and safety.

Content: TDC collection contains books and monographs (approximately 5,000), encyclopedias, subject and language dictionaries, various specialized guides, and approximately 250 technical journals; complete list of journals and years covered is available. Available on microfiche: dissertations, abstracts, standards material, product catalogs, back issues of the *Federal Register*, technical papers, reports, publications, material safety data sheets, and numerous publications from government agencies, e.g., National Bureau of Standards, National Institute for Occupational Safety and Health. TDC docket office maintains collection of OSHA rulemaking files, as well as transcripts of advisory committee meetings and impact statements. In-house computerized database, Technical Information Retrieval System includes docket office files, TDC collection, and card catalog. TDC distributes monthly compendium of table of contents of recent journals and publishes quarterly *TDC Information and Insight Bulletin.* Subject bibliographies prepared through manual and online searches available upon written request.

Compilation: TDC established in 1972. Collection compiled of published and unpublished documents acquired from various federal agencies, private industry, research organizations, and private standards setting organizations. Technical Information Retrieval System created in 1983; updated continuously. Subject bibliographies updated quarterly.

Access: Information regarding the use of Technical Data Center (TDC) reference materials and services is available upon request. In-house database may be used free of charge. TDC resources committed primarily to meeting needs of OSHA program activities in national office and field offices; however, non-government personnel may use center during office hours for reference purposes.

U.S. Industrial Outlook

Source: Industry Publications Division, Office of Industrial Assessment, International Trade Administration, Trade Development, U.S. Department of Commerce, 14th Street and Constitution Avenue, NW, Washington, DC 20230, 202-377-4356

Subject: Economic data and analyses of specific U.S. industries, including drugs, medical and dental instruments and supplies, and health and medical services.

Content: Each of nearly 70 chapters in this annual volume covers one or more Standard Industrial Classifications (SICs) of industry types. Chapters generally address each SIC's current situation, outlook for that year, and long-term prospects. Historical trends are given for each industry and type of product, and for international trade. Chapters relevant to medical technology include drugs (covering SICs for biologicals, medicinals and botanicals, and pharmaceutical preparations), medical and dental instruments and supplies (x-ray and electromedical equipment, surgical and medical instruments, surgical appliances and supplies, and dental equipment and supplies), and health and medical services. Chapters address such topics as industry production levels, domestic and foreign-based R&D expenditures, levels of innovation, international competition, areas of new product development, and impact of government regulations and policies.

Compilation: Published annually. The edition for any given year is written during the third quarter of the previous year, based on data that are generally two years old. Data for the intervening years are estimated, and data for the current year are forecasts. Data are compiled from Bureau of the Census sources, as well as other government and private sector sources appropriate for each industry.

Access: Can be purchased for $24 from U.S. Government Printing Office 202-783-3238, (order 003-008-00200-5); U.S. Department of Commerce federal bookstore; or local Commerce district offices. Inquiries about the content of the volume may be directed to the industry specialist whose name and telephone number appears at the end of each chapter or section.

WHO/LINFO Database on Health Technology Assessment

Source: Joint effort of Department of Computer and Information Science and Center for Medical Technology Assessment, Linköping University, S-581 83 Linköping, Sweden, (46-13) 28-19-69; and Regional Office for Europe, Hospital Programme, World Health Organization, 8 Scherfigsvej, DK-2100 Copenhagen, Denmark, (45-1) 29-06-19

Subject: Organizational based information about health technology assessment activities and reports.

Content: Information collected from more than 140 primarily European organizations. Records for descriptions of each assessment program include program name, contact person, address, telephone number, electronic mail address, type of institution (university, research institute, professional association, etc.), staff size, how assessments are initiated, types of technologies assessed (e.g., drugs, devices, procedures, etc.), list of assessments carried out, means of report dissemination, other services, organizational databases and means of accessing them, and availability of annual report. First product of information base is *WHO/LINFO Directory*, in which program descriptions are arranged by country and by type of technology usually assessed. Assessment reports records to include author, title, keywords or other indexing terms, abstract, and other bibliographic information.

Compilation: Database compiled by surveys of health related programs in Europe, Australia, Canada, and U.S. Planning and organizational based information collection initiated in late 1986; collection of bibliographic information for assessment reports initiated in 1987. Planning underway to initiate WHO/LINNET, a user network based on WHO/LINFO database.

Access: WHO/LINFO directory available from Linkping sources.

World Health Organization Publications

Source: World Health Organization (WHO), 1211 Geneva 27, Switzerland, (41-21) 91-21-11

Subject: Public health, including epidemiological data and statistical indicators.

Content: Books, reports, monographs, periodicals covering such topics as biologicals, pharmaceuticals, radiation and health, laboratories, health systems development, hospitals and health care facilities, human rights and medical ethics, immunology and immunization, health economics and expenditures, health statistics, cancer, cardiovascular diseases, chronic diseases, environmental health, health of the elderly. *Public Health Papers* focuses on modern trends and changing concepts in public health, *Technical Report Series* covers consensus findings and recommendations on medical and public health issues, quarterly journal *World Health Forum* presents new concepts in public health and new approaches to health problems, bimonthly *Bulletin of the World Health Organization* reviews progress in medical and related scientific research, *World Health Statistics Quarterly* assesses health situation worldwide and projects future trends, *Weekly Epidemiological Record* contains notifications of diseases and epidemiological data on diseases of international importance. Others include numerous regional publications, publications of the International Agency for Research on Cancer, and publications of the Council for International Organizations of Medical Sciences. Catalog contains author and subject index.

Compilation: WHO activities initiated in 1948. Information gathered from WHO programs, activities, and consensus reports of international groups of experts. WHO reports published continuously; new books featured in catalog issued every six months.

Access: Catalog of publications available upon request.

SUBJECT INDEX TO INFORMATION AND DATA RESOURCES

Part 4
Organizational Resources

Part 4: Organizational Resources

This part provides brief descriptions and contact information for 72 organizations that are active in affairs related to medical technology. Although most of these organizations do not generate technology assessment reports on a regular basis, they have memberships concerned with medical technologies, conduct relevant meetings and symposiums, publish conference proceedings and other documents of note, establish standards for technologies, or are active in government, regulatory, or other policy affairs relevant to the field.

The organizational descriptions are arranged alphabetically by organization name. Each includes name, address, and telephone number of the organization; contact person(s), and a brief narrative description of the organization. Beginning on page 603 is a subject index for identifying organizations involved in particular areas.

Alliance for Engineering in Medicine and Biology
1101 Connecticut Avenue, NW, Suite 700
Washington, DC 20036
202-857-1199

Contact: Patricia I. Horner, Executive Director

The Alliance for Engineering in Medicine and Biology (AEMB) was established in 1969 in response to a recognition among engineers, physicians, and other scientists that the development of the field of biomedical engineering needed improved linkages among those in medicine, the life sciences, engineering, and the physical sciences.

The alliance consists of 17 professional associations whose members are concerned with the introduction and use of advanced technology in life sciences research and in clinical practice. These associations are the: American Association for Medical Systems and Informatics, American Association of Physicists in Medicine, American College of Radiology, American Institute of Chemical Engineers, American Society for Artificial Internal Organs, American Society for Engineering Education, American Society for Hospital Engineering of the American Hospital Association, American Society for Testing and Materials, American Society of Agricultural Engineers, American Society of Mechanical Engineers, American Society of Civil Engineers, Biomedical Engineering Society, Institute of Electrical and Electronics Engineers, Instrument Society of America, Neuroelectric Society, RESNA—Association for the Advancement of Rehabilitation Technology, and SPIE—International Society for Optical Engineering. AEMB is the U.S. affiliate to the International Federation for Medical and Biological Engineering.

The alliance has conducted and participated in a number of significant programs, including an International Biomedical Engineering Workshop Series that resulted in a six-volume publication; a five-year medical ultrasound research and development agendum; a systems design for a clinical ultrasound facility; technology procurement in health care institutions; and an international technology transfer project in Cairo, Egypt, now a Middle East center for ultrasonography training and expertise.

The Annual Conference on Engineering in Medicine and Biology is a major national, interdisciplinary meeting; its published proceedings are an important reference for the field. AEMB sponsors a national honor society for biomedical engineering students.

American Academy of Dermatology

1567 Maple Avenue
PO Box 3116
Evanston, IL 60204-3116
312-869-3954

Contact: Raymond W. Cunningham, Jr., Director, Department of Dermatologic Practice

The 6,700-member American Academy of Dermatology (AAD) represents most practicing dermatologists in the U.S. The principle objective of the Association is the continuation of dermatologic education. AAD is committed to quality standards in continuing education and plays a role in formulating policies that can influence the quality of dermatologic care. The academy has developed programs that promote and advance the science and art of medicine and surgery related to the skin, hair and nails; promote standards in clinical practice, education and research in dermatology and related disciplines; support and enhance patient care; and promote public interest related to dermatology.

AAD is interested and aware of the many technological advances that have been made in the last few years. The AAD Council on Clinical and Laboratory Services is reviewing mechanisms to allow the academy to formally assess these technologies as they relate to dermatology. New technology requiring review and comment by the academy is now referred to the appropriate council, committee or task force germane to that particular issue.

American Academy of Orthopaedic Surgeons

222 South Prospect Avenue
Park Ridge, IL 60068-4058
312-823-7186

Contact: Rebecca M. Maron, Director, Department of Professional Affairs & Policy Analysis

The American Academy of Orthopaedic Surgeons (AAOS) is a nonprofit corporation founded in Chicago in 1933. With 12,181 members, the AAOS is the largest medical organization for musculoskeletal specialists. Members of the academy have completed up to five years of specialty study in orthopaedics in an accredited residency program, passed a comprehensive oral and written exam, and been certified by the American Board of Orthopaedic Surgery.

Educating its members to help assure a high level of skill and competence is the major function of the AAOS. Its educational programs include an appraisal of the effectiveness of relevant technology. Each year the academy offers more than 30 continuing medical education courses across the country.

The academy's annual meeting is its primary education program. It features the presentation of scientific papers, instructional courses, technical exhibits, audiovisual presentations, and symposia on a variety of topics.

The 50 committees of the academy address a myriad of technical subjects, sponsor education programs, and inform the membership and the public about the latest developments within orthopaedics. The academy is currently involved in a pilot project to develop minimum standards for orthopaedic care; these standards may or may not ultimately include technology assessments.

American Academy of Otolaryngology-Head and Neck Surgery

1101 Vermont Avenue, NW, Suite 302
Washington, DC 20005-3521
202-289-4607

Contact: Jerome C. Goldstein, M.D., Executive Vice President

The American Academy of Otolaryngology-Head and Neck Surgery (AAO-HNS) is a nonprofit medical association that provides governmental and socioeconomic support for otolaryngologists. It is intended to advance the science and art of medicine related to otolaryngology and provide educational services for the specialty. AAO-HNS conducts two scientific meetings per year and offers continuing education programs.

AAO-HNS relates to agencies of the federal government concerning matters relevant to otolaryngology such as ambulatory surgery, thyroid surgery, drug problems, hearing aids and other assistive devices, Medicare and Medicaid, noise, manpower, and technology assessment. It monitors legislative and regulatory activities and has activated a legislative network. Drawing from government publications and other sources, the academy keeps its members informed of advances in medical and surgical procedures, including new drug and device modalities.

The academy's 50 committees are involved with medical and surgical practices and procedures. These committees generate voluntary standards of care and develop policy statements. Several committees are working at developing guidelines for instruments, diagnostic tools and medical and surgical devices. One committee is concerned with safety standards for the use of lasers in surgery. The Hearing and Equilibrium Committee keeps abreast of standards for the manufacture and development of the cochlear implants and criteria for patient selection. Members of the Committee on National and International Standards work with the American National Standards Institute and the American Society of Testing and Materials in developing standards for medical equipment and devices and other standards for health care delivery. One committee has recently been developed to produce a manual for quality assurance.

American Academy of Physical Medicine and Rehabilitation

122 South Michigan Avenue, Suite 1300
Chicago, IL 60603-6107
312-922-9366

Contact: Ike A. Mayeda, Executive Director

Founded in 1938, the American Academy of Physical Medicine and Rehabilitation (AAPMR) is the national organization for physicians who have been certified through examination as specialists in physical medicine and rehabilitation by the American Board of Physical Medicine and Rehabilitation. This specialty focuses on patients who are disabled and whose functional abilities have been impaired to varying degrees.

These include disabilities and impairments from strokes, cerebral palsy or other birth defects; arthritis, cardiac disease, pulmonary disease, or from other paralyses; and injuries.

The academy is accredited by the Accreditation Council for Continuing Medical Education to sponsor CME programs, publishes study guides in nine areas related to physical medicine and rehabilitation, provides a self-assessment program for residents and practicing physicians to assess their knowledge, and works with other organizations in maintaining and improving educational standards for the profession.

The AAPMR Medical Practice Committee has various subcommittees for quality assurance and health care financing, facility standards, assessment of diagnostic and therapeutic modalities and devices. Other major activities include publication of the monthly journal *Archives of Physical Medicine and Rehabilitation*, annual meeting, and tracking legislative development and issues in physician medicine and rehabilitation practice, education and research.

American Association of Blood Banks

1117 North 19th Street, Suite 600
Arlington, VA 22209
703-528-8200

Contact: Jackie Campbell, Director of Communications

The American Association of Blood Banks (AABB) is a nonprofit professional, scientific and administrative association for individuals and institutions engaged in blood banking and transfusion medicine. The 7,000 individual members are physicians, medical technologists, nurses, administrators, donor recruiters, and others involved in blood banking. Institutional members are 2,400 community and hospital blood banks and hospital transfusion services that are responsible for collecting nearly half, and transfusing 80 percent, of the nation's blood supply.

AABB supports making available for patients a safe, adequate, economical and voluntary supply of blood and components; to encourage the voluntary donation of blood and other tissues and organs; to foster scientific investigation, clinical application, education and exchange of ideas; to encourage, advance and certify high standards of administrative and technical performance; to function as a clearinghouse for the exchange of blood and blood credits nationwide; and to plan for cooperation in times of disaster.

The AABB Committee on Standards sets standards for practice used world-wide in blood banks and transfusion services. The inspection and accreditation program strives to improve the safety and quality of transfusions and assists in determining whether methods, procedures and personnel meet established standards. AABB reference laboratories provide exchange of information and consultation on rare blood group antibodies and other advanced technical and scientific problems. The parentage testing program provides for accreditation in parentage testing and monitors advancements in the field. The autologous transfusion information file assists in planning programs and monitoring new techniques. AABB's annual meeting highlights new research and technology in the fields of blood banking, transfusion medicine, hematology, immunohematology and tissue/organ transplantation. AABB publishes several new books yearly on issues of significance in blood banking.

American Association for Medical Systems and Informatics

1101 Connecticut Avenue, NW, Suite 700
Washington, DC 20036
202-857-1189

Contact: Patricia I. Horner, Executive Director

The American Association for Medical Systems and Informatics (AAMSI) is a national professional medical society incorporated in 1981 in a merger of the Society for Computer Medicine and the Society for Advanced Medical Systems. In AAMSI, expertise is shared to ensure continued flow of information, research and education in the health care field.

Members are entitled to join one of 14 professional specialty groups that provide the opportunity to contribute, obtain, and exchange information about their professional areas of health care. AAMSI conducts its annual congress on the west coast each spring and a conference on the east coast in the fall. These meetings provide forums for sharing and teaching current developments and implementation of systems for health care and medical informatics in support of patient care, research and health administration.

AAMSI's two bimonthly journals are *Computers and Biomedical Research* and *M.D. Computing*. AAMSI makes available proceedings of the annual congress, a *Mental Health Systems Software Directory*, and a *Directory of Publications in Health Systems and Informatics*.

American Association of Tissue Banks

1117 North 19th Street, Suite 402
Arlington, Virginia 22209
703-528-0663

Contact: Jeanne C. Mowe, Executive Director

The American Association of Tissue Banks (AATB) is a nonprofit organization founded in 1976 in response to increased need for transplantable tissues. AATB has two principal goals: to establish standards for the collection, preservation, and distribution of tissues leading to the development of inspection and accreditation mechanisms for tissue collecting organizations, and to improve the efficiency of tissue banking by encouraging the development of regional tissue banks that collect and distribute a variety of tissues of high quality with maximum economy.

AATB is structured into councils in five areas: musculoskeletal, ocular, reproductive, skin, and tissue bank. Each council is responsible for development of guidelines and standards, and for scientific programs. In September 1984, the association published standards for tissue banking. Each of the councils has formulated, for its respective type of tissue, procedures for donor selection, retrieval procedures, maintenance of asepsis, storage conditions, quality control and record keeping. Based on these standards and procedures, AATB has developed a program of inspection and accreditation for organizations that retrieve, bank, and distribute tissues.

AATB acts as an information center regarding tissue retrieval and processing activities in the U.S. AATB collects and disseminates information regarding tissue banking and undertakes promotional and educational programs for stimulating tissue donation and encouraging efficiency of tissue banking. A program for training and certification of tissue bank personnel is currently under development.

American College of Emergency Physicians

1125 Executive Circle
Irving, TX 75038-2522
214-550-0911

Contact: Colin C. Rorrie, Jr., Ph.D., Executive Director

The American College of Emergency Physicians (ACEP) is a nonprofit professional medical association founded in 1968 to facilitate the exchange of information among physicians practicing emergency medicine. The college has more than 11,000 members, and is dedicated to the education and professional growth of emergency physicians and to the improvement of patient care.

ACEP conducts continuing medical education programs on clinical and non-clinical subjects through meetings, workshops, seminars, publications, cassettes, and courses. It provides such member services as monitoring federal legislation and regulations, programs related to pre-hospital emergency care, assistance to its state chapters, and liaison programs with government, third-party carriers, other medical associations, and various scientific and research organizations.

Although the college does not conduct technology assessment, the annual ACEP scientific meeting features more than 200 scientific and commercial exhibits. Technical information is sometimes addressed in articles in *Annals of Emergency Medicine*, the college's monthly clinical and scientific journal. For example, the journal has published articles on the effectiveness of different types of cervical immobilization collars and scientific studies comparing different techniques of drug administration.

American College of Gastroenterology

13 Elm Street
Manchester, ME 01944
617-927-8330

Contact: Thomas F. Fise, Executive Director

The American College of Gastroenterology (ACG) is an international nonprofit organization of over 2,000 members dedicated to serving the clinically oriented gastroenterologist. It is composed of gastroenterologists, surgeons, radiologists, hepatologists, pediatricians, and other physicians sharing an interest in the care of patients with digestive disease. ACG's purposes include promoting and advancing gastroenterology and allied subjects in medical schools and hospitals, and maintaining and promoting standards in medical education, practice, and research in gastroenterology. ACG endeavors to provide public education regarding digestive disease and develop and implement health care standards at the national and local level.

ACG is committed to clinical research and provides conceptual and financial support for investigative studies. Efforts in the area of technology assessment fall within the purview of the Committee on Research, which numbers 10 physicians engaged in teaching and patient care programs at major academic institutions and hospitals. Through this committee, competitive grants are awarded annually. In addition, national clinical research projects are supported through awards granted by the ACG board. The results of these and other ACG sponsored projects are presented at the national and local meetings. The emphasis on clinical relevance provides is intended to keep the practitioner abreast of trends in diagnosis and treatment modalities in gastroenterology, and serves to encourage clinical researcher-investigators by providing a forum for their work. Most recently ACG has provided grants in support of selected research programs on Barrett's esophagus and colon polyps.

ACG provides a broad spectrum of educational programs through meetings and courses with CME accreditation. Its annual meeting includes sessions, poster sessions, and symposia, and is held in conjunction with a postgraduate course and a large commercial exhibit covering the latest in gastrointestinal technology, therapy and literature. ACG also sponsors regional meetings.

American College of Nuclear Physicians

1101 Connecticut Avenue, NW, Suite 700
Washington, DC 20036
202-857-1135

Contact: Carol A. Lively, Executive Director

The American College of Nuclear Physicians (ACNP) represents over 1,200 physicians and scientists engaged in the practice or development of nuclear medicine. In support of the development and implementation of new and improved medical technology in the field of nuclear medicine, the college promotes funding for research and development, and works with federal agencies in addressing regulatory issues inherent in bringing nuclear medicine materials and instrumentation safely and efficiently to market and to medical practice and research.

The college's standing committees on nuclear medicine science, radiopharmaceuticals, and standardization of nuclear medicine instrumentation provide forums in which members can monitor and have input into the development of nuclear medicine technology.

As the need arises, the college establishes ad hoc task forces to address specific issues relevant to certain nuclear medicine technologies. For example, college members have participated in a joint task force with the Society of Nuclear Medicine to develop a comprehensive paper on the clinical utility of positron emission tomography, for purposes of recommending reimbursement under Medicare. college members have also promoted reimbursement for the use of dual photon absorptiometry in the diagnosis and monitoring of treatment of osteoporosis.

American College of Preventive Medicine

1015 Fifteenth Street, NW, Suite 403
Washington, DC 20005
202-789-0003

Contact: William M. Kane, Ph.D., Executive Director

The American College of Preventive Medicine (ACPM), established in 1954, is a society of physician specialists whose mission is to foster the professional standards, provide for scholarly exchanges, promote prevention-oriented medical care and research, and give national leadership in enhancing public awareness of benefits of health promotion, risk reduction and disease prevention.

Although the college does not engage directly in technology assessment, it has participated in the technology assessment activities of the American Medical Association and those conducted by the Council of Medical Specialty Societies. The college has identified a number of members with expertise in specific areas to work with both the AMA and CMSS. When issues related to preventive medicine procedures and technologies arise, the AMA and the CMSS refer these questions to selected ACPM members. In addition, the college has cooperated with the congressional Office of Technology Assessment.

American Council on Transplantation

700 North Fairfax Street
Suite 505
Alexandria, VA 22314-2040
703-836-4301

Contact: Nancy R. Holland, Executive Director

The American Council on Transplantation (ACT) was established in 1983 as a nonprofit, national federation to bring together organizations and individuals to improve the donation and delivery of organs and tissue transplantation. The council has over 800 organizational and individual members.

ACT provides a national public policy forum to address and seek consensus on social, psychological, ethical, and economic issues involved in organ and tissue recovery and transplantation. It provides the opportunity for individuals and organizations concerned with organ and tissue transplantation to have an active voice in the discussion and formulation of public policy regarding transplantation.

Among its activities, ACT encourages the availability of immunosuppressive drugs for patients on an outpatient basis; promotes the establishment of scientific registries for transplant recipients for ongoing scientific and clinical evaluations; promotes a national task force to evaluate the medical, ethical, legal, and economic and social issues of transplantation and to make recommendations for improvements; encourages the passage of require-request legislation; supports Medicare coverage of heart transplantation; and supports in principle the federal task force on organ transplantation.

Major avenues through which ACT's missions and objectives are carried out are its four forums on: organ retrieval and networking, patient and family issues, professional education, and public education.

The council publishes the bimonthly newsletter *Transplant Action*, which serves as the primary means of communicating with ACT membership. ACT holds annual meetings. The council responds to thousands of requests for information annually, which are made primarily through ACT's toll free number (1-800-ACT-GIVE).

American Geriatrics Society

770 Lexington Avenue, Suite 400
New York, NY 10021
212-308-1414

Contact: Carol S. Goodwin, Director of Executive Affairs

The American Geriatrics Society (AGS) is a nonprofit professional medical society founded in 1942 that attempts to provide optimal health care for the elderly through programs relating to graduate medical education, fellowship training, continuing medical education, and research and its practical applications. In addition, the society is active in issues related to long term care health policy and ethical problems in terminal care. The society's goals are defined by the health and social problems of the elderly.

The AGS is active in technology assessment through the following programs and activities.

- Publication of clinical investigations relating to technologies in the care of the elderly in the society's peer-reviewed *Journal of the American Geriatrics Society*.
- Preparation of an *amicus* brief relating to ethical problems in tube feeding of individuals in vegetative states.
- A project on clinical decision-making in catastrophic situations, including issues relating to ICU care.
- Preparation of material for the congressional Office of Technology Assessment concerning technologies in health care as related to the elderly.
- Preparation of policy statements on various issues in technologies in health care, such as drugs and devices.
- A summer research institute, sponsored jointly with the National Institute on Aging, intended to stimulate interest in careers in aging research.

The AGS conducts an annual scientific meeting on broad issues in the health care of the elderly, which includes presentations on new and established technologies and advances in all clinical fields concerned with geriatric care.

American Healthcare Institute

1919 Pennsylvania Avenue NW, Suite 703
Washington, DC 20006
202-293-2840

Contact: Merlin K. DuVal, M.D., President

The American Healthcare Institute (AHI) is a nonprofit organization that represents interests of its 31 members, each of which is a large, vertically integrated, nonprofit, multi-hospital system. Its constituent institutions number approximately 1,300 located in 44 states. The institute conducts an annual governance education conference for its members' trustees and corporate officers; sponsors research into the profiles and operation of multi-hospital systems; develops health policies supportive of development and growth of multi-hospital systems and the operation of not-for-profit hospitals generally; and promotes the implementation of those policies.

American Institute of Ultrasound in Medicine

4405 East-West Highway, Suite 504
Bethesda, MD 20814
301-656-6117

Contact: James S. Packer, Ph.D., Executive Director

The American Institute of Ultrasound in Medicine (AIUM) is a nonprofit medical society founded over 30 years ago to advance the art and science of ultrasonics in medicine and research. AIUM's membership of over 7,000 consists of physicians, scientists, engineers and sonographers as well as technicians, manufacturers, manufacturers' representatives and medical students. In addition to its annual convention featuring scientific sessions, educational courses, and exhibits, the AIUM makes available a variety of publications and videotapes on relevant ultrasound topics.

The AIUM Standards Committee and Manufacturers Commendation Committee are directly involved in activities related to technology assessment. The Standards Committee is responsible for developing standardized approaches to instrument performance measurements as well as presentation and labeling, phantoms, and nomenclature. The committee reviews documents, manuals, and standards produced by other organizations, government bodies, and individuals, especially as these documents relate to the physics, engineering, performance testing and clinical use of ultrasound equipment.

The Manufacturers Commendation Committee encourages manufacturers to make data on ultrasonic intensities and other parameters of their systems readily available to users by awarding certificates of commendation to manufacturers meeting the appropriate requirements. The requirements for commendation are based upon the guidelines established by a joint task force on standards sponsored by the AIUM and the National Electrical Manufacturers Association (NEMA).

In addition to these activities, the AIUM maintains liaison with other organizations developing standards for ultrasound equipment, including NEMA, International Electrochemical Commission, Acoustical Society of America and the Food and Drug Administration.

American Medical Care and Review Association

5410 Grosvenor Lane, Suite 210
Bethesda, MD 20814
301-493-9552

Contact: Charles Stellar, Director, Medical Issues

The American Medical Care and Review Association (AMCRA, formerly the American Association of Foundations for Medical Care) was founded in 1971. It is a national organization representing more than 600 individual practice associations (IPAs), IPA--type health maintenance organizations (HMOs), preferred provider organizations (PPOs), foundations for medical care (FMCs), peer review organizations (PROs), and other medical plans. AMCRA member plans work with industry, labor, insurance, and other organizations to develop and offer competitive health programs to emphasize quality of care and cost-effectiveness through utilization review programs.

AMCRA provides to its members a variety of educational programs, including those on data systems for claims processing, physician reimbursement, etc.; utilization review seminars; and medical issues meetings. Publications include an AMCRA newsletter and a PPO newsletter, and various bulletins, special surveys, and reports. Reports have covered such subjects as management information systems, drug and other ancillary coverages, marketing techniques, capital formation, premium comparisons, and reinsurance trends. AMCRA has a directory of PPOs and HMOs.

AMCRA cosponsors with the Group Health Association of America a National Committee for Quality Assurance, composed of HMO clinicians, that does quality assurance review under state and federal contracts. AMCRA is involved in monitoring, evaluating, and offering suggestions to federal and state policy makers and regulatory agencies.

AMCRA's nonprofit affiliate foundation, The AMCRA Foundation, is chartered to accept donations, initiate and manage research, and provide information to the HMO and PPO industry. It is sponsoring a patterns of treatment project involving peer review development of guidelines for 50 to 100 most common medical procedures to simplify claims management and to address outlier cases for peer review entities.

American Medical Peer Review Association

440 First Street NW, Suite 510
Washington, DC 20001
202-628-1853

Contact: Andrew Webber, Executive Vice President

The American Medical Peer Review Association (AMPRA) is an educational, nonprofit organization of parties interested in quality assurance and utilization review. The purposes of AMPRA are to improve the ability of its members to assess the quality of medical care services through the exchange of ideas, techniques and information; and assist in the development of methods for the monitoring of the appropriateness of medical care.

The institutional members of AMPRA are physician-directed organizations performing medical review services in the public and private sectors. Included in the AMPRA membership are the federally designated peer review organizations (PROs). The number of these organizations is increasing with the demand for cost-effective review programs from major purchasers of medical care in government, business, labor, and the insurance industry. AMPRA functions as an advocate for physician directed medical review services, acts as a liaison for government, private industry, consumer, and health care organizations; and serves as an information clearinghouse for organizations and individuals with an interest in the field.

In response to the need for standards for review of quality care, AMPRA acts as a clearinghouse for collecting and disseminating review criteria that will provide review groups with the tools to analyze and measure health care delivery performance. This effort is fostered through the conduct of regional conferences and the work of the AMPRA Quality Assurance and Data Committees.

American Medical Review Research Center

440 First Street, NW, Suite 510
Washington, DC 20001
202-639-8614

Contact: Carole J. Magoffin, M.S., Executive Director

The American Medical Review Research Center (AMRRC) is a nonprofit organization founded in 1985 by medical quality and utilization review physicians and professionals. AMRRC's central objective is to develop physician leadership and the tools to analyze medical practice patterns relative to their implications for quality medical care.

AMRRC seeks to provide a link between the research investigation of the development of quality evaluation methods and their application in quality-monitoring operational settings. AMRRC encourages provision of state-of-the-art information on current and developing quality review programs in all settings.

AMRRC's primary constituency includes peer review quality monitoring and educational organizations as well as quality assurance researchers and professionals in all settings. AMRRC facilitates physicians peer review involvement in academic research and development activities designed to improve the efficacy of physician quality monitoring programs.

AMRRC is interested in areawide, regional and national comparisons that yield medical practice variation data on quality patient outcomes. AMRRC and four peer review organizations are collaborating with George Washington University Medical Center on a project to develop quality measures for intensive care unit services. AMRRC has initiated a peer review outcome data project to aid peer review organizations in analyzing and responding to hospital-specific outcome data released by the Health Care Financing Administration. AMRRC publishes the newsletter *Quality Review News*.

American National Standards Institute

1430 Broadway
New York, NY 10018
212-354-3300

Contact: Joseph Tretler, Jr., Assistant Program Administrator, Medical Devices

The American National Standards Institute (ANSI) is the coordinating organization for the federated national standards system of the U.S. It is a private nonprofit organization founded in 1918 to coordinate standardization activities in the private sector. The federation consists of approximately 900 companies and 200 trade, technical, professional, labor, and consumer organizations.

In cooperation with its membership and through its councils, boards, and committees, ANSI coordinates the efforts of hundreds of U.S. organizations that develop consensus standards. ANSI does not develop the standards, but provides means for determining their need and ensures that appropriate organizations undertake standards development. Participating organizations submit standards to ANSI developed under their own procedures for recognition as national consensus standards, and often cooperate in the development of standards within committees that operate under ANSI procedures.

ANSI standards deal with dimensions, ratings, terminology and symbols, test methods, and performance and safety specifications. The standards are developed and used voluntarily; they become mandatory only when adopted or referenced by government.

There are some 10,000 sets of ANSI standards in many fields, among them electrical and electronics, information systems, and medical devices. Major categories of ANSI standards for medical and dental material, devices, and equipment include: anesthetic equipment, dental material, health care facilities, hearing aids, instrumentation, medical and surgical material, nuclear medicine, ophthalmics, and radiographic film equipment.

ANSI acts as a clearinghouse on standardization and the source of standards documents, including those of the International Organization for Standardization, International Electrotechnical Commission, and national standards bodies in other countries. ANSI makes available its own standards and those of many international standards organizations. It provides an annual catalog of ANSI standards with supplements and specialized listings, and a biweekly periodical *Standards Action*.

American Psychiatric Association

1400 K Street, NW
Washington, DC 20005
202-682-6138

Contact: Harold A. Pincus, M.D., Director, Office of Research

The American Psychiatric Association (APA) is a medical specialty society representing more than 33,000 psychiatrists nationwide. Its members share an interest in the continuing study of psychiatry and in the search for more effective ways to combat mental illnesses.

The association has a range of ongoing scientific assessment processes such as the development of the *Diagnostic and Statistical Manual of Mental Disorders*, as well as a task force on psychiatric treatments that is preparing a report on the utility of psychiatric treatments for specific disorders.

Issues pertaining to psychiatric research and technology assessment are addressed through the APA Office of Research and its Council on Research. In addition to the task force on treatments, the council is responsible for task forces on safety and performance standards for electroconvulsive therapy devices, use of laboratory tests, long-term effects of lithium on the kidney, sudden death, tardive dyskinesia, benzodiazepene dependency, and psychosocial treatment research.

The association also publishes the *American Journal of Psychiatry*, the *Journal of Hospital and Community Psychiatry*, and *Psychiatric News*. All of these report on new developments in diagnosis and treatment and on technological development within the field.

American Public Health Association

1015 15th Street, NW
Washington, DC 20005
202-789-5600

Contact: Seiko Baba Brodbeck, Associate Executive Director, Programs

The American Public Health Association (APHA), founded in 1872, is a membership organization representing 50,000 health workers. APHA is the oldest and largest organization of public health professionals in the world. APHA is organized by public health discipline. Its twenty-three sections and six special primary interest groups cover such areas as maternal and child health, occupational health and safety, radiological health, medical care, injury control and emergency health services, and health law.

APHA draws upon its members in accomplishing certain tasks, such as the development of books, monographs and technical reports. Among these diverse activities is the development of guidelines and technical standards. Examples include the following.

- The Committee on Laboratory Standards and Practices has developed publications on: methods for examination of water and wastewater, laboratory methods for sexually transmitted diseases, quality control for diagnostic microbiology, bacterial and viral diagnostic procedures, and quality assurance in health labs.
- The Task Force on Health Care in Prisons and Jails has published reports on standards for health services in correctional institutions.
- Program Development Board work groups have developed technical reports on the public health implications of the Bhopal disaster, and criteria for the development of health promotion and education programs.
- APHA was involved in the development and promotion of guidelines for abortion services in the U.S.
- APHA conducts various meetings and workshops throughout the year to address such issues as the role of nurses in meeting the health/mental health needs of the homeless.
- APHA public policy statements are used as the basis of its stand on legislative, legal and regulatory issues, and may stimulate scientific inquiry.

American Rheumatism Association

17 Executive Park Drive, NE, Suite 480
Atlanta, GA 30329
404-633-3777

Contact: Lynn M. Forbes, Director of Communications

The American Rheumatism Association (ARA) is a 3,000-member nonprofit medical organization founded in 1934. ARA members are clinical and research professionals concerned with the prevention, treatment, and eventual cure of rheumatic diseases, and provision of optimal care. ARA seeks to provide leadership for scientific research, education, and professional care of people with rheumatic diseases.

Yearly, ARA conducts a national and four regional educational symposia that present the latest research findings and clinical advances in the areas of humoral immunology, cellular immunology, inflammation, biochemistry, cartilage, molecular biology and genetics, mineral metabolism and bone, rheumatoid arthritis, systemic lupus erythematosus, scleroderma, osteoarthritis, spondylarthropathies, other rheumatic syndromes, pediatrics, orthopedics, health services, and rehabilitative rheumatology.

The Diagnostic and Therapeutic Criteria Committee of the ARA Research Council has been responsible for setting internationally accepted criteria for the classification of systemic lupus erythematosus, juvenile rheumatoid arthritis, osteoarthritis of the knee, rheumatoid arthritis, Reiter's Syndrome, gout, and scleroderma.

ARA publishes *Arthritis and Rheumatism*, a monthly journal of peer-reviewed articles covering all aspects of rheumatology. Other ARA publications include *Guidelines for Reviewers of Rheumatic Disease Care*, and the *Dictionary of the Rheumatic Diseases*.

American Society of Anesthesiologists

515 Busse Highway
Park Ridge, IL 60068
312-825-5586

Contact: John Andes, Executive Secretary (Park Ridge office), or G.W.N. Eggers, M.D., Vice President for Scientific Affairs, University of Missouri Medical Center, Columbia, MO 65201, 314-882-2568

Founded in 1905, the American Society of Anesthesiologists (ASA) is an organization of 24,000 physician and scientists engaged in the field of anesthesiology. It encourages specialization in the field, seeks to raise the standards of the specialty through education, research, and scientific progress in anesthesiology, recommends standards of postgraduate education in the field, and disseminates information in regard to the field.

The ASA is concerned with the safety and effectiveness of anesthetic drugs and adjunct drugs, mechanical anesthesia and ventilatory equipment, electrical and monitoring devices, and the operating room system. The ASA Section on Clinical Care addresses the anesthesia care team, acute medicine, ambulatory surgical, care, blood and blood products, equipment and standards, obstetrical anesthesia, occupational health of operating room personnel, pain therapy, pediatric anesthesia, respiratory care, and surgical anesthesia. ASA also has a Committee on Peer Review.

The society has issued statements, positions, guidelines, or standards in such areas as invasive monitoring in anesthesiology, monitored anesthesia care, delineation of privileges, ambulatory surgical facilities, delegation of technical functions to non-physician personnel, basic intra-operative monitoring, peer review, ethical practice, critical care, regional anesthesia, organization of an anesthesia department, physician DRGs, and records to facilitate medical audit. ASA publishes the journal *Anesthesiology*. In addition, it makes available a monthly newsletter, manpower reports, refresher course materials, and manuals in peer review and quality assurance.

ASA works with such organizations as the Joint Commission on Accreditation of Hospitals, American Board of Anesthesiology, American Medical Association, and American Society for Testing and Materials to maintain quality of care and training.

American Society of Clinical Pathologists

1101 Vermont Avenue, NW, Suite 604
Washington, DC 20005
202-371-0515

Contact: Robbi-Lynn Watnik, Legislative Assistant (Washington, DC office), or George F. Stevenson, M.D., Senior Vice President, 312-738-1336

The American Society of Clinical Pathologists (ASCP) is a nonprofit medical specialty society organized for educational and scientific purposes. Its membership numbers over 45,000 board-certified pathologists, other physicians, clinical scientists, and certified technologists and technicians. The society is intended to be a principal source of continuing education in pathology and a leading organization for the certification of laboratory personnel. ASCP's certifying board registers over 140,000 certified laboratory professionals annually.

The ASCP Commission on Continuing Education, composed of about 125 scientists representing all fields of laboratory medicine, annually conducts several hundred continuing education programs, many of which include extensive sections on new developments. It has formed a New Technology Committee that includes a section on communications technology and a section on laboratory technology. At least one content expert for each emerging technology is involved in the committee. The committee is considering subjects such as the CD-ROM interactive video disk, enhanced television for diagnosis of disease, flocytometry, DNA probes, and cutaneous sensor/monitoring devices. The ASCP Research Development and Strategic Planning Committee may consider an enhanced technology assessment role as it reviews the goals of the ASCP.

American Society of Internal Medicine

1101 Vermont Avenue, NW, Suite 500
Washington, DC 20005
202-289-1700

Contact: Robert Doherty, Vice President, Governmental Affairs and Public Policy

The American Society of Internal Medicine (ASIM) represents 20,000 physicians specializing in adult medical care. ASIM is concerned with social, political, and economic developments having an impact on the practice of internal medicine.

The society has a broad interest in issues relating to the use of technology in the delivery of medical care. ASIM has a strong interest in the pricing of new technologies. In 1983, the society adopted a policy calling for payments for new technology to be based on the resource costs associated with such technologies. ASIM is concerned about the disparity in payment between physicians' cognitive services and technologically-oriented services. ASIM has published several papers on the subject, including an issue of its journal *The Internist* and two white papers on reimbursement for physicians' cognitive and procedural services.

ASIM publishes *Guidelines on the Delineation of Hospital Medical Staff Privileges*, which includes recommendations on delineation of privileges to perform certain procedures. ASIM sponsors a proficiency testing program on medical laboratory evaluation to help improve the quality of physicians' office laboratory testing. The society also participates, along with the College of American Pathologists and the American Academy of Family Physicians, in the Commission on Office Lab Assessment, a voluntary initiative to develop quality standards for in-office labs. ASIM maintains liaison with government agencies and industry associations pertinent to its interests in medical technology.

American Society of Mechanical Engineers

345 East 47th Street
New York, NY 10017
212-705-7797

Contact: Julie Trunzo, Technical Administrator

The American Society of Mechanical Engineers (ASME) is an educational and technical society of mechanical engineers with a membership of 115,000. With 4,600 members, the ASME bioengineering division is a growing division of the society. It has technical committees on biomechanics, fluid mechanics, heat mass transfer, instrumentation and control, medical devices, and rehabilitation engineering. Members apply engineering concepts and technology to the design and development of instrumentation, substitutes for biological materials, diagnostic and therapeutic devices, and artificial organs. The division is also concerned with the issues of health care delivery, standards for medical devices, and government regulation of health care.

The Bioengineering division sponsors a full technical program at each ASME winter annual meeting, and several other technical meetings each year. In the summers of odd-numbered years, it sponsors a biomechanics symposium. The division publishes the quarterly *Journal of Biomechanical Engineering*, which addresses biocompatible materials, bioinstrumentation, biomechanics, and design and control of biological systems; *Advances in Bioengineering*, compiled from the annual meeting; *Biomechanics Symposium Proceedings*, and other special publications.

Other activities relevant to medical technology are conducted by the ASME Technology and Society division, which sponsors such sessions as social responsibility in technological development and applications, technology transfer, and biotechnology and society.

American Society for Parenteral and Enteral Nutrition

8605 Cameron Street, Suite 500
Silver Spring, MD 20910
301-587-6315

Contact: Sol Eskenazi, Research and Data Consultant

The American Society for Parenteral and Enteral Nutrition (ASPEN) was established in 1976 as a nonprofit, professional society to assist individuals in becoming more educated and knowledgeable about the field of parenteral and enteral nutrition. Through its membership of over 4,200 physicians, nurses, dietitians, pharmacists, and nutritionists, it promotes optimum nutrition for all patients, improved patient care by emphasizing the role of nutrition in rehabilitation and recovery, a multidisciplinary team approach to nutrition delivery, and professional education and scientific advancement in nutrition support.

ASPEN conducts continuing education programs, postgraduate courses, national and regional meetings, and scientific, clinical and educational workshops. Its two major publications are the *Journal of Parenteral and Enteral Nutrition* and *Nutrition in Clinical Practice.*

ASPEN has several activities related to technology assessment. The Research Workshop is conducted each year to examine important and controversial issues in the area of parenteral and enteral nutrition; the 1987 workshop dealt with nutrition in acute renal failure. The Research and Data Committee conducts programs and services to promote and support research and seeks to establish data resources for which analyses regarding the effectiveness of therapies can be assessed. ASPEN conducts an annual clinical congress in which events frequently focus on emerging devices, drugs, and techniques in providing nutritional care. In 1987 ASPEN convened a meeting to address how to assess the effectiveness of parenteral and enteral nutrition technology, and what further research is needed.

ASPEN is consulted by such organizations as the Office of Technology Assessment, the National Center for Health Services Research and Health Care Technology Assessment, and the Prospective Payment Assessment Commission regarding technological matters related to parenteral and enteral technologies.

American Society for Testing and Materials

1916 Race Street
Philadelphia, PA 19103
215-299-5400

Contact: Ray Sansone, Staff Manager for Medical and Surgical Materials and Devices

The American Society for Testing and Materials (ASTM) is a nonprofit organization in which producers, users, consumers, and representatives of government and academia develop voluntary consensus standards for materials, products, systems, and services. ASTM has 30,000 individual and organizational members worldwide.

ASTM has 140 technical committees and many subcommittees involved in standards writing for a wide variety of products from iron and steel to petroleum to textiles to medical devices. These address test methods, specifications, definitions, practices, and classifications.

The ASTM Committee on Medical and Surgical Materials and Devices is concerned with terminology and nomenclature, test methods, specifications, and performance standards. It includes 50 subcommittees on, e.g., orthopaedics, soft tissue replacement, electrodes, plastic and reconstructive surgery, mammary implants, urological materials and devices, surgical instruments, cardiovascular, neurosurgical, cranioplasty, device retrieval, and polymeric, metallurgical, and ceramic materials. ASTM also has committees on occupational health and safety; orthotics, external prosthetic, and mobility aids; anesthetic and respiratory equipment, emergency medical services; and health care services. Other ASTM committees have subcommittees in health-related areas, such as drug product packaging, medical thermometry, clinical laboratory systems, pharmacy automation, clinical data standards, and medical informatics.

The 66-volume *Annual Book of ASTM Standards* contains more than 8,000 sets of standards. The medical device standards volume addresses medical and surgical materials and devices, orthotics, external prosthetics, mobility aids, and forensic sciences. The quarterly *Journal of Forensic Sciences* covers instrumental analysis, measurement, and testing for forensic toxicology, pathology, psychiatry, immunology, odontology, and related topics. Other publications include standards adjuncts, special technical publications, data series, consumer publication series, and compilations of standards.

American Society of Transplant Physicians

Contact: Lawrence G. Hunsicker, M.D., President, Director, Bldg. 3, VA Medical Center, Iowa City, IA 52240, 319-338-0581

The American Society of Transplant Physicians (ASTP) is a professional society of physicians and immunologists with a commitment to clinical transplantation. The society's objectives are to promote education and research in transplantation medicine and immunology, to provide a scientific forum on transplantation medicine and immunology, and to provide for transplant physicians and immunologists a voice in dealing with governmental, medical, professional and private organizations.

ASTP deals with issues related to technology assessment in several forums. All recommendations of committees to establish policy relating to technology assessment are forwarded to the ASTP council for review and action. The Patient Care Standards Committee is charged with reviewing and recommending standards for the care of candidates for and recipients of organ transplants. This committee is preparing a pamphlet listing the information that potential transplant recipients should be able to obtain from their physicians to help them evaluate their medical care options.

The Committee on the Training of Transplant Physicians is charged with defining the role of transplant physicians in clinical practice, with establishing qualification criteria for use by such organizations as the National Organ Procurement and Transplantation Network, and with establishing requirements of and criteria for approval of programs for training transplant physicians.

Representatives of the ASTP Council serve on intersociety committees established for other specific purposes related to technology assessment. For example, the ASTP, American Society of Transplant Surgeons, American Society for Histocompatibility and Immunogenetics, and International Society for Heart Transplantation, drafted a 1986 consensus statement on criteria for designation of organ transplant centers.

ASTP conducts an annual scientific session focusing on new findings in the fields of the basic immunology of transplantation and advances in the clinical management of transplant patients.

American Society of Transplant Surgeons

Contact: Robert J. Corry, M.D., Professor and Chairman, Office of the Chairman, Department of Surgery, The University of Iowa Hospitals and Clinics, Iowa City, IA 52242, 319-356-2545

The American Society of Transplant Surgeons (ASTS) is a nonprofit professional society founded in 1974 consisting of surgeons trained in organ transplantation. Members of the society are limited to surgical specialists actively engaged in organ transplantation. Further qualifications consist of certification by American Boards or their foreign equivalent.

The purpose of the society is to promote and encourage education and research with respect to transplantation surgery. ASTS collaborates with public and private organizations to promote and encourage education and research in transplantation surgery, and participates in coordinating efforts or formulation of programs by physicians, agencies, and health personnel to provide maximum efficiency and optimal benefit to recipients of organ transplants.

ASTS holds a two-day annual meeting at which original scientific papers are presented. Papers at the annual meeting are published annually in the journal *Transplantation*. The society, often through its Advisory Committee on Issues, takes positions on ethical and societal issues involving organ transplantation.

American Urological Association
1120 North Charles Street
Baltimore, MD 21201
301-727-1100

Contact: Richard J. Hannigan, Executive Secretary

The American Urological Association (AUA) is a nonprofit medical society founded in 1902 with the goal of advancing the practice of urology and providing optimal care for persons with urological diseases and disorders. Its 6,100 members are physicians and scientists concerned with the clinical and basic sciences related to urology.

AUA receives requests from private insurers, federal agencies, and health care provider organizations regarding standard guidelines and appropriateness of urological procedures. Prior to replying to requests for information and opinions, AUA consults with panels of experts in the various facets of urology. Three complete sets of urological standards have been promulgated by the AUA since 1974. The 1987 edition of *Guidelines for Urologic Patient Care* is available from AUA.

AUA's official journal is the *Journal of Urology*, a monthly publication containing articles on the latest advancements in medicine and surgery pertaining to urology. AUA conducts an annual symposium focusing on recent advancements to urological care. Included is a biomedical engineering forum that concerns itself primarily with emerging modalities in urology. AUA conducts continuing medical education programs for urologists that include assessments of recent technological advances related to urology.

Association for the Advancement of Medical Instrumentation

1901 N. Fort Meyer Drive, Suite 602
Arlington, VA 22209-1699
703-525-4890

Contact: Elizabeth A. Bridgman, Director of Technical Programs

The Association for the Advancement of Medical Instrumentation (AAMI) is an alliance of individuals and organizations sharing interests in medical devices and instrumentation. Its 5,000 individual members include clinical and biomedical engineers and technicians, physicians, nurses, hospital administrators, educators, researchers, manufacturers, government representatives, and other health professionals. AAMI has 250 institutional members and 125 corporate members.

AAMI is a voluntary consensus standards organization accredited by the American National Standards Institute (ANSI). AAMI's technical committees and their sponsored programs produce several categories of documents. Standards and recommended practices are developed and voted on by technical committees. Medical device standards recommend to the manufacturer the labeling, safety, and performance requirements that the product should meet, and describe test methods for determining conformance with such requirements. Recommended practices for use, care, and processing devices and systems are directed primarily to users. Technical information reports disseminate new information on specific technologies. Monographs, technology assessment reports, technology updates, and technology analyses and reviews explore medical technology issues through articles written by experts, and are normally based on AAMI technical course or meeting proceedings.

AAMI's periodicals include the bimonthly peer-reviewed journal *Medical Instrumentation*, the newsletter *AAMI News*, and the magazine *Biomedical Technology Today*. ANSI standards on medical technology are available through AAMI. AAMI also provides biomedical engineering textbooks and reference materials, a membership directory, and annual meeting proceedings.

AAMI conducts an annual meeting, regional meetings, technology analysis and review conferences, and technical training seminars. It provides clinical engineering certification and biomedical equipment technician certification programs. AAMI provides to members free subscriptions to the BMEDSS (Biomedical Engineering Decision Support Services) electronic data base.

Association of Biotechnology Companies

1220 L Street, NW, Suite 615
Washington, DC 20005
202-842-2229

Contact: Bruce F. Mackler, Ph.D., J.D., General Counsel

The Association of Biotechnology Companies (ABC) is a nonprofit trade association in biotechnology. Formed in 1983, it has 180 member companies in eleven countries. Its purpose is to convene the companies on issues of common concern and to promote the growth of the biotechnology industry. Included among its major areas of interest are raising capital for the industry; trends in patenting biotechnology; regulatory policies of the Food and Drug Administration, U.S. Department of Agriculture, and Environmental Protection Agency; and public perceptions of biotechnology.

ABC has committees and working groups in insurance, import/export, and legislative and regulatory affairs. It acts as a liaison for the biotechnology industry to government, and has been active with regard to legislation relevant to the industry, such as regulations affecting export of biotechnology products, importation of cell lines and biological materials, environmental release of genetically engineered microorganisms, and patent protection of biotechnology products. ABC has developed a product and professional liability insurance program for its member companies. It publishes a bimonthly newsletter *Details*. It held its first international meeting in 1987, and holds regional regulatory workshops. In conjunction with the American Society of Testing and Materials, ABC will hold an October 1987 conference on worker and product safety related to biotechnology.

Association for Health Services Research

2100 M Street, NW, Suite 402
Washington, DC 20037
202-223-2477

Contact: Alice Hersh, Executive Director

The Association for Health Services Research (AHSR) is a national membership organization formed to represent the field of health services research. As such, AHSR promotes cooperative relationships between researchers and public and private decision makers, serves as a source of expertise and knowledge about health services research, and educates the public about the need for and contributions of the field.

As a national voice for health services research, AHSR monitors federal legislation and funding for health services research activities. It also serves to educate members of Congress and the Executive branch about the contributions of health services researchers.

The association's annual meeting provides a forum for researchers and health policy decision makers to discuss issues of common concern. This meeting also gives researchers the opportunity to discuss how health services research can be more effectively utilized in the decision making process.

The association publishes two newsletters—*HSR Update*, which keeps members current on federal policy initiatives and activities of major research centers, and *Focus on Mental Health Services Research*, which addresses developments in the mental health field. In 1985, the association published the *Directory of University-Based Health Services and Policy Research Centers*, and is updating this publication.

The Foundation for Health Services Research is the educational affiliate of the association. It conducts professional and educational activities such as the annual meeting, in addition to other conferences and workshops on topics important to the field.

Canadian Association of Manufacturers of Medical Devices

10 Four Seasons Place
Etobicoke (Tor.), Ontario M9B 6H7
Canada
416-620-1915

Contact: Margaret Guerrier, Director of Regulatory Affairs and Standards

Founded in 1972, the Canadian Association of Manufacturers of Medical Devices (CAMMD) is an organization of approximately 120 health product companies. The mission of the CAMMD is to encourage a business environment conducive to investment and growth of the Canadian health care industry by developing Canadian manufacturing and marketing capabilities, becoming involved in setting regulations governing medical devices, and writing of standards for these products.

CAMMD maintains contact with federal and provincial government agencies regarding regulations, trade development, occupational health and safety, and environmental issues. The association makes regulatory recommendations to the Canadian Health Protection Branch concerning such technologies as diagnostic pregnancy test kits, cardiac pacemakers, dental implants, AIDS test kits, intravenous therapy, and the reuse of disposable devices.

CAMMD has technical committees on diagnostic instrumentation and in-vitro products; general hospital equipment; implants, prosthetics, and sensory aids; orthopaedic equipment; radiation; and surgical supplies, sterile and disposable devices. Its members are active in committees of the Canadian Standards Association responsible for development of consensus standards, and certification standards. CAMMD holds an annual and semi-annual meeting.

Center for the Study of Drug Development

Tufts University
136 Harrison Avenue
Boston, MA 02111
617-956-0070

Contact: Kenneth I. Kaitin, Ph.D., Assistant Director

The Center for the Study of Drug Development (CSDD) is an independent nonprofit research organization affiliated with Tufts University. Its purpose is to explore scientific, economic, marketing, regulatory and other public policy issues that affect U.S. and international pharmaceutical research and development. It has an interdisciplinary perspective intended to involve government, industry, and the public.

Topics of current and recent projects include FDA use of outside advisors, new drug development by the U.S. pharmaceutical industry, new indications for already-approved drugs, post-approval research as a condition of approval, informed consent by patients for medication, and analysis of the 1984 generic drug and patent restoration legislation. Recent case studies have been conducted on such drugs as Bendectin, Depo-Provera, and AZT. International projects address such areas as development and introduction of new drugs in the U.S. and U.K., and the selection of drugs for the World Health Organization's model list of essential drugs.

CSDD has an in-house computerized library on drug development and regulation, including books, manuscripts, journal articles, government publications, articles from the news media, and trade publications. CSDD's New Chemical Entity (NCE) database includes information on drug development by the U.S. and European pharmaceutical industries. As some of the data are confidential, published analyses are in aggregate form only. Subjects of conferences recently sponsored by CSDD have included ibuprofen in its post-market stage, FDA use of foreign clinical trials data, maximizing the benefits of antibiotics, and therapeutic substitutions The center holds an annual five--day course on clinical pharmacology, drug development, and regulation.

The center responds to requests by industry, universities, and other outside parties for information from its library and NCE database. The center periodically sends out reprints and preprints of selected articles, as well as a newsletter with announcements of conferences and publications.

Council of Medical Specialty Societies

PO Box 70
Lake Forest, IL 60045
312-295-3456

Contact: Rebecca S. Rhine, Associate Executive Vice President

The Council of Medical Specialty Societies (CMSS) is a nonprofit scientific and educational organization. Founded in 1965 as the Tri-College Council by the American College of Obstetricians and Gynecologists, the American College of Physicians, and the American College of Surgeons, CMSS was established to provide a forum for the discussion by medical specialists of issues of mutual concern and national interest. In 1967, as other specialty societies joined, the CMSS adopted its current name. Today, 24 major specialties with certifying boards sanctioned by the American Board of Medical Specialties are represented on CMSS. The total active voting membership of the 24 CMSS member societies is more than 280,000.

Since 1978, CMSS has collected and disseminated to the public and private sectors information concerning the clinical appropriateness of various diagnostic and therapeutic procedures. The CMSS Program for Clinical Procedure Review provides for the evaluation by physician specialists of medical and surgical procedures and makes the results of these assessments available to all interested parties. The CMSS program draws upon its ability to bring together experts from major clinical disciplines to reach consensus on a procedures or modalities that apply to more than one specialty.

Employee Benefit Research Institute

2121 K Street, NW, Suite 860
Washington, DC 20037-2121
202-659-0670

Contact: Dallas Salisbury, President

The Employee Benefit Research Institute (EBRI) is an independent, nonprofit, public policy research organization established in 1978 to provide educational and research materials on employee benefits. Its work is intended to serve employers, employees, retired workers, public officials, news media, and academicians as they address health, welfare, and retirement issues. EBRI has a separate Education and Research Fund that performs the charitable, educational, and scientific functions of the institute.

EBRI publishes three periodicals: the monthly *Employee Benefit Notes* analyzes and discusses newly released employee benefits data and reviews a wide range policy issues, research, and publications. *EBRI Issues Briefs* summarize and analyze evolving current issues and trends; recent topics include features of employer health plans: cost containment, plan funding, and coverage continuation, and private initiatives to contain health care expenditures. The *EBRI Quarterly Pension Investment Report* tracks the flow and investment of private and public pensions. It provides historical data on net contributions to pension plans and the investment allocation of the contributions by plan type, examines pension plan earnings and rates of return by plan type, and looks at the portfolio allocation of pension funds.

EBRI provides other reports, seminars, and press statements, and it holds several policy forums each year on economic and social issues having impacts on health, welfare, and retirement programs. Policy studies and forum proceedings have addressed such topics as financing the elderly's health care, Medicare reform, and employer-provided health benefits coverage issues.

Federation of American Health Systems

1111 19th Street, NW, Suite 402
Washington, DC 20036
202-833-3090

Contact: Albert C. Baker, Deputy Director for Government Relations

The Federation of American Health Systems (FAHS, formerly the Federation of American Hospitals) acts as trade representative of the nation's 1,400 investor-owned hospitals, hospital management companies, and health systems and allied companies involved in the delivery of long-term care, home health care, and health insurance.

Members of the federation include such major hospital companies as Hospital Corporation of America, Humana, American Medical International, and National Medical Enterprises, as well as several hundred independent, free-standing hospitals.

The federation's primary objective is to monitor and influence federal legislative developments, and to inform and educate members of Congress, the Executive Branch and the national press about important issues in health care, particularly those issues relating to federal health programs.

In the medical technology arena, the federation's primary goal is to ensure that adequate federal funding is maintained for the research and development of new technologies. This is accomplished through the efforts of several FAHS committees, notably the Health Finance Committee and the Quality Care Task Force. Those committees work with leaders of government and industry to assess the impact of new technologies on the costs and quality of health care, as well as the impact of federal spending policies on the availability of important technologies.

Finnish Society of Technology Assessment in Health Care

c/o National Public Health Institute
Department of Epidemiology
Mannerheimintie 166
SF-00280 Helsinki
Finland
(358-0) 75-70-32-9

Contact: Seppo Leisti, M.D., President, or Jari Kankaanpää , M.D., Secretary

The Finnish Society of Technology Assessment in Health Care was founded in 1986. Its purpose is to promote communication, training, and research in health care technology assessment.

The society will provide a means to consider assessment needs, resource needs, and the organizational structure of assessment in Finland. It is intended to organize courses and conferences, publish articles and reports, support research, make initiatives toward the health care community, industry, and government, and act as a means for gathering and disseminating information about assessment.

The governing board includes representatives from the Ministry of Health and Social Affairs, National Public Health Institute, National Board of Health, Finnish Hospital League, State Technical Research Center, and City of Helsinki Department of Health, as well as hospitals and universities.

Generic Pharmaceutical Industry Association

200 Madison Avenue, Suite 2404
New York, NY 10016
212-683-1881

Contact: Dee Fensterer, President

The Generic Pharmaceutical Industry Association (GPIA) is a national association of independent manufacturers, distributors, and industry suppliers of generic prescription pharmaceuticals. The organization promotes increased acceptance and use of generic pharmaceuticals. It provides educational and technical information to physicians, pharmacists, consumers, legislators and government officials about the safety, efficacy, and therapeutic equivalence of generic pharmaceuticals.

GPIA monitors legislative developments in areas such as trade, intellectual property rights, and changes in regulatory technology requirements, and presents research materials and assessment reports to legislative committees and government agencies. Passage of the 1984 Drug Price Competition and Patent Term Restoration Act codified FDA approval requirements for generic pharmaceuticals via testing methodologies that compare the serum bioequivalence of generic pharmaceuticals to reference drug products. Increased use of bioequivalency testing technologies by generic pharmaceutical producers to meet federal approval requirements has led to further development of these technologies. Member firms and the association's Technical Committee prepare reports on such developments for publication and for presentation to regulatory bodies.

GPIA and its member firms also assist in the development of orphan drugs for rare diseases through sponsorship of product research and support of the National Organization for Rare Disorders (NORD), as well as NORD's Rare Disease Data Base, a computer-accessible library of current information for practitioners, researchers and patients. GPIA's Institute for Orphan Drugs monitors developments in technologies related to the development and testing of orphan drugs.

George Washington University Medical Center

Office of Research and Sponsored Programs
2300 Eye Street, NW
Washington, DC 20037
202-676-2995

Contact: Michael J. Jackson, Ph.D., Associate Dean for Research and Sponsored Programs

The George Washington University School of Medicine and Health Sciences is a private, nonprofit institution for education and research in fields related to health care. Technology assessment activities are concentrated mainly on a broadly based clinical research program. This program currently includes more than 400 projects directed to a wide range of new diagnostic or therapeutic modalities. Approximately 20 percent of the projects are institutionally sponsored, and the remainder are supported as collaborations between the institution and industrial, federal or private sponsors.

Oversight of the program is exercised by the Committee on Human Experimentation, consisting mainly of expert clinicians with specialist representation from the lay community as required by federal regulations. The committee reviews study protocols prior to initiation for subject safety and risk protection, study design and scientific value, and for provisions made for subject confidentiality and information.

Approved studies are reviewed at regular intervals for progress, incidence of adverse or unanticipated responses, and for compliance with required conditions. Protocols for proposed studies are submitted to the committee by members of the faculty of the school who assume responsibility for direction of approved studies. Reports on progress and final outcome of approved studies are provided to extramural sponsors by arrangement with the responsible faculty members.

Most projects in the program are directed to evaluation of safety and efficacy of new drugs and medical or surgical devices, but survey instruments, epidemiologic studies and expert opinions may be developed where appropriate. The program is fully supported by laboratory, inpatient, and ambulatory clinical care facilities.

Group Health Association of America

1129 20th Street, NW, Suite 600
Washington, DC 20036
202-778-3200

Contact: Margaret E. O'Kane, Director, Medical Directors Division

The Group Health Association of America (GHAA) is a national organization representing prepaid health care systems. GHAA currently represents more than 150 member health maintenance organizations (HMOs), including group, staff, network, individual practice association (IPA), and mixed models. GHAA represents the interests of the industry in Congress and with federal agencies, conducts conferences, seminars, and workshops, performs data collection and analysis, and maintains a comprehensive collection of published and unpublished work on prepaid managed care systems.

GHAA is involved in several activities relevant to technology assessment. Among its activities, the Medical Directors Division of GHAA responds to inquiries regarding coverage policies and disseminates information on NIH consensus development conferences, Office of Health Technology Assessment reviews, and other assessment findings.

GHAA research staff produce ad hoc studies of interest to the HMO industry. These have included issues in organ transplantation, alcoholism treatment, and supplemental benefits. The transplantation study assessed coverage for transplantation, volume of transplant procedures, HMO coverage compared to competition, role of formal HMO committees in decisions to cover and provide transplantation, and contractual arrangements for providing transplants. Also issued was an analysis of the integration of organ transplantation into HMO benefit structures. The research department generates an annual membership survey and, new in 1987, a national HMO industry survey. The latter uses a comparative data base of 410 HMOs to yield information describing benefits, coverage policies, and utilization. Included are data on coverage of such services as durable medical equipment, prosthetics, hospice care, in vitro fertilization, and organ transplantation, as well as enrollment profiles, premium structures, and other plan characteristics.

GHAA publishes *The Group Health Journal*, the monthly newsletter *Group Health News*, and an *HMO Managers Letter*.

Health Industry Manufacturers Association

1030 15th Street, NW, Suite 1100
Washington, DC 20005
202-452-8240

Contact: Paul Campbell, Director, Health Policy Research

The Health Industry Manufacturers Association (HIMA) includes over 300 companies that develop or manufacture more than 90 percent of the devices and diagnostic products used in the U.S. These products range from gauze bandages to artificial skin, from stethoscopes to computer assisted echocardiographs, and from surgical scalpels to CT scanners and magnetic resonance imaging scanners. HIMA's major policy initiative is to focus attention on the resources committed by the medical products industry to gaining FDA approval for marketing its products.

HIMA has three sections that address a wide range of issues affecting the medical product industry, including issues related to medical technology assessment. The Science and Technology Section has several committees and task forces which address topics such as product manufacture, safety, domestic and international standards, in vitro diagnostics, and biotechnology. The Legal and Regulatory Section focuses on the regulation and payment of medical devices and diagnostic products; it has proposed ways to streamline the FDA device approval process and the HCFA coverage process while assuring public safety and the integrity of industry's products. The Government and Public Affairs Section addresses public and private sector initiatives relating to health care financing and controlling health care costs.

HIMA conducts research and educational programs addressing medical technology assessment. HIMA contracted with Battelle Institute to develop a manual which gives companies a blueprint for conducting cost-effectiveness analyses. HIMA cosponsored two conferences with the National Center for Health Services Research that focused on use of patient classification systems for measuring health outcomes. HIMA contracted with Duke University's Center for Health Policy and Education for an analysis of the key medical technology assessment trends affecting the device industry. HIMA has also conducted research that documents health insurance and managed care industry trends affecting medical technology. A recent report outlines the current status of coverage and payment policies of Medicare and private payers.

Health Insurance Association of America

1025 Connecticut Avenue, NW
Washington, DC 20036
202-223-7836

Contact: Joel E. Miller, Deputy Director, Consumer and Professional Relations Division

The Health Insurance Association of America (HIAA) represents approximately 330 insurance companies responsible for over 85 percent of health care and disability benefit plans provided by insurance companies. HIAA conveys the industry's views to government, health care providers, news media, business, labor, and consumer groups. Member companies are kept apprised of government activities, trends and developments within the health care delivery system, and public opinion on health care issues. Technical assistance is provided to national, state, and local consumer and health care organizations.

Although HIAA does not have an internal mechanism to assess technologies, it serves as an information clearinghouse on assessments performed by public and private sector organizations. HIAA periodically publishes assessment findings from organizations such as the American Medical Association, American College of Physicians, and Office of Health Technology Assessment.

Through its Medical Relations Committee, HIAA serves as an intermediary between the Council of Medical Specialty Societies (CMSS) and HIAA member companies. HIAA forwards company inquiries to CMSS, evaluations or opinions on technologies are rendered, and this information is published in the HIAA's *Medical Appropriateness Compilation*, which is distributed to member companies. The Medical Relations Committee also monitors developments in the area of medical technology and related ethical, legal and economic considerations; and maintains liaison between the insurance industry and relevant organizations.

The Task Force on Health Care Technology Assessment of the Medical Relations Committee was established in 1983 to monitor public policy developments in the area of organ transplantation and technology assessment.

Institute for Alternative Futures

1405 King Street
Alexandria, VA 22314
703-684-5880

Contact: Clement Bezold, Ph.D., Executive Director

The Institute for Alternative Futures (IAF) is a nonprofit research and educational organization founded in 1977. It is primarily involved in futures research, using a variety of techniques related to environmental scanning and strategic planning. IAF attempts to assist organizations and communities in considering how they want the future to be shaped, and emphasizes community participation in evaluating technological impacts.

An emphasis of IAF's work has been in the health care field. With its for-profit consulting firm Alternative Futures Associates, IAF has prepared presentations and workshops on trends, alternative futures, and foresight for congressional staff and federal agencies, state governments, health professions organizations, hospitals, and health product manufacturers.

IAF has focused on the assessment of health care technology in a variety of ways. It has conducted forecasting projects on the development of new technologies such as the "hospital-on-the-wrist" and vaccines for cancer. IAF has conducted foresight seminars on biomedical issues intended to clarify the role of societal assumptions in technology assessment; these have addressed, for instance, the future of diagnostic testing, future of drugs and the elderly, future of organ transplantation, prospects for home health care, and pharmaceutical research and development for geriatric medicine and for vaccines and treatments for AIDS. Other futures projects have been conducted in nursing, mental health services, blood services, and artificial intelligence in health care. Examples of IAF publications are *Pharmacy in the 21st Century*, *Pharmaceuticals in the Year 2000*, and *The Future of Work and Health*.

Institute of Electrical and Electronics Engineers

1111 19th Street, NW, Suite 608
Washington, DC 20036
202-785-0017

Contact: Heidi Fauth James, Program Analyst (Washington, DC office), or Dr. Joseph D. Bronzino, Biomedical Engineering Program, Trinity College, Hartford, Connecticut 06106, 203-527-3151

The Institute of Electrical and Electronics Engineers, Inc. (IEEE) is the world's largest technical professional society with approximately 280,000 members, including 229,000 in the U.S. The organization's primary purpose is to serve as a forum for the dissemination of technical and scientific information through publications, conferences and educational programs. IEEE also serves, through its U.S. Activities Board and Technical Activities Board, as a resource for technology policy concerns to government.

IEEE is involved in technology assessment through numerous routes. It has 35 specialty societies with technical interests that span the scope of electrotechnology, including engineering in medicine and biology, computers, imaging, and social implications of technology. It maintains standing committees to gather and analyze information relative to specific topics, both technical and professional. The IEEE Standards Board issues voluntary standards developed by the members of IEEE societies and working groups. In the health care area, standards for the utilization of biomedical instruments and devices are established. IEEE societies hold hundreds of conferences each year on state-of-the-art applications of emerging technologies.

There are several IEEE societies that focus on health care related technologies and maintain an active interest in medical technology assessments. The IEEE Engineering in Medicine and Biology Society has the broadest scope. The Health Care Engineering Policy Committee consists of representatives from these societies to assist in formulation of health care legislation, regulation, and policy in the U.S. through the provision of technical and professional counsel.

Institute for the Future

2740 Sand Hill Road
Menlo Park, CA 94025-7097
415-854-6322

Contact: Roy Amara, Ph.D., President

The Institute for the Future (IFTF) attempts to assist organizations to plan their long-term futures. Typical project areas include environmental scanning, strategic planning assistance, policy analyses, and market outlooks and social impacts of emerging products and technologies. IFTF takes a futures orientation, with emphasis on structured workshops and other forms of networking, and use of environmental scenarios to identify and study organizational issues and options. It has conducted projects for insurers, manufacturers, federal and state agencies, and foundations and other nonprofit organizations.

IFTF's Health Care Outlook project is an ongoing forecasting and strategic planning service conducted with the Louis Harris survey firm to study structural change in the U.S. health care system and its impact on business strategy, product development, and marketing. Industry outlooks studies of the pharmaceutical and medical equipment industries were conducted for the California state government. Other efforts include studies of cost-effectiveness of clinical laboratories in Canada, and health futures workshops for trade associations and government and health care provider organizations.

Recent reports include *The Impact of New Diagnostic Technologies on the Practice of Medicine, 1982-95* (1985), *Twelve Emerging Technologies for the 1990s* (1986), and *Looking Ahead at American Health Care, Final Report* (1987).

International Federation for Medical and Biological Engineering

Contact: Dr. Jan Persson, Chairman, Joint Working Group, Implications and Assessment of Biomedical Innovations, c/o Dept. of Biomedical Engineering, University Hospital, S-581 85 Linköping, Sweden, (46-13) 19-24-56

The International Federation for Medical and Biological Engineering (IFMBE), founded in 1959, is a nonprofit scientific organization of independent affiliates in 30 countries. (The U.S. affiliate is the Alliance for Engineering in Medicine and Biology.)

IFMBE members include biomedical engineers, technologists and technicians, clinical engineers, rehabilitation engineers, physicians, medical physicists, and biologists. The objectives of the IFMBE are to generate and disseminate information to the international biomedical engineering community, provide a forum, encourage research and application of biomedical engineering knowledge in support of life quality and cost-effective health care, stimulate international cooperation in the field, and encourage educational programs in biomedical engineering.

IFMBE publishes the bimonthly *Journal of Medical and Biological Engineering and Computing*, the bimonthly news report *The MBEC News*, and the annual *IFMBE Directory* of affiliates and committees. In collaboration with the International Organization for Medical Physics, IFMBE organizes a world conference every three years; the next are in San Antonio, Texas in 1988 and Kyoto, Japan in 1991.

The IFMBE Joint Working Group on the Implications and Assessment of Biomedical Innovations seeks to convene engineers and medical scientists to explore social and economic influences of biomedical innovations, develop and apply assessment methods, and analyze means by which social and economic factors should influence engineering decisions.

IFMBE consults with the International Electric Commission and the International Measurement Confederation in developing standards, e.g., for digital imaging. IFMBE affiliates participate on technology assessment councils, standards and safety boards, and other efforts related to international standards in medical device safety.

International Federation of Voluntary Health Service Funds

15-17 Essex Street
London WC2R 3AD, England
United Kingdom
(44-1) 35-31-15-9

Contact: Kenneth N. Groom, Secretary General

The prime objective of the International Federation of Voluntary Health Service Funds (IFVHSF) is to promote the development and study of voluntary non-profit health services throughout the world in order to assist individuals in obtaining health services, and to strengthen the business capability of these services. The federation has 170 organizational members which together provide health care benefits for a total of 120 million people in twenty countries.

Voluntary health service funds exist to encourage the support and expansion of a private sector not-for-profit role in the financing and delivery of health care. The federation serves as a medium for the exchange of information on, and skills and experience in, voluntary non-profit health services; encourages research in voluntary non-profit health services; promotes and facilitates reciprocal arrangements among member funds for persons changing domicile between countries; organizes international conferences; and fosters relationships between organizations and persons carrying out, or interested in, voluntary non-profit health services in different countries.

The federation pursues its mission through a development program, meetings program, information program (conference and seminar proceedings, newsletters, and ad hoc publications), and a reciprocal services program among members.

The federation's role in health technology is to inform members in order to promote the assessment of new technology and to encourage the application of technologies that have proven cost-effectiveness. The federation provides international comparative information concerning voluntary health services. Other issues of the information program have included data processing, health education, health needs, and health economics. The federation has examined and made recommendations to the World Health Organization and the Pan American Health Organization regarding health care delivery systems of selected countries.

International Society of Technology Assessment in Health Care

Contact: Els Borst-Eilers, Secretary, and Vice Chairman, Health Council of the Netherlands, PO Box 90517, 2509 LM The Hague, Netherlands, (31-70) 47-14-41. Journal subscription and society membership: Cambridge University Press, 510 North Avenue, New Rochelle, New York 10501 (for U.S. and Canada), or Cambridge University Press, Edinburgh Building, Shaftesbury Road, Cambridge CB2 2RU, England (for U.K. and other countries)

The International Society of Technology Assessment in Health Care (ISTAHC) was organized in 1985 to encourage research, education, cooperation and the exchange of information concerning the clinical and social implications of technologies used in health care and to foster their optimal use.

The society has more than 400 members representing 30 countries. Members represent many disciplines, including physicians, nurses, biomedical engineers, economists, ethicists, policy analysts, sociologists, epidemiologists and hospital administrators. There are also representatives from health care insurers, the medical device industry, government, health policy institutes, universities and medical schools, and independent research organizations.

The society publishes the quarterly journal *International Journal of Technology Assessment in Health Care*. Themes of various issues have included technology and the elderly, advanced technology and home health care, magnetic resonance imaging, technology in prenatal care, organ transplantation, and the implantation of artificial organs.

The principal activity of the society is its annual meeting, held alternately on different sides of the Atlantic. The society plans to convene workshops and conferences to provide forums for exchange of data and information on specific topics of international interest and to foster international collaboration.

Technological issues of interest to the society include determination of evidence for safety and efficacy, cost and cost-effectiveness, ethical aspects and access, quality of care, legal and regulatory considerations, and comparison with competing technologies. Accordingly, the society is concerned with assessment of all the implications of health care technology and the use of assessment findings to provide a rational basis for the acquisition, diffusion and application of technology so as to foster and enhance the delivery of quality health care.

Maryland Hospital Association

1301 York Road, Suite 800
Lutherville, MD 21093
301-321-6200

Contact: Steven J. Summer, Vice President

The Maryland Hospital Association (MHA) is a nonprofit organization formed to encourage cooperation and communication among the state's 64 community acute care and special hospitals. MHA is governed by citizen volunteers who serve on hospital boards. MHA activities include advocacy, information, education, research, and programs to enhance the management efficiency and quality of care in Maryland hospitals. MHA also conducts educational programs through its affiliate, the Maryland Hospital Education Institute.

MHA's Maryland Council for Quality Health Care addresses the need for data collection and analysis to help member hospitals monitor and enhance the quality of care. Composed of hospital trustees, hospital medical staff representatives, and CEOs, the council's work is divided into four major areas:

- The Committee on Treatment and Technology is responsible for disseminating information to member hospitals on outcome studies, the efficacy of new treatment modalities, and emerging technology. It collects and distributes the results of clinical tests, assessments, and other materials concerning recently introduced technologies. It also considers related policy and payment implications for Maryland hospitals.
- The Committee on Practice Pattern Variations reviews geographic and medical practice variation data for surgical procedures and medical treatments. It promotes research through coordination with medical specialty groups and academic institutions.
- The Committee on Institutional Mortality Data initiates hospital review of mortality information generated by the association. It looks at trends and recommends in-house educational programs for hospital quality assurance.
- The Committee on Quality Indicators is responsible for overseeing the MHA Quality Indicator Project, currently testing nine quality indicators in seven Maryland hospitals.

National Advisory Council on Health Care Technology Assessment

National Center for Health Services Research and Health
Care Technology Assessment
Parklawn Building Room 18-05
5600 Fishers Lane
Rockville, MD 20857
301-443-5650

Contact: Nancy Blustein, Executive Secretary, and Special Assistant to the Director, National Center for Health Services Research and Health Care Technology Assessment

The Health Promotion and Disease Prevention Amendments of 1984 (P.L. 98-551) provided for the establishment of the National Advisory Council on Health Care Technology Assessment. The National Advisory Council is to advise the Secretary of the Department of Health and Human Services and the Director of the National Center for Health Services Research and Health Care Technology Assessment (NCHSR) with respect to the performance of NCHSR technology assessment activities. (P.L. 98-551 also provided for the establishment of the separate Council on Health Care Technology at the Institute of Medicine, National Academy of Sciences.)

The National Advisory Council's functions, as prescribed by law, include assisting the NCHSR Director in developing criteria and methods to be used in making coverage recommendations (particularly those of the NCHSR Office of Health Technology Assessment), and reviewing technology assessment research applications (particularly those administered by the NCHSR Division of Extramural Research) in excess of $50,000 in direct costs.

The National Advisory Council is composed of 12 voting members appointed by the Secretary. Six members are distinguished in medicine, engineering, and science, and four members represent individuals distinguished in law, ethics, economics, and management. Membership requirements provide for at least two physicians, two representatives of business engaged in the production or development of medical technology, one hospital administrator, one health insurance company or self-insured employer representative, and two individuals who represent the interests of health care consumers.

The National Advisory Council meets at least three times a year to review technology assessment research applications and to carry out its other advisory functions. Subcommittees are established by the National Advisory Council to conduct specific activities. For example, subcommittees have been utilized to prepare a preamble of over-arching principles to guide the technology assessment process, to develop recommended criteria to be utilized in performing technology assessments, and to study and make recommendations regarding the technology assessment process and the coverage process.

National Association of Health Data Organizations

316 Pennsylvania Avenue SE, Suite 202
Washington, DC 20003
202-546-5881

Contact: Marlene Larks, Executive Director

The National Association of Health Data Organizations (NAHDO) was established in 1986 by the Washington Business Group on Health to promote appropriate and accurate collection and analysis of health care data. Members include health data organizations that have legislative authority to collect and analyze health care data on a statewide or other jurisdictional basis, such as state health departments, health data commissions, rate setting commissions, hospital commissions, federal agencies, national associations, corporations, and individuals.

Through exchange of information between member organizations and educational programs, NAHDO seeks to improve the quality of health care data and data management. NAHDO intends to support the work of existing state data collection authorities, and to provide assistance to new and emerging health data organizations. To enhance this effort, the Intergovernmental Health Policy Project at George Washington University provides certain information and dissemination services to NAHDO.

NAHDO activities and projects underway include an annual meeting, technical seminars and other special meetings, a resource manual, the newsletter *NAHDO News*, an electronic bulletin board, circulation of health data organization reports, and a health data organization directory. One 1987 technical seminar, "Micro to Mainframe," addressed the collection, electronic transfer, and use of hospital discharge data. The NAHDO Ambulatory Data Committee addresses ambulatory data issues, and provides technical assistance to member organizations wanting to establish or modify their ambulatory data bases. NAHDO is conducting a two-year project to develop recommendations for an acute care uniform data set intended to minimize the number of different definitions imposed by data gatherers such as purchasers and insurers.

National Association of Manufacturers

1776 F Street, NW
Washington, DC 20006
202-637-3000

Contact: Sharon Canner, Director, Employee Benefits

The National Association of Manufacturers (NAM) is a nonprofit organization of over 13,500 corporations of many sizes and industrial classifications in every state. NAM represents members' interests to Congress and regulatory agencies. Members determine association policy through participation in 14 policy committees.

The Employee Benefits Committee is concerned with private sector retirement and health and welfare plans as well as federal health policy and legislation affecting individual company plans. Of special interest are Medicare's financing and benefit structure, the program's coverage decisions and their relationship to company medical plans for retirees. Other areas of focus are catastrophic insurance, the uninsured, health care data, and health care technology and its impact on corporate health care costs.

In 1984, NAM appointed a task force on technology. Concerns of this task force include issues related to technologies and health care costs, the role of the employer as purchaser and evaluator of efficacy and cost/benefits of the health services provided to workers under company plans, and the role of some employers in producing and marketing health care products. The committee is also concerned with the availability and utility of assessment information, appropriate utilization of technologies, and the impact of public and private sector policy on technological innovation and diffusion.

National Electrical Manufacturers Association

2101 L Street, NW, Suite 300
Washington, DC 20037
202-457-8432

Contact: Robert G. Britain, Manager, Diagnostic Imaging and Therapy Systems Division

The National Electrical Manufacturers Association (NEMA) is the principal national trade association of the electrical manufacturing industry. NEMA has 570 member manufacturing companies that are affiliated with one or more of its product divisions representing distinct industries.

NEMA's Diagnostic Imaging and Therapy Systems Division represents more than 95 percent of the market for manufacturers providing medical devices to the health care field in the areas of conventional medical and dental x-ray imaging, computed tomography, diagnostic ultrasound, nuclear imaging, radiation therapy, magnetic resonance, lithotripsy, and picture archiving and communication systems.

NEMA is especially concerned with the electrical equipment standards to facilitate uniform repetitive manufacture, and with product performance and safety. NEMA standards-writing activities are continuous. Standards are derived from industry-wide cooperative efforts with input from user organizations such as the American College of Radiology and regulatory agencies such as the FDA. Standards are approved by the NEMA Council for compliance with association policies and federal law prior to their adoption. NEMA standards are not sustained for more than five years without being revised, reaffirmed or rescinded. Performance characteristics of imaging equipment can be confirmed by users with the use of referee test procedures associated with NEMA standards.

National Health Council

1700 K Street, NW, Suite 1005
Washington, DC 20006
202-785-3913

Contact: Joseph C. Isaacs, Director of Government Relations

The National Health Council (NHC) is a nonprofit association that has served for nearly 70 years as an umbrella organization for many U.S. health groups. The council brings together such diverse organizations as charitable voluntaries, health care providers, insurers, manufacturers, and federal health agencies. Its current membership includes 65 such organizations.

The council's mission is to enhance the ability of its members to work together effectively to promote the health of all Americans and ensure accessibility to quality health care. Among its activities, the council monitors developments pertaining to a broad array of health policy issues, including technology assessment, management and innovation. As a service to its members and as a contribution to the policymaking process, the NHC has written reports and conducted seminars on technology issues and other topics of national interest. Additionally, it hosts an annual National Health Forum which addresses comprehensively a current or emerging health care system theme.

One of the long-standing traditions of the council is hosting breakfast briefings with leading federal policymakers. Several of these are sponsored each year to help professionals in the field obtain first-hand information on health care issues and the broad policy environment from key decisionmakers in Congress, the White House, and the various executive agencies.

Oley Foundation for Home Parenteral and Enteral Nutrition

214 Hun Memorial
Albany Medical Center
Albany, NY 12208
518-445-5079

Contact: Lenore Heaphey, Associate Director

Oley is a nonprofit research and education organization founded in 1983 for the purpose of promoting optimal care for those requiring long-term specialized nutritional therapy. The foundation has established a network of clinicians and patients throughout the U.S. and several other countries. This network is based on four major activities: an annual research registry of patients in the U.S. and Canada receiving home nutritional support, the publication of a bimonthly newsletter, an outreach system of patients, and coordination and oversight of multi-center research efforts related to long-term parenteral nutrition.

Oley has several mechanisms that relate to assessment of nutrition technology. It conducts research surveys to obtain patient product experience and evaluation. It disseminates information to clinicians and consumers through publications and conferences. Oley makes available consumer volunteers to provide feedback in the development of technology tailored for the ambulatory or home setting. Oley has affiliations with agencies developing and monitoring standards for specialized nutritional therapy in the home and nursing home. The foundation's Scientific Advisory Committee addresses a broad range of questions regarding the technology of home parenteral and enteral nutrition.

Pan American Health Organization

525 23rd Street, NW
Washington, DC 20037
202-861-3219

Contact: Jorge Peña Mohr, Regional Advisor on Health Technology, Health Policies Program

The Pan American Health Organization (PAHO) is an international organization of the Pan American System and the Regional Office of the World Health Organization. PAHO is supporting:

- A comprehensive research project on health technology development in seven countries including sixteen lines of study in four main topics: policy, supply, utilization, and impacts.

- A development and evaluation project on maternal and child health technology supported by the W. K. Kellogg Foundation.
- A technology information support system including regulatory, purchasing, and industrial development policy and decision making needs for member countries.

PAHO publishes the *Latin American Medical Index*, a scientific series, and other publications covering a large range of public health topics. More than 50 reports have been published on health technology issues; most of these reports are written in Spanish.

PAHO's health technology clearinghouse activity consists primarily of annotated bibliographies on technology development in health, as well as in the national economies, agriculture, manufacturing, and industrial sectors that encompass health. One technology evaluation report written in English, *Effectiveness of Cervical Cancer Screening Programs* (1986), is an annotated bibliography of 100 articles drawn from National Library of Medicine online information bases. The 22nd Pan American Sanitary Conference of PAHO included health technology as one of the six major priorities for the American Region.

Pharmaceutical Manufacturers Association

1100 15th Street, NW
Washington, DC 20005
202-835-3420

Contact: Gerald J. Mossinghoff, President

The Pharmaceutical Manufacturers Association (PMA) is a nonprofit scientific and professional organization of more than 100 firms that discover, develop and produce prescription drugs and biological products in the United States. The association's members produce most of the prescription drugs used in the U.S., and about half of the western world's supply of prescription drugs. PMA has a staff of approximately 90 and is governed by a 35-member board.

PMA has 13 Sections (with many subsections and committees) composed of representatives of member firms. The Sections are Biological, Financial, International, Law, Marketing, Medical, Personnel, Production, Engineering and Materials Management; Public Affairs, Quality Control, Research and Development, State Government Affairs, and Washington representatives. The sections identify issues and develop options and recommendations for the Board of Directors as well as relating with government agencies on legislative, regulatory and technical matters. Section meetings, seminars, workshops, and training courses deal with a wide variety of issues important to maintaining high standards of safety, efficacy and quality of prescription pharmaceuticals and other issues relating to quality of health care in this country.

PMA's regular publications include *The Annual Report*, the *Annual Statistical Fact Book and Survey*, a weekly newsletter, a quarterly bulletin, the biweekly *Trademark Bulletin*, a weekly *State Capital Report*, the monthly *Science and Technology Notes*, and periodic *Research Reports*. Other publications on policy and technical issues are published from time to time. A list of PMA publications may be obtained from the Communications Division.

Physician Payment Review Commission

2120 L Street, NW, Suite 510
Washington, DC 20037
202-653-7220

Contact: Paul B. Ginsburg, Ph.D., Executive Director

The Physician Payment Review Commission (PPRC) was created by Congress in 1986 to provide advice on reforms in the methods used to pay physicians for services to Medicare beneficiaries. PPRC began its work in November 1986. It is comprised of 13 members who represent a broad range of experience and perspectives on issues concerning physician payment.

The commission plays four roles. First, it serves as a source of independent expert advice to Congress and to the Secretary of Health and Human Services. Second, it provides opportunities for beneficiaries, physicians, and other interested parties to have their views considered in policy deliberations on physician payment issues. Third, PPRC conducts analyses to provide a basis for policy decisions to alter Medicare's method of paying physicians. Fourth, it performs design work necessary to implement major changes in physician payment.

PPRC is mandated to make recommendations to Congress by March 1 of each year regarding payment for physicians' services under Part B of the Medicare program. PPRC is required to address specific issues related to physician payment, including the variation in payment rates among specialties and geographic areas, the inherent reasonableness of charges for specific services or procedures, methods for developing a relative value scale for physicians' services, and physician participation in the Medicare program. The commission intends to consider both short-term improvements in the current payment system and alternatives for more fundamental long-term reform.

The title of PPRC's 1987 report to Congress is *Medicare Physician Payment: An Agenda for Reform*. The report outlines goals for physician payment policy, the commission's findings, a range of alternatives for physician payment reform, and a time frame for reform. Analyses and recommendations are also given for fee schedules, geographic variation in charges, inherent reasonableness, assignment and the participating physician program, the Medicare Economic Index, improving program administration, coding, data issues, and assistant at surgery.

Renal Physicians Association

1101 Vermont Avenue, NW, Suite 500
Washington, DC 20005-3457
202-898-1562

Contact: M. Eileen Widmer, Executive Director

The Renal Physicians Association (RPA) is a national organization of more than 1,200 physicians who care for patients with renal disease. Established in 1973 to represent the interests of physicians and their patients under the End Stage Renal Disease (ESRD) Program, RPA has since expanded its activities into various areas concerning treatment of renal disease.

RPA's goals are to ensure optimal care for patients with renal disease and related disorders, to act as a national representative for physicians in the field, and to serve as a resource for development of national health policy concerning renal disease. RPA monitors legislative and regulatory activity involving the ESRD program, and acts as an advocate for graduate medical education in nephrology. RPA supports various research activities and promotes funding for kidney disease research.

In cooperation with the Health Care Financing Administration and the Registry Committee of the European Dialysis and Transplant Association, RPA has undertaken a national random sample survey of ESRD patients in order to gauge the application and effectiveness of various modes of therapy for chronic renal failure. RPA also supports research efforts to improve and develop technologies for treatment of renal disease. The association has undertaken some informal and formal technology assessment activities including, most recently, a full-scale evaluation of the procedure of reprocessing dialyzers. RPA holds an annual three-day educational meeting on health policy and scientific issues. The association publishes the quarterly newsletter *RPA News*.

RESNA—Association for the Advancement of Rehabilitation Technology

1101 Connecticut Avenue, NW, Suite 700
Washington, DC 20036
202-857-1199

Contact: Patricia I. Horner, Executive Director

RESNA—Association for the Advancement of Rehabilitation Technology, formerly the Rehabilitation Engineering Society of North America, was renamed to better reflect the broad array of interests and skills within the organization. The organization was established in 1979, and membership includes rehabilitation professionals, providers, and consumers who are dedicated to putting technology to work for disabled persons.

RESNA annual conferences are held at various locations in North America. Other symposia and workshops are held periodically to seek answers to questions critical to the welfare of disabled persons. The proceedings of the conference are published, as well as a variety of other pertinent publications that emanate from the work of RESNA committees or from rehabilitation professionals.

Sixteen RESNA special interest groups respond to the need for a communication network within the rehabilitation community to address the diverse needs of consumers, providers, and industry. Regional conferences are being developed to provide members with the opportunity to meet more frequently to discuss their mutual interests.

RESNA has developed strategies to ensure interactions among relevant professions, and to develop consensus on definition of rehabilitative needs; funding requirements for R&D, education and training; monitoring legislation; working with industry to ensure high standards and to promote the marketing of new devices; and identifying funding sources for consumers.

Society for Medical Decision Making

One Main Street
PO Box 447
West Lebanon, NH 03784
603-298-9929

Contact: John Tomeny, Administrator

The Society for Medical Decision Making (SMDM) is a nonprofit professional society founded in 1979 for the purpose of advancing the teaching and scholarship in medical decision making. The 700 members of SMDM include physicians, public health scientists, economists, computer scientists, health services researchers, and cognitive scientists. Their interests revolve around clinical decision analysis, cost-effectiveness analysis, technology assessment, medical databases, and artificial intelligence. The SMDM conducts continuing education courses in decision analysis and technology assessment.

Medical Decision Making, an international journal of record in the field, is published quarterly by the society. SMDM holds an annual conference on decision making in the health sciences. This meeting is principally devoted to the presentation of abstracts, but hour lectures in decision science and technology assessment are staples of the conference.

Society of Non-Invasive Vascular Technology

1101 Connecticut Avenue, NW, Suite 700
Washington, DC 20036
202-857-1149

Contact: Patricia I. Horner, Executive Director

The Society of Non-Invasive Vascular Technology (SNIVT) is a nonprofit professional medical society founded in 1977 to provide education for the profession of noninvasive vascular technology and to represent the field among other health professions and to the public by providing information and education. Approximately 60 percent of the society's 2,700 members are practicing noninvasive vascular technologists or are technologists involved in supervision and/or education in a clinical setting. Physicians, other health care providers, researchers, and those involved in the sale and manufacture of equipment comprise the balance of the membership.

Through its publications, the *Journal of Vascular Technology* and newsletter *Spectrum*, and local and national meetings, the society attempts to meet the educational and professional needs of the technologists involved in vascular testing. In addition, SNIVT offers patient education pamphlets and training center directories.

SNIVT is a member of and maintains liaison with organizations whose goals are related to maintaining excellence in the field. These include the American Medical Association's Joint Review Committee on Education in Cardiovascular Technology, and the American Society of Allied Health Professions. SNIVT is represented on the AMA Panel of Consultants and the American Registry of Diagnostic Medical Sonographers (ARDMS).

In an effort to support the continuing education efforts of the registered vascular technologists, the society provides continuing education credits accepted by the ARDMS. SNIVT provides educational support for technologists preparing for the Vascular Technology Exam through its referenced study outlines.

Society of Nuclear Medicine

136 Madison Avenue
New York, NY 10016-6784
212-889-0717

Contact: Henry L. Ernstthal, Executive Director

The Society of Nuclear Medicine (SNM) is a multidisciplinary organization of physicians, physicists, chemists, radiopharmacists, technologists, and others interested in the diagnostic, therapeutic, and investigational use of radioactive and stable nuclides. Founded in 1954, it is the largest scientific organization dedicated to nuclear medicine with over 10,500 members world-wide.

The society has established special interest councils that function autonomously within the society. The Cardiovascular Council addresses performance and application of cardiovascular nuclear medicine procedures. The Computer Council is concerned with computer applications in diagnostic, therapeutic, and investigative areas of nuclear medicine. The Correlative Imaging Council is interested in developing and disseminating information on medical and physiological applications of various imaging modalities. The Instrumentation Council promotes advancement and dissemination of knowledge of instrumentation used in nuclear medicine. The Radioassay Council is concerned with the scientific, economic, and historic elements of the radioassay discipline. The Radiopharmaceutical Science Council addresses dissemination of information relating to the radiopharmaceutical sciences and encourages basic radiopharmaceutical research and development. The Academic Council promotes education in the field.

SNM has participated in technology assessments conducted by other institutions by forming ad hoc committees to address specific issues referred to it by such organizations as the American Medical Association and the Council of Medical Speciality Societies. The society recently formed a committee on positron emission tomography (PET) to examine the literature on PET scanning and to inquire as to its applications that improve patient management. Scientific data pertaining to assessment is published in SNM's *Journal of Nuclear Medicine* and as part of other ongoing educational activities through its annual and other meetings and publications.

Swedish National Center for Technology Assessment in Health Care

Drottning Gatan 16
11151 Stockholm
Sweden
(46-8) 24-05-65

Contact: Egon P. Jonsson, Ph.D., Director

The Swedish National Center for Medical Technology Assessment was established in 1987 and will begin operations in 1988. An independent government agency, it reports to the cabinet level of government, rather than being part of a particular ministry. The center's first-year budget is approximately $1.5 million.

The major purpose of the center is to enhance and coordinate health care technology assessment activities in Sweden. It was established in response to increased international interest in medical technology assessment and considerations of rising health care costs. Significant impetus to the center's formation arose from concern regarding the purportedly slow pace at which certain technologies have diffused in Sweden; an enhanced assessment capacity has been advanced as an appropriate means for enabling worthy technologies to diffuse more readily. Further, the center is intended to improve the transfer of information about medical technologies from the biomedical research community to health care providers and the public.

The governing board of the National center includes representation from the Ministry of Health, Medical Research Council, National Board of Health and Welfare, Federation of the County Councils, Swedish Planning and Rationalization Institute for the Health and Social Services (SPRI), Swedish Medical Association, and Swedish College of Physicians.

The center's program will address medical, economic, social, and ethical aspects of new and established technologies used for diagnosis and treatment. Assessments conducted by the center will largely involve syntheses of existing information, and it may purchase data from other organizations and encourage them to conduct assessments on certain topics. The center intends to coordinate its activities with similar organizations in other nations, such as the U.S. Office of Technology Assessment and the Council on Health Care Technology of the Institute of Medicine.

Technology Assessment and Forecast Program

U.S. Patent and Trademark Office
CM2-313
Washington, DC 20231
703-557-0433

Contact: Jane Myers, Office of Documentation

The U.S. Patent and Trademark Office (PTO) established the Technology Assessment and Forecast Program (TAF) to stimulate the use and enhance the usability of the patent file, and to assemble, analyze, and make available meaningful data about the file.

TAF uses the database in two principal ways. First, it periodically issues general distribution publications. One series of publications, the *Technology Assessment Forecast Reports*, have included reviews of highly active technological areas and areas experiencing high levels of patenting by foreign residents, profiles of the patenting patterns of the residents of selected foreign countries and U.S. states, reviews of the patent activity of the most active patent assignees, and comparisons of patent activity with economic activity in selected Standard Industrial Classification categories. Another series of publications, *Patent Profiles*, surveys the U.S. patenting activity in specific technologies.

One such profile is *Biotechnology: 1982 Update*; others address such topics as robots, telecommunications, and microelectronics. The second principal use of the TAF database is to prepare custom data reports tailored to individual needs. These reports, provided on a cost reimbursable basis, are used by government agencies and the private sector. One such custom report was a technology profile report on genetic engineering, an analysis of patent activity in this area from 1963 to 1986.

United States Pharmacopeial Convention

12601 Twinbrook Parkway
Rockville, MD 20852
301-881-0666

Contact: Diane M. McGinnis, Assistant Coordinator, Practitioner Reporting System

The U.S. Pharmacopeial Convention (USP) is an private, nonprofit body of 300 delegates representing state and national associations and colleges of medicine, nursing, and pharmacy; industry; and agencies of the federal government. Incorporated in 1900, the purposes of USP are to set standards for health care products in the U.S. and to collect and disseminate product use information to providers and consumers.

Every five years, USP publishes revised standards for drugs in *The United States Pharmacopeia* and *The National Formulary*. These standards are recognized as official by the federal government and are enforceable by the FDA. The standards include specifications pertaining to drug strength, quality, purity, packaging, and labeling.

USP provides official drug reference standards, which are highly characterized specimens of drugs, impurities, and degradation products. USP laboratories test and monitor these standards, and develop analytical procedures and tests of proposed revisions of tests and assays. USP publications include *USP DI Volume I: Drug Information for the Health Care Provider* and *USP DI Volume II: Advice for the Patient*. Other publications are the consumer edition of the reference volumes *About Your Medicines*, the bimonthly newsletter *About Your Medicines*, and various brochures and books.

The Drug Product Problem Reporting Program (DPPR) and the Medical Device and Laboratory Product Problem Reporting Program (PRP) are systems funded by the FDA for identifying and correcting problems associated with prescription and over-the-counter drugs and medical devices, laboratory products, radiopharmaceutical drugs, and radiological devices. Problem reports are usually submitted by practitioners to the USP via toll-free telephone or reporting forms, and are forwarded to the FDA and other appropriate government and industry agents for corrective action. Addressing product quality, DPPR is one of two FDA voluntary drug problem reporting programs (the other is the Drug Experience Reporting program for adverse drug reactions). PRP is the largest single source of device experience information for the FDA's Device Experience Reporting Network.

United Network for Organ Sharing

3001 Hungary Spring Road
PO Box 28010
Richmond, VA 23228
804-289-0600

Contact: Robert Bowie, Director of Communications

The United Network for Organ Sharing (UNOS) was incorporated in 1984 as a private non-profit organization, having grown out of the South-Eastern Organ Procurement Foundation. Its purpose is to provide the best possible organs to patients best suited to receive them, to the end that transplants may be successful and quality of life is sustained and improved.

The UNOS computer system has transplant-related data on 10,000 potential recipients, involving approximately 250 transplant centers, organ procurement organizations, and laboratories in the U.S. The system matches data on newly available organs and tissues with potential recipients. UNOS uses its database to study factors affecting recipients after they have received transplants, to evaluate transplant procedures, and to improve the computer system.

Linked to the computer system, the UNOS Organ Center assists procurement teams by providing information concerning potential placement of organs prior to procurement. With ties to transportation services, the Organ Center is the central point for organ distribution outside the U.S., and maintains relationships with transplant programs worldwide.

In 1984, the National Transplant Act mandated the establishment of a national computer transplant system. In 1986, UNOS received the federal contract to establish the national Organ Procurement and Transplantation Network (OPTN). Among its tasks, OPTN is to develop and implement a transplant information systems plan, develop and maintain a potential transplant recipient registration system, match donors and recipients, develop a telephone system, provide a transportation assistance system, develop organ procurement standards, conduct a high percent reactive antibodies patient transplant feasibility study, and improve professional education.

UNOS is developing a population-based Scientific Registry for Organ Transplantation for reporting to the federal government about transplantation and to study risk factors affecting transplantation outcomes. Requests by outside parties for access to the registry data will be considered by the UNOS scientific advisory committee. UNOS publishes the monthly newsletter *UNOS Update*.

University Hospital Consortium

One Mid America Plaza, Suite 624
Oakbrook Terrace, IL 60181
312-954-6766

Contact: Robert Baker, President

The University Hospital Consortium (UHC) is a nonprofit organization formed in 1984 to aid university teaching hospitals in their efforts to maintain and strengthen their positions in the marketplace. UHC includes 43 university hospitals in 24 states with a total of 23,000 beds, 775,000 admissions per year, and 25,300 medical school enrollees. UHC seeks to promote group efforts among academic teaching hospitals concerning access to information, alternative delivery systems, capital formation, insurance, research, marketing, and volume-purchasing.

UHC is considering methods through which its member hospitals can participate in alternative delivery systems by monitoring the development of such systems on a nationwide basis and making recommendations to its members. UHC is working to promote enhanced capital formation and improved malpractice insurance for its members. It is committed to sponsoring management research programs, information exchange, and sharing of marketing information. UHC's subsidiary, the University Hospital Consortium Services Corporation, develops agreements with providers to reduce costs to UHC institutions. It sponsors pharmacy, capital equipment, and supplies purchasing programs, and provides a management consulting pool.

UHC is developing a program to assist health product makers and venture capitalists to conduct multi-center technology assessments at its member institutions. Such a program may enhance universities' role in developing and testing technologies, and could provide a means of generating and gathering data for various assessment needs of government and the private sector.

SUBJECT INDEX TO ORGANIZATIONAL RESOURCES

Part 5
Index to Organizations

Part 5: Index to Organizations

This part includes an alphabetical listing with addresses and telephone numbers for all organizations described in the *Directory*, as well as a page index to the organizations beginning on page 622.

Organization Addresses and Telephone Numbers

Alcohol, Drug Abuse, and Mental Health Administration
Parklawn Building, Room 13C-05
5600 Fishers Lane
Rockville, MD 20857
301-443-3820

Alliance for Engineering in Medicine and Biology
1101 Connecticut Avenue NW, Suite 700
Washington, DC 20036
202-857-1199

American Academy of Dermatology
1567 Maple Avenue
PO Box 3116
Evanston, IL 60204-3116
312-869-3954

American Academy of Neurology
Practice Committee
2221 University Avenue SE, Suite 335
Minneapolis, MN 55414
612-623-8115

American Academy of Ophthalmology
Ophthalmic Procedures Assessment Program
PO Box 7424
655 Beach Street
San Francisco, CA 94120-7424
415-561-8500

American Academy of Orthopaedic Surgeons
222 South Prospect Avenue
Park Ridge, IL 60068-4058
312-823-7186

American Academy of Otolaryngology-Head and Neck Surgery
1101 Vermont Avenue NW, Suite 302
Washington, DC 20005-3521
202-289-4607

American Academy of Pediatrics
141 Northwest Point Boulevard
PO Box 927
Elk Grove Village, IL 60009-0927
312-228-5005

American Academy of Physical Medicine and Rehabilitation
122 South Michigan Avenue, Suite 1300
Chicago, IL 60603-6107
312-922-9366

American Association of Blood Banks
1117 North 19th Street, Suite 600
Arlington, VA 22209
703-528-8200

American Association for Medical Systems and Informatics
1101 Connecticut Avenue NW, Suite 700
Washington, DC 20036
202-857-1189

American Association of Tissue Banks
1117 North 19th Street, Suite 402
Arlington, VA 22209
703-528-0663

American College of Cardiology
1111 Old Georgetown Road
Bethesda, MD 20814
301-897-5400

American College of Emergency Physicians
1125 Executive Circle
Irving, TX 75038-2522
214-550-0911

American College of Gastroenterology
13 Elm Street
Manchester, ME 01944
617-927-8330

American College of Nuclear Physicians
1101 Connecticut Avenue NW, Suite 700
Washington, DC 20036
202-857-1135

American College of Obstetricians
and Gynecologists Committee Opinions
600 Maryland Avenue SW
Washington, DC 20024
202-638-5577

American College of Obstetricians
and Gynecologists
Committee on Technical Bulletins
600 Maryland Avenue SW
Washington, DC 20024
202-638-5577

American College of Physicians
Clinical Efficacy Assessment Project
4200 Pine Street
Philadelphia, PA 19104
215-243-1200; 800-523-1546

American College of Preventive Medicine
1015 15th Street NW, Suite 403
Washington, DC 20005
202-789-0003

American College of Radiology
Task Force on Breast Cancer
1891 Preston White Drive
Reston, VA 22091
703-648-8925

American Council on Transplantation
700 North Fairfax Street, Suite 505
Alexandria, VA 22314-2040
703-836-4301

American Dental Association
Council on Dental Materials, Instruments,
and Equipment
211 East Chicago Avenue
Chicago, IL 60611
312-440-2507

American Dental Association
Council on Dental Therapeutics
211 East Chicago Avenue
Chicago, IL 60611
312-440-2523

American Diabetes Association
1660 Duke Street
Alexandria, VA 22314
703-549-1500

American Gastroenterological Association
Patient Care Committee
c/o John Balint, M.D.
Chairman, Department of Medicine
Albany Medical College
47 New Scotland Avenue
Albany, NY 12208
518-445-5376

American Geriatrics Society
770 Lexington Avenue, Suite 400
New York, NY 10021
212-308-1414

American Healthcare Institute
1919 Pennsylvania Avenue NW, Suite 703
Washington, DC 20006
202-293-2840

American Heart Association
National Center
7320 Greenville Avenue
Dallas, TX 75231
214-373-6300

American Hospital Association
Hospital Data Center
Department of Special Studies
840 North Lake Shore Drive
Chicago, IL 60611
312-280-6520

American Hospital Association
Hospital Technology Series Program
Division of Clinical Services and Technology
840 North Lake Shore Drive
Chicago, IL 60611
312-280-6084

American Hospital Association
Office of Legal Communications
840 North Lake Shore Drive
Chicago, IL 60611
312-280-6679

American Hospital Association
Resource Center
840 North Lake Shore Drive
Chicago, IL 60611
312-280-6263

American Institute of Ultrasound In Medicine
4405 East-West Highway, Suite 504
Bethesda, MD 20814
301-656-6117

American Medical Association
Council on Scientific Affairs
535 North Dearborn Street
Chicago, IL 60610
312-645-5335

American Medical Association
Diagnostic and Therapeutic Technology Assessment
535 North Dearborn Street
Chicago, IL 60610
312-645-4530

American Medical Association
Drug Evaluations
535 North Dearborn Street
Chicago, IL 60610
312-645-4560

American Medical Care and Review Association
5410 Grosvenor Lane, Suite 210
Bethesda, MD 20814
301-493-9552

American Medical Peer Review Association
440 First Street NW, Suite 510
Washington, DC 20001
202-628-1853

American Medical Review Research Center
440 First Street NW, Suite 510
Washington, DC 20001
202-639-8614

American National Standards Institute
1430 Broadway
New York, NY 10018
212-354-3300

American Psychiatric Association
1400 K Street, NW
Washington, DC 20005
202-682-6138

American Public Health Association
1015 15th Street, NW
Washington, DC 20005
202-789-5600

American Rheumatism Association
17 Executive Park Drive NE, Suite 480
Atlanta, GA 30329
404-633-3777

American Society for Gastrointestinal Endoscopy
Committee on Technology Assessment
13 Elm Street
Manchester, MA 01944
617-927-8330

American Society of Anesthesiologists
515 Busse Highway
Park Ridge, IL 60068
312-825-5586

American Society of Clinical Pathologists
1101 Vermont Avenue NW, Suite 604
Washington, DC 20005
202-371-0515

American Society of Internal Medicine
1101 Vermont Avenue NW, Suite 500
Washington, DC 20005
202-289-1700

American Society of Mechanical Engineers
345 East 47th Street
New York, NY 10017
212-705-7797

American Society for Parenteral and Enteral Nutrition
8605 Cameron Street, Suite 500
Silver Spring, MD 20910
301-587-6315

American Society for Testing and Materials
1916 Race Street
Philadelphia, PA 19103
215-299-5400

American Society of Transplant Physicians
c/o Lawrence G. Hunsicker, M.D.
President, Director
VA Medical Center, Bldg. 3
Iowa City, IA 52240
319-338-0581

American Society of Transplant Surgeons
c/o Robert J. Corry, M.D.
Professor and Chairman
Office of the Chairman
Department of Surgery
The University of Iowa Hospitals and Clinics
Iowa City, IA 52242
319-356-2545

American Urological Association
1120 North Charles Street
Baltimore, MD 21201
301-727-1100

Association for the Advancement of Medical Instrumentation
1901 North Fort Meyer Drive, Suite 602
Arlington, VA 22209-1699
703-525-4890

Association of Biotechnology Companies
1220 L Street NW, Suite 615
Washington, DC 20005
202-842-2229

Association for Health Services Research
2100 M Street NW, Suite 402
Washington, DC 20037
202-223-2477

Battelle Medical Technology Assessment Program
2030 M Street NW
Washington, DC 20036
202-785-8400

Battelle Memorial Institute
Battelle Human Affairs Research Centers
4000 NE 41st Street
Seattle, WA 98105
206-525-3130

Bioethics Information Retrieval Project
Kennedy Institute of Ethics
Georgetown University
Washington, DC 20057
202-687-3885

Biomedical Business International
17722 Irvine Boulevard
Tustin, CA 92680
714-838-8350

Blue Cross and Blue Shield Association
Medical Necessity Program
676 North St. Clair Street, 11th Floor
Chicago, IL 60611
312-440-5577

Blue Cross and Blue Shield Association
Technology Evaluation and Coverage Program
676 North St. Clair Street, 11th Floor
Chicago, IL 60611
312-440-5577

Boston University Medical Center
400 Totten Pond Road
Waltham, MA 02154
617-890-1300

Brandeis University Health Policy Center
Organ Procurement Project
415 South Street
Waltham, MA 02254
617-736-3900

BRS Information Technologies
1200 Route 7
Latham, NY 12110
800-345-4277

BRS/Saunders
1290 Avenue of the Americas
New York, NY 10104
800-468-0908

California Medical Association
Medical Practice Opinion Program
PO Box 7690
San Francisco, CA 94120-7690
415-863-5522

Canadian Association of Manufacturers of Medical Devices
10 Four Seasons Place
Etobicoke (Tor.), Ontario M9B 6H7
Canada
416-620-1915

Center for Health Management Research
1423 South Grand Avenue
Los Angeles, CA 90015
213-742-6335

Center for the Study of Drug Development
Tufts University
136 Harrison Avenue
Boston, MA 02111
617-956-0070

Centers for Disease Control
Center for Environmental Health
Division of Birth Defects and Developmental Disabilities
1600 Clifton Road
Atlanta, GA 30333
404-454-4706

Centers for Disease Control
Center for Environmental Health
Division of Environmental Hazards and Health Effects
1600 Clifton Road
Atlanta, GA 30333
404-454-4772

Centers for Disease Control
Center for Environmental Health
Division of Environmental Health Laboratory Sciences
Chamblee 17/1103
1600 Clifton Road
Atlanta, GA 30333
404-452-4152

Centers for Disease Control
Center for Health Promotion and Education
1600 Clifton Road
Atlanta, GA 30333
404-321-2263

CBO (Centraal Begeleidingsorgaan voor de Intercollegiale Toetsing)
National Organization for Quality Assurance in Hospitals
Consensus Development Program
PO Box 20064, Churchilllaan 11
3502 LB Utrecht, The Netherlands
(31-30) 96-06-47

College of American Pathologists
Surveys Program
5202 Old Orchard Road
Skokie, IL 60077-1034
312-966-5700

Congress of the United States
Office of Technology Assessment Health Program
Washington, DC 20510
202-226-2070

Copenhagen Collaborating Center for the Study of Regional Variations in Health Care
Institute of Social Medicine
University of Copenhagen, Panum Institute
Blegdamsvej 3
2200 Copenhagen N., Denmark
(45-1) 35-79-00 Ext. 3011

Council of Medical Specialty Societies
PO Box 70
Lake Forest, IL 60045
312-295-3456

Commission on Professional and Hospital Activities
1968 Green Road
PO Box 1802
Ann Arbor, MI 48106
800-521-6210, 800-828-6762 in Michigan

Deutsches Institut für Medizinische
Dokumentation und Information
Welbhausstrasse 27
Postfach 42 05 80
D-5000 Cologne 41
Federal Republic of Germany
(49-221) 47-24-1

DIALOG Information Services, Inc.
3460 Hillview Avenue
Palo Alto, CA 94304
800-334-2564, 415-858-3785

Duke Comprehensive Cancer Center
Duke University Medical Center
PO Box 3153
Durham, NC 27710
919-684-2057

Duke University
Center for Health Policy Research and Education
Box GM, Duke Station
Durham, NC 27706
919-684-3023

ECRI Health Devices Program
5200 Butler Pike
Plymouth Meeting, PA 19462
215-825-6000

ECRI Technology Assessment Program
5200 Butler Pike
Plymouth Meeting, PA 19462
215-825-6000

Employee Benefit Research Institute
2121 K Street NW, Suite 860
Washington, DC 20037-2121
202-659-0670

F-D-C Reports, Inc.
5550 Friendship Boulevard, Suite One
Chevy Chase, MD 20815
301-657-9830

Federation of American Health Systems
1111 19th Street NW, Suite 402
Washington, DC 20036
202-833-3090

Finnish Society of Technology Assessment in
Health Care
c/o National Public Health Institute
Department of Epidemiology
Mannerheimintie 166
SF-00280 Helsinki
Finland
(358-0) 75-70-32-9

Food and Drug Administration
5600 Fishers Lane
Rockville, MD 20857
301-443-5470

Food and Drug Administration
Center for Devices and Radiological Health
12720 Twinbrook Parkway
Rockville, MD 20857
301-443-5807

Food and Drug Administration
Center for Devices and Radiological Health
HFZ-343
Division of Product Surveillance
Office of Compliance
8757 Georgia Avenue
Silver Spring, MD 20910
301-427-8100

Food and Drug Administration
Center for Drugs and Biologics
5600 Fishers Lane
Rockville, MD 20857
301-443-2894

Food and Drug Administration
Center for Food Safety and Applied Nutrition
Color for Drugs and Devices
200 C Street SW, HFF-214
Washington, DC 20204
202-485-0099

Food and Drug Administration
Center for Food Safety and Applied Nutrition
Special Purpose Infant Formulas
200 C Street SW, HFF-204
Washington, DC 20204
202-245-3117

Food and Drug Administration
Press Office
5600 Fishers Lane, HFI-20
Parklawn Building, Room 1505
Rockville, MD 20857
301-443-3285

Friedman, Eisenstein, Raemer, and Schwartz
Certified Public Accountants/Business and Personal Consultants
401 North Michigan Avenue
Chicago, IL 60611
312-644-6000

Generic Pharmaceutical Industry Association
200 Madison Avenue, Suite 2404
New York, NY 10016
212-683-1881

George Washington University Medical Center
Office of Research and Sponsored Programs
2300 Eye Street NW
Washington, DC 20037
202-676-2995

Georgetown University Medical Center
Institute for Health Policy Analysis
2121 Wisconsin Avenue NW, Suite 220
Washington, DC 20007
202-625-2115

Group Health Association of America
1129 20th Street NW, Suite 600
Washington, DC 20036
202-778-3200

Harvard School of Public Health
Institute for Health Research
677 Huntington Avenue
Boston, MA 02115
617-729-5657

Hastings Center
255 Elm Road
Briarcliff Manor, NY 10510
914-762-8500

Health Care Financing Administration
Bureau of Eligibility, Reimbursement, and Coverage
East Building, Room 401
6325 Security Boulevard
Baltimore, MD 21207
301-594-9690

Health Care Financing Administration
Office of Research and Demonstrations
Oak Meadows Building, Room 2-B-12
6325 Security Boulevard
Baltimore, MD 21207
301-597-1435

Health Council of The Netherlands
PO Box 90.517
2509 LM The Hague
The Netherlands
(31-70) 47-14-41

Health Data Institute
(subsidiary of Caremark, Inc.)
20 Maguire Road
Lexington, MA 02173
617-863-2000

Health Industry Manufacturers Association
1030 15th Street NW, Suite 1100
Washington, DC 20005
202-452-8240

Health Information Designs, Inc.
1616 North Fort Meyer Drive, Suite 1420
Arlington, VA 22209
703-528-2032

Health Insurance Association of America
1025 Connecticut Avenue, NW
Washington, DC 20036-3998
202-223-7836

Health and Welfare Canada
Health Services and Promotion Branch
Institutional and Professional Services Division
Guidelines for Institutional Programs
Ottawa, Ontario K1A 1B4
Canada
613-954-8623

HHS Evaluation Documentation Center
Office of the Assistant Secretary for Planning and Evaluation
U.S. Department of Health and Human Services
Humphrey Building, Room 438F
200 Independence Avenue SW
Washington, DC 20201
202-245-6445

IMS America Ltd.
660 West Germantown Pike
PO Box 905
Plymouth Meeting, PA 19462-0905
215-834-5000

Institute for Alternative Futures
1405 King Street
Alexandria, VA 22314
703-684-5880

Institute of Electrical and Electronics Engineers
1111 19th Street NW, Suite 608
Washington, DC 20036
202-785-0017

Institute for the Future
2740 Sand Hill Road
Menlo Park, CA 94025-7097
415-854-6322

International Federation for Medical and Biological Engineering
c/o Dr. Jan Persson, Chairman
Joint Working Group
Implications and Assessment of Biomedical Innovations
c/o Dept. of Biomedical Engineering
University Hospital
S-581 85 Linköping, Sweden
(46-13) 19-24-56

International Federation of Voluntary Health Service Funds
15-17 Essex Street
London WC2R 3AD, England
United Kingdom
(44-1) 35-31-15-9

International Resource Development, Inc.
6 Prowitt Street
Norwalk, CT 06855
203-866-7800

International Society of Technology Assessment in Health Care
c/o Els Borst-Eilers, Secretary, and Vice Chairman
Health Council of the Netherlands
PO Box 90517
2509 IM The Hague
The Netherlands
(31-70) 47-14-41

Johns Hopkins Program for Medical Technology and Practice Assessment
Center for Hospital Finance and Management
624 North Broadway, Room 305
Baltimore, MD 21205
301-955-2300

Joint effort of Department of Computer and Information Science and Center for Medical Technology Assessment
Linköping University
S-581 83 Linköping, Sweden
(46-13) 28-19-69

Kings Fund Centre for Service Development
Kings Fund Forum Consensus and Controversies in Medicine
126 Albert Street
London NWI, England
(44-1) 267-6111

Lewin and Associates, Inc.
Strategic Technology Group
1090 Vermont Avenue NW, Suite 700
Washington, DC 20005
202-842-2800

Linköping University
Center for Medical Technology Assessment
S-581 83 Linköping, Sweden
(46-13) 28-10-00, Ext. 2310

Maryland Hospital Association
1301 York Road, Suite 800
Lutherville, MD 21093
301-321-6200

Massachusetts Health Data Consortium, Inc.
400-1 Totten Pond Road
Waltham, MA 02154
617-890-6040

McGill University
Department of Epidemiology and Biostatistics
1020 Pine Avenue West
Montreal, Canada H3A 1A2
514-392-4740

McMaster University
Department of Clinical Epidemiology and Biostatistics
1200 Main Street
Hamilton, Ontario L8N 325
Canada
416-525-9140, Ext. 2425

Mead Data Central
PO Box 933
Dayton, OH 45401
800-227-4908, 513-865-6800

Medical Device Register, Inc.
655 Washington Boulevard
Stamford, CT 06901
800-222-3045, 203-348-6319 in Connecticut

Medical Engineering Department
Akron City Hospital
525 East Market Street
Akron, OH 44309-2090
216-375-3501

Medical Research Council
National Health and Welfare Canada
Jeanne Mance Building, Tunney's Pasture
Ottawa, Ontario K1A OW9
Canada
613-954-1959

Medical Technology and Practice Patterns Institute
National Health Services and Practice Patterns Survey
2233 Wisconsin Avenue NW, Suite 302
Washington, DC 20007
202-333-8841

MEDLINK
PO Box 9080
Waltham, MA 02254-9080
800-342-1338, 617-890-0385 in Massachusetts

National Advisory Council on Health Care Technology Assessment
National Center for Health Services Research and Health Care Technology Assessment
Parklawn Building, Room 18-05
5600 Fishers Lane
Rockville, MD 20857
301-443-5650

National Association of Health Data Organizations
316 Pennsylvania Avenue SE, Suite 202
Washington, DC 20003
202-546-5881

National Association of Manufacturers
1776 F Street NW
Washington, DC 20006
202-637-3000

National Cancer Institute
International Cancer Information Center
Office of International Affairs
Building 82, Room 103
Bethesda, MD 20892
301-496-7403

National Cancer Institute
National Institutes of Health
Surveillance, Epidemiology, and End Results Program
Surveillance and Operations Research Branch
Blair Building, Room 532
Bethesda, MD 20892-4200
301-427-8829

National Center for Health Services Research and Health Care Technology Assessment
Parklawn Building Room 18-05
5600 Fishers Lane
Rockville, MD 20857

National Center for Health Services Research and Health Care Technology Assessment
Division of Extramural Research
5600 Fishers Lane, Room 18A-19
Rockville, MD 20857
301-443-2080

National Center for Health Services Research and Health Care Technology Assessment
Office of Health Technology Assessment
5600 Fishers Lane, Room 18A-27
Rockville, MD 20857
301-443-4990

National Center for Health Statistics
Scientific Information Branch
Division of Data Services
3700 East-West Highway
Hyattsville, MD 20782
301-436-8500

National Electrical Manufacturers Association
2101 L Street NW, Suite 300
Washington, DC 20037
202-457-8432

National Health Council
1700 K Street NW, Suite 1005
Washington, DC 20006
202-785-3913

National Health Research and Development Program
Jeanne Mance Building, Room 513
Tunney's Pasture
Ottawa, Ontario K1A 1B4
Canada
613-954-8543

National Heart, Lung, and Blood Institute
Communications and Public Information Branch
Building 31, Room 4A-21
Bethesda, MD 20892
301-496-5343

National Heart, Lung, and Blood Institue
National Cholesterol Education Program/NHLBI Smoking Education Program Information Center
Office of Prevention, Education, and Control
Building 31, Room 4A-21
Bethesda, MD 20892
301-230-1340

National Heart, Lung, and Blood Institute
National Heart, Blood Vessel, Lung, and Blood Program
Office of Program Planning and Evaluation
National Institutes of Health
Building 31, Room 5A-11
9000 Rockville Pike
Bethesda, MD 20892
301-496-3620

National Heart, Lung, and Blood Institute
Office of Prevention, Education, and Control
120/80 National Institutes of Health
Bethesda, MD 20892
301-496-1809

National Institute of Child Health and Human Development
Office of Planning and Evaluation
Building 31, Room 2A10
9000 Rockville Pike
Bethesda, MD 20892
301-496-1877

National Institutes of Health
Consensus Development Program
Building 1, Room 210
9000 Rockville Pike
Bethesda, MD 20892
301-496-1143

National Institutes of Health
Statistics and Analysis Branch
Division of Research Grants
Bethesda, MD 20892
301-496-7543

National Library of Medicine
Building 38, Room 2S-18
8600 Rockville Pike
Bethesda, MD 20894
301-496-8834

National Library of Medicine
MEDLARS Management Section
Building 38, Room 4N421
8600 Rockville Pike
Bethesda, MD 20894
800-638-8480, 301-496-6193 in Maryland

National Perinatal Epidemiology Unit
Radcliffe Infirmary
Oxford OX2 6HE
England
(44-865) 81-68-76

National Technical Information Service
U.S. Department of Commerce
5285 Port Royal Road
Springfield, VA 22161
703-487-4650

Netherlands Organization for Applied Scientific Research
Medical Technology Unit
PO Box 188
2300 AD Leiden
The Netherlands
(31-71) 21-4441

New York State Center for Assessing Health Services
Health Services Center 4L 215
State University of New York at Stony Brook
Stony Brook, NY 11794
516-444-2101

Occupational Safety and Health Administration
U.S. Department of Labor
200 Constitution Avenue NW, Room N2439
Washington, DC 20210
202-523-9700

ODPHP National Health Information Center
Office of Disease Prevention and Health Promotion
U.S. Department of Health and Human Services
PO Box 1133
Washington, DC 20013-1133
800-336-4797, 202-429-9091

Oley Foundation for Home Parenteral and Enteral Nutrition
214 Hun Memorial
Albany Medical Center
Albany, NY 12208
518-445-5079

Pan American Health Organization
525 23rd Street NW
Washington, DC 20037
202-861-3219

Patent Depository Library Program Office
Patent and Trademark Office
U.S. Department of Commerce
Washington, DC 20231
703-557-9686

Pharmabooks, Ltd.
1775 Broadway, Suite 511
New York, NY 10019
212-262-8230

Pharmaceutical Manufacturers Association
1100 15th Street NW
Washington, DC 20005
202-835-3420

Pharmaprojects
18/20 Hill Rise
Richmond, Surrey, TW10 6UA
United Kingdom
(44-1) 94-83-26-2

Physician Payment Review Commission
2120 L Street NW, Suite 510
Washington, DC 20037
202-653-7220

Policy Analysis, Inc.
Medical Technology Cost-Effectiveness Program
1577 Beacon Street
Brookline, MA 02146
617-232-4400

Practitioner Reporting System
United States Pharmacopeial Convention, Inc.
12601 Twinbrook Parkway
Rockville, MD 20852
301-881-0666

Project HOPE
Center for Health Affairs
2 Wisconsin Circle, Suite 500
Chevy Chase, MD 20815
301-656-7401

Prospective Payment Assessment Commission
300 Seventh Street SW, Suite 301B
Washington, DC 20024
202-453-3986

Randomized Controlled Clinical Trials Report Collection
c/o Thomas C. Chalmers, M.D.
Harvard School of Public Health
677 Huntington Avenue
Kresge 4th Floor
Boston, MA 02115
617-732-1090

Renal Physicians Association
1101 Vermont Avenue NW, Suite 500
Washington, DC 20005-3457
202-898-1562

RESNA-Association for the Advancement of Rehabilitation Technology
1101 Connecticut Avenue NW, Suite 700
Washington, DC 20036
202-857-1199

Scrip
18/20 Hill Rise
Richmond, Surrey TW10 6UA
United Kingdom
(44-1) 94-83-26

Scrip World Pharmaceutical News
1775 Broadway, Suite 511
New York, NY 10019
212-262-8230

Society for Medical Decision Making
One Main Street
PO Box 447
West Lebanon, NH 03784
603-298-9929

Society of Non-Invasive Vascular Technology
1101 Connecticut Avenue NW, Suite 700
Washington, DC 20036
202-857-1149

Society of Nuclear Medicine
136 Madison Avenue
New York, NY 10016-6784
212-889-0717

SoftSearch, Inc.
1560 Broadway, Suite 900
Denver, CO 80202
303-832-7111, 800-426-2873

Steering Committee on Future Health Scenarios
Commission on Future Health Care Technology
Room BCB 203
PO Box 5406
2280 HK Rijwijk
The Netherlands
(31-70) 40-72-05

Swedish National Center for Technology Assessment in Health Care
Drottning Gatan 16
11151 Stockholm
Sweden
(46-8) 24-05-65

Swedish Planning and Rationalization Institute of the Health Services
Library and Research Report Bank
PO Box 27310
S-102
Stockholm, Sweden
(46-8) 63-05-60

Swedish Planning and Rationalization Institute of the Health Services
Technology Assessment and Health Economics
Box 27310
102 54 Stockholm, Sweden
(46-8) 663-05-60

Technology Assessment and Forecast Program
U.S. Patent and Trademark Office
CM2-313
Washington, DC 20231
703-557-0433

Theta Corporation
Theta Building
Middlefield, CT 06455
203-349-1054

United Kingdom Department of Health and Social Security
Supplies Technology Division
Medical Devices Evaluation Programme
14 Russell Square
London WC1B SEP
England
(44-1) 636-6811, Ext. 3248

United Network for Organ Sharing
3001 Hungary Spring Road
PO Box 28010
Richmond, VA 23228
804-289-0600

U.S. Administrators Inc.
Professional Policy Committee
5016 North Parkway Calabasas
Calabasas, CA 91302
800-872-7526, Ext. 173

U.S. Department of Commerce
Industry Publications Division
Office of Industrial Assessment
International Trade Administration
Trade Development
14th Street and Constitution Avenue NW
Washington, DC 20230
202-377-4356

U.S. Department of Commerce
Office of Commercial Information Management
Division of Market Analysis
14th Street and Constitution Avenue NW
Room 2012
Washington, DC 20230
202-377-4203

United States Pharmacopeial Convention
12601 Twinbrook Parkway
Rockville, MD 20852
301-881-0666

University of California, San Francisco
Institute for Health Policy Studies
1326 Third Avenue
San Francisco, CA 94143
415-476-4921

University Hospital Consortium
One Mid America Plaza, Suite 624
Oakbrook Terrace, IL 60181
312-954-6766

University of Lausanne
Institute of Social and Preventive Medicine
Evaluation of the Efficacy and Safety of Chorionic Villi Sampling
17 r. Bugnon
1005 Lausanne, Switzerland
(41-21) 41-28-66

University of Pennsylvania
Leonard Davis Institute of Health Economics
3641 Locust Walk
Philadelphia, PA 19104
215-898-6011

University of Pittsburgh School of Medicine
Section of Medical Informatics
Department of Medicine
190 Lothrop Street #165A
Pittsburgh, PA 15261
412-648-3190

Veterans Administration
Cooperative Studies Program (151 I)
Veterans Administration Medical Center
150 South Huntington Avenue
Boston, MA 02130
617-739-3479

Veterans Administration
Health Services Research and Development Service (152)
810 Vermont Avenue NW
Washington, DC 20420
In collaboration with:
Special Projects Office
VA Medical Center (152)
Perry Point, MD 21902
301-642-2411

World Health Organization (WHO)
1211 Geneva 27
Switzerland
(41-21) 91-21-11

INDEX TO ORGANIZATIONS

Appendices

Appendix A

About the Council on Health Care Technology

Rosters of Council and Panels

ABOUT THE COUNCIL ON HEALTH CARE TECHNOLOGY

The National Academy of Sciences (NAS) is a private, non-profit organization established by federal charter in 1863 to provide advice to the government on matters of science. The Institute of Medicine (IOM) was established under the NAS charter in 1970 to conduct studies of policy issues related to health and medicine, acting both as an advisor to the federal government and on its own initiative. It is the responsibility of the IOM for establishing and operating the Council on Health Care Technology.

The Council on Health Care Technology (CHCT) was established within the IOM in 1986 to promote the development and application of technology assessment in health care and to review health care technologies for their appropriate use. The council was mandated by the U.S. Congress in the Health Promotion and Disease Prevention Amendments of 1984 (P.L. 98-551) and by technical amendments made in 1985 (P.L. 99-117).

The functions of the council are: to serve as a clearinghouse for data and information sources related to health care technologies and technology assessments; to improve the methodologies, techniques, and procedures of technology assessment; to identify needs in assessment of technologies and the criteria for setting priorities among assessment needs; to stimulate, coordinate, and commission the assessment of health care technologies; and to promote related education, training, and technical assistance.

The federal government provided the IOM with initial funding for the council in December 1985. The IOM appointed the council in March 1986, which met for the first time in April 1986. The council consists of 16 people who are experts on the safety, efficacy, effectiveness, appropriateness, and cost of health care technology, and who represent health professionals, hospitals and other health care providers, health care insurers, employers, consumers, and manufacturers of products for health care.

The council established four panels, each of which has as many as 18 members with appropriate ranges of expertise, to help fulfill the council's responsibilities. The Evaluation Panel was established to address the council functions to identify and set priorities among assessment needs and to stimulate, coordinate, and commission assessments. The Information Panel oversees the development and operation of the information clearinghouse for health care technologies and assessments. The Methods Panel was established to improve the methods, techniques, and procedures of technology assessment and to promote education and training in the use of these approaches. The Federal Liaison Panel was established to maintain a strong relationship between the council and federal agencies with assessment programs and interests. Federal Liaison Panel members participate in activities of the council and other panels. Except for the

Federal Liaison Panel, at least two members of the council serve on each of the panels. Council and panel members and their respective organizational affiliations are shown in the appendices.

In addition to the activities of the panels, the council sponsors other matters of interest to the assessment community. The council's forum series consists of two-day symposiums linked by a common concern for major health policy issues that cut across the public and private sectors. They are invitational conferences held two or three times annually, organized to promote interaction among speakers and audience to encourage the exchange of differing views without pressure to resolve differences. Themes for the first two forums in 1987 were *Quality of Care and Technology Assessment* and *Care of the Elderly Patient: Policy Issues and Research Opportunities*. Also in 1987, the IOM cosponsored with the National Academy of Engineering a symposium entitled *New Medical Devices: Factors Influencing Invention, Development, and Use*. It addressed key economic, technical, and political factors expected to influence development and appropriate use of innovative medical devices during the coming decade. Published proceedings of that symposium will be available in early 1988.

The council published its first issues of its *CHCT Newsletter* during 1986, and plans to continue publication quarterly. The newsletter reports current council activities, lists forthcoming conferences and events of interest to the assessment community, and describes recent report releases and other publications, and related developments of interest to the assessment community. Most issues include a profile of an assessment program similar to those in Part 1 of this *Directory*. The first annual report of the council, to cover activities through 1987, will be available in early 1988.

The council is supported by contributions and grants from the private sector and by federal matching grants. Public Law 98-551 set aside up to $500,000 for the first year, $750,000 for the second year, and $750,000 for the third year in federal grants for initial, partial support of the council. These amounts were earmarked for the council in annual appropriations made by Congress for the National Center for Health Services Research and Health Care Technology Assessment (NCHSR), a component of the U.S. Public Health Service. According to the statute, granting of any portion or all of these funds was subject to matching requirements for financial support from the private sector. First year federal grant funds had to be matched by half their amount from other sources, i.e. two federal dollars for every non-federal dollar. Second and third year federal grants for operation of the council were to be matched by twice these amounts from private sector sources, i.e. one federal dollar for every two non-federal dollars. Thus, the activities of the council, including production of this *Directory*, have been supported in part by grant number HS 05526 from the NCHSR.

Private sector contributors to the council include health insurers, medical professions organizations, health product makers, hospitals, health maintenance organizations, business groups, and other organizations served by the council and that participate in its activities. Other non-federal grant support is to include some cost-recovery on council products and services, such as this *Directory*. Also, the National Research Council, a component of the NAS, has provided program initiation support for certain activities. A list of contributors to the council is shown in Appendix B.

In December 1987, the President signed the Public Health Service Amendments of 1987, (P.L. 100-177). These amendments to the Public Health Service Act pertain in part to the Council on Health Care Technology, and extend the authority of the NCHSR, the National Center for Health Statistics, and other Public Health Service programs for fiscal years 1988, 1989, and 1990.

The 1987 amendments affecting the council provide for the Secretary of Health and Human Services to make available up to $750,000 for the support and operation of the council in each of the three fiscal years. Awarding of these federal funds is contingent upon matching support from non-federal sources. The matching requirement for fiscal 1988 and 1989 is one federal dollar for one non-federal dollar; in fiscal 1990, the ratio is one federal dollar for every two non-federal dollars.

In support of the 1987 legislation, the report of the Senate Committee on Labor and Human Resources stated: "The Committee continues to support this program which it believes provides an important forum for joint government and private cooperation to promote the development of methods of health care technology assessment." The House Committee on Energy and Commerce stated: "The Committee wishes to reaffirm its support for the Council and its expectation that the Council will play a vital role in the development of health policy and improvements in the delivery of health care services. Federal health programs, and their beneficiaries, stand to benefit immensely from the activities of the Council, and the Federal government should continue to be an effective participant in the activities and funding of the Council."

COUNCIL ON HEALTH CARE TECHNOLOGY

WILLIAM N. HUBBARD, JR.
former President, The Upjohn Company, Hickory Corners, Michigan *(Chairman)*

JEREMIAH A. BARONDESS
Irene F. and I. Roy Psaty Distinguished Professor of Clinical Medicine, Cornell University Medical College, New York, New York *(Co-Chairman)*

HERBERT L. ABRAMS
Professor of Radiology, Stanford University School of Medicine, Stanford, California

RICHARD E. BEHRMAN
Dean, School of Medicine, Case Western Reserve University, Cleveland, Ohio

PAUL A. EBERT
Director, American College of Surgeons, Chicago, Illinois

PAUL S. ENTMACHER
Senior Vice President and Chief Medical Director, Metropolitan Life Insurance Company, New York, New York

MELVIN A. GLASSER
Director, Health Security Action Council, Washington, D.C.

GERALD D. LAUBACH
President, Pfizer Inc., New York, New York

WALTER B. MAHER
Director, Employee Benefits and Health Services, Chrysler Corporation, Detroit, Michigan

ROBERT H. McCAFFREY
Chairman and Chief Executive Officer, C.R. Bard Inc., Murray Hill, New Jersey

LAWRENCE C. MORRIS
Senior Vice President, Health Benefits Management, Blue Cross and Blue Shield Association, Chicago, Illinois

FREDERICK MOSTELLER
Roger I. Lee Professor, Harvard School of Public Health, Boston, Massachusetts

MARY O. MUNDINGER
Dean, School of Nursing, Columbia University, New York, New York

ANNE A. SCITOVSKY
Chief, Health Economics Department, Palo Alto Medical Foundation, Palo Alto, California

C. THOMAS SMITH
President, Yale-New Haven Hospital, New Haven, Connecticut

GAIL L. WARDEN
President and Chief Executive Officer, Group Health Cooperative of Puget Sound, Seattle, Washington

EVALUATION PANEL OF THE COUNCIL ON HEALTH CARE TECHNOLOGY

GEORGE E. THIBAULT
Associate Chief of Medicine, Department of Medicine, Massachusetts General Hospital, Boston, Massachusetts *(Chairman)*

CHERYL F. AUSTEIN
Director, Division of Science and Public Health Policy, Office of Assistant Secretary for Planning and Evaluation, Department of Health and Human Services, Washington, D.C.

JEREMIAH A. BARONDESS
Irene F. and I. Roy Psaty Distinguished Professor of Clinical Medicine, Cornell University Medical College, New York, New York

KATHLEEN BUTO
Deputy Director, Bureau of Eligibility, Reimbursement, and Coverage, Health Care Financing Administration, Baltimore, Maryland

H. TRISTRAM ENGELHARDT, JR.
Professor of Medicine and Community Medicine, Center for Ethics, Medicine and Public Issues, Baylor College of Medicine, Houston, Texas

PAUL S. ENTMACHER
Senior Vice President and Chief Medical Director, Metropolitan Life Insurance Company, New York, New York

BERNADINE HEALY
Chairman, Research Institute, The Cleveland Clinic Foundation, Cleveland, Ohio

ROGER C. HERDMAN
Assistant Director, Health and Life Sciences Division, Office of Technology Assessment, U.S. Congress, Washington, D.C.

GERALD D. LAUBACH
President, Pfizer Inc., New York, New York

ROBERT H. McCAFFREY
Chairman and Chief Executive Officer, C.R. Bard Inc., Murray Hill, New Jersey

MARY O. MUNDINGER
Dean, School of Nursing, Columbia University, New York, New York

SEYMOUR PERRY
Deputy Director, Institute for Health Policy Analysis, Georgetown University Medical Center, Washington, D.C.

CHARLES E. PHELPS
Professor of Political Science, Director, Public Policy Analysis Program, Department of Political Science, University of Rochester, Rochester, New York

MICHAEL F. ROIZEN
Professor and Chairperson, Department of Anesthesia and Critical Care, University of Chicago, Chicago, Illinois

HAROLD C. SOX
Associate Chief of Staff for Ambulatory Care, Veterans Administration Medical Center, Palo Alto, California

EARL P. STEINBERG
Assistant Professor of Medicine, Johns Hopkins University School of Medicine, The Johns Hopkins Hospital, Baltimore, Maryland

JOHN C. VILLFORTH
Director, Center for Devices and Radiological Health, Food and Drug Administration, Rockville, Maryland

DONALD A. YOUNG
Executive Director, Prospective Payment Assessment Commission, Washington, D.C.

INFORMATION PANEL OF THE COUNCIL ON HEALTH CARE TECHNOLOGY

LAWRENCE C. MORRIS
Senior Vice President, Health Benefits Management, Blue Cross and Blue Shield Association, Chicago, Illinois *(Chairman)*

GAIL L. WARDEN
President and Chief Executive Officer, Group Health Cooperative of Puget Sound, Seattle, Washington *(Co-Chairman)*

MORRIS F. COLLEN
Consultant, Division of Research, Kaiser Permanente Medical Care Program, Oakland, California

RICHARD C. FARMER
Chairman, Division of Medicine, The Cleveland Clinic Foundation, Cleveland, Ohio

MELVIN A. GLASSER
Director, Health Security Action Council, Washington, D.C.

G. MAX K. HUGHES
Vice President, Systems and Communication, Pfizer Pharmaceuticals, New York, New York

RICHARD J. JOHNS
Massey Professor and Director, Department of Biomedical Engineering, Johns Hopkins University and Hospital, Baltimore, Maryland

DONALD A.B. LINDBERG
Director, National Library of Medicine, National Institutes of Health, Bethesda, Maryland

WALTER B. MAHER
Director, Employee Benefits and Health Services, Chrysler Corporation, Detroit, Michigan

JOHN H. MOXLEY, III
President, MetaMedical Inc., Beverly Hills, California

C. THOMAS SMITH
President, Yale-New Haven Hospital, New Haven, Connecticut

GEORGE E.T. STEBBING
Director, Professional Activities, Office of the Secretary of Defense, Health Affairs, Washington, D.C.

METHODS PANEL OF THE COUNCIL ON HEALTH CARE TECHNOLOGY

FREDERICK MOSTELLER
Roger I. Lee Professor, Harvard School of Public Health, Boston, Massachusetts *(Chairman)*

HERBERT L. ABRAMS
Professor of Radiology, Stanford University School of Medicine, Stanford, California *(Chairman)*

RICHARD E. BEHRMAN
Dean, School of Medicine, Case Western Reserve University, Cleveland, Ohio

PAUL A. EBERT
Director, American College of Surgeons, Chicago, Illinois

DAVID M. EDDY
Center for Health Policy Research and Education, Duke University, Durham, North Carolina

SUSAN D. HORN
Associate Director, Center for Hospital Finance and Management, Johns Hopkins University School of Hygiene and Public Health, Baltimore, Maryland

BRYAN LUCE
Senior Research Scientist, Battelle Human Affairs Research Centers, Washington, D.C.

JAY MOSKOWITZ
Associate Director for Program Planning and Evaluation, National Institutes of Health, Bethesda, Maryland

ANNE A. SCITOVSKY
Chief, Health Economics Department, Palo Alto Medical Foundation, Palo Alto, California

WALTER O. SPITZER
Professor and Chair, Department of Epidemiology and Biostatistics, McGill University, Montreal, Quebec

STEPHEN B. THACKER
Assistant Director for Science, Center for Environmental Health, Centers for Disease Control, Atlanta, Georgia

ELEANOR TRAVERS
Chairman, Task Force on Technology Assessment, Veterans Administration, Washington, D.C.

NORMAN W. WEISSMAN
Director, Division of Extramural Research, National Center for Health Services Research and Health Care Technology Assessment, Rockville, Maryland

FEDERAL LIAISON PANEL OF THE COUNCIL ON HEALTH CARE TECHNOLOGY

ROGER C. HERDMAN
Assistant Director, Health and Life Sciences Division, Office of Technology Assessment, U.S. Congress, Washington, D.C. *(Chairman)*

CHERYL F. AUSTEIN
Director, Division of Science and Public Health Policy, Office of Assistant Secretary for Planning and Evaluation, Department of Health and Human Services, Washington, D.C.

KATHLEEN BUTO
Deputy Director, Bureau of Eligibility, Reimbursement, and Coverage, Health Care Financing Administration, Baltimore, Maryland

J. MICHAEL FITZMAURICE
Director, National Center for Health Services Research and Health Care Technology Assessment, Rockville, Maryland

JANET KLINE
Director, Health Section, Congressional Research Service, Library of Congress, Washington, D.C.

DONALD A.B. LINDBERG
Director, National Library of Medicine, National Institutes of Health, Bethesda, Maryland

JAY MOSKOWITZ
Associate Director for Program Planning and Evaluation, National Institutes of Health, Bethesda, Maryland

GEORGE E.T. STEBBING
Director, Professional Activities, Office of the Secretary of Defense, Health Affairs, Washington, D.C.

STEPHEN B. THACKER
Assistant Director for Science, Center for Environmental Health, Centers for Disease Control, Atlanta, Georgia

ELEANOR TRAVERS
Chairman, Task Force on Technology Assessment, Veterans Administration, Washington, D.C.

JOHN C. VILLFORTH
Director, Center for Devices and Radiological Health, Food and Drug Administration, Rockville, Maryland

DONALD A. YOUNG
Executive Director, Prospective Payment Assessment Commission, Washington, D.C.

Appendix B

Funding Sources for the Council on Health Care Technology

CONTRIBUTORS TO THE COUNCIL ON HEALTH CARE TECHNOLOGY

The Council on Health Care Technology is supported by contributions and grants from the private sector and by federal matching grants made as described in the preceding discussion about the council. These federal matching grants have been provided by grant number HS 05526 from the National Center for Health Services Research and Health Care Technology Assessment.

Private sector contributors to the council through 1987 include the following.

$10,000 and More

American Academy of Pediatrics
American College of Cardiology
American College of Physicians
American Hospital Association
American Medical Association
Baxter Travenol Foundation
Blue Cross and Blue Shield Association
CIGNA Corporation
Equicor, Inc.
Ford Motor Company Fund
The HCA Foundation
Health Industry Manufacturers Association
Hoffman-La Roche, Inc.
Kaiser Foundation Hospitals
Metropolitan Life Foundation
National Research Council Fund
The Prudential Foundation
Squibb Corporation
The Upjohn Company

$5,000 to $9,999

American Academy of Ophthalmology
General Mills Foundation
John Hancock Mutual Life Insurance Company
Pfizer Inc.
Provident Life and Accident Insurance Company

Under $5,000

Aid Association for Lutherans
American Chambers Life Insurance company
American College of Radiology
American Community Mutual Insurance Company
American General Corporation
American Hardware Mutual Insurance Company
Association Life Insurance Company
Benefit Trust Life Foundation
Boston Mutual Life Insurance Company
Business Men's Assurance Company of America
The Canada Life Assurance Company
Central Life Assurance Company
Central States Health and Life Co. of Omaha

Under $5,000 continued

CNA Insurance Companies
Cologne Life Reinsurance Company
Colonial Life and Accident Insurance Company
The Colonial Penn Life Insurance Company
Continental Casualty Company
Country Life Insurance Company
Educators Mutual Life Insurance Company
Family Health Plan, Inc.
Farm Bureau Insurance
Farm Family Life Insurance Company
Federal Home Companies
Federal Life Insurance Company (Mutual)
Federated Mutual Insurance Company
First Colony Life Insurance Company
General American Life Insurance Company
General Reassurance Corporation
Great American Reserve Insurance Company
Great-West Life Assurance Company
Group Health Association
Group Health Plan of Southeast Michigan
Guarantee Mutual Life Company
Guarantee Trust Life Insurance Company
The Guardian Life Trust
The Hartford Insurance Group
Health Care Plus of America, Inc.
HMO of Western Pennsylvania
IBA Health and Life Assurance Company
J.C. Penney Life Insurance Company
Jefferson Pilot Life Insurance Company
Lamar Life Insurance Company
Liberty Mutual Insurance Company
Life Insurance Company of Georgia
The Life Insurance Company of Virginia
Lincoln National Life Insurance Company
Lutheran Brotherhood
Massachusetts Mutual Life Insurance Company
Ministers Life
Monarch Capital Corporation
Munich American Reassurance Company
Mutual Benefit Life
The Mutual Life Insurance Company of New York
Mutual of Omaha
National Travelers Life Company
Nationwide Life Insurance Company
The New England
New York Life Insurance Company
North American Life and Casualty Company
Northwestern Mutual Life Insurance Company
Northwestern National Life Insurance Company
The Ohio National Life Insurance Company
Pacific Mutual Foundation
Pan-American Life Insurance Company
The Paul Revere Life Insurance Company
Peak Health Plan, Ohio Region
Phoenix Mutual Life Insurance Company
Prime Health
Principal Mutual Life Insurance Company
Protective Life Insurance Company
Reserve Life Insurance Company
Shelter Life Insurance Company
Shenandoah Life Insurance Company
State Farm Mutual Automobile Insurance Company
Teachers Insurance and Annuity Association/ College Retirement Equities Fund
Time Insurance Company
Transamerica Occidental Life Insurance Company
The Union Central Life Insurance Company
Washington National Insurance Company
Wausau Insurance Companies
Western Life Insurance Company
Wisconsin National Life Insurance Company
Woodmen Accident and Life Company

Appendix C

Survey of Organizations with an Ongoing Medical Technology Assessment Program

Name of person completing survey ______________________

Telephone: ______________________

Survey of Organizations With an Ongoing Medical Technology Assessment Program

The purpose of this survey is to compile a directory of **organizations** with an **ongoing program** of **medical technology assessment**. For purposes of this survey:

an organization may be a professional, trade, or other association, university or other not-for-profit entity, government agency, or for-profit corporation

an ongoing program is a structure or process within the organization, if not the entire organization, that assesses medical technologies and generates assessment reports

a medical technology assessment is any study or inquiry the objective of which is to provide information regarding the effects of a technology designed to maintain or improve health or be used as part of an intervention for such purpose, whether or not the study evaluates the effects

an assessment may be made by any one or a combination of methods, e.g., panel of experts, information synthesis, empirical study

the report of results may be published by the organization/program, in a journal, or other vehicle. However, for the organization/program to be eligible for inclusion in this survey, the report must be available to others outside of the organization.

This survey is **not** for organizations that: may have conducted medical technology assessments but do not have any ongoing program; catalog, index, or evaluate assessments but do not produce them; conduct assessments but do not make results available to anyone outside of the organization. Information on these types of activities may be incorporated into the directory using other collection instruments.

If your organization contains two or more programs that qualify for inclusion, please complete a separate survey form for each one. Additional copies, and information, may be obtained from Pamela Simerly on 202/334-2319.

Please complete and return this survey by ______________ using the envelopes provided or mail to **Pamela Simerly, IOM Council on Health Care Technology, 2101 Constitution Avenue, N.W., JH 751, Washington, DC 20418.**

Instructions for Completing the Survey

This survey consists of four parts.

- Part I asks you to describe your organization.
- Part II consists of categorized checklists that ask you to select one or more response categories to describe your program.
- Part III is a series of open-ended questions that ask you to describe your program in a brief narrative format.
- Part IV requests listings of completed, ongoing, and planned assessment reports.

If an item is not applicable, please note "NA" (rather than leaving the answer space blank).

In completing this survey, if more convenient, you may type answers on separate sheets and append them to the survey form. If you do append sheets, be sure that you have keyed them to the question, responded to all survey items, and completed structured items on the survey form.

Please provide a current example of a medical technology assessment report published by your program. **By providing the report you are consenting to its reproduction in**

the directory as a sample assessment, if the IOM chooses to include it. If you produce different types of assessment reports, please append a current example of each type; key the report to the type of assessment.

If your organization has two or more assessment programs, please complete a separate survey form for each one (Parts II, III, and IV).

If your program conducts two or more types of medical technology assessment, please complete a separate survey form for each one (Parts II, III, and IV).

Does your organization have two or more assessment **programs**?

____ yes (**If yes**, please list the separate programs below, and complete a separate survey form for each one. You may copy survey formats or request additional copies from Pamela Simerly, 202/334-2319.)

____ no

List of programs (only if your organization has two or more distinct programs that assess medical technology).

1. ____________________

2. ____________________

3. ____________________

4. ____________________

Does your program conduct two or more **types of assessment** that differ materially with respect to purpose, subject selection, method of assessment, or assessment process or methods? Check **one**:

____ yes (**If yes**, please list the separate types of assessment below and complete a separate survey form for each one. You may copy survey formats or request additional copies from Pamela Simerly, 202/334-2319.)

____ no (A "**no**" response implies that your program and its assessments are uniform with respect to purpose, subject selection, method of assessment, and assessment process, even though some slight variation may occur to suit individual assessments.)

List separate types of assessment (only if your program conducts two or more types).

1. ____________________

2. ____________________

3. ____________________

4. ____________________

To the extent possible, please provide publication titles and citations in *Index Medicus* style. Examples follow:

Journal

1. Standard Journal Article (List all authors when six or less; when seven or more, list only first three and add et al.)
   Soter NA, Wasserman SI, Austen KF. Cold urticaria: release into the circulation of histamine and eosinophil chemotactic factor of anaphylaxis during cold challenge. N Engl J Med 1976;294:687–90.
2. Corporate Author
   The Committee on Enzymes of the Scandinavian Society for Clinical Chemistry and Clinical Physiology. Recommended method for the determination of gammaglutamyltransferase in blood. Scnd J Clin Lab Invest 1976;36:119–25.

   Anonymous. Epidemiology for primary health care. Int J Epidemiol 1976;5:224–5.

Books and Other Monographs

3. Personal Author(s)
   Osler AG. Complement: mechanisms and functions. Englewood Cliffs: Prentice-Hall, 1976.
4. Corporate Author
   American Medical Association Department of Drugs. AMA drug evaluations. 3rd ed. Littleton: Publishing Sciences Group, 1977.
5. Editor, Compiler, Chairman as Author
   Rhodes AJ, Van Rooyen CD, comps. Textbook of virology: for students and practitioners of medicine and other health sciences. 5th ed. Baltimore: Williams & Wilkins, 1968.
6. Chapter in Book
   Weinstein L, Swartz MN. Pathogenic properties of invading microorganisms. In: Sodeman WA Jr, Sodeman WA, eds. Pathologic physiology: mechanisms of disease. Philadelphia: WB Sauders, 1974:457–72.
7. Agency Publication
   National Center for Health Statistics. Acute conditions: incidence and associated disability, United States July 1968–June 1969. Rockville, Md.: National Center for Health Statistics, 1972. (Vital and health statistics. Series 10: Data from the National Health Survey, no. 69) (DHEW publication no. (HSM)72-1036).

Other Articles

8. Newspaper Article
   Shaffer RA. Advances in chemistry are starting to unlock mysteries of the brain: discoveries could help cure alcoholism and insomnia, explain mental illness. How the messengers work. Wall Street Journal 1977 Aug 12:1(col. 1), 10(col. 1).
9. Magazine Article
   Roueche B. Annals of medicine: the Santa Claus culture. The New Yorker 1971 Sep 4:66–81.

Part I. Description of Parent Organization

Please complete a separate survey form for each program/type of assessment conducted. For each, please specify the program/type of assessment covered by this survey format.	Program: ______ Type of assessment: ______

A. For the parent organization to the assessment program, please describe the following.

1. **Name, address, telephone**

   Name: ______

   Address: ______

   ______

   Telephone: ______

2. **What is the organization's purpose?**

3. **Who are its sponsors, owners, stockholders?**

4. **What products or services does the organization provide?**

B. Which of the following categories best describes your organization?
Circle **one** number.

Government agency
1. federal
2. state/local
3. international

Not-for-profit
4. university
5. research institute
6. foundation

Association
7. professional
8. trade/industry
9. labor union

For-profit corporation
10. business

Other, specify: ______

Part II. Type of Assessment Program

Please complete a separate survey form for each program/ type of assessment conducted. For each, please specify the program/type of assessment covered by this survey format.	Program: ______________ Type of assessment: ______________

A. Who are the primary intended users of your assessments? **Check** all that apply.

_____ General public
_____ People concerned about their health
_____ Patients
_____ Providers, generally
_____ Physicians
_____ Acute facility administrators
_____ Long-term care facility administrators
_____ Other care givers
_____ Health product (drugs, devices, equipment) manufacturers
_____ Health/medical professional associations
_____ Health industry associations
_____ Consumer associations
_____ Employers
_____ Unions and other employee organizations
_____ Third party payers
_____ Government regulators
_____ Voluntary associations, organizations
_____ Biomedical researchers
_____ Financial analysts, consultants
_____ Reporters, writers, news media
_____ Information/computer industry
_____ Labs, blood banks, etc.
_____ Public policy-makers, legislators
_____ Policy research organizations
_____ Lawyers
_____ Liability, malpractice insurers
_____ Other, specify: ______________

____

____

B. Which of the following technologies does your program assess? **Check** all that apply. **Circle** the **one** assessed most often.

_____ 1. **Drug**: any chemical or biological substance that may be applied to, ingested by, or injected in order to prevent, treat, or diagnose disease or other medical conditions. Included are biologicals such as vaccines and blood products, medicinals and botanicals, and pharmaceutical preparations.

_____ 2. **Device**: any physical item, excluding drugs, used in medical care. Included are diagnostic and therapeutic equipment, prostheses, surgical and medical instruments and supplies, dental equipment and supplies, ophthalmic goods, and *in vitro* diagnostic products-reagents, instruments, and systems used in the collection, preparation, and examination of specimens taken from the human body to determine the state of a patient's health.

_____ 3. **Medical or surgical procedure**: a practice of a health care provider that generally involves a combination, often quite complex, of special skills or abilities with drugs, devices, or both. In some cases, the drugs or devices involved are not predominant factors in a procedure. Instead, the technique of the provider performing the procedure is most important, such as in the performance of a surgical procedure facilitated by the use of scalpels, clamps, and drugs against infection. Psychotherapy or prescription of a special diet are examples of procedures which may not involve drugs or devices.

_____ 4. **Support system**: a system that provides the environment for and otherwise facilitates the provision of health care, but is not the focal technology in a medical regimen, surgical procedure, or other form of health care. Examples are laboratory and radiology services, medical information systems, blood banking services, hospital infection control programs, food services, laundry, hospital facilities, and physical plant. Many of these are often referred to as ancillary services.

_____ 5. **Organizational or administrative system**: used in management and administration to ensure that health care is delivered effectively. Included are alternative delivery modes or settings (e.g., health maintenance organizations (HMOs), area-wide emergency care systems, and home health delivery), and payment systems (e.g., prospective payment using diagnosis-related groups).

_____ 6. **Other**, specify: ______________

____

____

C. Which of the following phases of technological intervention does your program normally assess? **Check** all that apply. **Circle** the **one** assessed most often.

_____ 1. **Prevention**: designed to prevent a disease from occurring, reduce the risk of its occurrence, or promote health and welfare.

_____ 2. **Diagnosis**: designed to identify an individual at high-risk (of a disease) or who has the disease (whether or not clinical signs and symptoms are present).

_____ 3. **Treatment**: designed to restore, maintain or improve health status, encompassing cure (of an acute disease), care (of a chronic disease), or avoidance of further deterioration (of a degenerative process).

_____ 4. **Rehabilitation**: designed to restore, maintain, or improve a person's ability to function without necessarily affecting health status.

_____ 5. **Other**, specify: ______________________

____

____

D. At what stages in the life-cycle of technologies do you carry out your assessments? **Check** all that apply. **Circle** the **one** assessed most often.

_____ 1. **Emerging**: in the applied research or development stage, at about the time of initial clinical testing; once the prototype has been built (device) or described (procedure) but prior to the point were the technology can be readily used by practitioners other than its developers.

_____ 2. **New**: initial use of the defined by practitioners other than its developers but not in widespread use; the beginnings of diffusion.

_____ 3. **Established or widespread practice**: when practitioners generally consider the technology to be accepted or standard practice.

_____ 4. **Obsolete**: when one or more other technologies (or using no technology) have superseded the technology as established practice, but it continues to be used by some practitioners.

_____ 5. **Other**, specify: ______________________

____

____

E. What properties (or attributes) of a technology do you assess? **Check** all that apply. **Circle** the **one** usually emphasized.

_____ 1. **Safety**: a judgment of the acceptability of risk in a specified situation, e.g., for a given medical problem, by a provider with specified training, at a specified type of facility.

_____ 2. **Efficacy**: health benefit for a specified population with a given medical problem under ideal conditions of use (i.e., a special case of effectiveness).

_____ 3. **Effectiveness**: the health benefit for a specified population with a given medical problem under average conditions of use.

_____ 4. **Cost**: of using the technology for an individual application (e.g., direct and indirect/overhead costs) including charges or prices.

_____ 5. **Cost-benefit**: the costs of a technological application compared to the resultant benefits, with both costs and benefits expressed in the same (usually monetary) units.

_____ 6. **Cost-effectiveness**: the costs of a technological application compared to the resultant benefits, with cost and benefits/effectiveness not expressed by the same unit. Costs are usually expressed in monetary units, but benefits/effectiveness are ordinarily expressed in such terms as lives saved, disability avoided, quality-adjusted life years or other similar measures.

_____ 7. **Service requirements**: for using the technology in practice, such as its placement and distribution within a health care system, organizational arrangements within a facility, need for technologists or staff training.

_____ 8. **Acceptance/adoption level**: actual/projected level of a technology's acceptability among providers, extent of diffusion/use, stage in lifecycle, etc.

_____ 9. **System impact**: beyond clinical effectiveness, the actual/projected impact on medical practice patterns, health care delivery organization/systems.

_____ 10. **Economic implications**: the cost of the technology in the aggregate, and its impact on factor prices, medical costs, alternative uses of national or industrial resources, etc.

_____ 11. **Ethical, legal, social implications**: of using the technology, including, e.g., its impact on moral values, challenges to legal principals, and effects on society.

____ 12. **Other**, specify: ____________________

____

____ 8. **Bench testing** in the laboratory; non-clinical, *in vitro* testing, experiments, or related observations.

F. Which of the following broad categories of assessment methods do you employ to conduct an assessment? **Check** all that apply. **Circle** the **one** relied on primarily.

____ 1. **Information syntheses**: summarizing, integrating, and interpreting findings reported in the literature. May include unstructured literature reviews as well as various systematic and quantitative procedures such as meta-analysis.

____ 2. **Expert opinion**: consultation with individual experts who may be involved in drafting, editing, reviewing assessments but who do not interact as a group.

____ 3. **Group judgment**: a process in which a group of experts interact in assessing a technology and formulate findings by vote or other process of reaching general agreement. It is necessary that group members have the opportunity to interact in formulating and reviewing each other's and the group's observations and findings.

____ 4. **Modeling**: use of simulations or models to test or evaluate proposed interventions, often undertaken when evaluation of the actual intervention would be impractical.

____ 5. **Cost analyses**: analyses, including cost-benefit and cost-effectiveness analyses, that identify, measure, and compare both the benefits and costs of medical technologies. Analyses may vary in terms of perspective (i.e., the parties to whom the benefits and costs accrue) and the choice and valuation of the benefits and costs considered.

____ 6. **Epidemiological and other observational methods**: excludes the more rigorous experimental design studies such as randomized clinical trials. Included are such studies known as quasi-experiments, including those with historical cohorts, series, case studies, cohort studies, natural experiments, descriptive surveys and certain cross-sectional, case control, and longitudinal methods.

____ 7. **Clinical trials**: prospective clinical experiments designed to test the safety and efficacy of a technology in which people are assigned to experimental or control groups and outcomes are compared. Includes randomized controlled clinical trials, in which people are randomly assigned to experimental and control groups.

G. Which of the following items/topics are included/addressed in most or all of your assessment reports? **Check** all that apply.

____ 1. Abstract

____ 2. The assessment's intended audience

____ 3. The purpose of the assessment (i.e., why it was conducted)

____ 4. Relationship of this assessment to prior or concurrent assessments of the technology or other technologies intended for similar purposes

____ 5. Who sponsored/commissioned/supported the assessment

____ 6. Who conducted the assessment (including, e.g., identity of subcontractors or support agencies, assessors' types of expertise)

____ 7. Description of the technology (including, e.g., intended purpose, target patients/populations, indications/contraindications, competing technologies for the same type intervention)

____ 8. Stage of life-cycle of technology when assessed

____ 9. Properties assessed (e.g., safety, effectiveness, efficacy, service arrangements, economic, ethical, legal, social implications)

____ 10. Procedure used for the assessment

____ 11. Sources of data/information (e.g., patient groups studied, types of experts surveyed)

____ 12. Methods for collecting data/information

____ 13. Methods for analyzing/synthesizing data/information

____ 14. Results (quantitative and/or qualitative)

____ 15. Findings or conclusions

____ 16. Limitations of findings

____ 17. Implications of findings for practice

____ 18. Recommendations for practice, future assessments, technology development, research

_____ 19. How much the assessment cost

_____ 20. How the technology works, including theory, principles

_____ 21. Development of the technology (including, e.g., its development, evolution, prospects for further development)

_____ 22. Procurement/deployment information (e.g., manufacturer name, how to order, cost, availability, delivery, installation, staffing/training requirements, quality control procedures, maintenance)

_____ 23. Where technology is in use

_____ 24. Regulatory agency approval status (e.g., status of premarketing approval or 510(k) application, supplemental approvals, regulatory agency product identification/docket numbers, certificate-of-need status)

_____ 25. Coverage/reimbursement status of the technology (e.g., which payers cover the technology and how much is paid for it, diagnosis-related group status)

_____ 26. Product recall history, liability actions

_____ 27. Other, specify: _______________

____

____

H. How do you disseminate technology assessment results? Check **all** that apply. **Circle** the **one** relied on primarily.

_____ 1. Printed reports (excluding journal articles)

_____ 2. Journal articles

_____ 3. Advisories to members/constituents

_____ 4. Press conferences/news releases, TV/radio broadcasts, video products

_____ 5. Clearinghouses; data/citation bases; on-line services; specify which: _______________

____

____

_____ 6. Other, specify: _______________

____

____

I. What is your assessment program's approximate annual budget (excluding value of in-kind services)? What percentage of the budget is met by each of the following sources?

Approximate annual budget: U.S. $_______________

Sources (total = equal 100%; figures may be approximate)	**Percent**
Parent organization (for programs that are part of government agencies, this line would likely be 100%)	_____ %
Government grants/contracts	_____ %
Foundations, other private grants	_____ %
Sponsors/members dues, contributions	_____ %
Sales of assessments, consultant services, etc.	_____ %
Other (specify source, percentage)	
_______________	_____ %
_______________	_____ %
Total	100%

Part III. Description of Assessment Program

Please complete a separate survey form for each program/type of assessment conducted. For each, please specify the program/type of assessment covered by this survey format.	Program: ______ Type of assessment: ______

This section of the survey is for **brief narrative** descriptions of selected aspects of your assessment program. These descriptions will enable a better understanding of your program than can be conveyed alone by the categorical checklists in the previous section. Many of the selected aspects below are accompanied by questions and other items that may be used as guides to your descriptions. Some of these may not be applicable to your program; if so, simply indicate "NA."

The descriptions for this section need not be detailed. It is sufficient to complete the items in the space provided. You may use more words if appropriate, but please try not to exceed 250 words per item. Should you require extra space for your answers or the requested citations, please append extra sheets, keying your answers to the item in the survey.

A. Identification and access

Program name: ______

Type of assessment: ______

Director: ______

Contact person and title: ______

______

Address: ______

______

______

Telephone: ______

Telex: ______

Telefax: ______

Other access information (e.g., alternative contact persons, publications office, special inquiries)

______

______

______

B. Program origin/chronology

C. What is the purpose of the assessment program?

D. What types of technologies are assessed?

E. During what stages of their life-cycles are technologies assessed?

F. What properties or attributes of technologies are assessed?

G. Selection process for assessment topic

1. Who can request that an assessment be conducted?

2. How are requests for assessment made?

3. How and by whom are assessment topic priorities set?

4. What, if any, provisions are made for reassessing technologies?

H. Assessment process

1. What methods are used to conduct assessments?

2. How is the assessment process conducted?

3. What are areas of expertise of the assessors?

4. What is the approximate (e.g., average or range of) turnaround time from selection of assessment topic to reporting of findings?

5. What is the approximate cost per assessment?

I. Assessment products and dissemination

1. What are the types of assessment products?

2. How are assessment results disseminated?

3. How does one acquire copies of your assessments?

J. Use of assessments

1. How does the parent organization use the program's assessment reports?

2. Who else uses the reports and for what purposes? How do you know?

3. Please describe briefly any documented instances of use of your assessment reports and their impact, citing any pertinent published documents.

4. Please list any citations in the published literature (journal articles and other publicly available documents) to the program.

5. Please list any citations in the published literature to individual assessment reports from your program.

K. **Assessment program evaluations**. Please briefly describe below any evaluations that have been made of your assessment program. If more than one evaluation has been conducted, please provide information separately for each one.

1. What was the purpose of the evaluation? Who requested that it be conducted? Who funded it?

2. How was it conducted?

3. Who conducted it?

4. During what period (starting and ending dates) was it conducted?

5. What were the findings?

6. How were the findings used to modify the assessment program?

7. Please list citations to published documents about the evaluation or its findings.

L. **Related Activities**. If appropriate, please describe (in 250 words or less) activities other than, but related to, technology assessment with which your program is involved. These activities could include conferences, symposia, newsletters, special panels or committees, etc.

Part IV. Listing of Assessment Reports

Please complete a separate survey form for each program/ type of assessment conducted. For each, please specify the program/type of assessment covered by this survey format.	Program: ______________________ Type of assessment: ______________________

This section asks you to append lists of citations for the assessment reports that your program has completed, has in progress, and is planning; and to note the primary assessment method(s) used for each. When appending these lists, please key them to the appropriate section.

To indicate the primary assessment method used to produce each report, please complete the following steps.

1. **Check below the method you usually rely on for conducting assessments.** If you generally use two or more methods for conducting each assessment, you may check the corresponding methods listed (although we would prefer you check only one—the method primarily relied upon for producing the assessment). **Definitions of methods may be found in Part II of the survey (Question F).**

2. **For assessment reports produced using a method other than that indicated in step 1 above,** as your usual method for assessing a technology, indicate the method used in the particular case by writing (in parenthesis following the report title) the letter (from the following list) corresponding to the assessment method actually used. Thus, you have only to indicate exceptions to your usual method for conducting assessments.

If you have never deviated from your usual method for conducting an assessment, which you described in step 1 above, then you would have nothing to add after any of your assessment report titles.

General category of assessment method

_____ A. Information syntheses

_____ B. Expert opinion

_____ C. Group judgment

_____ D. Modeling

_____ E. Cost analyses

_____ F. Epidemiological and other observational methods

_____ G. Clinical trials

_____ H. Bench testing

A. **Completed reports. Please append a list of all medical technology assessment reports that your program has published from its inception to the present.**

If your reports are only published elsewhere, e.g., in a journal, please provide the citation. If you publish the report **and** permit collateral journal publication, listing your publication is sufficient, although you may list both together if you choose.

If you already have a list of publications or journal citations, please check that it is current, and that it specifies clearly the technologies assessed.

To the extent possible, provide publication titles and citations in *Index Medicus* style. (See page 2 of the instructions for examples.) Please provide at minimum the report title, date of publication, other citation information such as volume, number, and publisher where appropriate; and primary assessment method(s) as described above.

We would appreciate receiving an **abstract** of each assessment, **if available**. We are **not** asking that you create abstracts if none are available presently, unless you want to do so.

B. **List of ongoing assessments. Please append a list of all medical technology assessments that your program is conducting presently or are in the process of being published and their expected publication dates.**

To the extent possible, provide (anticipated) publication titles and citations in *Index Medicus* style. Please provide where possible the (anticipated) report title, date of publication, other citation information such as volume, number, and publisher where appropriate; and primary assessment method(s) as described above.

If you already have a list of anticipated reports, please check that it is current, and that it specifies clearly the technologies being assessed.

C. **List of planned assessments. Please append a list of any medical technology assessments that your program is planning to conduct within the next three years.** A planned study is one that is not being conducted presently, but that you have identified as needed and have or will set aside resources to conduct it, whether or not a starting date has been set.

To the extent possible, provide (planned) publication titles and citations in *Index Medicus* style. Please provide where possible the (planned) report title, date of publication, other citation information such as volume, number, and publisher where appropriate; and primary assessment method(s) as described above.

If you already have a list of planned reports, please check that it is current, and that it specifies clearly the technologies to be assessed.

Other information, comments. Please provide below any other information you think is relevant to the purpose of this survey or any comments you may have about the survey. Thank you very much for completing it.

6|5|4 → 15.

(0,5) (5,2)

3+

No. 9 -63